Handbook of
ORTHOPAEDIC SURGERY

ALFRED RIVES SHANDS, Jr., B.A., M.D., F.A.C.S.
    Medical Director of the Alfred I. duPont Institute of the Nemours Foundation, Wilmington, Del.; Visiting Professor of Orthopaedic Surgery, University of Pennsylvania School of Medicine, Philadelphia, Pa.

RICHARD BEVERLY RANEY, B.A., M.D., F.A.C.S.
    Professor of Orthopaedic Surgery, University of North Carolina School of Medicine, Chapel Hill, N. C.

With the collaboration of
H. ROBERT BRASHEAR, B.A., M.D., F.A.C.S.
    Associate Professor of Orthopaedic Surgery, University of North Carolina School of Medicine, Chapel Hill, N. C.

With 277 illustrations and a bibliography

SIXTH EDITION

THE C. V. MOSBY COMPANY
    Saint Louis   1963

SIXTH EDITION
Copyright © 1963 by
THE C. V. MOSBY COMPANY

Second printing
All rights reserved
Previous editions copyrighted 1937, 1940, 1948, 1952, 1957
Printed in the United States of America
Library of Congress Catalog Card Number 63-12116
Distributed in Great Britain by Henry Kimpton, London

To WILLIAM STEVENSON BAER
1872-1931

Preface to sixth edition

The subject matter of orthopaedics undergoes constant change as new information on bone and joint affections is added to existing knowledge. Advances in prophylaxis and treatment lessen the prevalence and seriousness of some disease entities, while newly acquired facts and technics increase the importance of others. To reflect the changing emphases of the past several years, the sixth edition of the *Handbook of Orthopaedic Surgery* has been extensively revised and in part rewritten. Such alterations, additions, and deletions have been made as seemed advisable in continuing the purpose of earlier editions: to present the fundamental facts and principles of orthopaedics in brief, readily available form.

Approach toward this objective has been made easier by help from many confreres. In 1959 a letter requesting criticism of the *Handbook* was sent to orthopaedic teachers in the United States and in Canada. The replies contained many constructive ideas. Although some of these suggestions could not be implemented in the sixth edition, many were utilized, and for all most grateful appreciation is expressed.

The plan of dividing the subject matter into chapters accommodating a weekly schedule of study has again been followed. Several major changes, however, have been made in the text. In keeping with the decreased incidence of serious infections, the two chapters on osteomyelitis and pyogenic arthritis have been condensed into one, and a single chapter replaces the two on tuberculosis of bones and joints. Thus space has been gained for a subject of increasing importance to orthopaedics, amputations and prostheses, and in this new chapter a brief presentation of the principles of bracing has been included. A discussion of fracture principles has been added as an Appendix in order that the student of nontraumatic orthopaedics may also have at hand an introduction to the terminology and rationale used in the management of bone injuries. The chapters on chronic arthritis and that on tumors have undergone detailed revision, and the section on lumbar disk lesions and affections of the hand have been greatly expanded. Anatomic nomenclature has been modernized.

A number of illustrations appearing in the last edition have been replaced by new ones, several old illustrations have been deleted, and forty-seven new illustrations, mostly photographs and roentgenograms, have been added.

The bibliography has been revised by the deletion of certain older references and the addition of selected titles appearing in the orthopaedic literature published in English prior to June, 1963.

Grateful acknowledgment is expressed to Dr. H. Robert Brashear, whose collaboration in producing the sixth edition of the *Handbook* has been close and invaluable. Dr. Howard Hatcher's suggestions, based on detailed consideration of the fifth edition, have been most helpful. Too numerous for individual mention are the faculty members of the University of North Carolina School of Medicine who have assisted with advice in specialized fields, as well as the orthopaedic residents at the North Carolina Memorial Hospital who have contributed their assistance; to all of them warm appreciation is expressed. The Medical Illustration Department of the University of North Carolina School of Medicine has been most cooperative in the preparation of illustrations, and Mrs. Martha Thomas has been very patient and efficient in producing the typescript.

A. R. Shands, Jr.
R. Beverly Raney

Preface to first edition

The purpose of this book is to present for the consideration of the medical student and the general practitioner the fundamental facts and principles of orthopaedic surgery as concisely as possible and yet in sufficient detail to convey a well-rounded knowledge of the subject.

An attempt has been made to present, not the views of one man or of one school, but the consensus of opinion as recorded in the orthopaedic textbooks and in the more recent orthopaedic literature, criticized and tempered with the experience and thought of twenty-four teachers of orthopaedic surgery and allied subjects representing eighteen different medical schools. It was believed to be unfair to ask any one man or group of men to criticize the whole text. To obviate the labor which this would necessarily impose upon a few individuals, various sections of manuscript were sent to these authorities for their criticism. This has been productive of most helpful suggestions for the betterment of the text. Each chapter has been reviewed by more than one authority. When there were conflicting opinions, the author has reserved the right to choose the subject matter which he thinks most suitable. Because of limitation of space certain important parts of orthopaedic teaching have been omitted; among these are the subjects of fresh fractures, plaster technic, and orthopaedic apparatus, as well as certain forms of treatment which in the past have been widely used but which are not generally accepted today. On the other hand, it may appear to some readers that too much material has been included for an elementary textbook. In the bibliography are grouped most of the outstanding American and English articles on the various orthopaedic subjects, and the reader who is desirous of gaining further knowledge will find these an excellent source of detailed and authoritative information.

Illustrations which are clear and to the point are used. Those taken from textbooks and journals have been redrawn. The majority of the illustrations are original pen and ink drawings, many of which were made from specimens provided by the author's collection of pathologic bones. No photographs or roentgenograms have been reproduced directly; all have been redrawn to emphasize their characteristic features. The drawings of operative technic have been chosen to illustrate certain principles of orthopaedic surgery. A great many surgical procedures which are described in the text have not been illustrated because of limitation of space.

The subject matter of the text has been divided into twenty-four chapters in accordance with a report of the Committee on Undergraduate Instruction in Orthopaedic Surgery of the American Orthopaedic Association, which in 1934 called attention to the fact that in several of the leading medical schools approximately twenty-four class periods of an hour's duration are profitably employed for undergraduate orthopaedic instruction. Sixteen of the chapters are arranged upon the basis of pathology; seven chapters are arranged according to anatomical region, and include disease entities which do not fall readily into the pathology grouping. It is realized that this arrangement is imperfect; nevertheless it has seemed to the author that such an organization of the subject matter provides an approach to completeness, at the same time reducing unnecessary repetition to a minimum.

While the value of a historical background is appreciated, it is believed that the student should not be confused with the names of too many individuals. Experience in teaching has shown that it is advisable to emphasize the principles of diagnosis and treatment rather than the identity of the originator; therefore, first importance has been given to the description of orthopaedic entities, and individual credit for their original presentation has in most cases been acknowledged as a secondary consideration.

The first chapter on chronic arthritis (Chapter X) has been taken from the *Arthritic Primer,* prepared by the American Committee for the Study and Control of Rheumatism. This Primer treats most ably the entire subject of chronic arthritis and presents the mature opinion of authorities who are most interested in this subject and best qualified to discuss it. The chapter on the low back (Chapter XIX) is a modification of Dr. Steindler's presentation of this subject in his text, *Diseases and Deformities of the Spine and Thorax.*

Most sincere appreciation is expressed to the following for their invaluable criticisms of various sections of the text: Dr. Lloyd T. Aycock, Boston, Mass.; Dr. G. E. Bennett, Baltimore, Md.; Dr. Willis C. Campbell, Memphis, Tenn.; Dr. W. B. Carrell, Dallas, Texas; Dr. F. A. Chandler, Chicago, Ill.; Dr. H. Earle Conwell, Birmingham, Ala.; Dr. R. S. Crispell, Durham, N. C.; Dr. A. H. Freiberg, Cincinnati, Ohio; Dr. J. A. Freiberg, Cincinnati, Ohio; Dr. R. V. Funsten, University, Va.; Dr. Ralph K. Ghormley, Rochester, Minn.; Dr. A. Bruce Gill, Philadelphia, Pa.; Dr. R. W. Johnson, Jr., Baltimore, Md.; Dr. J. Albert Key, St. Louis, Mo.; Dr. Richard Kovacs, New York, N. Y.; Dr. Arthur Krida, New York, N. Y.; Dr. Arthur T. Legg, Boston, Mass.; Dr. Leo Mayer, New York, N. Y.; Dr. J. R. Moore, Philadelphia, Pa.; Dr. J. J. Morton, Rochester, N. Y.; Dr. I. W. Nachlas, Baltimore, Md.;

Preface to first edition

Dr. Robert B. Osgood, Boston, Mass.; Dr. W. M. Phelps, Baltimore, Md.; Dr. Robert D. Schrock, Omaha, Neb.; Dr. R. Plato Schwartz, Rochester, N. Y.; Dr. Arthur Steindler, Iowa City, Iowa; Dr. John C. Wilson, Los Angeles, Calif.; and Dr. Philip D. Wilson, New York, N. Y.

Appreciation is expressed to Dr. W. M. Roberts, of the North Carolina Orthopaedic Hospital, and to Dr. O. L. Miller, of Charlotte, for the use of their case records and roentgenograms. Sincere thanks are extended to Dr. D. C. Hetherington for his criticism of construction and syntax. Appreciation is expressed also to the Radiological Division of Duke Hospital and to various members of the staff who have offered many helpful suggestions in their special fields of work. We also feel indebted to the following who have so kindly made suggestions regarding certain of the drawings: Dr. Toufick Nicola and Dr. Isadore Zadek, of New York; Dr. Irvine M. Flinn, Jr., of Wilmington, Del.; Dr. I. W. Nachlas, Dr. G. E. Bennett and Dr. R. E. Lenhard, of Baltimore; and Dr. J. Warren White, of Greenville, S. C.

Without the splendid work of the artists the value of the book would be greatly impaired. The author feels deeply indebted to Mr. Jack Bonacker Wilson, who has done a major part of the illustrative work, to Mr. Elon Clark, and to Mrs. E. M. Collins, who drew many of the preliminary sketches, and to Miss Elizabeth Brödel, whose illustrations of arthritic spines have proved most useful. For valuable stenographic aid appreciation is expressed to Mrs. Lucille Lyon and to Miss Henrietta Fagan and her associates.

It is hoped that this short textbook will assist in the teaching of orthopaedic surgery, and that it may find a permanent place of usefulness in this special field of medicine.

A. R. Shands, Jr., M.D.
Durham, North Carolina

Contents

CHAPTER 1

Introduction, 21

General considerations of bone and joint affections, 22; Embryology, anatomy, and physiology, 22; Etiology, 26; Physical diagnosis, 27; Roentgenographic diagnosis, 34; Laboratory diagnosis, 34; Treatment, 35; Rehabilitation, 36.

CHAPTER 2

Congenital deformities, 37

Congenital talipes, 38; Congenital talipes equinovarus (congenital clubfoot), 39; Other forms of congenital talipes, 45; Talipes calcaneovalgus, 45; Talipes valgus, 45; Talipes calcaneus, 45; Talipes varus, 45; Talipes equinus, 45; Metatarsus varus (metatarsus adductus), 46; Congenital vertical talus, 47; Congenital clubhand, 47; Congenital defects of individual bones, 49; Humerus, 50; Radius, 50; Ulna, 50; Femur, 51; Tibia, 51; Fibula, 51; Patella, 52; Congenital radioulnar synostosis, 52; Congenital contractures, 53; Congenital abnormalities of fingers and toes, 53; Syndactyly (webbed fingers or toes), 53; Macrodactyly, 54; Polydactyly, 54; Cleft hand and cleft foot, 55; Arachnodactyly (Marfan's syndrome), 56; Congenital amputations and constricting bands, 56; Asymmetrical development (congenital hemihypertrophy, hemimacrosomia), 56; Arthrogryposis multiplex congenita (amyoplasia congenita), 57; Cleidocranial dysostosis, 58; Congenital elevation of the scapula (congenital high scapula, Sprengel's deformity), 59; Congenital synostosis of the cervical spine (Klippel-Feil syndrome), 61.

CHAPTER 3

Congenital deformities—cont'd, 63

Congenital dysplasia of the hip, 63; Acetabular dysplasia and subluxation of the hip, 64; Congenital dislocation of the hip, 65; Congenital dislocation of other joints, 79; Knee, 79; Patella, 80; Shoulder, 80; Elbow, 80; Wrist, 80.

CHAPTER 4

General affections of the skeleton, 81

Affections caused by abnormalities of diet or metabolism, 84; Skeletal changes associated with vitamin disturbances, 84; Rickets (infantile rickets), 85; Genu varum (bowleg), 89; Genu valgum (knock-knee), 92; Scurvy, 94; Metabolic affections simulating rickets, 95; Fanconi's syndrome, 97; Renal dwarfism (renal rickets, renal osteodystrophy), 97; Osteomalacia (adult rickets), 98; Reticuloendotheliosis (histiocytosis), 100; Eosinophilic granuloma, 100; Hand-Schüller-Christian disease, 101; Letterer-Siwe disease, 102; Gaucher's disease, 102.

CHAPTER 5

General affections of the skeleton—cont'd, 104

Affections caused by congenital developmental abnormalities, 104; Achondroplasia (chondrodystrophia foetalis), 104; Dyschondroplasia (diaphyseal or metaphyseal aclasis), 105; Morquio's disease (Morquio-Brailsford chondro-osteodystrophy), 109; Hurler's syndrome (gargoylism, lipochondro-osteodystrophy), 110; Osteogenesis imperfecta (fragilitas ossium, idiopathic osteopsathyrosis, brittle bones), 111; Fibrous dysplasia, 113; Polyostotic fibrous dysplasia, 113; Monostotic fibrous dysplasia, 115; Osteosclerosis, 116; Osteopetrosis (Albers-Schönberg disease, marble bones), 116; Osteopathia striata, 116; Osteopoikilosis (spotted bones), 117; Melorheostosis, 117; Progressive diaphyseal dysplasia (Engelmann's disease), 117; Progressive myositis ossificans, 119; Affections caused by endocrine abnormalities, 120; Hypopituitary dwarfism, 120; Hyperpituitarism, 121; Gigantism, 121; Acromegaly, 121; Cretinism (hypothyroidism), 122; Hyperparathyroidism (generalized osteitis fibrosa cystica, von Recklinghausen's disease of bone), 123; Affections caused by unknown acquired abnormalities, 124; Osteitis deformans, 124; Senile osteoporosis, 127; Secondary hypertrophic pulmonary osteoarthropathy (Bamberger-Marie disease), 129; Infantile cortical hyperostosis (Caffey's disease), 130; Posttraumatic painful osteoporosis (Sudeck's atrophy, posttraumatic or reflex sympathetic dystrophy), 132.

CHAPTER 6

Infections of bones and joints (exclusive of tuberculosis), 133

Pyogenic or suppurative osteomyelitis, 133; Brodie's abscess, 140; Sclerosing osteitis (Garré's osteitis), 141; Osteitis pubis, 141; Pyogenic or suppurative arthritis, 142; Pyogenic arthritis of the hip in infants, 144; Pneumococcal arthritis, 144; Gonococcal arthritis, 144; Salmonella osteomyelitis and arthritis, 145; Brucella osteomyelitis and arthritis, 145; Fungus infections of bones and joints, 146; Echinococcus cyst, 146; Syphilis of bones and joints, 146; Osteochondritis, 147; Localized periostitis, 147; Diffuse periostitis and osteoperiostitis, 147; Symmetrical serous synovitis, 147; Gummatous arthritis, 148.

CHAPTER 7

Tuberculosis of bones and joints, 149

Tuberculosis of the spine, 154; Tuberculosis of the sacroiliac joint, 160; Tuberculosis of the hip, 161; Tuberculosis of other joints, 164.

Contents 15

CHAPTER 8
Chronic arthritis, 166

Rheumatoid arthritis (atrophic arthritis, proliferative arthritis), 167; Osteoarthritis (degenerative joint disease), 175; Gout, 179.

CHAPTER 9
Chronic arthritis of individual joints—ankylosis and arthroplasty, 182

Chronic arthritis of the spine, 182; Rheumatoid arthritis, 182; Strümpell-Marie arthritis (ankylosing spondylitis), 183; Osteoarthritis, 186; Treatment of chronic arthritis of the spine, 188; Chronic arthritis of the hip, 189; Malum coxae senilis, 189; Chronic arthritis of the knee, 192; Ankylosis, 194; Optimum positions of joint fixation, 197; Arthroplasty, 200.

CHAPTER 10
Neuromuscular disabilities—poliomyelitis, 203

Operations for the correction of deformities of long standing, 213; Muscle and tendon transplantations, 215; Operations to increase the stability of joints, 218; Leg equalization operations, 222.

CHAPTER 11
Neuromuscular disabilities (exclusive of poliomyelitis)—involvement of the brain and spinal cord, 224

Involvement of the brain, 224; Cerebral palsy, 224; Neuromuscular disabilities of psychiatric origin (hysterical paralysis), 232; Involvement of the spinal cord, 233; Progressive muscular atrophy (Aran-Duchenne type), 233; Infantile spinal muscular atrophy (amyotonia congenita), 233; Friedreich's ataxia, 234; Subacute combined sclerosis, 234; Neuropathic disease of bones and joints, 235; Spina bifida, 237.

CHAPTER 12
Neuromuscular disabilities (exclusive of poliomyelitis)—involvement of peripheral nerves and of muscles, 241

Involvement of peripheral nerves, 241; Peripheral nerve injuries, 241; Injuries of individual nerves, 246; Accessory nerve (eleventh cranial nerve), 246; Brachial plexus, 247; Obstetric paralysis, 247; Paralysis following dislocation of the shoulder, 250; Axillary nerve, 251; Long thoracic nerve, 251; Radial nerve, 251; Ulnar nerve, 252; Median nerve, 254; Lumbosacral plexus and cauda equina, 255; Lumbosacral plexus, 255; Cauda equina and conus medullaris, 255; Sciatic nerve, 256; Common peroneal nerve, 256; Tibial nerve, 257; Femoral nerve and obturator nerve, 257; Neuritis, 257; Traumatic neuritis, 257; Toxic neuritis, 258; Serum neuritis, 258; Guillain-Barré syndrome, 259; Neuralgia, 259; Hereditary muscular atrophy of peroneal type (Charcot-Marie-Tooth disease), 260; Involvement of muscles, 260; Progressive muscular dystrophy (primary myopathy), 260.

CHAPTER 13
Tumors, 263

Tumors and tumorlike affections of bone, 263; Benign tumors and tumorlike affections of bone, 265; Osteoma, chondroma, and osteochondroma, 265; Osteoma, 265; Chondroma, 265; Osteochondroma, 266; Osteoid-osteoma, 267; Nonosteogenic fibroma (nonossifying fibroma), 268; Giant cell tumor (osteoclastoma), 270; Bone cyst, 271; Malignant tumors of bone, 272; Osteogenic sarcoma (osteosarcoma), 272; Chondrosarcoma, 275; Ewing's sarcoma, 276; Multiple myeloma, 277; Tumors metastasizing to bone, 279; Tumors of joints, tendons, tendon sheaths, and bursae, 282; Tumors of muscles and fasciae, 283; Fibroma, lipoma, and angioma, 283; Fibrosarcoma, 283; Tumors of nerves, 284; Solitary neurofibroma, 285; Neurofibromatosis (von Recklinghausen's disease), 285.

CHAPTER 14
Fracture deformities, 286

Repair of fractures, 286; Delayed union, 289; Nonunion, 291; Congenital fractures and nonunion, 296; The treatment of massive defects of the long bones, 297; Nonunion of individual bones, 298; Neck of the femur, 298; Shaft of the femur, 300; Patella, 300; Tibia and fibula, 300; Clavicle, 301; Humerus, 302; Radius and ulna, 302; Carpus and metacarpus, 302; Malunion, 303; Malunion of individual bones, 303; Femur, 303; Patella, 303; Tibia and fibula, 304; Ankle, 305; Talus, 306; Calcaneus, 307; Metatarsus, 307; Clavicle and scapula, 307; Humerus, 307; Radius and ulna, 309; Wrist, 310; Hand, 311; Pelvis, 312; Spine, 312; Comment, 313.

CHAPTER 15
Amputations, prostheses, and braces, 314

Amputations and prostheses, 314; Indications, 314; Amputations of the upper extremity, 316; Amputations of the lower extremity, 318; Amputations in children, 321; Preparation for the prosthesis, 322; Disabilities of the amputation stump, 322; Braces, 323.

CHAPTER 16
Affections of the spine and thorax, 327

Affections of the spine, 327; Scoliosis, 327; Kyphosis (round back), 338; Vertebral epiphysitis (Scheuermann's disease, adolescent kyphosis), 338; Vertebral osteochondritis (vertebra plana, Calvé's disease), 341; Adult round back, 341; Lordosis (hollow back), 343; Faulty posture, 343; Deformities of the thorax, 346; Pigeon breast (pectus carinatum), 346; Funnel chest (pectus excavatum), 346.

CHAPTER 17
Affections of the low back, 348

Ligamentous and muscular strains of the normal low back, 349; Abnormalities of the bony structure of the low back, 354; Sacralization of the last lumbar vertebra, 355; Elongation of the transverse process of the last lumbar vertebra, 355; Defects of the laminae (spina bifida occulta), 356; Variations of the spinous processes, 356; Variations of the lumbosacral angle, 357; Variations of the articular facets, 357; Constitutional variations, 358; Isthmus defects, 358; Spondylolisthesis, 358; Lesions of the lumbar intervertebral disks, 360; Other lesions of muscle and fascia, 367; Myofascitis, 367; Herniation of fascial fat, 367; Common osteoarticular lesions of infectious, neoplastic, or traumatic nature, 367; Visceral lesions that may cause low back pain, 368; Gastrointestinal diseases, 368; Urologic diseases, 368; Gynecologic diseases, 368; Lesions of the central nervous system, 369; Sciatic neuritis, 369; Lesions of the retroperitoneal structures, 369; Generalized infectious diseases, 369; Vascular lesions, 369; Coccygodynia, 369; Comment, 370.

CHAPTER 18

Affections of the hip, 372

Coxa plana (Legg-Calvé-Perthes disease, avascular necrosis of the capital femoral epiphysis), 374; Coxa vara, 378; Congenital coxa vara, 380; Slipping of the capital femoral epiphysis (epiphyseal or adolescent coxa vara), 381; Coxa valga, 387; Pathologic dislocation of the hip, 387; Intrapelvic protrusion of the acetabulum (arthrokatadysis, Otto pelvis, protrusio acetabuli), 388; Transient synovitis of the hip, 389; Bursitis in the region of the hip, 389; Iliopectineal or iliopsoas bursa, 389; Deep trochanteric bursa, 390; Superficial trochanteric bursa, 391; Ischiogluteal bursa, 391; Snapping hip, 391.

CHAPTER 19

Affections of the knee, 392

Internal derangements of the knee joint, 393; Lesions of the semilunar cartilages, 393; Injuries of the medial semilunar cartilage, 393; Injuries of the lateral semilunar cartilage, 396; Cysts of the semilunar cartilages, 398; Discoid cartilages, 398; Rupture of the tibial and fibular collateral ligaments, 399; Rupture of the cruciate ligaments, 400; Fracture of the tibial spine, 401; Loose bodies, 401; Hypertrophy and pinching of the infrapatellar fat pad and the synovial membrane, 404; Infrapatellar fat pad, 404; Synovial membrane, 405; Exostoses, 405; Osgood-Schlatter disease (partial separation of the tibial tuberosity, apophysitis of the tibial tuberosity), 405; Recurrent or habitual dislocation of the patella (slipping patella), 407; Chondromalacia of the patella, 408; Ossification of the tibial collateral ligament (Pellegrini-Stieda disease), 409; Rupture of the quadriceps tendon and of the patellar ligament, 409; Snapping knee, 410; Intermittent hydrarthrosis (intermittent synovitis), 410; Bursitis, 411; Prepatellar bursa, 411; Deep infrapatellar bursa, 411; Superficial pretibial bursa, 412; Popliteal bursae, 412; Variable bursae beneath the tibial collateral ligament, 412; Involvement of joints in hemophilia, 412.

CHAPTER 20

Affections of the ankle and foot, 415

Foot strain, 417; Flexible flatfoot (pes planus), 418; In children, 418; In adults, 419; Spastic flatfoot, 419; Shortening of the Achilles tendon, 421; Clawfoot, 421; Köhler's disease (avascular necrosis or osteochondritis of the navicular bone), 424; Anterior metatarsalgia, 425; Morton's toe (plantar neuroma), 427; Stress fracture of a metatarsal bone (march or fatigue fracture) 428; Freiberg's disease (avascular necrosis or osteochondritis of a metatarsal head), 428; Hallux valgus, 428; Hallux varus, 431; Hallux rigidus, 431; Hammer toe, 431; Overlapping or dorsal displacement of the toes, 432; Pigeon-toe, 432; Affections of the heel, 433; Inflammation and injury about the insertion of the Achilles

18   Contents

tendon, 433; Tenosynovitis, 433; Bursitis, 433; Periostitis, 433; Calcaneal apophysitis or epiphysitis, 433; Partial or complete rupture of the Achilles or plantaris tendon, 434; Inflammation and injury under the calcaneus, 434; Exostoses of the bones of the foot, 435; Accessory bones of the foot, 436; Displacement of the peroneal tendons, 436.

CHAPTER 21

Affections of the neck, shoulder, and jaw, 437

Affections of the neck, 437; Torticollis (wry neck), 437; Congenital torticollis, 437; Acquired torticollis, 440; Spasmodic torticollis, 441; Cervical root syndrome, 441; Cervical rib and the scalenus syndrome, 444; Affections of the shoulder, 446; Minor injuries: traumatic synovitis, sprain, and strain, 447; Subacromial bursitis, 448; Subcoracoid bursitis, 451; Bicipital tenosynovitis, 451; Frozen shoulder (adhesive capsulitis, periarthritis), 452; Rupture of the supraspinatus tendon and tears of the musculotendinous cuff, 453; The shoulder-hand syndrome, 455; Rupture of the biceps brachii, 455; Snapping shoulder, 456; Recurrent dislocation of the shoulder, 457; Old dislocation of the shoulder, 458; Old acromioclavicular dislocation, 459; Old sternoclavicular dislocation, 459; Affections of the jaw, 460; Snapping jaw, 460; Ankylosis of the jaw, 461.

CHAPTER 22

Affections of the elbow, wrist, and hand, 462

Affections of the elbow, 462; Strains and sprains, 462; Olecranon bursitis, 463; Radiohumeral bursitis (tennis elbow, epicondylitis), 464; Bicipitoradial bursitis, 465; Radiohumeral subluxation in children, 465; Old dislocation of the elbow, 465; Volkmann's ischemic contracture, 466; Traumatic myositis ossificans, 468; Affections of the wrist and hand, 470; Affections of tendons and tendon sheaths, 471; Tendon lacerations, 471; Tendon ruptures, 472; Rupture of the extensor pollicis longus tendon, 472; Rupture of the central extensor slip, 473; Mallet finger (baseball or dropped finger), 473; Tenosynovitis, 474; Traumatic tenosynovitis, 474; Stenosing tenosynovitis, 475; Snapping finger or thumb, 475; Acute suppurative tenosynovitis, 475; Tuberculous tenosynovitis, 476; Acute calcific tendinitis, 476; Ganglion, 477; Contractures of the wrist and hand, 478; Skin contractures, 478; Metacarpophalangeal and interphalangeal contractures, 478; Intrinsic contracture of the hand, 479; Dupuytren's contracture, 479; Affections of the bones of the wrist and hand, 481; Avascular necrosis of the carpal bones, 481; Old dislocation of the lunate bone, 482; Accessory bones of the wrist and hand, 483; Madelung's deformity, 483.

APPENDIX

Fracture principles, 485

Definitions, 485; Diagnosis, 485; Principles of fracture treatment, 489; Open (compound) fractures, 500; Fractures in children, 500.

Bibliography, 502

Handbook of
ORTHOPAEDIC SURGERY

CHAPTER 1

Introduction

THE DEVELOPMENT of orthopaedic surgery as a specialized division of medical practice has been a long and gradual process. It was early recognized that the problems peculiar to this field of work should be grouped together as one subject for study and that these problems are best handled by individuals especially trained and experienced in their diagnosis and treatment. This principle can be observed in the works accredited to Hippocrates in the fifth century B.C., which contain many excellent descriptions of affections of the bones and joints. The first work devoted exclusively to the subject of orthopaedics, Andry's *L'Orthopédie*, was published in 1741. It provided an impetus for the frank separation of orthopaedics as a specialized branch of medical science. With the accelerated development of surgical technic one hundred years later, orthopaedic surgery finally became separated from the general field of surgery and established as a specialty. With the introduction of anesthesia and asepsis, rapid progress was made in the development of surgery of the bones and joints. Operations could be performed successfully, which in earlier years had been impossible because of the extreme suffering of the patients and the severe infection that often followed the opening of joints and the exposure of bones. Recent developments in anesthesiology and anesthetic technics have led to further advances in the surgical treatment of bone and joint affections. The development and widespread use of roentgenography in visualizing bone and joint lesions increased greatly the accuracy of diagnosis and the effectiveness of surgical treatment. With the advent of modern industrial machinery and the automobile and airplane, the incidence of traumatic orthopaedic problems rapidly increased. The care of large numbers of men crippled by injuries during the first and second world wars led to an increased development of orthopaedic surgery. In recent decades attention has been focused on the importance of the care and treatment of the crippled child, and as a result there have been instituted extensive state and national programs for the medical care of the crippled child and his restoration to normal living. Still more recently, special programs for the orthopaedic rehabilitation of the crippled adult have been inaugurated and expanded.

In definitions of orthopaedic surgery emphasis is placed equally upon the prevention and the correction of deformity and disability. Certain phases of orthopaedics can be interpreted as representing a mechanical aspect of preventive medicine; for example, the deformity that might follow a crippling disease can often be prevented by the orthopaedic measure of using braces, splints, traction, or similar devices. This concept of prevention dates back to the original orthopaedic textbook, written by Nicholas Andry of the University of Paris. The term "orthopaedic" has been adopted from the title of Andry's work; he originated it by combining two Greek words: *orthos*, meaning "straight," and *pais*, "child." Andry stated that the purpose of his book was "to teach the different methods of preventing and correcting the deformities of children." From this definition has been expanded the modern interpretation of orthopaedic surgery as applying to patients of all ages.

The subject matter of orthopaedic surgery includes the injuries, diseases, and deformities of bones and joints and of their related structures—the muscles, tendons, ligaments, and nerves. Of the many definitions of orthopaedic surgery, that adopted by the American Academy of Orthopaedic Surgeons is most descriptive: "Orthopaedic Surgery is the medical specialty that includes the investigation, preservation, restoration, and development of the form and function of the extremities, spine, and associated structures by medical, surgical, and physical methods."

In this textbook of orthopaedic surgery, etiologically related entities have, insofar as possible, been placed together. Affections that cannot be satisfactorily classified in this manner have been grouped under headings that indicate the anatomic regions involved. It is hoped that this arrangement will enable the physician and student unfamiliar with orthopaedic surgery to obtain a clear understanding of the relationships between its different entities.

GENERAL CONSIDERATIONS OF BONE AND JOINT AFFECTIONS

Embryology, anatomy, and physiology. Bone is derived from the mesenchyme or primitive connective tissue. In its development it passes through either a membranous or a cartilaginous phase. In membranous bone formation there is gradual replacement of the primitive connective tissue by osteoid matrix, which calcifies promptly to become mature bone. Only a few of the flat bones of the skull undergo this type of development initially, but it occurs in the growth, reconstruction, and remodeling of all bones throughout life. In the cartilaginous or endochondral type of development, hyaline cartilage models of the bones are formed in the mesenchymal tissue during embryonic life; the cartilage is replaced by osteoid matrix that calcifies to form bone. The long bones, spine, scapulae, ribs, sternum, and pelvis develop in this manner.

Grossly, bones are of three shapes: flat, irregular, and long. Except for the haversian systems contained in the compact portion of long bones, all bone is histologically similar. The flat and the irregular bones consist of an inner and an outer plate of compact bone, between which is situated a cancellous or spongy portion. Each long bone comprises, from within out-

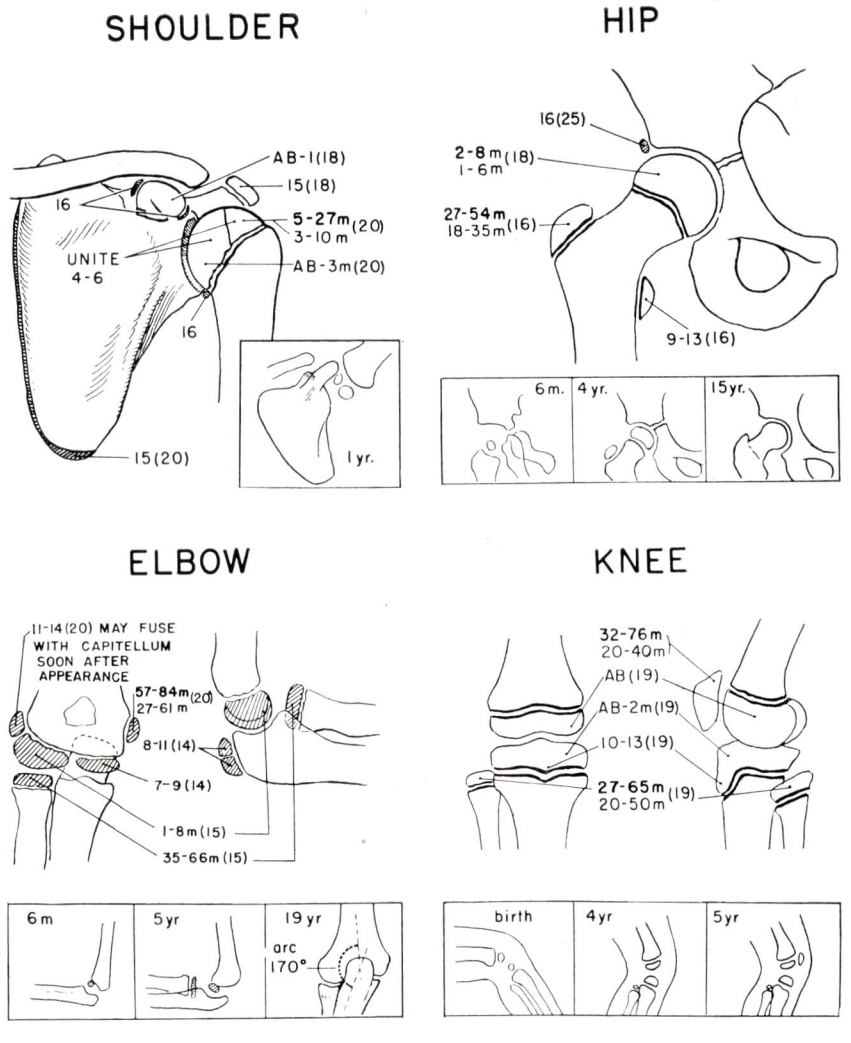

Fig. 1. Epiphyseal development at several major joints, showing the age at which these secondary ossification centers appear in roentgenograms and the age (in parentheses) at which union occurs. Age is expressed in months (m) or in years; when two sets of age figures appear, that in heavy type refers to males and that in lighter type to females; **AB** signifies at birth. The inset diagrams show average development at sample ages. (Original chart in Camp, J. D., and Cilley, E. I. L.: Am. J. Roentgenol. **26**:905, 1931; copyright, 1951, by Thomas Nelson & Sons. Chart that appears here revised by Dr. Bertram B. Girdany [Radiological Service of the Babies Hospital, New York] for Dr. D. C. Pugh's chapter entitled "The roentgenologic diagnosis of diseases of bones," which appeared in Diagnostic roentgenology [Golden, R., editor], Baltimore, 1959, Williams & Wilkins Co.)

ward, an elongated medullary canal; a fine layer of connective tissue called the endosteum; the cancellous or spongy portion at either end, which in children is the epiphysis; the compact layers, with their numerous haversian systems, which form the diaphysis or shaft; and the outer fibrous covering called the periosteum. The periosteum is firmly bound to the compact layer of bone, or cortex, by anchoring fibers called Sharpey's fibers.

Bone formation in the diaphyses, from primary centers of ossification, is well developed by the time of birth. Ossification of the epiphyses, which proceeds from secondary centers, is a much slower process. At birth, ossification centers are not usually visible roentgenographically in any epiphyses except those of the lower end of the femora. Thereafter, ossification appears in the various epiphyses in orderly chronologic sequence (Fig. 1). Between epiphysis and diaphysis is the epiphyseal cartilaginous plate, which is silhouetted in roentgenograms as the epiphyseal line. Long bones increase in length by growth at the epiphyseal plates; their shafts thicken by appositional growth beneath the periosteum. As local skeletal maturity is reached, the thinned epiphyseal plate is replaced by fusion between diaphysis and epiphysis. Certain of the vertebral epiphyses are last to fuse, doing so at about 25 years of age.

Bone is a highly specialized form of connective tissue composed of branching cells in an organic calcified matrix. The chief components of the matrix are collagen fibers and a ground substance. The hardness of bone results from the deposition of a complex mineral substance composed of calcium, phosphate, and carbonate in the soft matrix. The ground substance contains mucopolysaccharides, which include hyaluronic acid and chondroitin sulfates; it is the extracellular and interfibrillar component that permits the exchange of inorganic calcium, phosphorus, and other substances between the blood and the bone. The collagen fibers are composed of mixed proteins; the small quantities of reticular fibers also present are glycoproteins.

Osteoblasts, osteocytes, and osteoclasts are the cellular components of bone, each having its specific function: (1) the osteoblast is to form bone; (2) the osteoclast, to destroy or resorb bone; and (3) the osteocyte, to maintain bone as a living tissue. During active bone growth and the healing of fractures, frequent transformations of these cells from one to another probably occur, while at the same time each cell retains characteristics common to all three.

The haversian systems, or *osteones,* of compact bone (Fig. 2) can be considered as long, patent columns, irregularly parallel to the long axis of the shaft of the bone. The central space of the column is known as the haversian canal; surrounding it are concentric layers of calcified intercellular substance, called lamellae. Within the lamellae are spaces called lacunae, occupied by the bone cells or osteocytes. The lacunae are connected with one another and with the haversian canal by tiny irregular channels, termed canaliculi, which contain the processes of the osteocytes. From the haversian canals arise Volkmann's canals, which are broad irregular channels perpen-

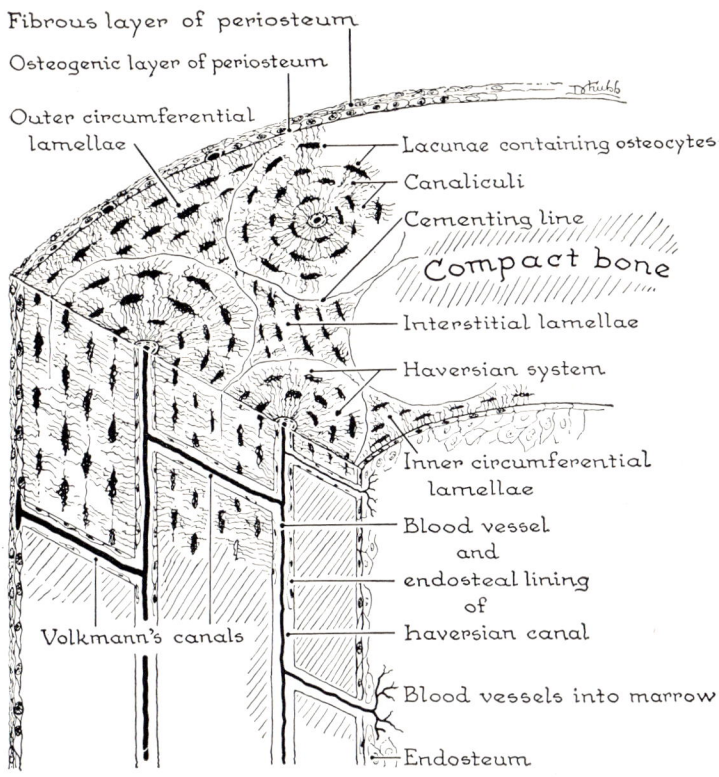

Fig. 2. Schematic drawing of a section of the cortex of a long bone. Note especially the several types of lamellae and the several kinds of vascular channels. (From Ham, A. W., and Leeson, T. S.: Histology, ed. 4, Philadelphia, 1961, J. B. Lippincott Co.)

dicularly placed; they transmit the vascular supply from the periosteum to the osteones and thence to the medullary canal.

The bone receives its nourishment from blood circulating through the nutrient arteries and the periosteal vessels. The nutrient arteries of the long bones enter the shafts, usually obliquely, through nutrient foramina situated in most cases near the middle of the shaft; they send branches to the ends of the diaphysis where they form an abundant capillary bed close to the epiphyseal plate. Vessels from the nutrient arteries supply also the marrow and endosteum. The periosteum is supplied from the outside, and from its dense arterial network numerous small vessels pass into minute orifices in the compact bone and run through the haversian canals. Other vessels pass from the periosteum through orifices in the compact bone to supply its spongy portion. The epiphysis is nourished by branches of the anastomotic vessels surrounding the joint. Lymphatic vessels are present in the periosteum; although they have been traced into the bone substance, bone essentially has no lymphatic circulation. Nerves are distributed freely to the periosteum; nonmedullated fibers accompany the nutrient arteries into the interior of the bone.

A joint is made up of the contacting articular surfaces of two or more bones, surrounded by a capsule and held in place by ligaments and muscles. The cancellous ends of the long bones are covered by a thin layer of compact bone and a layer of hyaline cartilage. The cartilage contains no blood vessels and is nourished through the joint fluid, arteries of the subjacent bone, and small vessels in the region of the attachment of the synovial membrane. For articular cartilage to maintain its normal state, it is necessary that the joint function normally.

The lining of the joint cavity is a delicate serous membrane called the synovial membrane, which in the embryo covers the articular cartilage but which disappears from the cartilaginous surfaces when growth and joint motion take place. Within the joint is the synovial fluid, a clear, light yellow, viscid liquid consisting of a plasma dialysate plus other substances, chiefly mucin, which are added by the synovial membrane. The lubricating properties of the synovial fluid depend chiefly upon its hyaluronic acid content. Nerve fibers are not present in articular cartilage but are contained in the capsule and the synovial membrane and there mediate the pain of joint reactions.

The synovial membrane is surrounded by a strong fibrous capsule. Flexible but inelastic ligaments thicken and reinforce the capsule and, in turn, are partly covered by muscles and muscle attachments. In addition, certain joints, such as the knee and the jaw, possess intra-articular fibrocartilages that decrease shock, facilitate joint motion, and provide increased stability. Fibrocartilaginous disks between the bodies of adjacent vertebrae perform a similar function. The motion in joints is brought about by muscle activity. In order to function properly, a joint requires normal tone, strength, and correlated action in the muscles by which it is moved.

About the joints are bursae, which are closed sacs lined by specialized connective tissue and containing synovial fluid. Bursae are usually found over bony prominences, especially where a muscle or tendon moves over a projection of bone. The function of bursae is to facilitate gliding movements by diminishing friction.

Etiology. The most common causes of pathologic changes in bones and joints are congenital anomalies, trauma, infection, metabolic disorders, endocrine disorders, tumors, circulatory disorders, neurologic disorders, and psychologic disorders.

Congenital anomalies. Deformities of prenatal development, or congenital anomalies, may be either primary or secondary. Primary abnormalities, which are the more common, arise from genetic causes and defects in the fertilized ovum and from intrinsic irregularities in its development during the first few weeks of embryonic life. Nongenetic causes include endocrine disturbances, excessive irradiation, certain toxic drugs, and virus infections of the embryo. Secondary congenital defects develop in a previously normal fetus as the result of extraembryonic influences exerted during intrauterine life, usually during the last two trimesters of pregnancy.

Trauma. Mechanical injury may be acute, like a sudden blow or wrench, or chronic, such as the stress on the knee joint that may accompany flatfoot.

Infection. Pathogenic organisms may enter the bone or joint by way of the blood stream, directly through a lacerating wound, or by direct extension from a neighboring focus. The most common sources of blood stream infection are boils and infected abrasions, tonsils, teeth, or lymph nodes. Bacteria in bone or joint may cause osteomyelitis or pyogenic arthritis.

Metabolic disorders. Numerous changes take place in and about the bones and joints as a result of disturbances of metabolism. Gouty arthritis, occasioned by a disturbance of purine metabolism, is an example.

Endocrine disorders. Extensive changes in the bones may take place as a result of abnormalities of the endocrine glands. An example is the absorption of bone salts and development of bone cysts associated with the excessive production of parathormone in hyperparathyroidism.

Tumors. Benign bone tumors are common and amenable to treatment; malignant bone tumors have a lower incidence and a far more serious prognosis. Tumors of joints, muscles, and tendons are uncommon.

Circulatory disorders. Disturbances that decrease the blood supply of certain epiphyses are believed to cause profound changes in these growing areas. Lesions of this type have been termed aseptic, ischemic, or avascular necrosis. Changes sometimes observed in the head of the femur, tarsal navicular, distal end of the second metatarsal, lunate, and certain other bones are examples of avascular necrosis. Disturbances that increase the blood supply to an epiphysis, such as a healing fracture of the femoral shaft, may cause an increase in bone length.

Neurologic disorders. Neurologic disorders, a large and varied group, make up a considerable part of orthopaedic practice: (1) lesions located in the brain may cause cerebral palsy; (2) lesions in the spinal cord may cause affections such as paraplegia, poliomyelitis, progressive muscular atrophy, and neuropathic joint disease; and (3) lesions in the peripheral nerves may cause obstetric palsy and other forms of localized paralysis.

Psychologic disorders. Psychiatric disorders sometimes lead to joint lesions, such as contractures. Most orthopaedic affections may be aggravated by psychologic disorders. Neuromuscular manifestations of hysteria often simulate primary orthopaedic affections.

Physical diagnosis.[*] Every student of orthopaedic surgery must gain an accurate understanding of the physical diagnosis of orthopaedic affections. Such knowledge is best acquired by careful study of the history and the examination of each patient.

History. When taking a history, record the age, sex, occupation, racial background, and economic status of the patient. Then make a careful

---

[*]For more detailed information on orthopaedic physical diagnosis, the reader is referred to the *Manual of orthopaedic surgery* (published by the American Orthopaedic Association with the cooperation of the American Academy of Orthopaedic Surgeons, 29 E. Madison St., Chicago 2, Ill.).

analysis of the presenting complaint. It is necessary to determine whether the complaint concerns a new symptom or the recurrence of an old one. Gain an accurate understanding of the time and manner of onset. It is important to determine whether the onset was (1) gradual or sudden, (2) associated with an injury or strain, and (3) accompanied by constitutional symptoms such as chills, fever, and malaise. A gradual onset may indicate a static disability such as that which may accompany arch strain; the sudden onset of disability suggests a traumatic lesion or, if accompanied by febrile symptoms, an acute bone or joint infection.

In orthopaedic patients the presenting complaint usually concerns pain, deformity, or paralysis. In analysis of the character and type of *pain*, determination of the following points is important: (1) the severity of the pain and whether it is aching or sharp, (2) whether the pain is becoming progressively worse or is diminishing, (3) whether it is less severe in the morning after rest and worse at night, (4) whether activity and cold or damp weather increase its severity, (5) whether radiation of the pain occurs (and in what course), and (6) whether any pain is present in other parts of the body. The extent of disability produced by the pain should be ascertained, as well as the character and result of previous treatment. Pain, although always an important symptom, is variable and, as far as possible, must be analyzed with full appreciation of the patient's psychic stability and tolerance of discomfort. Sharp pain may indicate bone injury with muscle spasm, or a purulent exudate under pressure within a closed cavity; increasing pain may indicate progression of an infectious process; pain that becomes worse with activity during the day may indicate joint strain; pain that is worse in bad weather and is felt in more than one part of the body may be associated with chronic arthritis; and radiating pain frequently accompanies rupture of an intervertebral disk and pressure on a nerve root.

If *deformity* is present, the following points should be ascertained: (1) the patient's concept of the deformity, (2) when and by whom it was first noted, (3) whether its onset was associated with known injury or disease, (4) whether the deformity appears to be increasing, and (5) the degree of disability experienced by the patient. Deformity, unless immediately associated with trauma, is seldom recognized first by the patient. Lateral curvature of the spine, for example, is often first called to the attention of the child's parents during the fitting of a dress.

If there has been *paralysis*, one should note these factors: (1) the time and mode of onset, (2) the distribution and degree of paralysis, (3) the improvement or the increase of symptoms, (4) the presence of sensory disturbance, (5) the presence of trophic changes, and (6) any disturbance in the control of bladder or bowel.

When reviewing the past history, pay careful attention to whether there have been previous orthopaedic disabilities, such as a short leg; a limp when growing up, which might indicate a coxa plana or mild slipping of the upper femoral epiphysis; and sprains, fractures, or dislocations. Note also whether the patient has had diabetes, a venereal disease, abscessed teeth, a series of furuncles, or a chest complaint that might indicate pulmonary tuberculosis. It is essential to be always on the lookout for psychic disorders, misleading subjective exaggeration of the symptoms, and malingering, especially in conditions involving the spine. The family history is of significance, particularly in reference to tuberculosis, hemophilia, malignancy, and congenital anomalies.

Examination. Whenever possible a thorough physical examination should be done initially, with the patient undressed, in addition to a careful study of the area of local complaint. This is especially important in conditions marked by low back pain, since the possibility of referred pain must be considered. A comprehensive physical examination is always indicated in the search for contributing factors, such as visceral neoplasms that may have metastasized to bone. In order to obtain the confidence of the patient, which is so important, especially with children, the examiner should proceed quietly and gently. In addition to the routine physical examination, there should be careful observation of the patient as he stands and walks, since abnormalities of posture and gait are often helpful in suggesting the diagnosis. Whether the patient is of slender or stocky build should be noted and whether his muscles are overdeveloped, normal, or underdeveloped. In

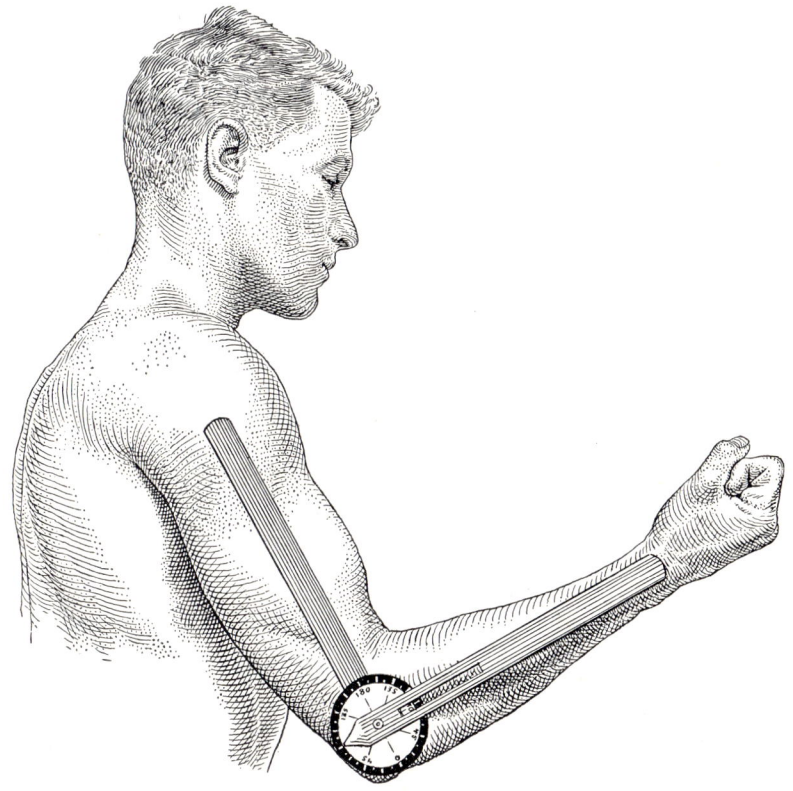

Fig. 3. Goniometer for measuring the range of joint motion.

a child, overdevelopment of certain muscles may indicate pseudohypertrophic muscular dystrophy. Underdeveloped muscles and faulty posture may underlie backache and foot pain.

Often a tentative diagnosis can be made on the basis of gait alone, such as the "duck waddle" associated with congenitally dislocated hips, coxa vara, and progressive muscular dystrophy, or the unilateral sway associated with a weak gluteus medius after poliomyelitis.

Careful inspection of the affected region should be made, and any dissimilarity as compared with a corresponding normal area should be observed. Any redness, swelling, atrophy, or other visible abnormality should be noted. Muscular atrophy is frequently a valuable confirmatory sign of disuse and local disability. Following inspection, a careful palpation of the affected region should be performed in an attempt to determine the presence of increased local heat, tenderness, crepitation, changes in consistency, or abnormal masses.

Both active and passive motion of the joint or joints should be observed carefully. It is important to compare the range of motion of the pathologic joint with that of the corresponding normal joint. The range of motion should be measured with a *goniometer* wherever possible (Fig. 3); if such an instrument is not available, an approximation of the range of joint motion should be made.

The terminology of joint motions has not been standardized, but progress toward this goal is being made. At the shoulder, for example, the terminology long in use (Fig. 4) describes certain end positions adequately but is confusing when applied to intermediate positions. A committee of the American Academy of Orthopaedic Surgeons, of which Rowe is chairman,

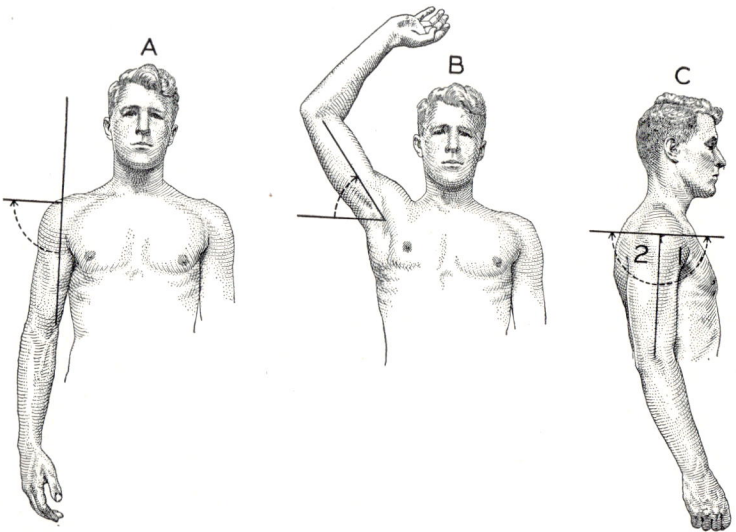

Fig. 4. Terminology of shoulder motion. Arrows indicate direction of **A**, abduction; **B**, elevation; **C**, flexion (**1**) and extension (**2**). (After Cave and Roberts.)

Introduction 31

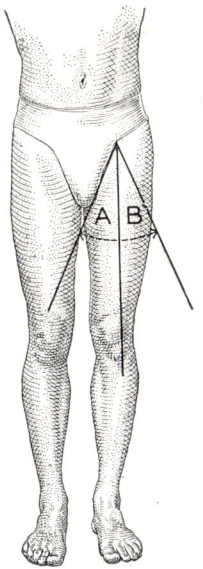

Fig. 5. Terminology of hip motion. Arrows indicate direction of **A**, adduction, and **B**, abduction. (After Cave and Roberts.)

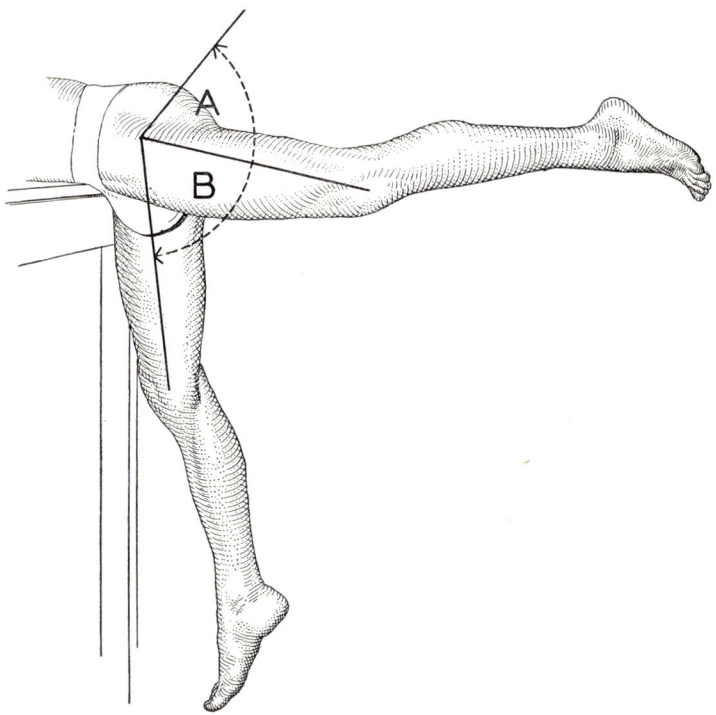

Fig. 6. Terminology of hip motion. Arrows indicate direction of **A**, hyperextension, and **B**, flexion. (After Cave and Roberts.)

has developed a system of terminology, based on earlier work by Cave and Roberts, which is applicable to all joint positions.* In this system mobility is expressed in degrees of deviation from a defined "neutral zero" position for each joint. The neutral zero position of the elbow, wrist, fingers, hip (Figs. 5 and 6), knee, and toes, for example, is that of the extended extremity or anatomic position. Motion from the neutral position (Fig. 7) and limitation of motion (Fig. 8) are expressed in degrees. The medical student should learn this terminology and use it for describing joint mobility in the records of his patients.

During the examination of joint motion, the presence of muscle spasm and of crepitus should be noted. A joint which has a normal range of smooth, painless, active motion can be presumed to be free of any advanced lesion. It is often desirable to measure the length of the extremities and their circumference at corresponding levels. In determining the length of the lower extremities, one should take the following measurements: (1) the distance between the lower margin of the anterior superior iliac spine and the tibial malleolus (actual length) and (2) the distance between the umbilicus and the tibial malleolus (apparent length). Such measurements of the lower extremities approach accuracy only when made with the patient lying relaxed on a table, with his pelvis level, his hips and knees fully extended, and both hips equally abducted or adducted. To determine the length of the upper extremities, take measurements from the tip of the acromion to the tip of the middle finger while the shoulder is adducted, the elbow is extended, the wrist is in the neutral position, and the fingers are extended. About the hip it may be useful to determine the relationship of the greater trochanter to *Nélaton's line* (the line from the anterior superior iliac spine to the tuberosity of the ischium) and to note the length of *Bryant's line* (the distance between lines projected perpendicular to the long axis of the body at the anterior superior spine and at the greater trochanter). Displacement of the tip of the greater trochanter above Nélaton's line and shortening of Bryant's line indicate a lesion of the head or neck of the femur. One should become acquainted with conventional methods of expressing deformity and the degree of limitation of motion. The following will serve as an example. In deformities of the hip, routine examination sometimes fails to demonstrate the degree of hip flexion in the presence of a lordosis or hyperextension of the lumbar spine (Fig. 9). In such cases the examiner should flex the patient's normal hip fully on the abdomen. This procedure will flatten the lumbar spine against the examining table, and an accurate determination of the amount of flexion contracture of the affected hip can then be made. At times it is difficult to ascertain abnormal limitation of motion of the spine. There is great variation in the flexibility of the spinal column in different individuals. Abnormal limitation of motion is usually present when there are tenderness and evidence of muscle spasm; stiffness of long standing may be present in the absence of pain, tenderness, and spasm.

*Available in booklet form from the American Academy of Orthopaedic Surgeons, 29 E. Madison St., Chicago 2, Ill., and also printed in the *Manual of orthopaedic surgery* (see footnote, p. 27).

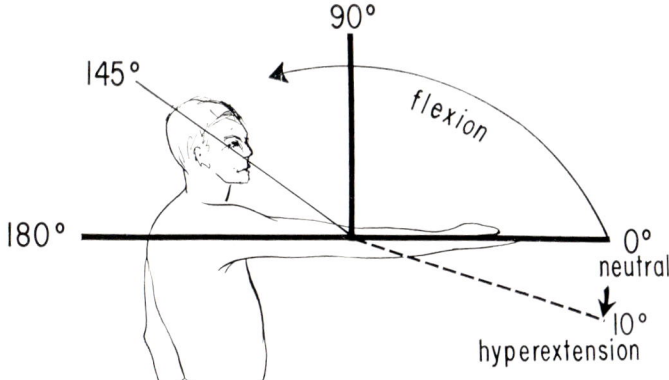

Fig. 7. Terminology of elbow motion. Range of motion is expressed in number of degrees of flexion and of hyperextension from the straight, or neutral zero, position. (After Rowe.)

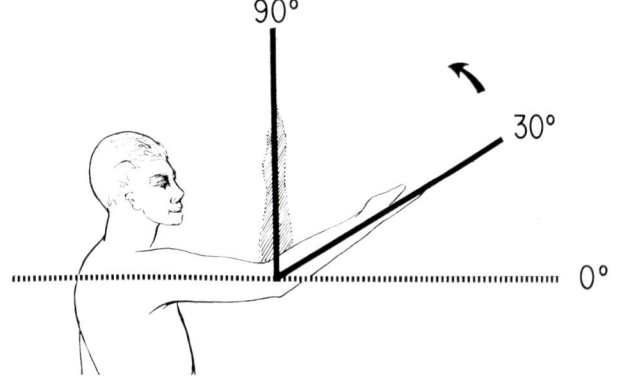

Fig. 8. Terminology of limited motion in the elbow joint. In this instance motion is present from 30 degrees to 90 degrees. This may be expressed also as "a flexion deformity of 30 degrees with further flexion to 90 degrees." (After Rowe.)

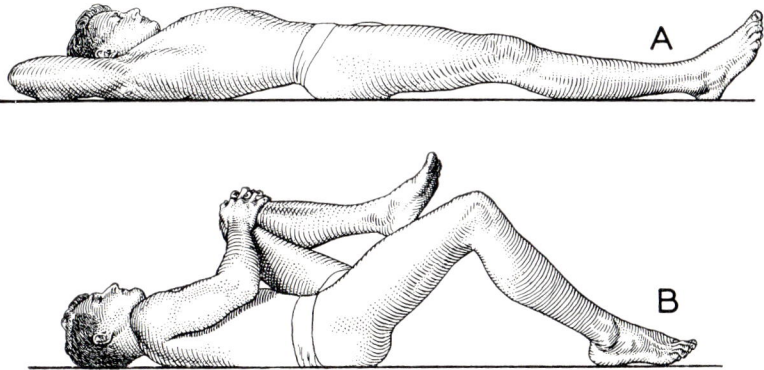

Fig. 9. Test for flexion contracture of right hip. **A,** With patient supine, flexion of right hip is concealed by arching of lumbar spine. **B,** With normal left hip held in extreme flexion to flatten the lumbar lordosis, flexion contracture of right hip is evident.

Occasionally auscultation of joints, especially in the case of the knee, is helpful in determining whether crepitation is present.

A careful neurologic examination is necessary when a neuromuscular disturbance is suspected. The type and distribution of motor paralysis should be determined, the character of the reflexes should be recorded, any change in sensation should be charted, and the presence of atrophy should be noted. In cases of paralysis it is most important to estimate the power of each muscle or muscle group. Muscle testing should be done with great care, and the findings should be recorded in detail. It is convenient to use the following scale, which was introduced by the National Foundation for Infantile Paralysis:

100%	5	N	Normal	Complete range of motion against gravity with full resistance
75%	4	G	Good	Complete range of motion against gravity with some resistance
50%	3	F	Fair	Complete range of motion against gravity
25%	2	P	Poor	Complete range of motion with gravity eliminated
10%	1	T	Trace	Evidence of slight contractility, but no joint motion
0	0	0	Zero	No evidence of contractility
S	or	SS	Spasm	Spasm or severe spasm
C	or	CC	Contracture	Contracture or severe contracture

Congenital abnormalities should be recorded. Static deformities should be noted, as well as abnormalities of posture, and especially those which may be associated with unequal lengths of the legs, flatfeet, or knock-knees. As a rule such postural abnormalities can be recognized without difficulty.

Roentgenographic diagnosis. Roentgenographic examination of the bones and joints is frequently necessary to clarify or confirm the clinical diagnosis. The roentgen-ray findings may include bone atrophy or hypertrophy, erosion or increased density, change in bone relationships, change in joint contour, or change in the soft tissues. For interpretation of roentgenograms the student or practitioner should not rely on the roentgenologist's report but should himself examine and interpret every film in the light of the clinical findings. Comparison of roentgenograms of the involved structure with films of the opposite, normal side is often essential, particularly in children because of normal variations of the epiphyses incident to growth. In children, roentgenograms of the carpal bones may be indicated to determine bone or physiologic age. Certain cases may require, in addition to routine anteroposterior and lateral roentgenograms, films made in oblique positions, stereoscopic films, or laminagrams. Roentgenograms made after the injection of contrast media often provide useful diagnostic data.

Laboratory diagnosis. The clinical examination of the patient should be supplemented, whenever indicated, by laboratory studies of the blood, urine, synovial fluid, spinal fluid, aspirates, or other material, which often reveal facts essential to the diagnosis and treatment. In many bone diseases it is important to have a determination of the serum proteins, calcium, phosphorus, and phosphatase. Microscopic examination of pathologic tissue is especially indicated when the presence of tuberculosis or of malignancy is suspected. Joint cultures and inoculation of guinea pigs with joint fluid are often essential in establishing the presence of tuberculosis. Often the intracutaneous tuberculin test is of considerable diagnostic value. Tests of thyroid function, an electrocardiogram, or an electroencephalogram may be indicated.

Treatment. Orthopaedic treatment may be divided into nonoperative and operative types. Nonoperative treatment comprises such procedures as rest and support, secured by strapping, braces, splints, traction, and plaster casts; physical therapy, including the use of selected exercises, heat, and massage; occupational therapy; and medical treatment, such as the administration of drugs and the prescription of diets. Operative treatment may be classified as closed or open. The closed operations consist of manipulative procedures, such as the reduction of dislocations and fractures, and the stretching of contractures. The most frequently performed open operations are tenotomy, osteotomy, arthrotomy, arthrodesis, arthroplasty, and the open reduction of fractures. Tendon and muscle transference, nerve transference or resection, and bone grafting are indicated less frequently. The object of all operative treatment is to improve function. Operation should never be performed at the risk of decreasing function, lessening needed stability, or leading to pain.

The treatment of orthopaedic patients frequently requires consultation with one or several other specialists. The consultants' advice should be carefully considered with the orthopaedic findings before the final decision concerning treatment is made. The orthopaedic surgeon who fails to obtain a consultation when it is needed may be embarrassed by finding, after weeks or months of unsuccessful treatment, that the diagnosis is not primarily orthopaedic.

Lesions of the bones, joints, and allied structures often require a longer time for healing than do those of other tissues of the body; hence the convalescence of the average orthopaedic patient is notably slow. Because of the long period often necessary for treatment, the patient may become disheartened, lose morale, and develop a mental attitude that acts as a psychologic barrier to normal convalescence. To offset this, patience and optimism are required of the physician, and a well-rounded program of rehabilitation should be started early in the course of treatment. The rehabilitation program should include intelligently planned physical and mental activities. Too quick a recovery cannot be expected and should not be promised. Because of the slowness of the improvement often encountered in orthopaedic patients, they may change from doctor to doctor and from one form of treatment to another and may ultimately find themselves in the hands of an unethical practitioner or cultist. For the best understanding between patient and doctor, a frank and honest statement should be made early by the doctor to the patient, to the family, or to both, explaining in detail as much as is known about the cause of the complaint, the treatment, and the prognosis. Consultation with other physicians should be encouraged if the diagnosis is uncertain or the results of treatment are slow.

Rehabilitation. In recent years increased emphasis has been placed on the physician's part in restoration of the patient to normal living following his illness or injury. This phase of medicine, which has always been a part of good, comprehensive medical care, is termed rehabilitation. Programs of rehabilitation are designed (1) to separate the patient from bed and hospital as soon as possible, (2) to restore the patient to maximum functional activity as quickly as possible, and (3) to facilitate the patient's early adjustment to work, home, and community.

The orthopaedic patients most often requiring long-term rehabilitation are those with paraplegia, cerebral palsy, poliomyelitis, low back pain, arthritis, fresh fractures, fracture deformities, and amputations. The orthopaedic surgeon, who deals predominantly with chronic disabilities, has always included rehabilitation as an essential part of orthopaedic treatment. Effective rehabilitation in orthopaedic cases often requires a team composed of representatives from various disciplines and including, in addition to the orthopaedic surgeon, a physiatrist, physical therapist, occupational therapist, vocational counselor, and social worker. It is important to the patient's welfare that his attending physician—who in orthopaedic cases is usually the orthopaedic surgeon—plan, direct, and interpret the rehabilitative procedures.

In hospital, rehabilitation should start when the patient is admitted. The orthopaedist should explain to the adult patient the nature of his illness or injury, what is to be its treatment, and what is to be the patient's own part in getting well. A physical conditioning program, occupational therapy, planned recreational activity, and vocational counseling may be indicated. If on discharge from hospital the patient will obviously be unable to resume his former occupation, the orthopaedist should consider sending him to a rehabilitation facility where, after an evaluation of interests, aptitudes, and capacities, the patient can learn a suitable occupation. The orthopaedic surgeon should work with the state rehabilitation counselor in obtaining vocational training for his handicapped patients and as a rule should follow all of his patients at intervals until their occupational and social readjustments have been achieved.

NOTE: Anyone further interested in these subjects should make use of the bibliography (p. 502) for more extended reading. The bibliography is by no means exhaustive; an attempt has been made, however, to select as references the most authoritative orthopaedic textbooks and the most informative articles written in English.

CHAPTER 2

Congenital deformities

CONGENITAL DEFORMITIES are abnormalities of development present at birth. They are frequently observed in all orthopaedic clinics, particularly on the crippled children's services. There are many different types of anomalies and numerous minor variations, which may involve any bone or joint structure. Congenital deformities vary in significance from very minor abnormalities, such as webbing of the toes, to serious and disabling defects, such as absence of the major portion of an extremity.

In recent years much progress has been made in study of the causes of congenital anomalies. Anomalies are believed to result from abnormal genetic factors, alterations in the environment of the developing fetus, or both. Recently it has been demonstrated that individuals affected with certain congenital syndromes such as mongolism possess an abnormal number or type of chromosomes. Genetically determined defects may result from such chromosomal aberrations or from mutations of genes in recent or distant ancestors. New hereditary defects appear as the result of either small point mutations or larger chromosomal disorders. Animal experimentation has shown that mutations can be brought about by exposing the germ cells to ionizing radiations or to any of a great variety of chemical agents. This fact is of considerable importance in an age when human exposure to radiation and chemicals in the environment is of increasing occurrence. According to Fraser, however, only about 10% of all human congenital deformities can be definitely classed as hereditary in origin.

Harmful influences in the environment of the developing fetus possibly account for the majority of congenital defects. Factors shown to have an adverse effect on the human fetus are heavy irradiation, the folic acid antagonist aminopterin, rubella, toxoplasmosis, and certain androgenic hormones. Probably many other agents can injure the human fetus. All of these produce damage during the first trimester of pregnancy. The incidence of congenital defects increases as maternal age increases. Maternal diabetes also has an unfavorable influence on the fetus.

Congenital defects have been produced experimentally in many animals, including mammals. Defects of the nervous system, cleft palate, clubfoot, polydactyly, syndactyly, and many other deformities have been produced in the laboratory by a variety of means. Agents capable of inducing congenital abnormalities include deficient diets, x-rays, hypothermia, hypoxia, certain viruses, and many chemicals. Hormones such as androgens, insulin, and cortisone, when injected into animals during early pregnancy, have also produced a variety of defects. These teratogenic agents are not specific in their action. The type of congenital defect depends greatly upon the stage of fetal development at which the agent is applied.

Largely because of their uncertain etiology, congenital deformities are generally not preventable, but it is possible that improved care of the health of the expectant mother may lessen their incidence. Treatment, when indicated, should in most instances be started quite early in infancy, before abnormal changes in the affected tissues become more advanced and fixed by increasing age and trauma and before they lead to deforming secondary changes in adjacent structures. The effectiveness of treatment in reducing disability and disfigurement varies widely with the type of anomaly and with the promptness with which the treatment is instituted.

The two most common and important congenital anomalies are clubfoot and dislocation of the hip. Congenital dislocations are considered in Chapter 3. In the present chapter, congenital clubfoot and a number of other congenital deformities are described. Several additional types of congenital anomaly, including cervical rib, torticollis, and lumbosacral variations, are discussed in subsequent chapters, dealing with individual regions of the body.

CONGENITAL TALIPES

The term "talipes" is used in connection with many foot deformities, whether congenital or acquired. It is derived from the Latin *talus*, meaning ankle, and *pes*, meaning foot, and was originally used to designate a foot

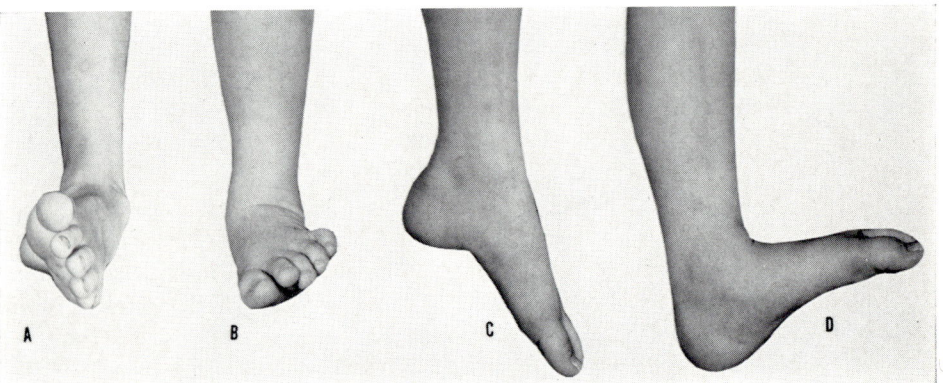

Fig. 10. Four cardinal positions of foot deformity. **A**, Varus. **B**, Valgus. **C**, Equinus. **D**, Calcaneus.

deformity that caused the patient to walk on the ankle. Deformities of the foot and ankle are conventionally described according to the position of the foot. The four cardinal positions (Fig. 10) are (1) *varus,* or inversion, (2) *valgus,* or eversion, (3) *equinus,* or plantar flexion, and (4) *calcaneus,* or dorsiflexion. Of the congenital deformities of the foot, the combination of equinus and varus is the most common, and that of calcaneus and valgus next. The equinovarus foot has a clublike appearance and is the classical type of congenital clubfoot.

CONGENITAL TALIPES EQUINOVARUS (CONGENITAL CLUBFOOT)

Etiology. A hereditary factor is often concerned in the etiology of clubfoot, its presence being observed in from 5 to 22% of the cases in reported series. The most widely accepted hypotheses of the pathogenesis of clubfoot are the following:

1. Arrested or anomalous development of this particular part of the germ plasm in the first trimester of pregnancy may be the cause. This theory receives indirect support from the statistical fact that between 4 and 12% of the patients with congenital clubfoot in reported series have other congenital anomalies as well.

2. At about the third month of intrauterine life the foot occupies normally an equinovarus position. As the fetus develops, inward rotation of the leg normally takes place, and by the seventh month the foot is no longer in the equinovarus position. If inward rotation fails to occur, however, the foot remains in equinovarus, and the child is born with a clubfoot. By some embryologists, however, this hypothesis is not accepted.

3. Recent investigations of pathologic changes in the soft tissues in congenital clubfoot have shown abnormalities in the relative maturity and length of the muscles, as well as variations in their tendon insertions. These findings suggest that muscle imbalance may play a considerable part in the causation of congenital clubfoot.

Incidence. Talipes equinovarus is one of the most common congenital anomalies of the foot. It is twice as common in boys as in girls. The statistics of most clinics have shown that it is observed in a single foot more frequently than in both, but a few reports have shown the reverse. Occasionally there is talipes equinovarus on one side, with talipes calcaneovalgus on the other.

Pathology. All degrees of talipes equinovarus, from a very mild deformity to one in which the toes touch the medial side of the lower leg, are found. The Achilles tendon is always shortened. The anterior and posterior tibial tendons are contracted in proportion to the degree of varus deformity. In some cases degenerative changes in the fibers of certain muscles and anomalous insertions of tendons in the foot have been demonstrated. The ligaments and joint capsules on the medial side of the foot are thickened and contracted.

In most instances the individual bones of the foot are normal at birth, and only their relationships to each other are altered. The calcaneus is rolled in under the talus, and the navicular is medially displaced on the head of the talus. As the child grows, adaptive changes take place in these bones. The talus may be wedge-shaped, with only its posterior surface apposed to the tibia. Its neck is elongated, depressed, and deflected medially, and its head is flattened. A small portion of the navicular bone articulates with the inner border of the head of the talus. The calcaneus points downward and is tilted in such fashion that its medial process approaches the tibial malleolus. The anterior extremity of the calcaneus is pointed medially and follows the direction of the neck of the talus. The calcaneus lies more nearly under the talus than normally. The distal portions of the tibia and fibula usually show slight inward rotation; this deformity of the tibia is called *tibial torsion*. Structural changes are found in all other bones of the foot but are less extreme in degree. The anatomic changes vary according to the degree of the deformity; in the mild clubfoot the bony changes may be minimal.

In older, untreated patients proliferative bone changes due to weight bearing take place about the edges of the articulating surfaces. The articular cartilage undergoes atrophy. New bone is practically always formed around the greatly thickened and broadened proximal end of the fifth metatarsal bone. A large bursa forms over the weight-bearing surface on the lateral portion of the dorsum of the foot and may contain a semisolid gelatinous material. In the older cases genu valgum is frequently associated.

Clinical picture. The heel is drawn up, the entire foot below the talus is inverted, and the anterior half of the foot is adducted (Fig. 11). The medial border of the foot is concave, the lateral is convex, and there is a transverse crease across the sole at the level of the mediotarsal joint. When the infant starts to walk, he suffers a tremendous handicap because of his inability to bear weight normally. The muscles of the leg quickly become fatigued and soon show marked atrophy. Pain is experienced only by the adult patient in whom arthritic changes have developed.

Unilateral clubfoot causes a marked limp. The child with bilateral clubfoot deformity exhibits a typical gait called the "reel walk," in which considerable wobbling from side to side takes place.

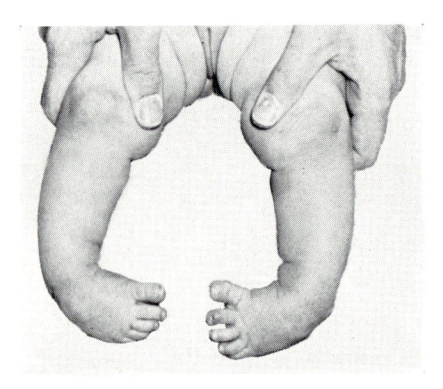

Fig. 11. Bilateral talipes equinovarus (clubfeet) in 2-month-old infant.

In extreme talipes equinovarus the weight is borne upon a bursa which rapidly develops over the cuboid and proximal end of the fifth metatarsal bone when the child begins to walk. This pad acts to absorb shock in the same manner as does the heel cushion of the normal foot.

Diagnosis. In infants the diagnosis of congenital clubfoot is made with ease, but in older children and adults it is sometimes difficult to exclude paralysis as a cause of the deformity. Clubfoot is seen frequently in association with paralytic changes in the lower extremities in spina bifida, cerebral palsy, and poliomyelitis. Often the first sign of the peroneal type of progressive muscular atrophy is the development of slight equinovarus. Occasionally in progressive muscular dystrophy the foot has a similar appearance. Old injury of the lower tibial epiphysis, osteomyelitis, and fracture in the region of the ankle joint are other causes of equinovarus deformity.

Prognosis. The earlier the treatment is started, the better the result. When treatment is begun within the first three months of life there is an excellent chance that the deformity may be completely corrected by nonoperative procedures in a relatively short time. The course of treatment may be long, however, requiring several years. According to Kite, from 10 to 15% of the patients tend later to relapse and require a second period of treatment. In the case of a patient who is treated late—i.e., after the first year—the prognosis for a normally functioning foot is poor. In untreated cases the deformity usually increases until the patient walks upon the lateral portion of the dorsum of the foot, and the disability becomes greater as the patient grows older.

Treatment. Treatment should be started as soon as the deformity is recognized. If treatment is begun immediately after birth, the problem of correcting the deformity is simple as contrasted with the difficulty encountered in older infants or children.

The treatment is divided into three stages: (1) correction of the deformity, (2) maintenance of correction until normal muscle balance has been regained, and (3) observation for several years in order to forestall any recurrence of the deformity.

It is most important that the first stage of treatment be continued until a position of marked overcorrection has been reached. Anything short of this constitutes inadequate treatment. The position of dorsiflexion and eversion of the foot and abduction of the forefoot is the goal of every form of treatment.

It is generally agreed that the functional result is far better if the final position can be obtained without the trauma of forceful manipulation and without radical surgery, either of which may be followed by bone changes and stiffness of the joints of the foot. Lengthening of the Achilles tendon and posterior capsulotomy of the ankle joint, however, usually produce no unfavorable effects if unaccompanied by forceful manipulation.

The ease with which correction may be obtained and the choice of method in the *first stage of treatment* vary according to the age of the patient. In young infants a series of plaster casts, applied without manipulation other than holding the foot in a position of as much correction as can be ob-

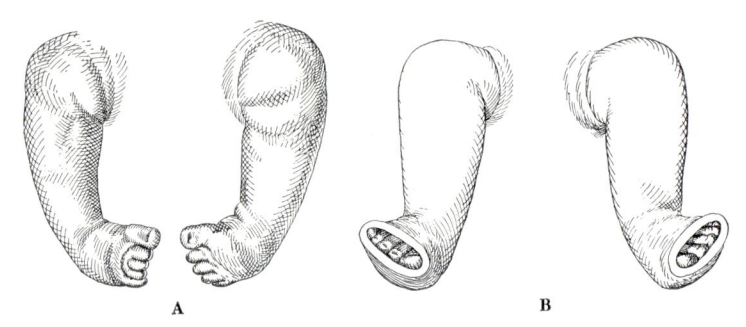

Fig. 12. Bilateral talipes equinovarus in infant. **A,** Before correction. **B,** Undergoing correction in plaster casts.

tained without the use of force, is usually effective (Fig. 12). Painting the skin with a nonirritating, adhesive liquid helps to prevent slipping of the cast and loss of the corrected position. The cast should be changed at intervals of from three to fourteen days. Successive casts provide an opportunity for the tight structures on the medial side of the foot to stretch and for the lax structures on the lateral side of the foot to contract. In this way a gradual correction of the deformity is obtained without the application of excessive force. The casts should be padded, particularly over bony prominences, and usually should extend above the flexed knee to allow effective correction of the rotation deformity. It is often convenient to use the technic of wedging the cast instead of changing the entire cast. A wedge of plaster is taken out over that aspect of the foot toward which correction is desired, the sides of the wedge are brought together, and plaster is applied in circular fashion over the closed-in wedge.

The adduction deformity should be corrected first; this phase of the treatment must be continued until the navicular bone is brought directly in front of the head of the talus. Next, the inversion deformity is corrected; care must be taken to continue this until there is no inversion of the calcaneus. Complete correction of the relationship between the talus and the calcaneus may be verified by an anteroposterior roentgenogram of the foot showing anterior divergence of their long axes. Finally, the plantar flexion or equinus is corrected by gradually increased dorsiflexion of the ankle. Attempts to correct simultaneously all three elements of the deformity may produce a misshapen "rocker-bottom" foot. If necessary, correction of the equinus may be aided by (1) lengthening of the Achilles tendon and (2) posterior capsulotomy of the ankle joint. The final cast is often left on for a period of four to eight weeks to allow thorough accommodation to the new position. It may be necessary, for many months, to use a night splint to hold the foot in the overcorrected position.

An alternative method of correcting the deformity of congenital clubfoot is the use of the Denis Browne splint. This splint (Fig. 13) consists of two padded metal plates that are securely fastened with adhesive tape to the infant's feet and are then connected by a crossbar. The stretching of contracted structures is accelerated by the infant's kicking. The footplates can

Congenital deformities 43

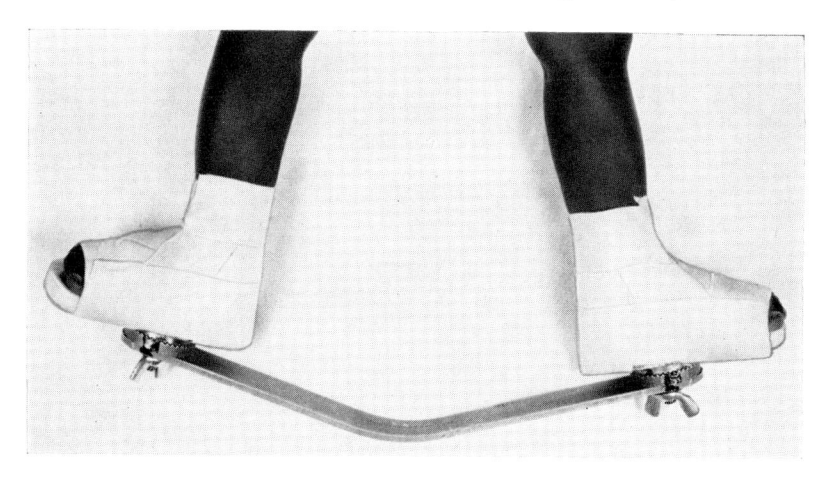

Fig. 13. Denis Browne splint for correction of clubfoot. Felt-padded plates are strapped to the feet in corrected position with adhesive tape. The control of rotation, eversion, and dorsiflexion is adjustable.

be so rotated outward on the crossbar that progressive correction of the adduction and later of the equinus may be obtained.

After full overcorrection of the deformity in all planes has been secured by means of casts or the Denis Browne splint, measures are taken to maintain the correction and to encourage the development of normal muscle balance. A clubfoot shoe to hold the corrected position should be used. This shoe has a lateral deviation of its anterior half and a slight raise ($\frac{1}{8}$ to $\frac{1}{4}$ inch) of its entire lateral border (Fig. 14). When special clubfoot shoes cannot be obtained, ordinary shoes can be altered to aid in preventing a recurrence of the deformity. Corrective night shoes and splints are also useful. The Denis Browne splint may be applied by means of shoes and used to maintain correction (Fig. 15). Walking should be encouraged in order to strengthen the weakened muscles. If the patient is old enough to cooperate in muscle training, exercises to strengthen the muscles of abduction, eversion, and dorsiflexion of the foot and ankle may be helpful.

In certain of the more difficult cases, casts alone may prove inadequate for correcting the deformity within a reasonable length of time. This is particularly true in older children and in cases of recurrent clubfoot. For such patients surgical treatment should be considered. If the child is less than 8 to 10 years old, operation should usually be limited to the soft tissues. The simplest and most frequently used operation is lengthening of the Achilles tendon to lessen the equinus deformity. Often this should be accompanied by section of the posterior capsule of the ankle joint, which may be tightly contracted. Surgical correction of the varus and forefoot adduction is more difficult. Various soft tissue releases may be used. They usually involve cutting the tendinous and ligamentous structures on the medial side of the foot. All such surgical procedures must be followed by further attempts at overcorrection by plaster casts.

44   *Handbook of orthopaedic surgery*

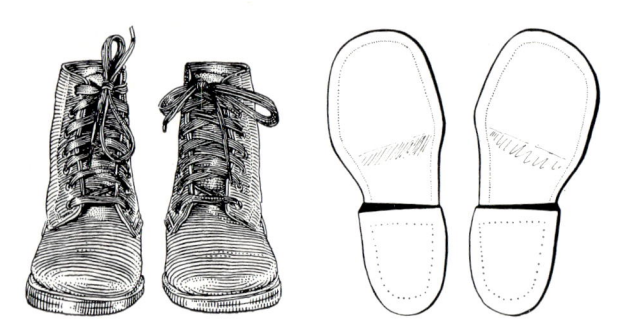

Fig. 14. Clubfoot shoes. The lateral side of the soles and heels is raised to maintain correction of varus deformity, and the front half of the shoes is turned out to maintain correction of forefoot adduction.

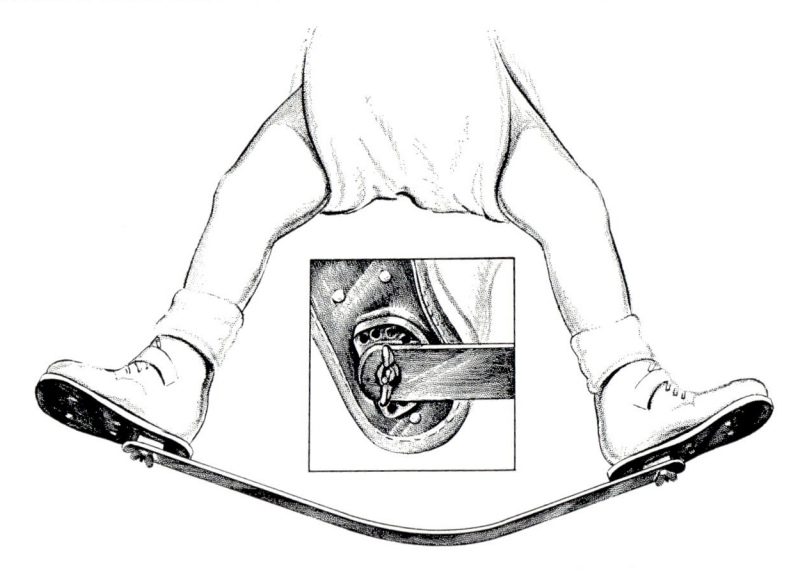

Fig. 15. Denis Browne splint worn day and night, or at night only, to assist in maintaining corrected position after full overcorrection of clubfoot deformity has been accomplished by earlier treatment. Note dorsiflexion of ankles and external rotation. Attachment of footplate to crossbar, shown in inset, allows adjustment of rotation. Bending the crossbar increases dorsiflexion.

The correction of a clubfoot deformity in a child more than 10 years old or in an adult usually requires operation upon the tarsal bones. A *wedge osteotomy,* the base of the wedge being on the dorsal and lateral aspect of the foot, is frequently indicated. As much bone as is necessary to correct the deformity completely is removed from the region of the mediotarsal joint. At the same time the subtalar joint is usually fused. While such operations stiffen one or more of the abnormal tarsal joints, they usually improve the function, endurance, and appearance of the foot.

After either nonoperative or surgical treatment, the corrected clubfoot should be observed until the child has reached adolescence, or in the case of older patients for at least several years. During this period any tendency toward recurrence of the deformity should be promptly and thoroughly treated. A recurrent deformity is usually more difficult to treat than the original clubfoot. Lateral transference of the anterior tibial tendon, as advocated by Garceau, is often helpful in preventing a recurrence of the varus and adduction deformity.

OTHER FORMS OF CONGENITAL TALIPES

In comparison with talipes equinovarus, other forms of congenital talipes are less common and less difficult to treat.

Talipes calcaneovalgus

Talipes calcaneovalgus, a congenital deformity characterized by eversion of the foot, increased dorsiflexion of the ankle, and apparent lengthening of the Achilles tendon, is seen frequently. It is often of mild degree and, unlike congenital equinovarus, is not fixed but can be easily overcorrected by stretching. It is most noticeable immediately after birth. As the child begins to use his muscles and kick his legs, the condition becomes less marked and often seems to disappear completely. When the infant later begins to stand, however, persistent changes in the affected foot or feet may be evidenced by excessive pronation.

Mild degrees of calcaneovalgus require no treatment. Moderate ones may be improved by gentle stretching exercises applied by the mother. Feet severely deformed at birth should be held in light corrective casts for at least several weeks. A Denis Browne splint holding the feet in an equinovarus position for several months is sometimes indicated. Every foot that has shown an early calcaneovalgus deformity should be fitted with a strong shoe with a ⅛-inch raise of its medial border when the infant begins to stand and walk; usually the shoe modification should be continued for several years.

Talipes valgus

At times a valgus deformity is seen without calcaneus. The treatment is identical with that of talipes calcaneovalgus.

Talipes calcaneus

Simple calcaneus deformity is treated in the manner outlined for talipes calcaneovalgus.

Talipes varus

Talipes varus is usually an incomplete form of congenital equinovarus deformity; it sometimes resembles a relapsed equinovarus foot. The treatment is the same as that described for talipes equinovarus.

Talipes equinus

Congenital talipes equinus is about half as common as talipes varus. It should be treated at birth or soon thereafter by corrective casts. In the

46   Handbook of orthopaedic surgery

older child it is often necessary to lengthen the Achilles tendon and to perform a posterior capsulotomy of the ankle joint before the equinus can be fully corrected. Operation should be followed by a plaster cast for from four to six weeks.

Metatarsus varus (metatarsus adductus)

The deformity known by these names is quite common, being seen more frequently than talipes equinovarus. It consists of adduction of the forefoot at the tarsometatarsal joints; sometimes inversion is present also (Fig. 16). The condition has at times been called "skewfoot." Many observers, among them Kite, report that the incidence of this deformity is increasing. It may involve one or both feet; when unilateral it is sometimes associated with clubfoot of the opposite extremity. At times it may be a residual deformity resulting from an old congenital talipes equinovarus. Metatarsus varus may also be of acquired type, in which case it is usually combined with valgus deformity of the posterior portion of the foot. The deformity is obvious on inspection. If it is untreated until after walking has begun, the mother will usually complain that the child "toes in," walks clumsily, and trips over his feet. Metatarsus varus is one of the causes of pigeon-toe.

Treatment in very mild cases may involve only stretching exercises carried out by the mother five or six times a day. The exercise is simple, consisting of stretching the forefoot gently into abduction. If the deformity is more than minimal, cast treatment is indicated. The earlier such treatment is started, the better the end result. A bootee cast extending from the toes to just above the ankle is sufficient. As the plaster begins to set, the forefoot is molded into a position of abduction. The cast is changed at intervals of a week or two. Overcorrection of the deformity is desired. If the

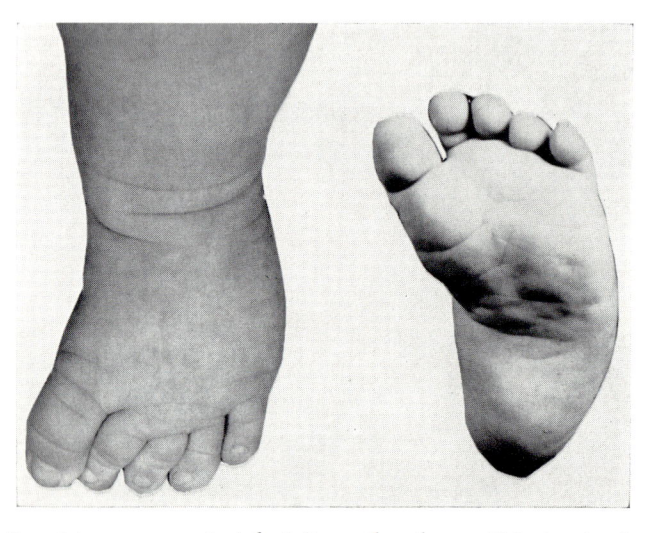

Fig. 16. Left metatarsus varus in infant 3 months of age. Note turning-in of anterior part of the foot.

treatment is early and adequate, the results are usually quite satisfactory. After the correction, special shoes with outswung soles are sometimes prescribed. In severe or late cases, complete correction may not be obtained. Severe metatarsus varus in older children can be improved by surgical treatment.

Congenital vertical talus

A rare and severe form of flatfoot, congenital vertical talus is characterized by a marked plantar flexion of the talus (Fig. 17). Since the forefoot is dorsiflexed, the diagnosis of talipes calcaneovalgus may be mistakenly made. Actually the heel is in equinus and the foot simulates the "rocker-bot-

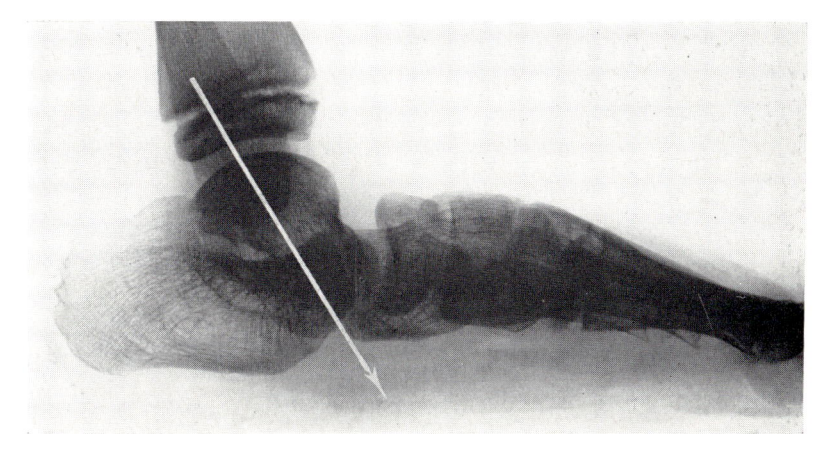

Fig. 17. Congenital vertical talus. Note downward pointing of talar head, subluxation of talonavicular and talocalcaneal joints, equinus position of calcaneus, and loss of longitudinal arch.

tom" foot of inadequately treated clubfoot. The treatment of this rigid foot is most difficult. In infants, alignment of the forefoot with the plantar-flexed talus by a series of casts may be attempted. Early open reduction has sometimes been successful, but if the foot later becomes painful, it may be necessary to reconstruct the bony architecture of the foot surgically in middle childhood or later.

CONGENITAL CLUBHAND

Clubhand is a rare congenital malformation usually associated with complete or partial absence of one of the bones of the forearm. It is sometimes hereditary and may be bilateral (Fig. 18). The hand may be in a flexed, extended, adducted, or abducted position. Of these the most common type is abduction or radial deviation of the hand, associated with defective development or complete absence of the radius (Fig. 19). The thumb is usually very small or completely absent. In this type of deformity the ulna is practically always bowed, with its concavity directed toward the radial side. The forearm is shortened in the unilateral case. The hand and upper

48   Handbook of orthopaedic surgery

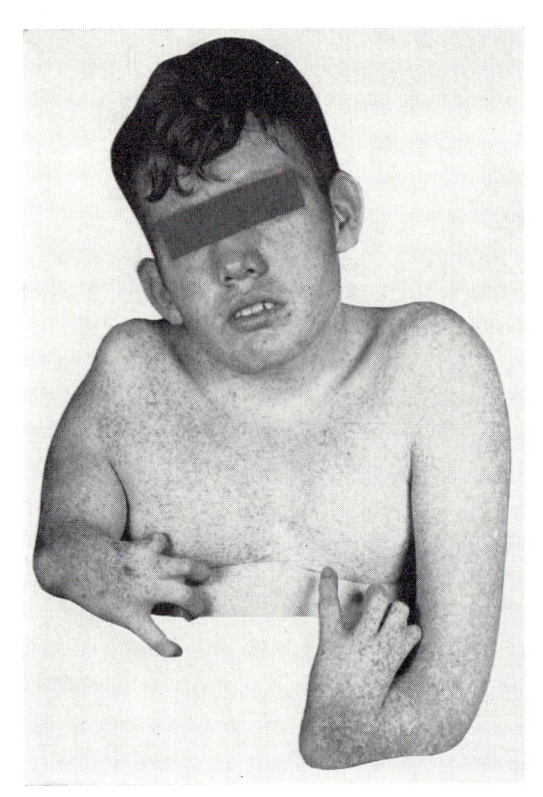

Fig. 18. Bilateral clubhand in a boy 14 years of age. Note turning-in of hands and shortness of forearms. This patient showed bilateral complete absence of the radius, bilateral absence of the thumb, and absence of the proximal two-thirds of the right humerus.

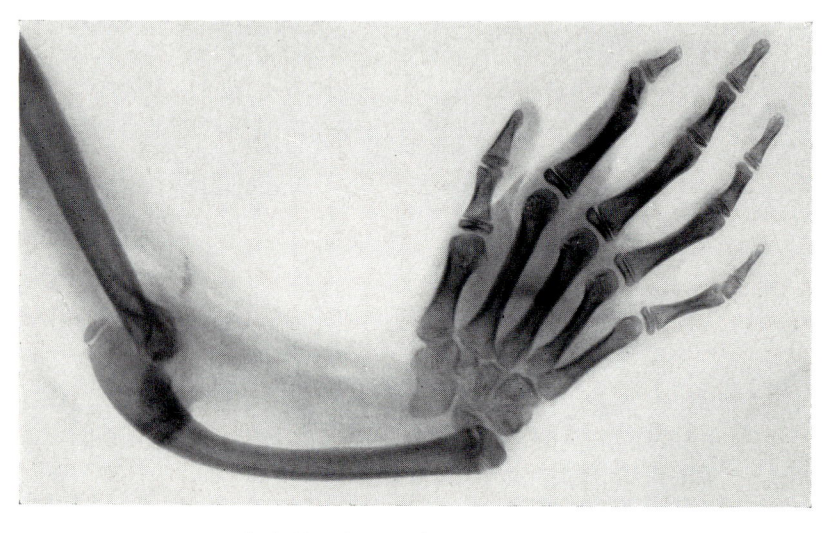

Fig. 19. Roentgenogram of clubhand in girl 10 years of age. Note the turning-in of hand, absence of radius, bowing of ulnar shaft, and prominence of distal end of ulna.

arm are small, and the shoulder girdle is underdeveloped. The right side is affected twice as often as the left. Clubhand with radial deviation is often associated with the presence of a cervical rib. In some instances the radial nerve or the artery has been absent. Despite the deformity, the hand is ordinarily quite useful.

Treatment. If the patient is in infancy or early childhood, an attempt should be made to improve the deformity by means of a series of corrective casts. A brace or splint should be used to maintain the corrected position. Several operative procedures for correction of the deformity have been devised. When the radius is absent, one of the most useful methods consists of beveling the end of the ulna anteriorly and posteriorly and inserting it into a longitudinal split made in the carpus. When the ulna is defective, an analogous operation on the radius may be indicated. The results of these operations are not always satisfactory, especially in younger children. Usually the functional result is better than the cosmetic result.

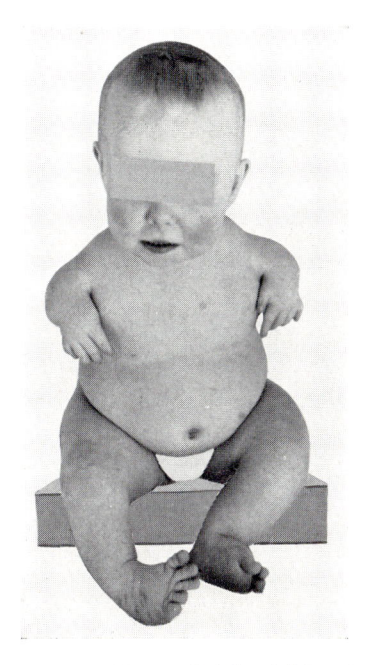

Fig. 20. Phocomelia of upper extremities and right clubfoot in an infant of 11 months.

CONGENITAL DEFECTS OF INDIVIDUAL BONES

Congenital partial absence of a long bone is seen more frequently than total absence. Defects in the bones of the upper extremity are more often bilateral than those occurring in the lower extremity. Complete absence of a

50   Handbook of orthopaedic surgery

middle or intercalary segment of a limb is called *phocomelia* (Fig. 20). Congenital bone defects are often associated with other anomalies. In many instances they form a most difficult therapeutic problem.

Humerus

Humeral defects associated with other anomalies in the upper limb are uncommon; isolated defects of the humerus are rare.

Radius

Partial absence of the radius is observed more often than complete absence, the upper end being most often missing. Clubhand is nearly always associated with this deformity. In 40% of the cases of clubhand associated with a defect of the radius, the condition is bilateral.

Ulna

Defects of the ulna are not so common as those of the radius. Clubhand associated with deficiency of the ulna exhibits a bowing of the forearm, with its concavity directed medially.

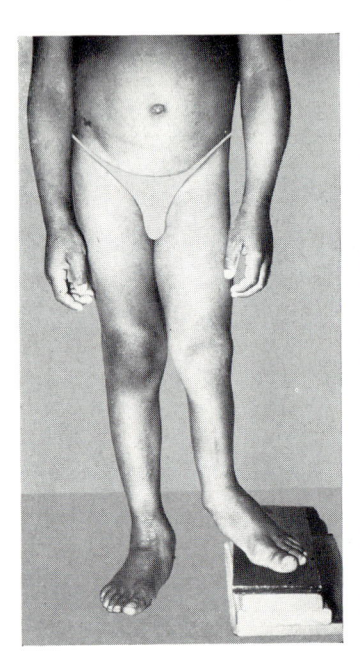

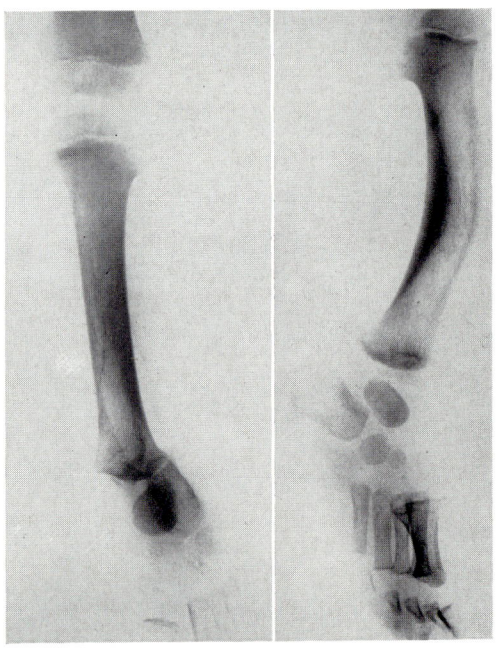

Fig. 21

Fig. 22

Fig. 21. Congenital absence of left fibula in boy 4 years of age. Note shortness of left lower extremity, external rotation of leg and foot, and valgus deformity of foot. The shortness measured 3 inches.

Fig. 22. Anteroposterior and lateral roentgenograms of left lower extremity of the patient shown in Fig. 21. Note absence of fibula, bowing of short and thick tibia, lateral displacement of foot, and equinovalgus deformity.

Congenital deformities 51

Femur

Underdevelopment or partial absence of the femur, especially of its upper third, is much more common than complete absence. With partial absence of the femur are often associated complete absence of the patella and anomalies of the pelvis on the affected side.

Tibia

Absence of the tibia is rare. The limb exhibits a characteristic deformity. The thigh is rotated externally and adducted, the knee is flexed, and the upper end of the fibula is displaced laterally and backward from the femur. The fibula is bowed, with its concavity directed medially, and the foot is in a varus or equinovarus position. It is possible to correct the deformity of the foot surgically and to fuse the upper end of the fibula to the femur. The end results, however, have not always been satisfactory, and amputation at or just above the knee is usually preferable.

Fibula

Congenital absence of the fibula is more common than that of any other long bone. Total absence (Figs. 21 and 22) is observed more fre-

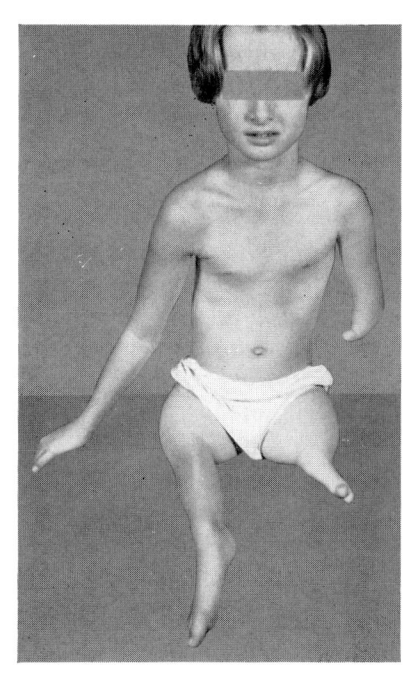

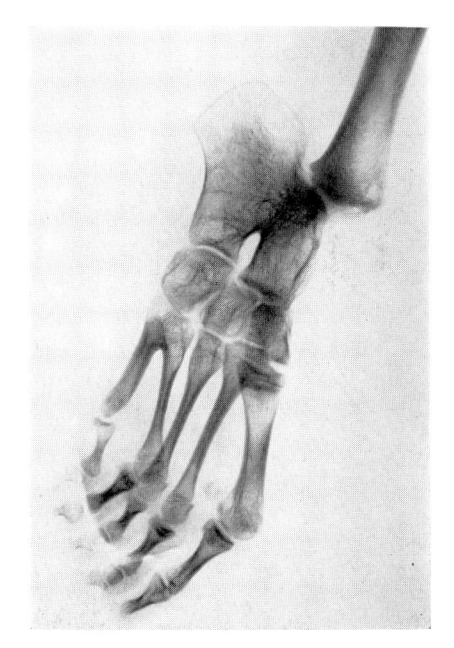

Fig. 23   Fig. 24

Fig. 23. Multiple congenital deformities in girl 9 years of age. Note absence of major parts of left upper and lower extremities, apparent absence of right knee, and severe equinus of right foot.

Fig. 24. Roentgenogram of the right foot of the patient in Fig. 23, showing absence of fibula, severe equinus, and synostosis of calcaneus, talus, and navicular bone.

quently than partial absence. The tibia is usually bowed anteriorly; the foot is short, occupies an equinovalgus position, and may show deformities of the toes. The whole lower extremity is short. Congenital absence of the fibula may occur in association with other congenital anomalies (Figs. 23 and 24). The treatment of congenital absence of the fibula involves correction of the foot deformity and of the tibial bowing. Osteotomy of the tibia is sometimes necessary. A strong fibrous band may be present in the region of the missing fibula; excision of this band may be helpful. When the shortening is not too great, an elevated shoe and brace may be used to equalize the leg length. In some instances the shortening is quite marked and amputation may be indicated to permit the fitting of a conventional prosthesis.

Patella

The development of the patella may be delayed or imperfect, or the bone may be completely absent. Occasionally, an ossification center in the upper and lateral segment fails to fuse with the remainder of the bone, producing a *bipartite patella*. This condition is usually bilateral and ordinarily causes no symptoms. Partial or complete absence of the patella is usually associated with underdevelopment of the quadriceps tendon and occasionally with congenital dislocation of the knee. Clubfoot, dislocation of the hip, and other congenital anomalies are sometimes associated. Deformity and weakness of the knee depend more upon the associated anomalies than upon the defect of the patella.

CONGENITAL RADIOULNAR SYNOSTOSIS

An infrequent congenital anomaly, usually bilateral, is radioulnar synostosis. It occurs as a rule at the proximal end of the radius and ulna (Fig. 25). Sometimes there is only a small bridge of connecting bone. There is practically always a fibrous union between the bones in the lower third of the forearm. The head of the radius is sometimes dislocated. Occasionally there is fusion of the radius, ulna, and humerus, with absence of the elbow joint. The forearm may be fixed in a position of pronation or in one that is midway between pronation and supination. Extension of the elbow is

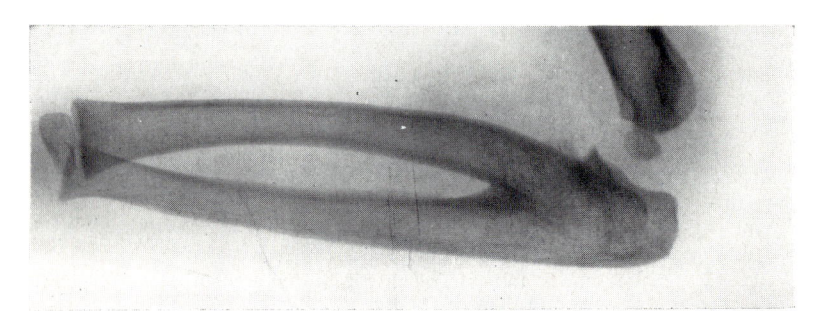

Fig. 25. Roentgenogram showing congenital synostosis of the radius and ulna. Note that their proximal ends have failed to develop separately.

limited. Since the patient learns to compensate for his loss of forearm rotation by increased use of the shoulder, the disability is slight.

Treatment. The whole upper end of the radius may be resected, or only the bone between the radius and ulna, and the space so formed may be filled with fat, muscle, or fascia. Rarely, however, do these operative procedures meet with success. The disappointing postoperative results have been ascribed to the persistence of fibrous bands between the bones in the distal part of the forearm and to the congenital absence of muscles that control rotation of the forearm.

CONGENITAL CONTRACTURES

Congenital contractures may involve any of the joints. When present at the ankle or the wrist, they produce clubfoot or clubhand, respectively. They are usually associated with other congenital malformations. Flexion contracture of the little finger is common and frequently bilateral. Congenital contracture of the elbow is usually associated with a flexion deformity of the wrist. The shoulder often suffers a limitation of abduction. Congenital hip flexion contracture is rare; it may be associated with flexion of the knee. When the knee is flexed, there may be redundant skin in the popliteal space. It is thought that these contractures of the knee and of the hip may result from a long-continued position of flexion in utero.

Treatment. Congenital contractures are treated by (1) gradual manipulation into the corrected position, (2) exercises to develop the weak muscles, usually the extensors, and (3) the use of retention splints. Occasionally it may be desirable to incise the tight skin and underlying resistant bands; it may be necessary to graft skin over resulting denuded areas.

CONGENITAL ABNORMALITIES OF FINGERS AND TOES

Deformities of the hand or foot occur approximately once in every 600 live births; most of them affect only the fingers or toes.

Syndactyly (debbed fingers or toes)

Syndactyly (Fig. 26, A) occurs twice as often in boys as in girls and more often in the hand than in the foot. In the hand the fingers on the ulnar side are more often affected than those on the radial side, and the thumb is seldom involved. The union between the affected parts may consist only of skin and connective tissue or may include bone. Webbing is sometimes associated with polydactyly, and both of these conditions may be hereditary. Syndactyly is often associated with multiple congenital deformities of the hands and feet. Syndactyly of the hands and sometimes of the feet, associated with a pointing of the head in the region of the anterior fontanel, was described in 1906 by Apert and is called Apert's syndrome (acrocephalosyndactyly).

Separation of the involved fingers or toes is accomplished by dividing the soft tissues and bony structures and should be done between the sec-

54 *Handbook of orthopaedic surgery*

ond and the sixth year. Many plastic procedures have been devised; the results are usually satisfactory.

Macrodactyly

Macrodactyly is an overdevelopment of one or more fingers or toes (Fig. 26, B). It is due presumably to an abnormal growth capacity of the germ plasm forming this part. In some cases lesions of local nerve trunks have been found, suggesting neurofibromatosis. The usual treatment is amputation, but occasionally a plastic operation to effect a reduction in size is preferable.

Polydactyly

Supernumerary digits are the commonest deformity of the hand (Fig. 26, C). They occur in the hand and foot with about equal frequency. The

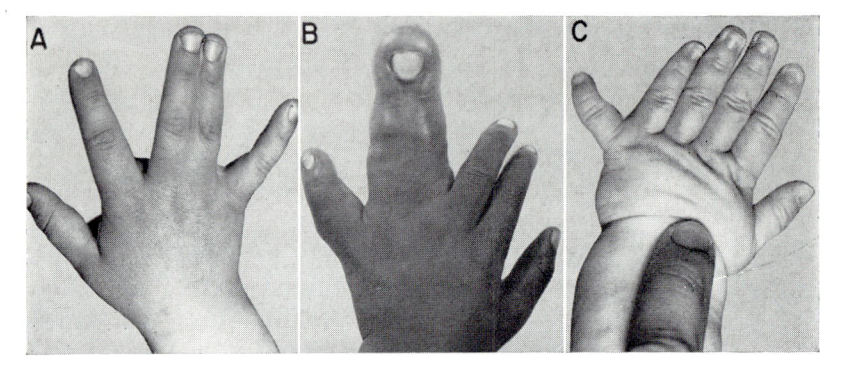

Fig. 26. Congenital deformities of the hand. **A,** Syndactyly. **B,** Macrodactyly. **C,** Polydactyly.

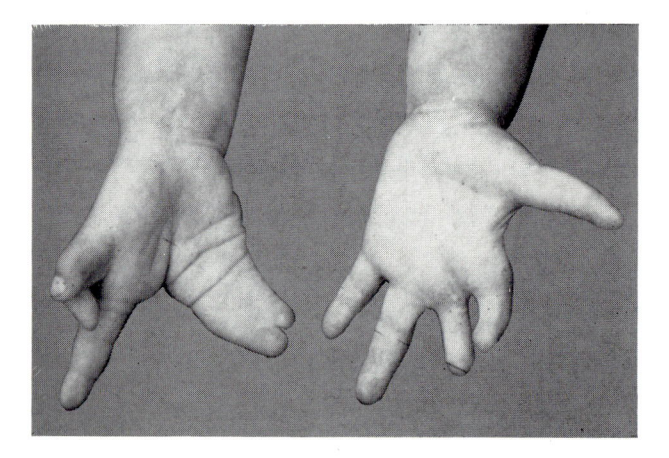

Fig. 27. Cleft hand and finger deformities in infant 2½ years of age. In right hand, note mid-palmar cleft, syndactyly of ring and little fingers, and deformity of index finger and thumb. In left hand, note abnormally long thumb and congenital amputations of distal phalanges of index and middle fingers.

Congenital deformities 55

condition is often bilateral and may be combined with syndactyly. Amputation of the extra finger or toe is indicated.

Cleft hand and cleft foot

This anomaly consists of a cleft or division in the middle of the hand or foot, which results in the formation of large digits or parts (Fig. 27). It is spoken of as the "lobster claw" hand or foot and is sometimes associated with syndactyly or polydactyly. These hands and feet are unsightly but often function satisfactorily. They are sometimes treated surgically for cosmetic improvement.

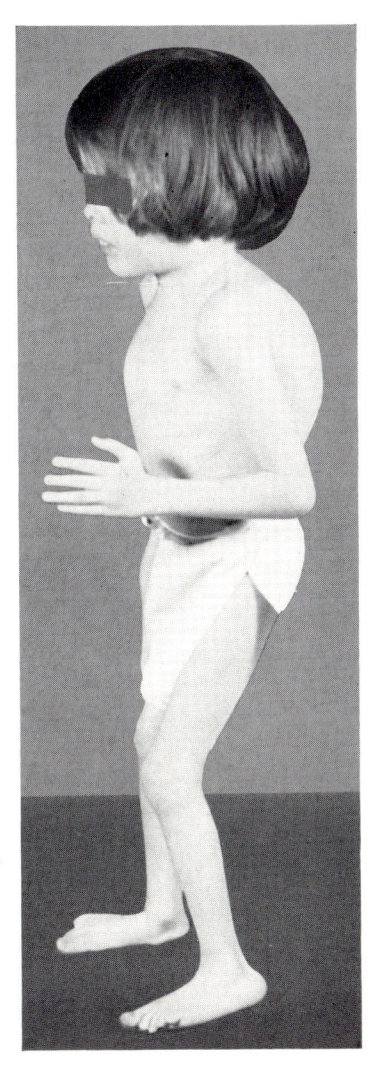

Fig. 28. Marfan's syndrome in a girl of 6 years. Note the long, thin fingers and toes, so-called "spider fingers and toes," the barrel-shaped thorax with kyphosis, and the thin upper and lower extremities with marked pronation of the feet.

ARACHNODACTYLY (MARFAN'S SYNDROME)

This uncommon congenital and usually hereditary condition, which occurs in tall and slender individuals, is characterized by thin fingers and toes with elongated phalanges, metacarpals, and metatarsals (Fig. 28). It is sometimes spoken of as "spider fingers and toes." In approximately 80% of the cases, there is an asymmetry of the skull. About half of the patients have eye deformities with dislocation of the lens, and approximately a third have a congenital heart lesion. There are marked atrophy and weakness of all muscles, with a lack of normal muscle development, and hypermobility of joints due to laxity of the ligaments. There may be a coxa vara and a lateral curvature of the spine that increases as the child grows older. Arachnodactyly is to be differentiated from the Ehlers-Danlos syndrome, which also is characterized by hypermobility of the joints but includes increased elasticity of the skin and fragility of the walls of the blood vessels.

Treatment. There is no specific therapy. Individual deformities or disabilities should be treated as indicated.

CONGENITAL AMPUTATIONS AND CONSTRICTING BANDS

Congenital amputations (Fig. 27), once thought to be caused by constriction in utero, are now considered to be, as a rule, primary congenital defects due to abnormal constitution of the germ plasm. Often there is a deep circular constriction about the arm or leg without actual amputation. The constriction may occur in any portion of the arm or leg. Beyond it the distal portion of the extremity may be enlarged.

Treatment. The treatment of congenital amputations is discussed in Chapter 15. When a deep indented band is associated with disturbance of the distal circulation, it may be necessary to dissect out the band through a Z-plasty incision. The operation may be done in two or three stages to avoid increasing the circulatory embarrassment. Occasionally it may be desirable to complete the amputation.

ASYMMETRICAL DEVELOPMENT (CONGENITAL HEMIHYPERTROPHY, HEMIMACROSOMIA)

In the normal individual there are often slight differences between the development of the two lateral halves of the body. This condition, however, is sometimes severe and of congenital origin. It may be caused by an increased blood supply to one side of the body, resulting from a primary developmental abnormality of the circulatory system. It has also been regarded as the result of an asymmetrical growth capacity of the germ plasm. Neurofibromatosis may occasionally produce a similar appearance. Hemihypertrophy may at times resemble a unilateral elephantiasis, the redundant tissue being of fibrous and fatty nature. The increase in size usually ceases at the end of the growth period, but the disproportion constitutes a permanent deformity. Sometimes one extremity only is involved. Occasionally

Congenital deformities 57

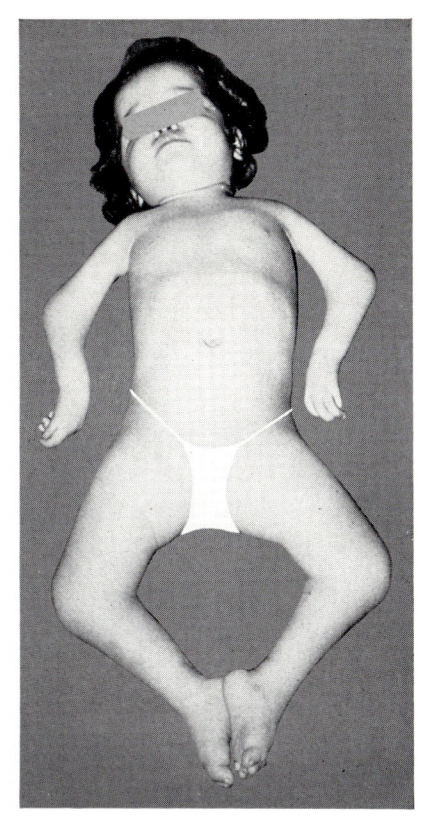

Fig. 29. Arthrogryposis multiplex congenita in girl 2 years of age. Note internal rotation of arms and hands, flexion contracture and thickening of elbows, external rotation of lower extremities, flexion of knees, and equinus of feet. Kissing feet and hoop-shaped lower extremities are terms applied to these deformities.

an arteriovenous fistula may be the cause. Treatment is not uniformly effective, but cosmetic operative procedures, such as shortening the longer leg, are indicated in selected cases.

ARTHROGRYPOSIS MULTIPLEX CONGENITA (AMYOPLASIA CONGENITA)

Arthrogryposis multiplex congenita is an incomplete congenital fibrous ankylosis of many or all of the joints, except those of the spine and jaw, and is usually symmetrical. The spine may show a lateral curvature. The condition is thought to be caused by a primary aplasia or failure of muscle development early in embryonic life. The joints appear enlarged, and the periarticular tissues show contractures and fail to develop normally. In contour the extremities may resemble stuffed sausages (Fig. 29).

The typical patient shows internal rotation of the arms and flexion contractures of the wrists. The elbows and knees have a fusiform appearance and may be hyperextended. The hips may be flexed. The thighs are ro-

58   *Handbook of orthopaedic surgery*

tated outward and the tibiae twisted on the femora. The patellae are sometimes absent. There are usually associated clubfeet and sometimes clubhands. The hands show contractures of the palms and have been likened to "walrus flippers." Numerous other congenital anomalies, such as syndactyly and polydactyly, may be present.

Treatment. Because of the muscle deficiency and the tendency for the deformities to recur after correction, the treatment is seldom satisfactory. The feet are in general more amenable to treatment than the hands. Gentle manipulations performed several times a day may be helpful. Elastic splinting for the hands, traction for the hips and knees, and corrective casts for the feet are indicated in selected cases. Hip dislocation associated with arthrogryposis is more resistant to treatment than is uncomplicated congenital dislocation. The position of the arms and legs may be improved with tenotomies and myotomies; osteotomies to correct deformities of the long bones and arthroplasties of the joints may be done in older patients. Following these procedures physical therapy should be diligently carried out for a long period of time.

CLEIDOCRANIAL DYSOSTOSIS

Cleiodocranial dysostosis (Figs. 30 and 31) is a partial or complete absence of both clavicles, together with changes in the skull. It is uncommon and is of hereditary origin in about two-thirds of the cases. The sexes are affected with equal frequency.

Pathology. The characteristic changes are a partial or complete absence of both clavicles and an exaggerated development of the transverse diameter of the cranium with delayed ossification of the fontanels. The muscles attached to the clavicle and chest develop in an anomalous manner. Often

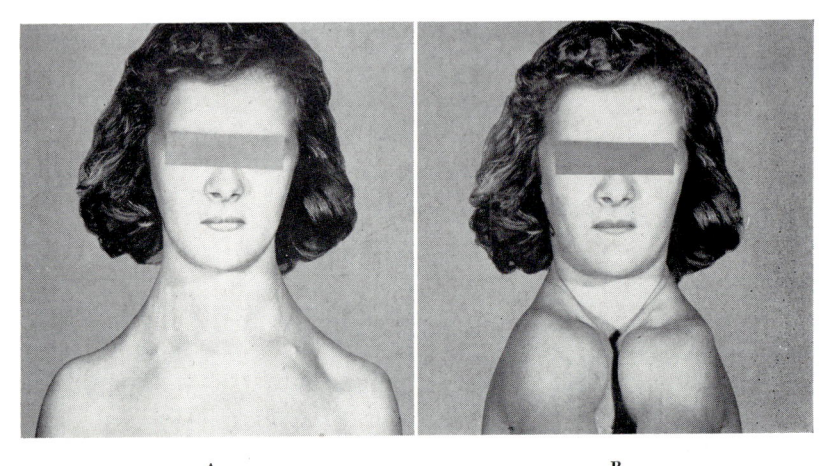

Fig. 30. Cleidocranial dysostosis. **A**, Note long neck and low shoulders. A depression in the middle of the forehead and a broadening of the occiput due to delay in fontanel closure are also characteristic. **B**, Absence of the clavicles allows anterior approximation of the shoulders.

Congenital deformities 59

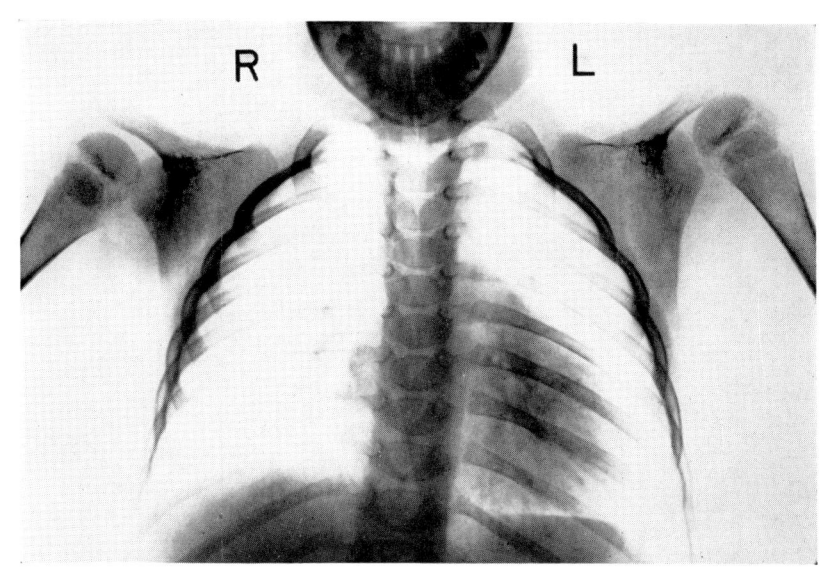

Fig. 31. Roentgenogram of boy 10 years of age with cleidocranial dysostosis, showing complete absence of clavicles.

other congenital malformations are associated, such as coxa vara and imperfect pubic ossification and spinal segmentation.

Clinical picture. Usually the patient is brought to the physician because it has been found adventitiously that there is something wrong with one or both shoulders. A defect of the clavicle is demonstrable clinically. Because of the extreme relaxation of the shoulder girdle the patient can often bring the tips of the shoulders together below the chin (Fig. 30, *B*).

Treatment. As a rule there is little disability and no treatment is indicated. If the patient complains of pain, however, one or both ends of the clavicles, if present, may be removed.

CONGENITAL ELEVATION OF THE SCAPULA (CONGENITAL HIGH SCAPULA, SPRENGEL'S DEFORMITY)

In this uncommon congenital anomaly, which was first described by Eulenburg in 1863, the scapula is elevated from 1 to 4 inches above its normal position, and usually its inferior angle is rotated medially (Fig. 32). The deformity is sometimes bilateral. It is often associated with other congenital anomalies, and particularly with defective development of the cervical vertebrae and upper ribs.

Etiology. Congenital elevation of the scapula is believed to be the result of failure of the scapula to descend to normal position from its high level in the early weeks of gestation.

Pathology. The affected scapula is small. Usually its vertical length is decreased and its width relatively increased. Its upper portion tends to hook forward. The cervical muscles are shortened on the affected side and are changed in direction. In about one-fourth of the cases there is

60   Handbook of orthopaedic surgery

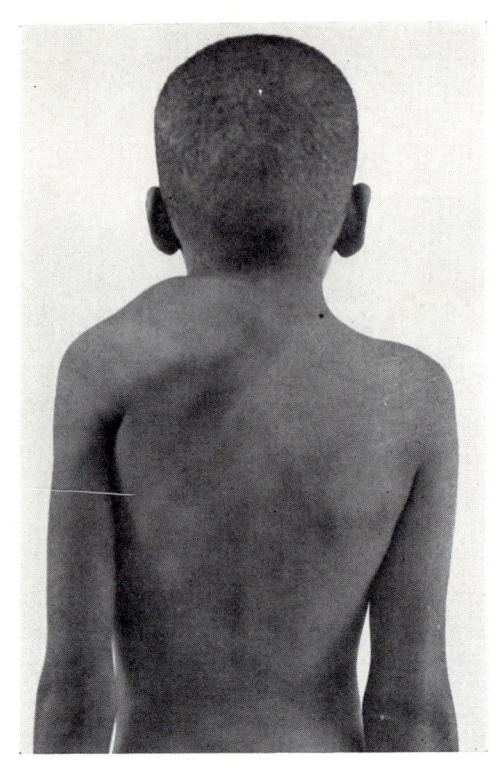

Fig. 32. Congenital elevation of left scapula in a boy 13 years of age. Abduction of left shoulder was limited at 60 degrees.

union between one of the lower cervical vertebrae and the scapula; such union may consist of bone, cartilage, or fibrous tissue. When a bony connection is present, it extends from the spinous process, lamina, or transverse process of one or more vertebrae to the upper part of the vertebral border of the scapula. Such an osseous bridge is spoken of as an *omovertebral bone.*

Clinical picture. Asymmetry of the shoulder is often the first evidence of abnormality. In most of the cases abduction of the shoulder is markedly restricted. In 10% of the cases torticollis is present, together with lateral curvature of the spine. In bilateral cases the neck appears shortened.

Diagnosis. The diagnosis is made from the physical signs and the roentgenogram. Congenital elevation of the scapula must be differentiated from paralysis of the serratus anterior muscle and from obstetric paralysis.

Prognosis. Without operation no improvement of the deformity is to be anticipated. Surgical treatment is often followed by moderately improved function and appearance.

Treatment. Postural training and exercise of the shoulder may increase the joint function. In cases in which motion is markedly limited and the deformity is unsightly, operative measures may be indicated. If an omovertebral bone is present, it should be resected.

Subperiosteal transplantation of the scapula, within its muscular envelope, downward to the desired level, and its anchorage to one of the ribs by fascia or wire, as described by Schrock, may be indicated. To be effective, the operation must be performed in childhood, preferably before the age of 5 years.

CONGENITAL SYNOSTOSIS OF THE CERVICAL SPINE (KLIPPEL-FEIL SYNDROME)

Congenital synostosis of the cervical spine is a rare malformation resulting from an arrest of development. The outstanding pathologic change is fusion of all or of only the lower cervical vertebrae into one homogeneous mass of bone. The posterior portion of some or all of the laminal arches is not developed, resulting in spina bifida which usually involves the lower cervical vertebrae and one or two of the upper dorsal vertebrae. Cervical ribs, crowding of the upper ribs, and congenital anomalies in other parts of the body are often associated. Roentgenograms show the anomalies of the cervical spine, including the clefts in its vertebral arches.

Clinical picture. Abnormal shortness of the neck is the most noticeable feature, sometimes causing the head to seem to rest directly on the trunk (Fig. 33). There is painless restriction of neck motion in all directions. Occasionally there may be associated neurologic changes due to spinal cord or nerve root compression. Flexion and extension of the cervical spine, which may take place wholly at the joints between occiput and atlas,

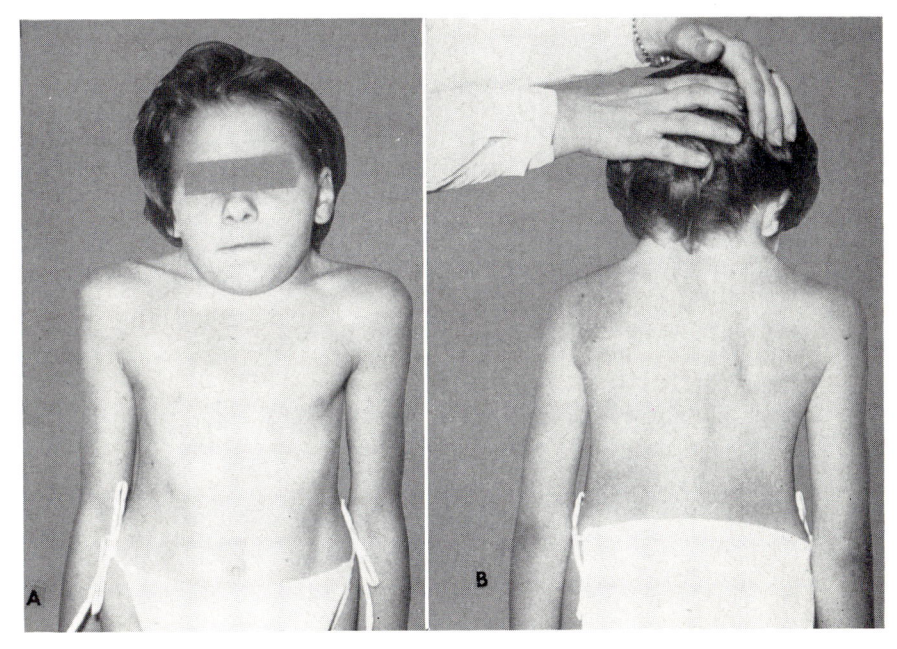

Fig. 33. Klippel-Feil syndrome in girl 7 years of age. **A,** Note short neck with chin resting on chest. **B,** Note short, thick neck and lateral webbing from head to shoulders, which is termed web neck or pterygium colli.

are better preserved than is lateral motion. The head and neck may be held in an oblique position which simulates that of congenital torticollis. Occasionally the trapezius muscles stretch winglike from the mastoid processes to the shoulders, suggesting the term of pterygium colli or "web neck."

Treatment. As a rule, no treatment is indicated. However, sometimes a plastic surgical operation to release the webbing of the neck is followed by increased motion. In early childhood a neck brace is occasionally helpful. Attempts to increase mobility by manipulation have proved harmful.

CHAPTER 3

Congenital deformities—cont'd

OF the orthopaedic congenital deformities, dislocations form an important group. By far the most common and serious congenital dislocation is that affecting the hip joint.

CONGENITAL DYSPLASIA OF THE HIP

Congenital dysplasia is a malformation of the hip joint that may lead to subluxation or to complete dislocation of the hip at the time of birth or shortly thereafter. Three degrees or phases of congenital dysplasia are recognized: (1) acetabular dysplasia, (2) subluxation, and (3) dislocation. Acetabular dysplasia or preluxation is the mildest form of hip dysplasia; in it there is neither subluxation nor dislocation. The femoral head remains seated in its socket, but the acetabulum is shallow. This phase merges imperceptibly into the second, that of subluxation, in which the femoral head, although in contact with the acetabulum, is no longer well seated but begins to ride upward and outward. The third and most advanced phase is that of complete dislocation, in which the femoral head is no longer in contact with the acetabulum. The difference between subluxation and dislocation may be dependent upon the position of the fibrocartilaginous labrum or limbus. If the femoral head lies within the limbus, it is in contact with the acetabulum and only subluxation exists. In some cases this difference can be determined only by arthrograms or at open surgery.

Incidence. Dysplasia of the hip is one of the more common congenital deformities. It is seen with great frequency in certain areas of the world, particularly in the Latin races. The incidence is high, for example, in northern Italy, and also in Japan. Hip dysplasia is seldom observed in Negroes. It is six to eight times as common in girls as in boys. Complete dislocation is more frequently a unilateral than a bilateral condition.

Etiology. The exact cause of hip dysplasia is unknown. Heredity is a factor. Various attempts have been made to explain the origin of the dislocation. Its higher incidence in girls has led to the thought that the wider female pelvis, with its more vertical walls, associated with excessive hip flexion and adduction in utero may cause dislocation. This idea is not generally accepted. The condition may arise from a primary developmental defect which causes imperfect formation of the posterosuperior margin of the acetabulum. It may be the result of some teratogenic factor which adversely affects the embryo at a critical stage in the development of this portion of the skeleton. This view is supported by the fact that other congenital defects are frequently associated with dysplasia of the hip.

ACETABULAR DYSPLASIA AND SUBLUXATION OF THE HIP

Clinical picture. Acetabular dysplasia and subluxation of the hip are frequently discovered shortly after birth by the examining physician. The most important finding is limitation of abduction of the flexed hip or hips (Fig. 34). Another commonly noted sign is asymmetry of the gluteal folds. Neither of these findings is sufficient to establish the diagnosis, but either should alert the doctor to look more closely. Looking for these signs takes but a moment or two and should be part of the routine examination of every newborn child. Another important finding in congenital subluxation of the hip is the snapping sign *(Ortolani's sign)*. If traction is applied to the subluxated hip while abduction is being tested, a definite click will be felt as the femoral head slips into its socket. The presence of this sign suggests strongly that the subluxation will progress to dislocation if untreated. Obvious shortening and instability of the hip as demonstrated by the telescoping test are not found in subluxation but are indicative of dislocation. When dysplasia in the newborn infant remains untreated, the mother may observe in succeeding months that the hip is abnormal, that she has difficulty spread-

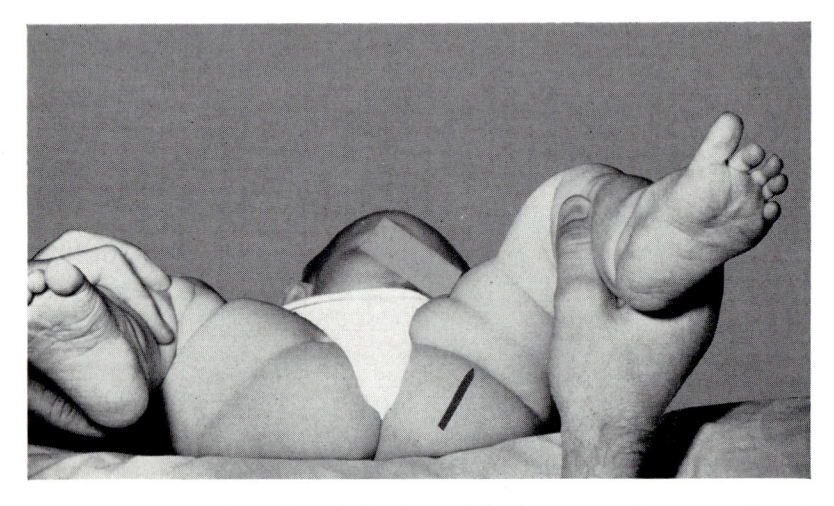

Fig. 34. Abduction test for unilateral dysplasia of the hip in an infant 8 months of age, who has subluxation on the left. When the test is positive, the thigh on the dysplastic side cannot be abducted so far as the thigh on the side with a normal hip. Note deepening of proximal fold in left thigh, which also suggests dysplasia.

ing the infant's thighs to put on diapers, or that the thigh creases are unequal.

Roentgenographic picture. The roentgenographic findings of acetabular dysplasia may not be obvious at birth. The most readily observable change is an increase in the obliquity of the acetabular roof. A slight upward and lateral displacement of the femur from the acetabulum may also be seen in early subluxation. At 2 to 6 months of age, delay in the appearance of the ossification center of the femoral head will become evident. As pointed out by Caffey, however, some of these radiologic signs can be seen in children with normal hips. The diagnosis must therefore be based on a combination of physical and roentgenographic findings.

Treatment. The treatment of congenital subluxation of the hip is to maintain the head of the femur as deeply as possible within the acetabulum until there is roentgenographic evidence of an adequate, well-developed socket. This is accomplished by maintaining the hips in an abducted or frog-leg position by means of a brace or pillow splint. The treatment may require a few months to more than a year. With early treatment the prognosis is excellent. Some of the milder degrees of dysplasia may improve without treatment. Since there is no method of determining which subluxations will persist or progress to cause degenerative hip changes in later years, it is far better to institute the rather simple treatment than to risk the development of serious sequelae.

CONGENITAL DISLOCATION OF THE HIP

In 1826 Dupuytren first described accurately the pathologic changes in congenital dislocation of the hip, but not until 1888 did Paci suggest reduction of the dislocation as a means of treatment. Until then such deformities of the hip had been considered incurable. The suggestions made by Paci were first popularized in 1895 by Lorenz. It is now generally agreed that if a congenitally dislocated hip can be reduced early, and if the corrected position can be maintained for an adequate period of time by means of a plaster cast or brace, a stable joint with satisfactory function will often result.

Pathology. The pathologic changes are characteristic and vary with age, being minimal in the early case and increasing with the duration of the dislocation. The acetabulum is usually shallow with an oblique superior and posterior surface. It may be filled with fat and fibrous tissue. The head of the femur is nearly always displaced upward and backward upon the ilium. Anterior dislocation is uncommon. When the epiphysis of the femoral head appears in roentgenograms, it is smaller than that of a normal hip; this is believed to be due to decreased functional stimulation. The head of the femur becomes flattened and later mushroom-shaped. The neck of the femur is short and thick and, with continued dislocation, may show an increase in its angle with the shaft (coxa valga). The whole upper portion of the femur usually develops a structural alteration, as a result of which the neck or shaft and neck undergo torsion, assuming a more anterior position in relation to the lower end of the femur (antetorsion or anteversion). The capsule over the head, which on weight bearing acts as a suspensory ligament, becomes elongated, thick, and fibrous; it may become constricted in the middle and assume an hourglass shape. The ligamentum teres may be extremely thin, ribbonlike, and atrophic and may even be absent; in some cases, however, it is broad and thick. The muscles about the joint, especially the adductor group, become shortened and contracted.

With continued weight bearing a shallow secondary acetabulum may develop on the wing of the ilium. The pelvis is underdeveloped on the affected side, and a postural deviation of the lumbar spine toward this side takes place. Forward tilting of the pelvis and increase of the lumbar lordosis develop to a slight degree in unilateral dislocation and to a much greater degree in bilateral dislocation (Fig. 35).

Clinical picture. It may be difficult to recognize dislocation of the hip in early infancy. In a unilateral case the mother may notice that the affected hip

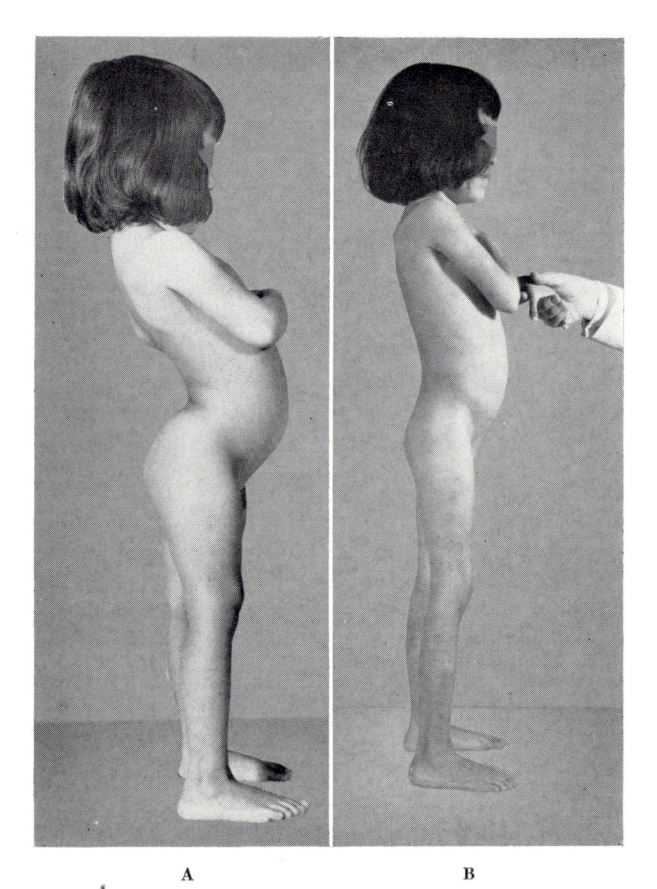

Fig. 35. Bilateral congenital dislocation of the hip in a girl 3½ years of age. **A**, Note extreme lumbar lordosis and protrusion of the abdomen. **B**, One year following reduction. Note normal curve of lumbar spine and improvement of abdominal protrusion.

Congenital deformities 67

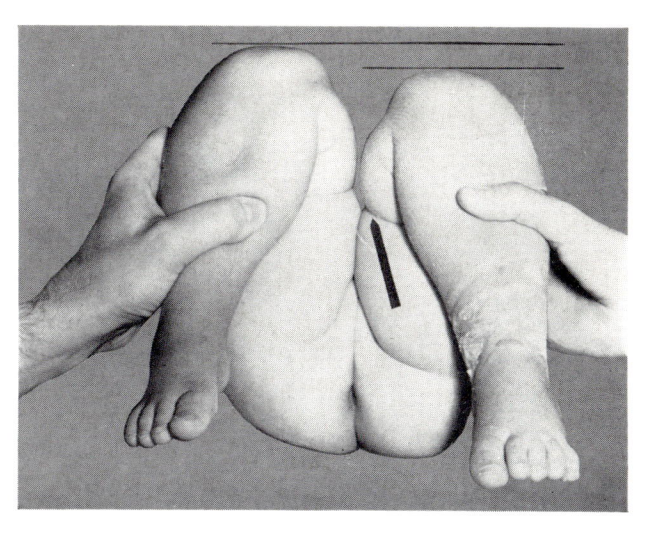

Fig. 36. Knee level test (Allis' sign) for unilateral congenital dislocation of hip in girl 2½ years of age. With infant supine on a hard surface, hips and knees are fully flexed. When test is positive, knee on dislocated side is lower. Note increased depth of left thigh fold, which also suggests dislocation. (Same patient as shown in Figs. 39 and 40.)

is prominent laterally and that the extremity is short. By placing the child supine on a hard examining table and then flexing both of the child's hips and knees to a right angle, the examiner can see that on the affected side the knee is lower than on the normal side (Allis' sign, Fig. 36). Then by abducting the flexed hip as far as possible, the examiner will note restriction of motion on the side of the dislocation or subluxation (Fig. 34); the restriction is caused primarily by adductor tightness. If the extended thigh is first pushed toward the patient's head and then pulled distally, the greater trochanter and head of the femur can be felt to move up and down in the buttock. This is commonly called "telescoping" or "piston mobility." The instability may sometimes be recognized more easily by testing with the hip and knee flexed to 90 degrees. In the unilateral case the skin folds of the thighs are usually asymmetric (Figs. 34 and 36), and the trochanter is more prominent than normal. Instability of the hip on weight bearing delays the child in learning to stand and walk and causes a characteristic limp. In young children there are no other complaints, and function is usually good. In older children fatigue may be present on exertion, and pain may develop after activity. Sometimes, even in adult patients, there is no complaint of pain.

In bilateral dislocation the gait is especially characteristic: the patient, because of the instability of his hips, sways from side to side, exhibiting a "duck waddle" gait. This gait is present in less marked degree in unilateral dislocation. In bilateral dislocation the perineum is wide, the buttocks are broad, and the transverse gluteal folds are altered (Fig. 37). The normal lordosis of the lumbar spine is increased, and there is marked protrusion of the abdomen (Fig. 35). In both unilateral and bilateral cases the greater

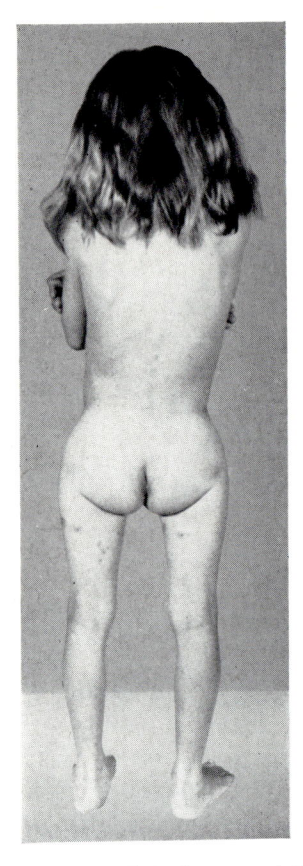

Fig. 37. Bilateral congenital dislocation of the hip in girl 5 years of age. Note widening of perineum and broadening of the buttocks.

trochanter is prominent and appears above Nélaton's line (the line from anterior superior iliac spine to tuberosity of the ischium). When the patient stands, bearing weight on the affected hip, the pelvis is tilted downward on the normal side (positive Trendelenburg sign) instead of tilting upward as it would if the hip being tested possessed normal stability (Fig. 38). The femoral head can usually be felt outside of the acetabulum and forward on external rotation. The range of abduction and of external rotation may be decreased. In older children a flexion deformity of the hip can be demonstrated upon flattening the lumbar spine on the examining table.

Diagnosis. In the infant it may be impossible to make a diagnosis with certainty until roentgenograms of the hip have been examined. These should be taken first with the knees together and the patellae pointing forward and second with the hips in maximum abduction and internal rotation. If Shenton's line is disrupted, the diagnosis is strongly suggested (Figs. 39 and 40). Outstanding roentgenographic findings in older children are increased displacement of the femur, continued underdevelopment of the femoral

Congenital deformities 69

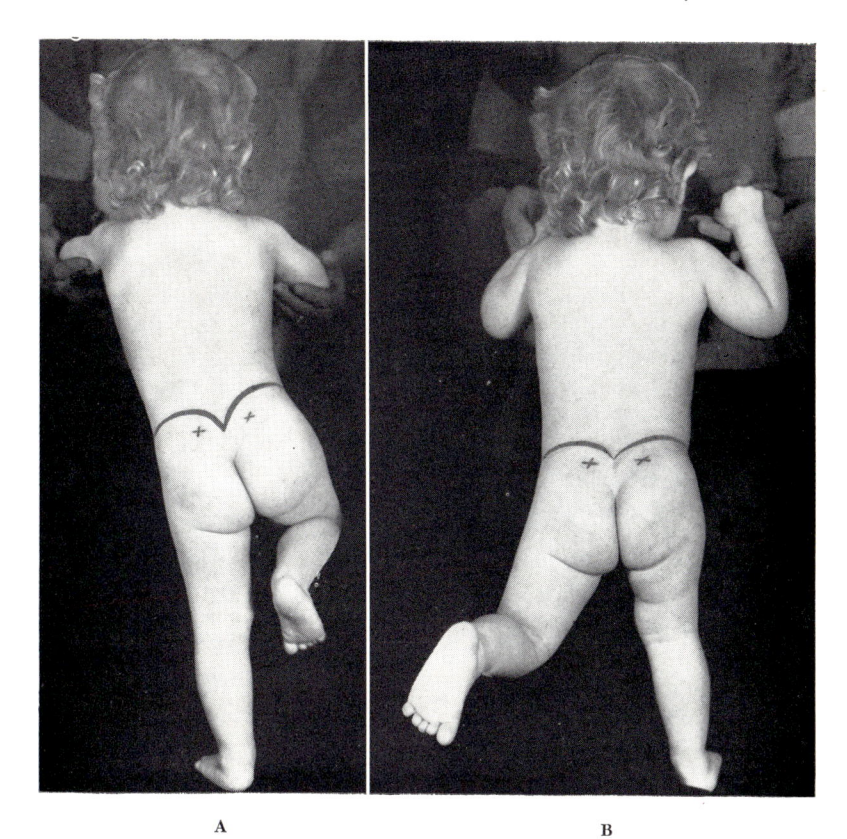

Fig. 38. Trendelenburg test for instability of hip in unilateral congenital dislocation in child 2½ years of age. **A,** When child bears weight on normal left hip, opposite side of pelvis is elevated to maintain balance (negative test). **B,** When weight is borne on dislocated right hip, opposite side of pelvis cannot be normally elevated (positive test).

head, and obliquity of the acetabular roof (Figs. 41 and 42). Aside from the roentgenogram, the diagnosis depends upon eliciting the signs previously described, particularly palpation of the femoral head in an abnormal position. Because of the waddling gait of patients with either unilateral or bilateral congenital dislocation of the hip, the initial diagnosis may be confused with that of coxa vara, excessive lumbar lordosis, rickets with muscular hypotonia, tuberculosis of the lumbar spine, poliomyelitis with weakness of the gluteus medius, and early progressive muscular dystrophy.

Treatment. Treatment should be begun as soon as the dislocation is recognized, for the earlier it is started the more favorable should be the ultimate result. The treatment varies with the age of the patient and may be considered in four age categories: (1) under 1 year, (2) between 1 and 3 years, (3) between 3 and 6 years, and (4) over 6 years.

First age period—under 1 year. In the infant under 12 months of age, it has been shown that if the dislocated hip is brought to full abduction and held in this position there is a definite tendency for the dislocation to be-

70 *Handbook of orthopaedic surgery*

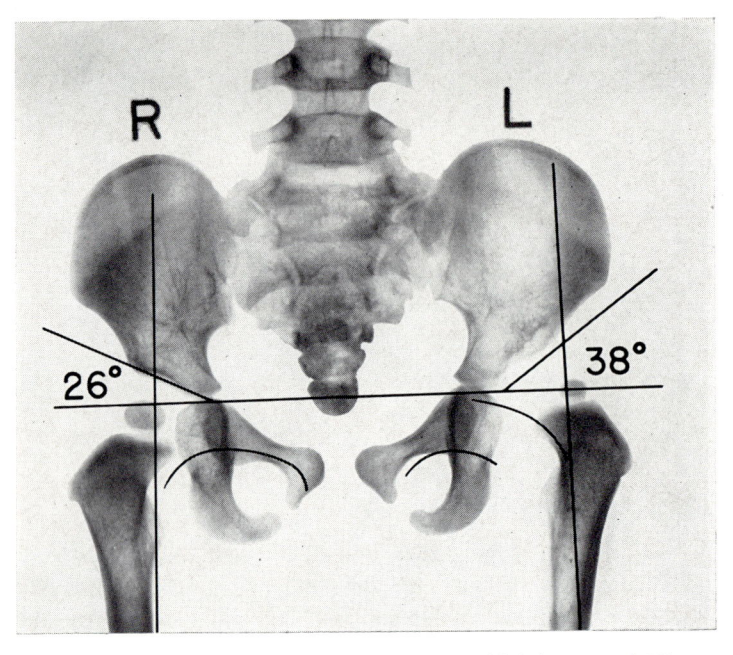

Fig. 39. Roentgenogram showing congenital dislocation of left hip in girl 2½ years of age. Note upward and lateral displacement of left femoral head, underdevelopment of left capital epiphysis, increased obliquity of superior margin of left acetabulum, and disruption of left obturator-coxofemoral line (Shenton's line). (Same patient as shown in Fig. 36.)

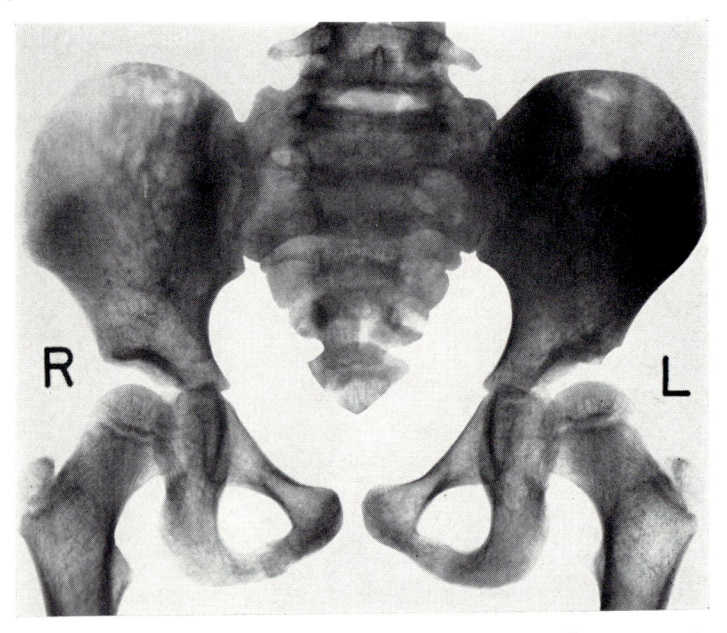

Fig. 40. Roentgenogram of same patient as shown in Fig. 39, three years after closed reduction. Note that left hip shows well-rounded, normally trabeculated capital epiphysis and well-developed acetabulum, and that Shenton's line is intact.

Congenital deformities 71

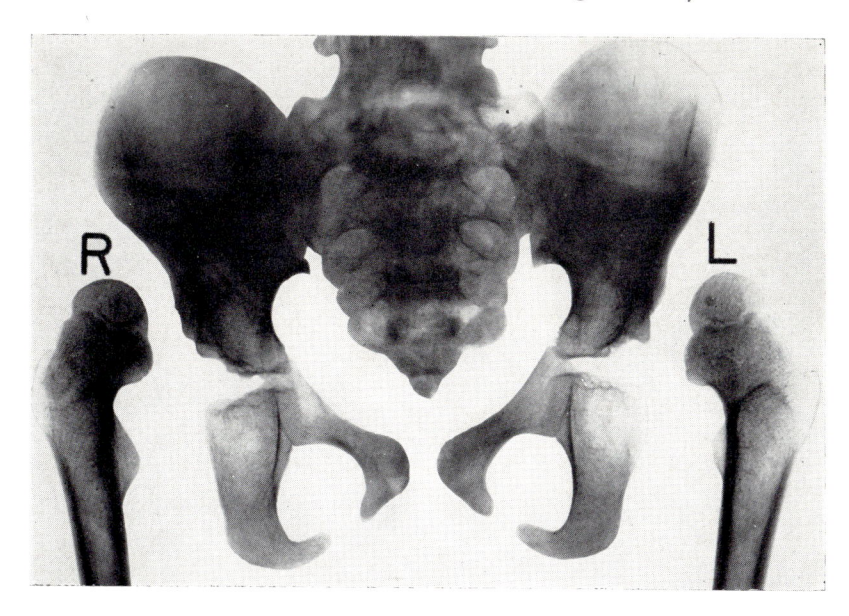

Fig. 41. Roentgenogram of bilateral dislocation of the hip in 5-year-old girl shown in Fig. 37. Note upward displacement of proximal end of femora and almost complete absence of acetabula.

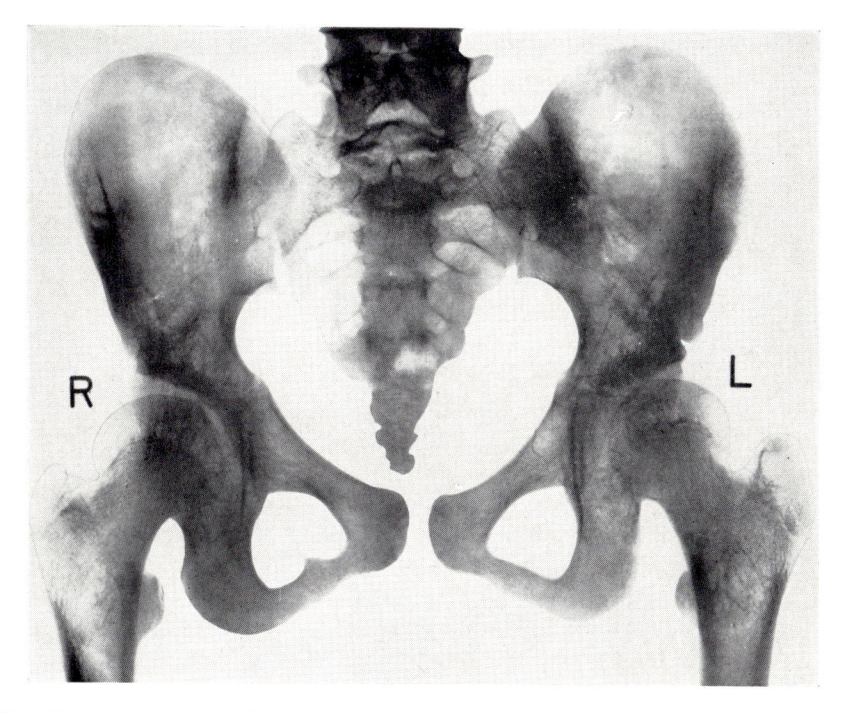

Fig. 42. Roentgenogram of same patient as shown in Fig. 41, seven years after closed reductions. Now 12 years old, patient has a perfect functional result. Note that femoral heads are well rounded and normal in appearance but that left acetabulum is not so deeply developed as the right.

72   Handbook of orthopaedic surgery

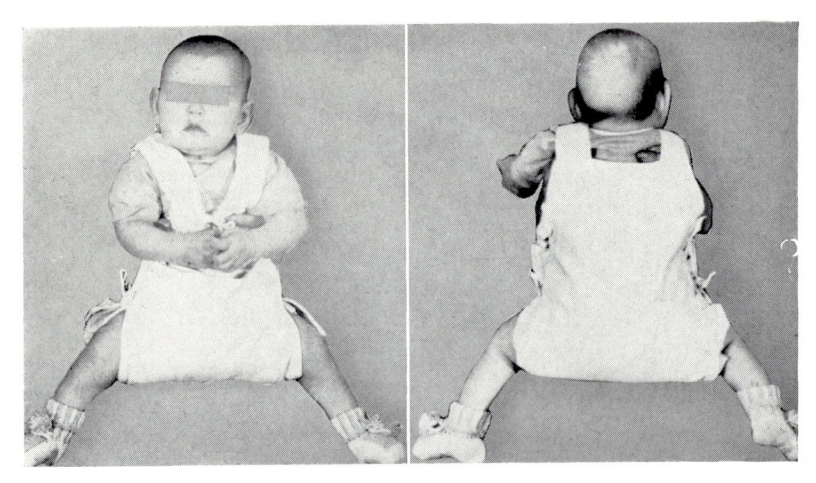

Fig. 43. Pillow splint (Frejka) used to maintain abduction of the hips. (Courtesy Dr. V. L. Hart.)

come reduced and for a normal acetabulum to form. The treatment is often begun with from one to three weeks of skin traction in increasing abduction. Putti advocated the use of a triangular abduction splint, in which the amount of abduction could be gradually increased. This can be accomplished also by using lower extremity casts joined by turnbuckles or by using shoes attached to an adjustable spreader bar. Having been secured by other means, wide abduction can be maintained by a brace or a Frejka pillow splint (Fig. 43). Gradual resumption of hip adduction is allowed after clinical and roentgenographic examination shows sufficient stability to prevent redislocation. Many hips treated by the abduction method during the first year of life will be reduced by the normal time for walking.

Second age period—1 to 3 years. Often a congenital dislocation of the hip is not recognized until the child begins to walk at about 1 year of age. At this age treatment by closed reduction is indicated. Manipulative reduction should be preceded by a period of skin or skeletal traction. Traction should be continued until the head of the femur has been pulled down to a point opposite or below the level of the center of the acetabulum. The soft tissue structures about the hip, which may have been contracted, become stretched, and the danger of trauma to the head of the femur with manipulation is minimized. With sufficient traction on the hip in wide abduction, extension, and internal rotation, closed reduction can often be obtained without manipulation.

Manipulative reduction is done with the child under general anesthesia and supine on a hard surface. Gentleness is essential. Careful, thorough stretching of the muscles and ligaments about the hip is effected by gradual flexion, extension, abduction, and adduction to extremes. The hip and knee are then flexed to 90 degrees and the hip is externally rotated slightly; then gradually and slowly the thigh is abducted and further externally rotated, while a forward pressure is exerted on the head and greater trochanter of the femur through the buttock. As the dislocation is reduced, the head of the femur can be felt to slip over the posterior acetabular rim into the acetabulum, usually with a click. In a successful reduction, the head of the femur will be well placed in the acetabulum when approximately 90 degrees of abduction are reached. If it has not been possible adequately to stretch the adductor muscles preceding reduction, an adductor tenotomy should be done; by allowing a greater amount of abduction this will often lead to successful reduction. A method of determining whether a hip is reduced is to decrease gradually the abduction, flexion, and external rotation; at a certain point the head of the femur will be felt to slip out of the acetabulum. Following the reduction a bilateral hip spica cast should be applied to support the lower extremities with the hips in approximately 90 degrees of abduction, 90 degrees of external rotation, and 90 degrees of flexion, the knees in 90 degrees of flexion, and the ankles in neutral zero position. This is the "frog-leg" position (Fig. 44). A double hip spica should be applied for the unilateral case as well as the bilateral. The infant's mother should be instructed concerning methods of keeping the cast clean and dry.

In different clinics the length of time the frog-leg cast is left on varies from three to nine months. The immobilization period varies also according to the stability of the individual patient's hip; six months is usually advisable. Following this a bilateral hip spica is applied with the hips brought down into 45 degrees of abduction, 45 degrees of external rotation, and 45 degrees

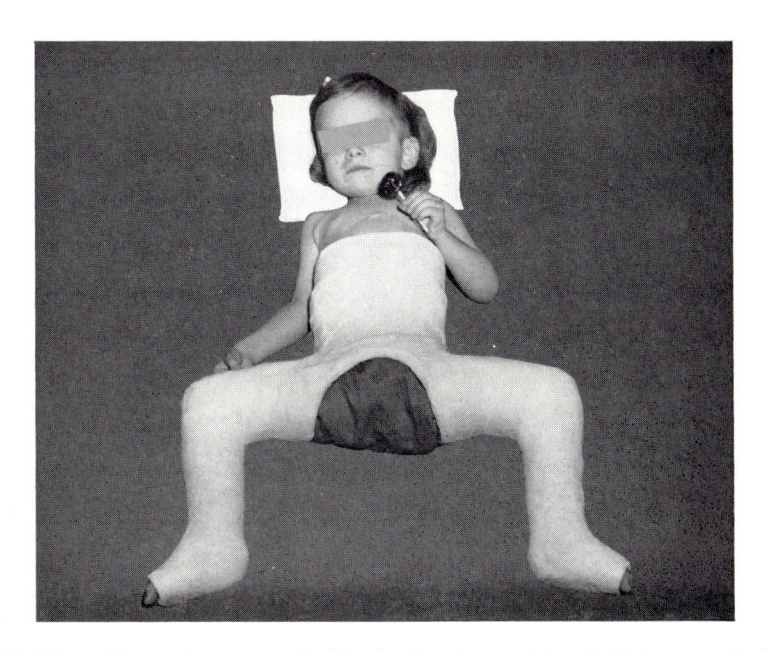

Fig. 44. Bilateral hip spica cast applied in the frog-leg position of 90 degrees of abduction, 90 degrees of external rotation, and 90 degrees of flexion of the hips, and 90 degrees of flexion of the knees, in a girl 1 year 9 months of age with bilateral dislocation of the hip.

of flexion; this cast is left on for two to three months. After removal of the cast, the child is allowed to move around in bed for about one week. Physical therapy is then started; it should include pool or tank therapy if available. Walking is allowed as soon as the legs will return to a normal standing position; this is usually several weeks after removal of the plaster. Roentgenograms of the hips should be made at long intervals while the child is in plaster, since redislocation sometimes occurs in spite of all precautions. After redislocation, either a second attempt at closed reduction should be made or an open reduction should be done.

When closed reduction has been unsuccessful, an open reduction should be performed. This usually consists of an anterior approach to the hip joint, incision of the capsule, and placing the head of the femur in the acetabulum with the extremity in an abducted and internally rotated position. The more common obstacles to closed reduction which may necessitate an open reduction are capsular thickening and constriction, interposition of the acetabular limbus, hypertrophy of the ligamentum teres, deformities of the femoral head, and aplasias. Some orthopaedic surgeons perform open reductions more freely than others, believing that with open reduction there is less damage to the circulation of the hip joint and to the head of the femur than with manipulative closed reduction. Most, however, are of the opinion that open reduction is not the treatment of choice in this age group.

In recent years many orthopaedic surgeons have discarded closed manipulative reduction under anesthesia, followed by a frog-leg cast, in

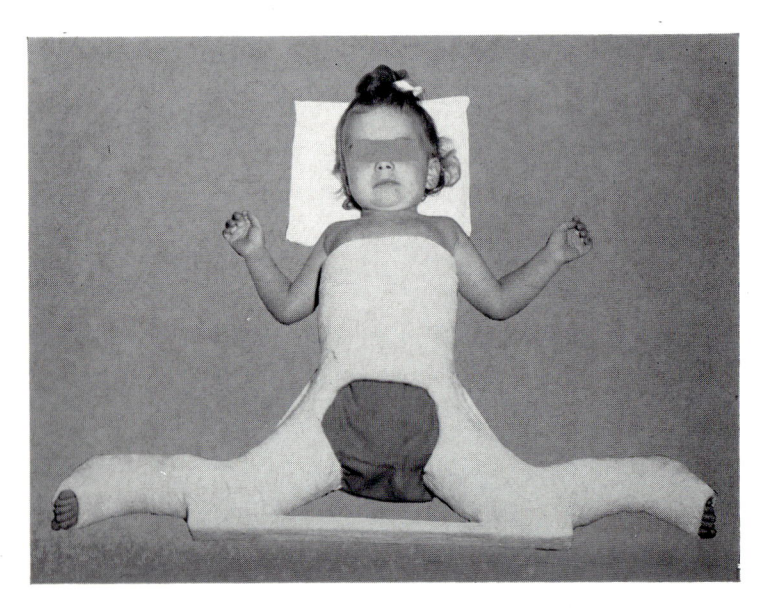

Fig. 45. Bilateral hip spica cast applied in a position of abduction and full internal rotation. This is the same patient as shown in Fig. 44. Her dislocations recurred in this position but remained perfectly reduced in the frog-leg position.

favor of the less traumatic method of reducing the dislocation by skeletal traction in abduction and internal rotation and immobilizing the hip in this position (Fig. 45). This has been called the "functional attitude." Recently this method of plaster immobilization has been modified by flexing the knee and attaching a walking pylon to the unilateral hip spica cast. When the child stands and walks on this pylon, upward pressure on the shaft of the femur theoretically results in a deeper and better acetabulum. After approximately six months of walking on the cast a derotation osteotomy is performed. This method is applicable to both the second and third age groups.

After open reduction the period of immobilization should not be less than three months. Physical therapy, including pool therapy, can be started immediately after removal of the plaster. A bilateral, long leg brace, which has a waistband to include the pelvis and which holds the hips in abduction, has been used both after closed and after open reduction. It is believed that walking in an abduction brace tends to improve and deepen the acetabulum. For a year or more following removal of the plaster cast it is frequently desirable for the patient to use a night splint which maintains the hips in wide abduction by means of a long bar between the shoes.

An increase in the normal anteversion of the neck, sometimes called *antetorsion* of the femur, is present in nearly all cases of congenital dislocation of the hip, usually measuring from 30 to 90 degrees. This is an important factor in hip dislocations and in explaining unsatisfactory therapeutic results. In order to correct excessive anteversion, many surgeons advocate in nearly all cases a derotation femoral osteotomy either below the greater trochanter or above the condyles. In the young child, especially when under 3 years of age, much of the excessive anteversion may undergo spontaneous correction and a derotation osteotomy may not be necessary. When osteotomy is to be done, the amount of anteversion should be determined before operation as accurately as possible by one of various roentgenographic technics. The method of measuring anteversion developed at the Alfred I. duPont Institute *(Dunlap method)* is believed not to have more than a 10% error.

The percentage of satisfactory results after manipulative treatment of congenital dislocation of the hip in patients under 3 years of age has been reported as from 60 to 80%, and in patients under 6 years, from 40 to 60%.

Third age period—3 to 6 years. After skeletal traction for at least three weeks, during which the head of the femur has been pulled down to a point opposite or below the center of the acetabulum, a closed manipulative reduction may be attempted if the hip has not been reduced with abduction, internal rotation, and traction alone. The size of the child and the tightness of the structures about the hip should be taken into consideration in making a decision concerning a manipulative reduction. Excessive force in closed reduction undoubtedly will injure the epiphysis of the femur and its blood supply and is always contraindicated. An adductor tenotomy

76 *Handbook of orthopaedic surgery*

is usually indicated when a closed reduction is to be done in this age group. If a closed reduction is not possible, an open reduction is indicated. In patients from 3 to 8 years of age, Colonna has reported successful results following an arthroplastic procedure; this consists of enlarging or deepening the acetabulum, covering the head of the femur with the elongated capsule, and placing it deeply in the acetabulum. The hip is then immobilized in plaster in abduction and internal rotation, and several weeks later a derotation osteotomy is performed.

Fourth age period—over 6 years of age. In some of the smaller children with minimal displacement, open reduction may be indicated. However, because of the marked upward displacement of the head of the femur in most of this group, an operative procedure to replace the head in an acetabulum is seldom successful. The treatment of the dislocation in older children and adults forms an entirely different and more difficult problem.

It has been found that reduction is usually impracticable because of

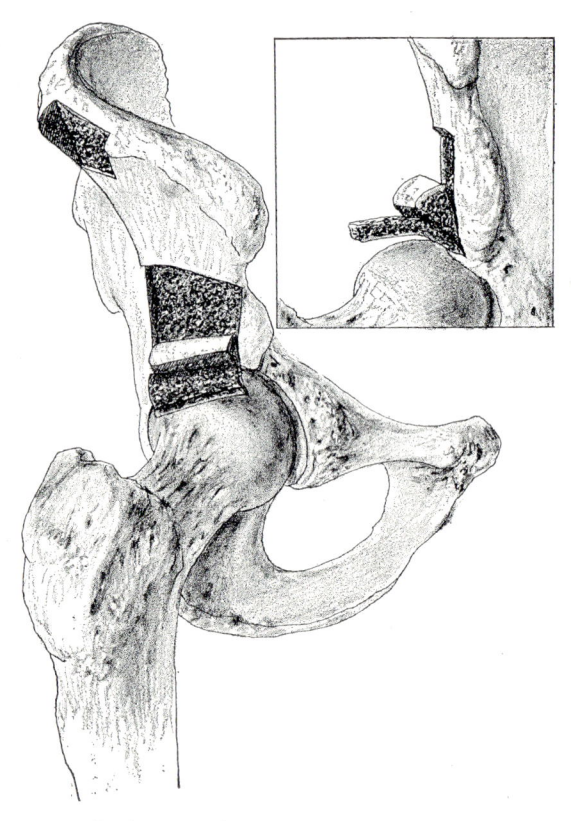

Fig. 46. Shelf operation for late unreduced congenital dislocation or subluxation of the hip. A procedure of this type may be used when it is impossible to effect reduction or is difficult to maintain reduction because of shallowness of the acetabulum. A shelf of bone is turned down from the ilium and held in place by a triangular wedge of bone taken from the iliac crest.

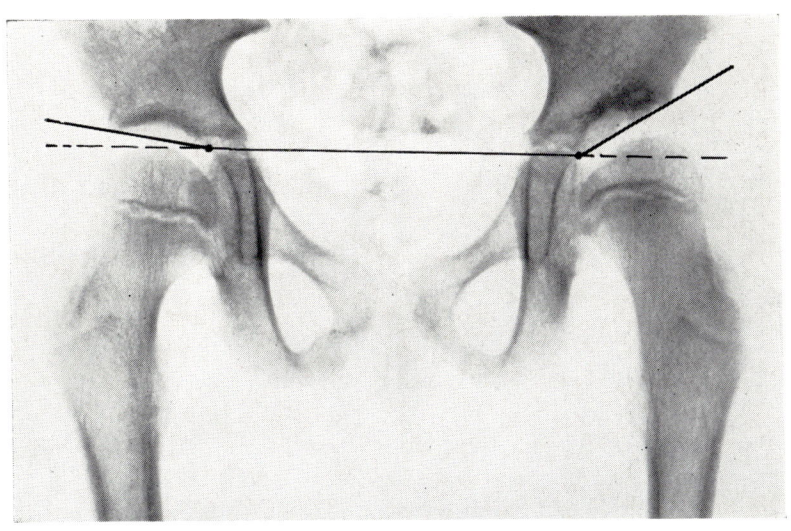

Congenital deformities 77

Fig. 47. Roentgenogram showing dysplastic changes in left hip of a 6-year-old boy, four years after closed reduction of congenital dislocation. Note density changes and increased obliquity of superior margin of left acetabulum. Left acetabular angle is 30 degrees; normal right acetabular angle, 10 degrees. Superior portion of left acetabulum does not cover femoral head so completely as in normal right hip. Left capital epiphysis has "jockey-cap" shape. Note bilateral coxa valga (155 degrees).

the shape of the head of the femur, the acetabular changes, the thickened and contracted capsule, and the shortening of the muscles. Three operative procedures that provide increased stability and at the same time preserve a useful amount of motion are most commonly used: (1) the shelf operation, (2) subtrochanteric osteotomy, and (3) the bifurcation operation.

1. The shelf operation is indicated when there is an upward subluxation because of failure of the upper lip of the acetabulum to develop satisfactorily. It consists of improving the acetabular socket by constructing a ledge of bone over the head of the femur after it has been pulled down as far as possible. This may be done by turning down a bone flap from the ilium and reinforcing the back of this ledge with bone chips or a triangular piece of bone from the iliac crest (Fig. 46), or by inserting tibial grafts into the ilium over the head of the femur. If the head is in the acetabulum, the shelf of bone should be created at the superior acetabular margin and should constitute an extension of the roof of the acetabulum over the head of the femur. This type of operation was advised by Gill for the symptoms sometimes associated with persistent acetabular dysplasia after the reduction of a congenital dislocation (Fig. 47).

2. The subtrochanteric osteotomy of Schanz may be advisable when there is a marked upward dislocation of the head of the femur with considerable instability. This operation permits the shaft of the femur to be placed in abduction while its upper portion lies against the pelvis in such fashion as to provide greatly increased stability; it also allows the femur

to be shifted anteriorly and hyperextended, which decreases the pelvic tilt and the strain on the lumbar spine.

3. The bifurcation operation of Lorenz is sometimes indicated in the older cases when marked adduction and flexion are present. In this operation an oblique osteotomy of the femur is performed below the level of the lesser trochanter. The proximal end of the lower fragment is placed in the old acetabulum. The upper fragment is then allowed to unite with the lower fragment in its new position.

In older cases marked by instability, stiffness, and pain, an arthrodesis of the hip may be advisable for relief of the symptoms.

In the older untreated cases, a high cork sole under the shortened leg will sometimes relieve the strain. When back pain due to strain is present, a corset or snugly fitting back brace should be applied.

Complications. Avascular necrosis of the epiphysis of the head of the femur is a common complication in age groups up to about 12 years and affects the end result of treatment. Reports have shown the incidence of aseptic necrosis to vary between 18 and 64%. Such changes are much more common in older patients than in younger ones. Avascular necrosis is probably caused by circulatory changes incident to the reduction; some observers believe it may be the result of vascular occlusion associated with the frog-leg position. When the epiphysis begins to show evidence of disintegration, it is often best to put the hip at rest by discontinuing weight bearing. This avascular necrosis is in many ways similar to that seen in coxa plana. In addition to the epiphyseal changes there is often an associated coxa vara; in these cases transtrochanteric osteotomies are sometimes recommended to increase the angle of the neck of the femur to the shaft (angle of inclination). Avascular necrosis of the head of the femur may be associated with excessive anteversion. Hips showing avascular necrosis usually develop flattening and irregularity of the femoral head and in later life osteoarthritis.

Gill and others have shown that disability from subluxation or redislocation of the hip frequently develops years after an apparently successful closed or open reduction. Patients with reduced dislocations should be kept under observation for many years; roentgenograms should be taken at long intervals, and no patient should be discharged as cured until the roentgenographic appearance of the acetabulum and femoral head has become normal.

Prognosis. In congenital dislocation of the hip, the prognosis for good joint function is excellent if treatment is started before the third year of age and if late redislocation or subluxation is prevented. In older patients good results are much less certain. Circulatory changes in the femoral head sometimes lead to local deformity and impairment of function. The patient with an incomplete reduction is likely to complain of weakness and early fatigue and, later in life, of pain on weight bearing. Secondary hypertrophic bone changes which gradually develop in the hip region and the lumbar spine may cause considerable pain of a chronic type. A completely unreduced dislocation causes deformity, limping, and hip and low back discomfort, all of which tend to increase as the patient grows older.

CONGENITAL DISLOCATION OF OTHER JOINTS

These entities, in sharp contrast to congenital dislocation of the hip, are rare. In many instances they are more correctly considered subluxations or relaxations of the joint ligaments than true dislocations.

Knee

Two types of congenital luxation are encountered. One is a hyperextension of the knee or congenital genu recurvatum (Fig. 48); this is more common than true dislocation. The second type exhibits an actual complete or incomplete posterior displacement of the condyles of the femur on those of the tibia, constituting an anterior dislocation of the knee joint. The most plausible explanation for the origin of these conditions is an abnormal position of the knee in utero, because when the deformity is corrected the knee usually develops in normal fashion.

Clinical picture. In true congenital dislocation of the knee the leg may be brought to a straight line but will not flex beyond this point, because of contracture of the quadriceps muscle and the patellar ligament. Often the patella is absent, or it may be very small. There is usually a wrinkling of the skin over the patella, and there may be an associated varus or valgus deformity of the knee. Lateral instability is often present.

Treatment. As soon as dislocation of the knee is recognized, an attempt should be made to correct the displacement. This can be done usually either by gentle manipulation of the joint and stretching the quadriceps

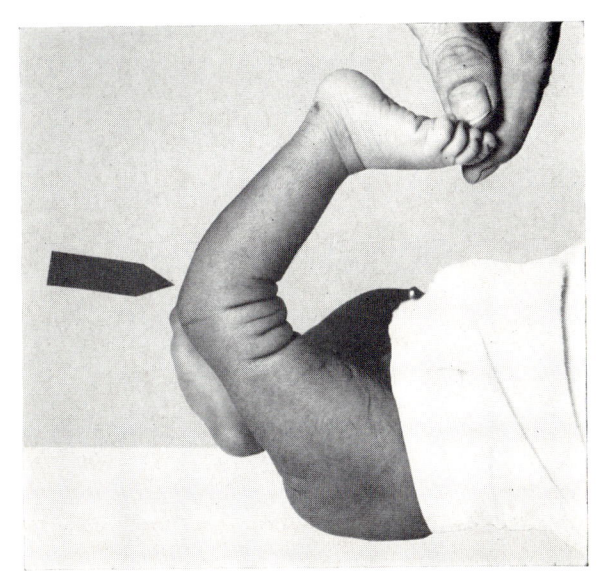

Fig. 48. Congenital luxation of the left knee in infant. Note extreme hyperextension (genu recurvatum) of the knee when the leg is held up.

tendon or by wedged casts. Massage of the anterior muscles may relax them and facilitate the manipulation. After reduction the knee should be kept in a flexed position by means of a posterior splint. This position should be maintained until the flexors of the knee are strong enough to prevent a recurrence of the deformity. It is sometimes necessary to lengthen the quadriceps tendon, and occasionally the iliotibial band must be released, before satisfactory reduction can be obtained.

Patella

Congenital dislocation of the patella rarely occurs. It may be bilateral and is usually associated with genu recurvatum and genu valgum. The patella is usually displaced laterally. An attempt should be made to replace the patella, and a dressing should be applied to maintain the corrected position. If the correction cannot be held, an operative procedure such as that described for recurrent dislocation of the patella (p. 407) is indicated when the child has become older.

Shoulder

Congenital dislocation of the shoulder is extremely rare. The head of the humerus may lie beneath the spine of the scapula with the arm in a position of abduction and internal rotation. The condition may be associated with other congenital malformations. Congenital dislocation of the shoulder must be differentiated from dislocation caused by trauma at birth and from subluxation secondary to obstetric paralysis.

Treatment. Manipulative reposition of the head of the humerus should be done as early as possible. If the result is unsatisfactory, it may be necessary to carry out later an arthrodesis of the shoulder joint.

Elbow

Congenital dislocation of the elbow is also a rare condition. Partial luxation of the head of the radius sometimes occurs. If the radial head is displaced posteriorly, extension of the elbow is usually limited. If both ulna and radius are dislocated posteriorly on the humerus, flexion is usually restricted. Congenital dislocation of the elbow may be associated with an elongation of the upper third of the radius or with a radioulnar synostosis.

Wrist

Congenital dislocation of the wrist is usually associated with clubhand and defective development of the bones of the forearm. Posterior luxation of the lower end of the ulna is spoken of as *Madelung's deformity* (Fig. 270, p. 483). This is an acquired deformity but is believed by some orthopaedic surgeons to develop on the basis of an underlying congenital abnormality which may result in a growth defect in the lower end of the radius.

CHAPTER 4

General affections of the skeleton

B Y ITS PHYSICAL PROPERTIES of strength, resilience, and lightness, bone is admirably adapted to its major function as the supporting framework of the body. Bone is not on this account to be regarded as an inert structural material, however; it is an actively living tissue and like other tissues is constantly undergoing the simultaneous processes of destruction and regeneration.

Functional adaptations of bone. With this continuous breaking down and rebuilding is associated an adaptive remodeling of the bones in response to functional demands that are placed upon them. This far-reaching principle, formulated by Julius Wolff in 1868 and known as *Wolff's law*, holds that: "Every change in the form and the function of bones, or in their function alone, is followed by certain definite changes in their internal architecture, and equally definite changes in their external conformation, in accordance with mathematical laws."

Increased functional demands cause the physicochemical processes of bone regeneration to outdistance those of resorption, and *bone hypertrophy* results. The thick, heavy bones of athletes and laborers, as contrasted with the lighter bones of sedentary individuals, are illustrative of bone hypertrophy. Of greater clinical concern, however, is the converse condition, *bone atrophy,* which results from a predominance of the catabolic and resorptive processes over those of regeneration. In neither hypertrophy nor atrophy of a bone is its general conformation usually altered.

Bone atrophy, in accordance with Wolff's law, may be caused by disuse (Fig. 49). The bone atrophy which constantly develops during therapeutic immobilization of an extremity is a classical example. The cortical bone becomes thinned and the medullary cavity widened, slight narrowing of the shaft occurs, and generalized porosity and loss of weight may become very marked. These bone changes appear to represent merely a quantitative variation, however, since the chemical composition undergoes no demonstrable alteration, the breaking strength in relation to weight is normal, and

82   *Handbook of orthopaedic surgery*

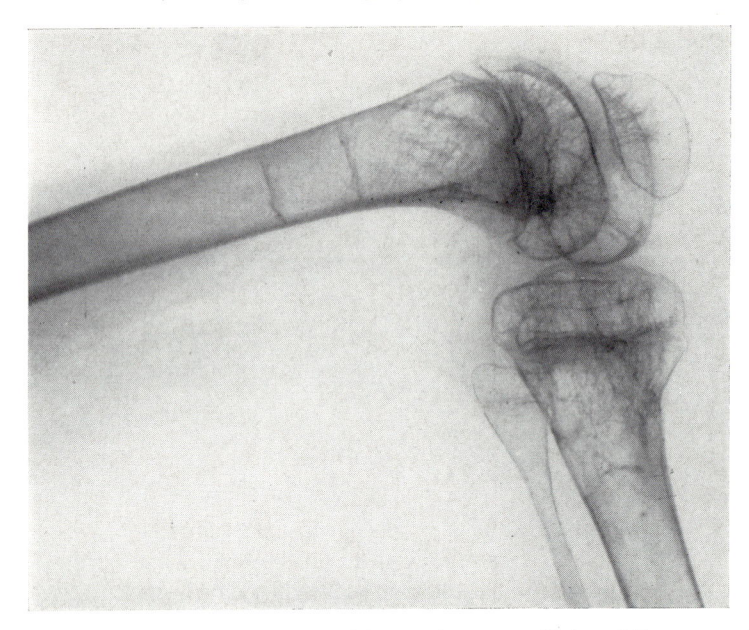

Fig. 49. Bone atrophy. Roentgenogram of knee of 12-year-old boy following prolonged bed rest after excision of a spinal cord tumor. Note decreased density of all bones, narrowed cortices, and pathologic fracture in upper end of tibia.

the power of repair after fracture is retained. Extreme bone atrophy is of particular importance when it involves the growing bones of childhood, since atrophic bones may grow slowly and may never attain full size.

Bone atrophy appears in roentgenograms as a loss of density of the bone shadow as compared with that of the soft tissues. Narrowing of the cortex and attenuation of the bony trabeculae are frequently pronounced. It must be remembered that roentgenographic density is simply an index of the total lime salt content of the bones and gives no information regarding the pathologic changes that may be taking place in their organic constituents. Little is known of the physiology of the organic compounds in bone, or of their part in metabolism and bone formation. Further research in this field may lead to an understanding of many unusual bone conditions about which little information is available at this time.

Since the bony skeleton is a living and continually changing tissue, it is, like other tissues, subject to characteristic disorders. These diseases are alike in producing widespread skeletal changes but vary markedly in etiology. Some, such as *rickets* and *scurvy*, are of dietetic origin; others, such as *cretinism* and *acromegaly*, are the result of endocrine disturbances; several others—for example, *fibrous dysplasia, osteitis deformans,* and *senile osteoporosis*—may be grouped together as of unknown etiology. In the past few decades much has been accomplished toward defining the causation of bone diseases; the role of the parathyroid glands in producing the extensive bone changes of *hyperparathyroidism* is one comparatively recent discovery. Such advances suggest that the causation of other members of this group of diseases will be learned and that with discovery of the etiologic factors will come improvement in methods of prevention and treatment.

Classification of general skeletal affections. Since the cause of many of the general affections of the skeleton is still unknown or debatable, no final etiologic grouping can be constructed. Accordingly, the following classification, which has been considerably modified from that of Fairbank, is subject to further change as additional information on the more obscure entities becomes available.

I. **Caused by abnormalities of diet or metabolism**
   A. Vitamin disturbances
      1. General
         (a) Rickets (infantile rickets)
         (b) Scurvy
   B. Metabolic affections simulating rickets
      1. Fanconi's syndrome
      2. Renal dwarfism (renal rickets, renal osteodystrophy)
   C. Osteomalacia (adult rickets)
   D. Reticuloendotheliosis (histiocytosis)
      1. Eosinophilic granuloma
      2. Hand-Schüller-Christian disease
      3. Letterer-Siwe disease
   E. Gaucher's disease

II. **Caused by congenital developmental abnormalities**
   A. Achondroplasia (chondrodystrophia foetalis)
   B. Dyschondroplasia (diaphyseal or metaphyseal aclasis)
   C. Chondro-osteodystrophy
      1. Morquio's disease (Morquio-Brailsford chondro-osteodystrophy)
      2. Hurler's syndrome (gargoylism, lipochondro-osteodystrophy)
   D. Osteogenesis imperfecta (fragilitas ossium, idiopathic osteopsathyrosis, brittle bones)
   E. Fibrous dysplasia
      1. Polyostotic
         (a) Albright's syndrome
      2. Monostotic
   F. Osteosclerosis
      1. Osteopetrosis (Albers-Schönberg disease, marble bones)
      2. Osteopathia striata
      3. Osteopoikilosis (spotted bones)
      4. Melorheostosis
   G. Progressive diaphyseal dysplasia (Engelmann's disease)
   H. Progressive myositis ossificans

III. **Caused by endocrine abnormalities**
   A. Pituitary
      1. Hypopituitary dwarfism
      2. Hyperpituitarism
         (a) Gigantism
         (b) Acromegaly
   B. Thyroid
      1. Cretinism (hypothyroidism)
   C. Parathyroid
      1. Hyperparathyroidism (generalized osteitis fibrosa cystica, von Recklinghausen's disease of bone)

IV. **Caused by unknown acquired abnormalities**
   A. Osteitis deformans
   B. Senile osteoporosis
   C. Secondary hypertrophic pulmonary osteoarthropathy (Bamberger-Marie disease)
   D. Infantile cortical hyperostosis (Caffey's disease)
   E. Posttraumatic painful osteoporosis (Sudeck's atrophy, posttraumatic or reflex sympathetic dystrophy)

Affections caused by abnormalities of diet or metabolism

SKELETAL CHANGES ASSOCIATED WITH VITAMIN DISTURBANCES

Bone is most affected by the presence or absence of vitamins during its stage of formation. Important effects of the better-known vitamins on the skeletal system may be summarized as follows.

Vitamin A. Vitamin A has a specific effect on the osteoblasts, osteoclasts, and epiphyseal chondroblasts of growing bone. It affects the pattern of bone growth. Thick, short bones may result from either a lack or an excess of this vitamin.

Chronic hypervitaminosis A, caused by excessive administration of the vitamin, produces an elevation of the periosteum followed by a subperiosteal calcification similar to that seen in scurvy. These changes, together with pain in the extremities and irritability, usually appear in children between the ages of 1 and 3 years. The serum vitamin A level is greatly elevated. The prognosis is excellent after the excessive vitamin A dosage has been recognized and discontinued. Hypervitaminosis A may be confused not only with scurvy but also with *infantile cortical hyperostosis (Caffey's disease)*, which is usually accompanied by swelling of the jaw and occurs in infants 1 to 4 months of age (p. 130), and with *progressive diaphyseal dysplasia (Engelmann's disease)*, which is extremely rare, occurs in the older child and young adult, and is associated with a waddling gait and muscular weakness (p. 117).

Vitamin B complex. It has been shown by Warkany that, in rats, a lack of riboflavin in early pregnancy causes a high incidence of congenital deformities. This has not been proved in human beings. Experimentally it has been shown also that lack of the B complex may cause thinning of epiphyseal cartilage plates and cessation of growth. Nicotinic acid is thought by some observers to stimulate callus formation and the consolidation of fractures by means of its ability to activate phosphatase.

Vitamin C (ascorbic acid). Vitamin C promotes the formation of collagen and maintains the intercellular substance. A deficiency causes the activity of the osteoblasts and chondroblasts to cease, resulting in resorption and rarefaction of bone. The periosteum may be elevated by subperiosteal hemorrhages. There is a marked widening of the epiphyseal cartilages. Scurvy, which is caused by a deficiency of ascorbic acid, is discussed as an entity on p. 94.

Vitamin D. The principal physiologic action of vitamin D is regulation of the calcium and phosphorus in the blood. It regulates also the deposition of these salts in the osteoid matrix or protein framework of bone that has been laid down by the osteoblasts. The organic salts of calcium and phosphorus in the blood stream are changed by vitamin D into inorganic salts, which are deposited in the osteoid tissue. A deficiency of this vitamin produces rickets in the young (see below) and osteomalacia in adults (p. 98).

Hypervitaminosis D, a rare affection resulting from extremely large doses of the vitamin, is characterized by hypercalcemia, widespread deposition of calcium in the soft tissues, and slowly progressive deossification of the skeleton. In periarticular tissues, bursae, and tendon sheaths the calcium deposits may reach several centimeters in diameter; in the kidneys they may lead to insufficiency and uremia. Hypervitaminosis D in several respects simulates hyperparathyroidism; the normal or slightly elevated serum phosphorus in hypervitaminosis D is helpful in differential diagnosis.

RICKETS (INFANTILE RICKETS)

Rickets is a constitutional disease of infancy and childhood caused by a lack of vitamin D and evidenced by bony deformities, which may be striking in degree and widespread in distribution. The orthopaedic problems of rickets are always secondary to the pediatric ones. With improved nutrition and pediatric care, the severe cases of infantile rickets which were formerly so common have become rare in highly developed parts of the world.

Etiology. Underlying the rachitic syndrome is a disorder of calcium metabolism, the exact mechanism of which remains obscure. Three factors are generally considered to be important in the prevention of rickets: (1) the antirachitic vitamin D, (2) adequate amounts of calcium and phosphorus in the diet, and (3) sunlight or artificial ultraviolet irradiation.

Pathology. The chief characteristic of the pathologic changes is subnormal calcification and a relative increase of osteoid tissue throughout the skeleton. This results in an increased plasticity of the bones that allows them to undergo changes in shape and to become deformed by gravitational and physiologic stresses which would be withstood by bony structures of normal strength. At the epiphyseal lines ossification is delayed and disordered, and the epiphyseal cartilages become thickened and abnormally vascularized.

In active rickets, characteristic blood chemistry findings include a normal or low calcium content, decreased phosphorus, and increased phosphatase.

Roentgenographic picture. The pathologic changes cause the roentgenographic appearance of a rachitic bone to undergo a cycle of typical alterations as the disease pursues its course.

In the early stages the metaphysis is widened and concave and presents an irregular and indistinct margin (Fig. 50). The epiphyseal line is broad. The epiphysis is obscurely outlined and contains one or more indistinct areas of ossification; as growth proceeds, the epiphysis assumes a vaguely

86   *Handbook of orthopaedic surgery*

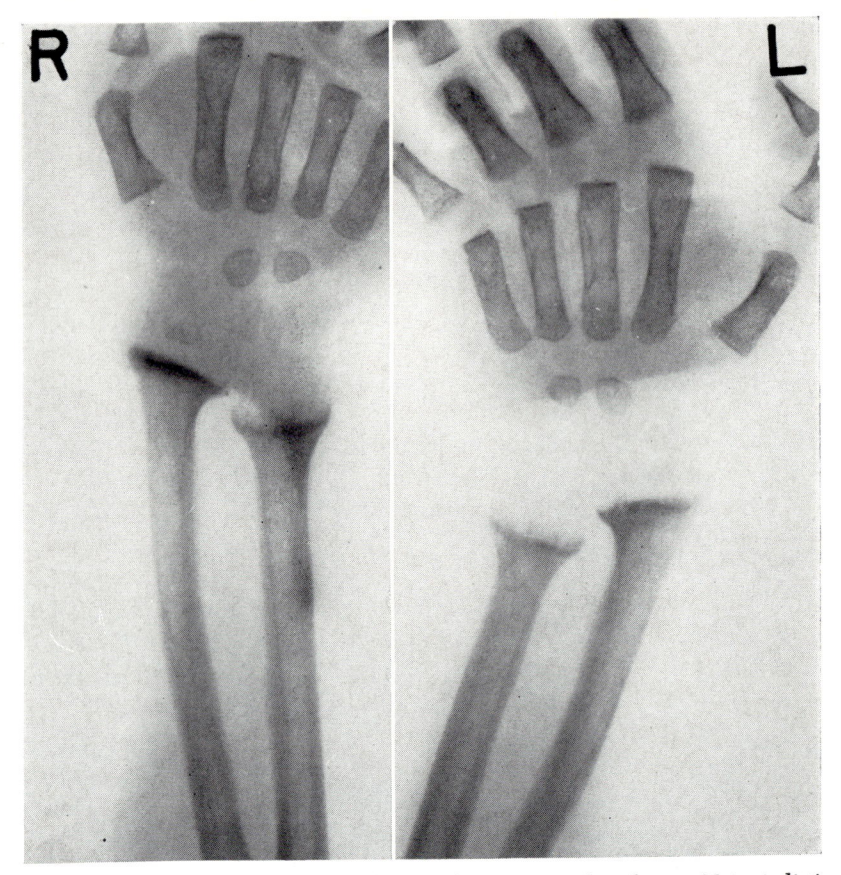

Fig. 50. Roentgenograms of active rickets in boy 10 months of age. Note indistinct, oblique epiphyses with increased calcification on the diaphyseal side of the epiphyseal lines of the radius and ulna, and the cupping of the ulnar metaphyses.

mottled appearance. The shaft may show periosteal thickening and occasionally a fracture line.

In later stages (Fig. 51), the end of the diaphysis loses most of its concavity but remains widened. The epiphysis becomes more distinct in outline and more homogeneous in density. The shaft shows an increased calcium content. Abnormal curvature, with thickening of the cortex on the side of the concavity, is a characteristic finding (Fig. 52).

Clinical picture. Rickets is usually first recognizable near the end of the first year of life. The early symptoms are of pediatric rather than orthopaedic interest and are not pathognomonic. The clinical picture of the more advanced case, however, is characteristic. The typical rachitic patient has a pale skin, flabby subcutaneous tissue, and poorly developed musculature. The joints, because of changes in the epiphyses, are slightly enlarged. The liver and spleen are likely to be increased in size, and the abdomen is prominent. The thorax may be of grossly abnormal shape and may show the *rachitic rosary,* due to enlargement of the costochondral junctions, or *Harri-*

General affections of the skeleton 87

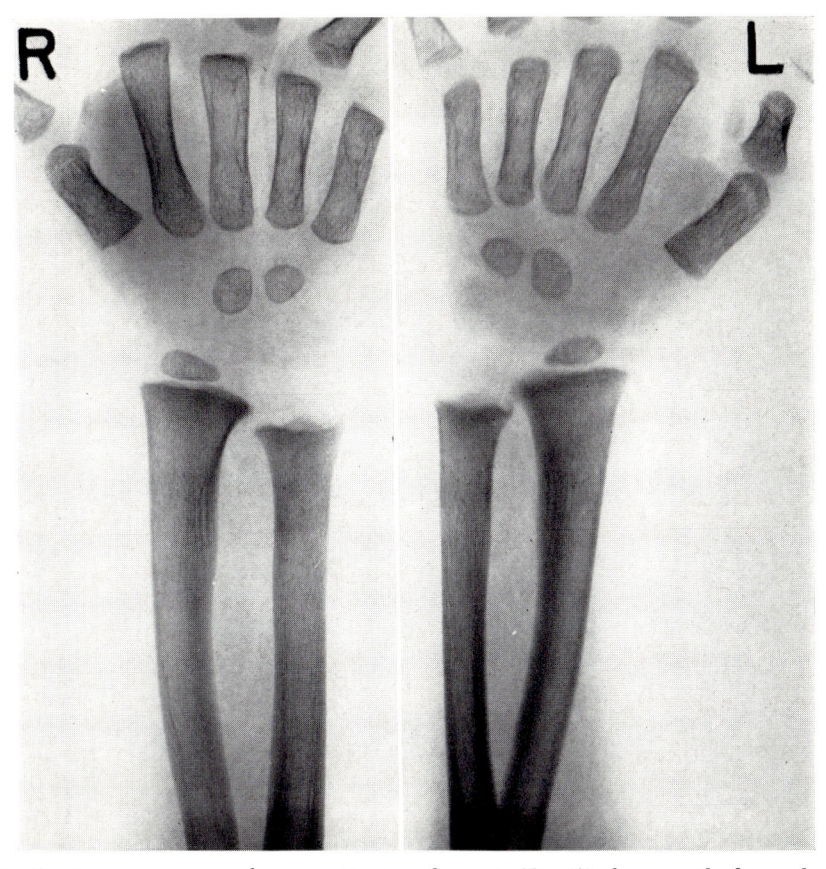

Fig. 51. Roentgenograms of same patient as shown in Fig. 50, four months later, showing inactive rickets. Note more uniform bone density, and improvement of obliquity and cupping.

son's groove, a transverse sulcus across the lower portion of the chest, thought to be due to the pull of the diaphragm. The skull is large and because of its imperfect calcification may be soft and exhibit a delicate crepitation on palpation, a condition known as *craniotabes*. There is noticeable delay in closure of the fontanels, in development of the teeth, and in acquisition of the ability to stand. Bowleg, knock-knee, coxa vara, scoliosis, and other deformities of the bones occur with great frequency in rickets.

Treatment. Of chief importance in the prevention of rickets and in the treatment of its active stage are adequate dietary calcium, phosphorus, and vitamin D, together with an abundance of sunshine and general hygienic care. An ample intake of vitamin D must be assured by supplementary medication with a concentrate of cod-liver oil.

When the disease is established and still in its active stage, orthopaedic measures should be added. For the prevention of deformity, weight bearing and sitting with the legs crossed should be avoided. It is occasionally advisable to keep the patient recumbent. Slight degrees of

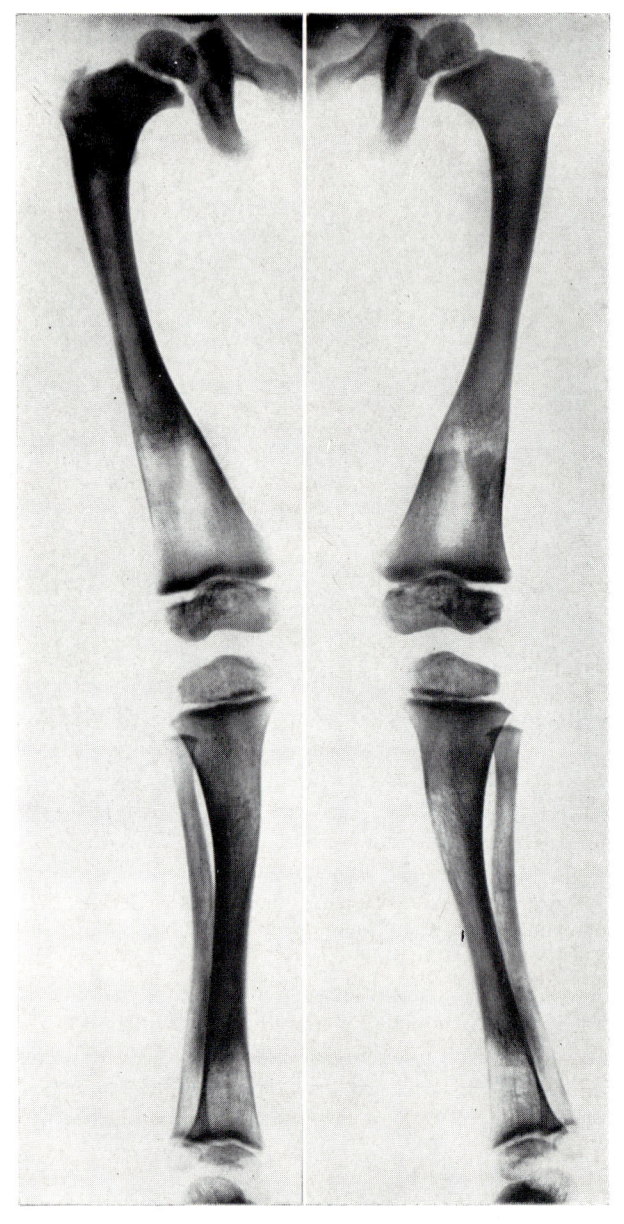

Fig. 52. Healed rickets in patient 6 years of age. Note widening of epiphyseal lines, distortion of tibiae and lower end of femora, and bilateral genu valgum and coxa vara.

deformity in the relatively plastic long bones of infants may sometimes be corrected gradually by the use of wedged casts. However, when rickets is controlled by medical treatment, most rachitic deformities in infants will be corrected by growth alone.

Osteoclasis, or fracture without operative exposure, has been used frequently in the past for the correction of deformity of the long bones in infants and young children but is now seldom employed.

Osteotomy, or operative section of a bone, is the procedure of choice for persistent, severe bowing of the long bones after inadequately treated rickets. Osteotomy is a quick, simple, and accurate procedure requiring a relatively short incision and obviating contusion of the soft tissues. The exact level and degree of the desired correction should be determined preoperatively from analysis of the roentgenograms. Following closure a well-padded plaster cast is applied with the extremity in a slightly overcorrected position. It is sometimes advantageous to do a first-stage, incomplete osteotomy and to follow it after three weeks by a second-stage osteoclasis, as described by J. R. Moore. Immobilization is continued for from six to twelve weeks or until there is satisfactory union, as indicated by adequate callus shown in the roentgenogram and by absence of mobility at the site of osteotomy. Gradual return to weight bearing is then carried out under observation.

GENU VARUM (BOWLEG)

Deforming curvature of the legs, sometimes found in association with rickets, occurs so commonly as to merit consideration as an entity. A very frequent deformity of this kind is *genu varum*, or *bowleg*, in which the major convexity of the limb is disposed laterally. Curvature in which the major convexity lies anteriorly is occasionally seen and is called *anterior bowleg*.

Etiology and pathology. Mild to moderate bowleg may be normal for most infants and will persist to approximately the twenty-fourth month, following which the legs will become straight (Figs. 53 and 54) or even develop knock-knees. In rickets, bowleg is caused by the gradual bending of pathologically softened bone under the influence of weight-bearing and postural stresses. A bowleg may result from a change in the upper tibial epiphysis, at which growth does not take place normally on the medial side of the epiphyseal plate. This is an epiphyseal dysplasia sometimes termed *tibia vara* (Blount's disease). Some observers believe it is caused by a medial epiphyseal injury. Infection of the medial side of the tibial or femoral epiphysis may lead to premature growth arrest and unilateral bowleg. Rarely the healed fractures of osteogenesis imperfecta may lead to similar deformities; in differential diagnosis the roentgenograms are of value. The *saber shin* of congenital syphilis is differentiated from anterior bowleg by collateral clinical evidence of syphilis, a positive complement fixation reaction, and the roentgenographic findings. In adults bowleg may occur from the changes of osteitis deformans, osteomalacia, hyperparathyroidism, malunited fracture, or destructive disease of the knee joint.

The curvature may be present in only one leg or in both. It may involve the tibia alone, the tibia and femur equally, or rarely the femur alone; sometimes it is the result of a lateral yielding at the knee joint while the shafts of the femur and tibia remain straight. As the three-cornered column of the tibial shaft bends, torsion necessarily takes place, and the lower end of the

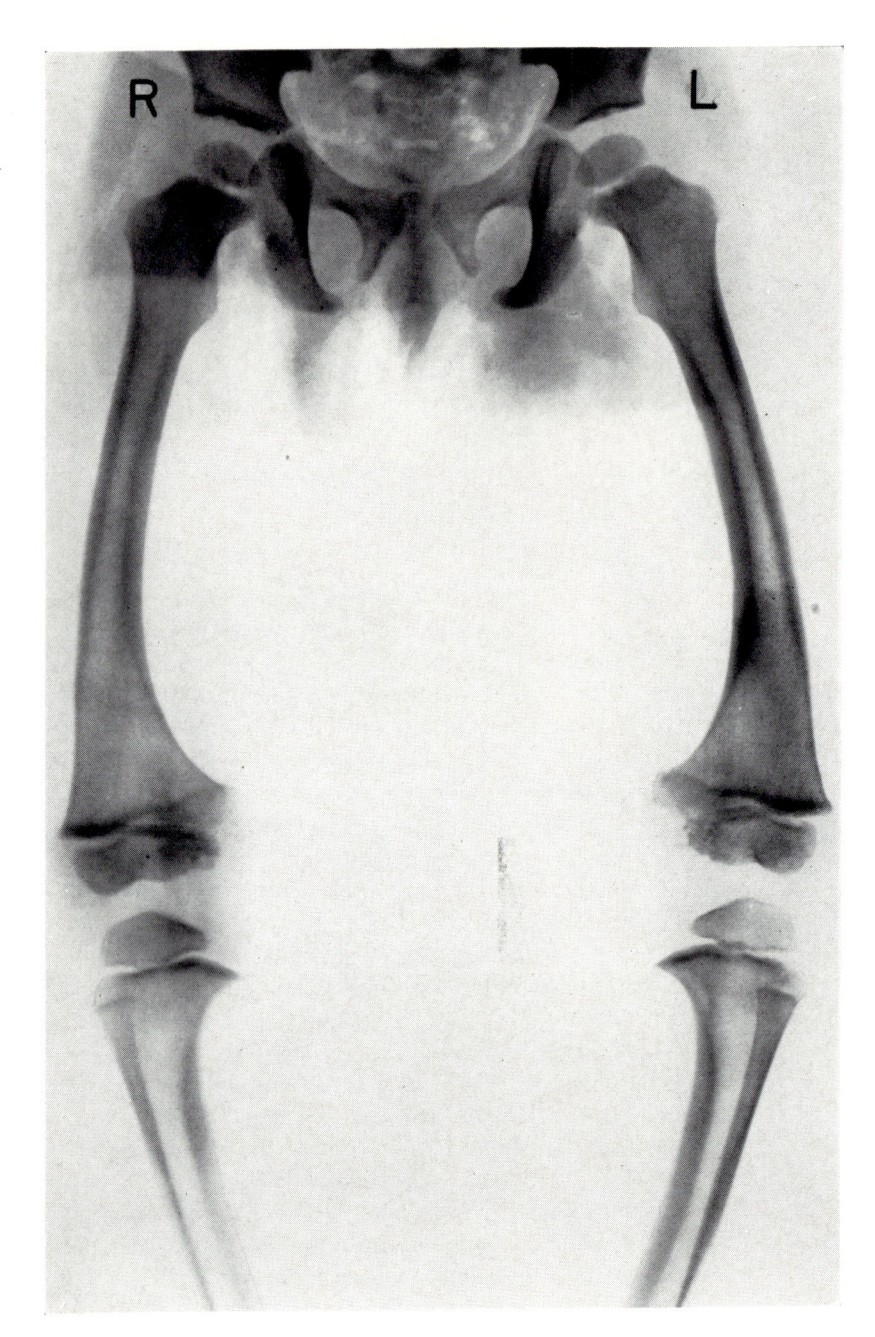

Fig. 53. Bilateral genu varum. Roentgenogram of child 24 months of age, showing marked bowing of femora and tibiae with lipping of the medial margins of the femoral and tibial metaphyses at the knees.

General affections of the skeleton 91

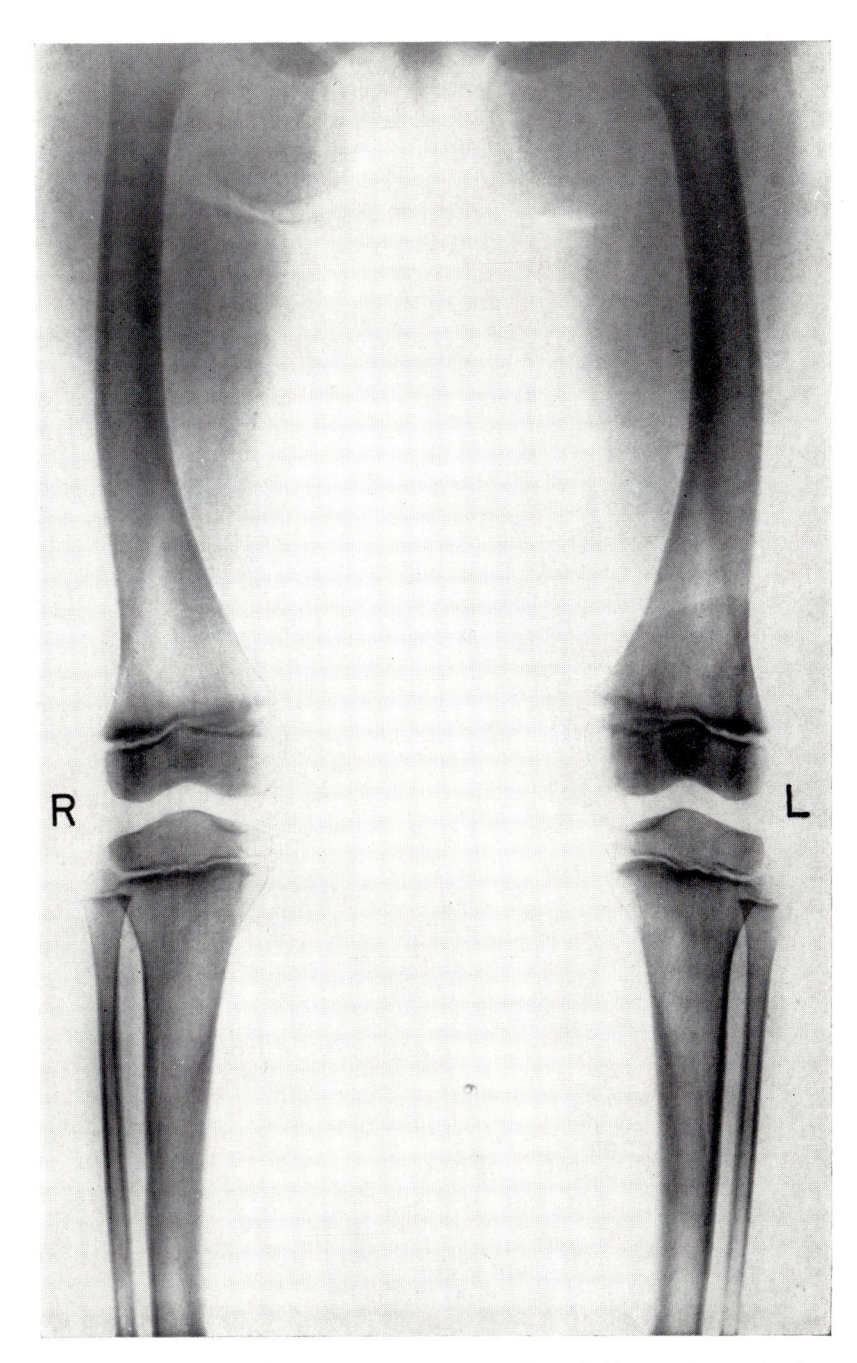

Fig. 54. Same patient as shown in Fig. 53, two and one-half years later. The femoral and tibial bowing has improved greatly, and clinically the lower extremities are straight. Surgical treatment was not required.

tibia becomes internally rotated. Anterior bowleg may exist independently or in association with the lateral form.

Clinical picture. Bowleg is present if the extended knees are separated when the medial malleoli of the ankles are approximated. Measurements of the space between the knees, other elements of the position being unchanged, provide a ready clinical estimation of the degree of deformity and of its progress. Because of the outward bowing at the knee and the inward rotation at the ankle, the child tends to walk with the feet widely separated and the toes turned in; this may lead to considerable lateral shift of the body weight with each step and thus to a waddling type of gait.

Treatment. The stage at which the patient is first seen influences the treatment. Antirachitic treatment should be instituted if any degree of active rickets is suspected. The patient should be re-examined at intervals for a long period, since spontaneous correction of the many nonrachitic cases usually occurs with growth. Rarely are braces indicated. Persistent bowleg may require correction by *osteotomy*. As a rule, osteotomy should not be done before the age of 3 years and not unless the knees are separated 1½ inches or more when the ankles are approximated with the child supine. At osteotomy any internal rotation can be corrected along with the bowing.

GENU VALGUM (KNOCK-KNEE)

In genu valgum, or knock-knee, there is an abnormal curvature of the leg, with the apex of the convexity disposed medially at the level of the knee (Fig. 55). Knock-knee may occur in one or both legs; it may be present in one leg while a bowleg deformity exists in the other; or elements of knock-knee and bowleg may be present at different levels of the same extremity.

Etiology and pathology. Normally the medial femoral condyle is slightly longer than the lateral, thus maintaining the horizontal plane of the knee joint despite the obliquity of the femur. The axis of weight bearing at the knee, however, passes lateral to the center of the joint, so that the lateral condyle bears more weight than the medial. With the bone-softening changes of rickets, a gradual depression of the lateral tibial condyle may therefore occur, leading to various degrees of valgus deformity. With increasing knock-knee, external rotation of the tibia takes place from the pull of the lateral hamstring muscles. The foot usually develops marked pronation; in occasional cases, however, compensatory adduction of the anterior part of the foot occurs and leads to a position of varus. Knock-knee is sometimes associated not with obliquity of the joint line but rather with curvature of the tibial or femoral shaft.

In many parts of the world, rickets is no longer a frequent cause of genu valgum in children. Nonrachitic children, when standing, sometimes show a knock-knee deformity that is not the result of bony changes in the tibia or the femur but is associated with eversion of the foot and is exaggerated by relaxation of the collateral ligaments of the knee joint. In other cases genu valgum of slow development may be caused by an impairment

General affections of the skeleton 93

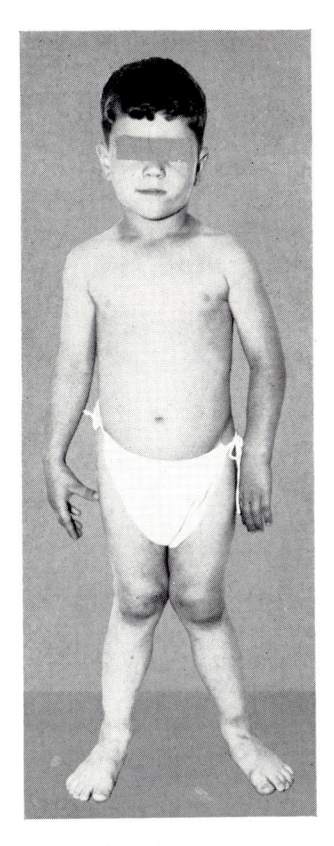

Fig. 55. Rachitic knock-knee (genu valgum) in a boy 5 years of age. The deformities were corrected by supracondylar osteotomies.

of bone growth in the lateral half of the epiphyseal plate as a result of trauma or infection. Genu valgum may also occur in advanced tuberculosis of the knee, after severe poliomyelitic paralysis, and after "bumper fractures" of the tibia with uncorrected depression of the lateral condyle.

Clinical picture. As in bowleg, the diagnosis of knock-knee deformity is made on inspection of the extended knee. On flexion the valgus deformity of rachitic knock-knee disappears, since the posterior portion of the femoral condyles is not deformed, and in this position an abnormal length of the anterior portion of the medial femoral condyle, as compared with the lateral, may be evident. The child, as viewed from the front, may stand with the knees overlapping. The gait is altered by an internal rotation of the leg and foot to prevent the knees from striking each other while passing and by an increased lateral sway of the body to carry its weight to a position directly over the foot.

Treatment. Knock-knee from rickets requires dietetic and medical treatment of the underlying disease. Most nonrachitic knock-knees undergo spontaneous correction with growth. In young children, a ⅛-inch raise of the medial border of the heel may be helpful. Rarely are braces indicated.

In later cases *osteotomy* is the procedure of choice. The level of section, determined after roentgenographic analysis of the deformity, is usually in the supracondylar region of the femur, but at times tibial and fibular osteotomy is preferable. In older patients the removal of a small wedge of bone may be helpful. Care must be taken to overcorrect slightly the valgus deformity. The external rotation, estimated from the position of the foot with respect to the patella, can often be corrected by the same osteotomy.

SCURVY

Scurvy is an acquired constitutional disease caused by an abnormality of nutrition and manifested chiefly by signs related to the bones.

Etiology and pathology. The cause of scurvy is a dietary lack of the antiscorbutic vitamin C. This vitamin occurs in largest amount in the citrus fruits, unboiled milk, and fresh vegetables.

The pathologic changes involve an alteration in certain intercellular materials throughout the tissues, resulting particularly in subperiosteal and submucous hemorrhages.

Clinical picture. Like rickets, scurvy usually makes its clinical appearance in infants between 6 and 18 months of age. Adult cases caused by the same dietary deficiency, however, have in the past been common among sailors and others whose diets have been abnormally restricted, and sporadic cases of scurvy in adults are still occasionally seen.

The scorbutic infant, who often has rickets also, is poorly nourished and irritable and experiences extreme pain on motion of the joints and on slightest pressure over the affected bones. In well-marked cases, subperiosteal hemorrhage (Fig. 56) causes a palpable thickening of the bone. This thickening may be visible in the roentgenograms but often does not appear until calcification has taken place following dietetic treatment. It must be differentiated from similar roentgenographic changes seen in hypervitaminosis A, Caffey's disease, and syphilis. The metaphyseal margin at the epiphyseal line may be dense; beneath it may appear a narrow radiolucent band, the so-called white line of scurvy. Examination of the blood may show the absence of ascorbic acid. In extreme cases there may be loosening of the epiphyses from the shafts, resulting in an obvious crepitation on clinical examination. Slipping of an epiphysis, followed by a deformity with subsequent growth, is a rare complication. In adult cases, and in infantile scurvy when the teeth have already appeared, the gums are likely to be swollen, spongy, and hemorrhagic.

Treatment and prognosis. The treatment of scurvy is primarily of pediatric nature and consists chiefly of the administration of ascorbic acid and foods, such as orange juice, which contain relatively large quantities of vitamin C. Clinical improvement is usually rapid, and the prognosis for complete cure is excellent. The orthopaedic treatment of scurvy is largely of symptomatic type. During the acute stage, recumbency is indicated for protection of the affected bones, and occasionally simple splints are useful to relieve pain and minimize further subperiosteal hemorrhage.

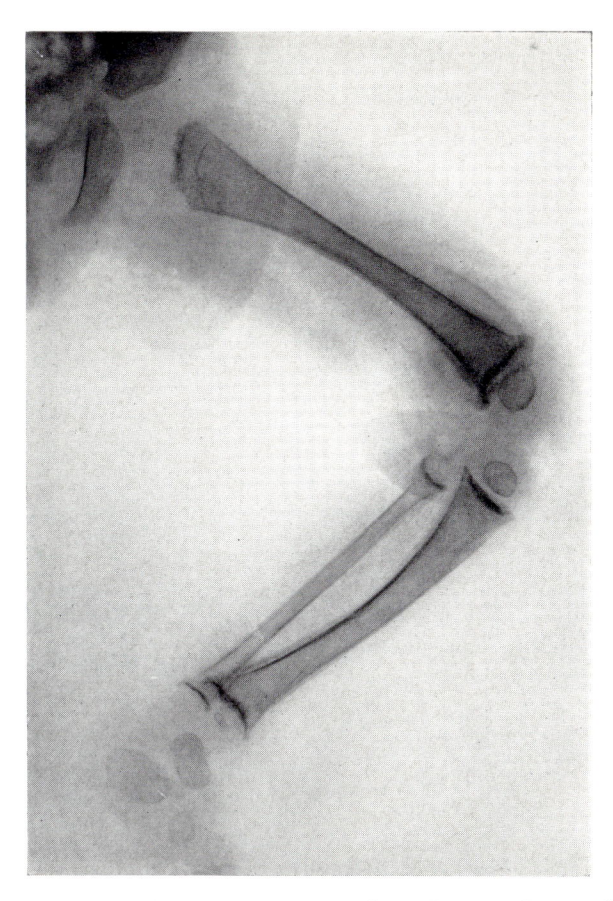

Fig. 56. Roentgenogram of lower extremity in infant, showing changes due to scurvy. Note generalized osteoporosis, calcification in subperiosteal hemorrhages about femur and tibia, and increased, irregular calcification at metaphyseal margins of epiphyseal lines.

METABOLIC AFFECTIONS SIMULATING RICKETS

Disturbances of ossification similar to those occurring in infantile rickets are seen in a number of disorders characterized by defective kidney function and abnormal calcium-phosphorus metabolism.

In this group probably belongs the affection, frequently hereditary or familial, which has been called *vitamin-resistant rickets*, in which the rachitic bone changes can often be cured by enormous daily doses of vitamin D. The dosage should be great enough to maintain a 1 plus or 2 plus Sulkowitch urine reaction. Overdosage of vitamin D, manifested by nausea, weight loss, and hematuria due to hypercalcemia, must be avoided. The typical deformities of rickets may develop (Fig. 57). If they persist to adolescence despite medical treatment, orthopaedic treatment like that described for rickets (p. 87) may be indicated.

The term "late rickets" or "adolescent rickets" has been applied to cases

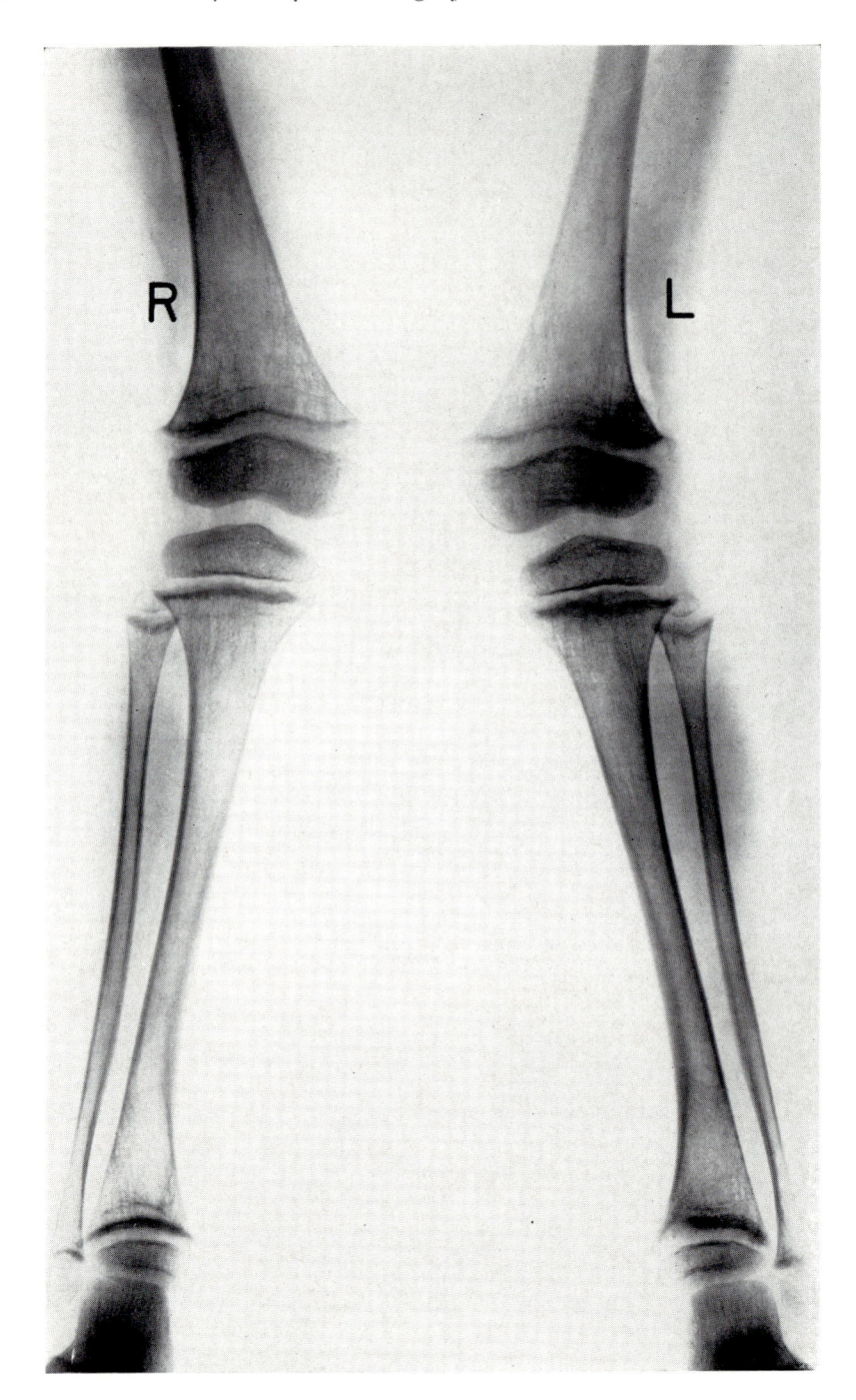

Fig. 57. Roentgenogram of vitamin-resistant rickets in child 5 years of age. Note widening of epiphyseal lines, increased calcification on the diaphyseal side of epiphyseal lines, and marked genu valgum.

in which symptoms, bone changes, and deformities of rachitic type make their appearance in late childhood, usually limited to one or two bones. It seems likely that this designation has included syndromes primarily renal in origin, as well as cases of osteomalacia. The treatment is that of the underlying metabolic abnormality, supplemented by orthopaedic measures such as osteotomy when indicated.

Among additional members of this group of metabolic diseases are two that warrant individual description: Fanconi's syndrome and renal dwarfism.

Fanconi's syndrome

Fanconi's syndrome is a rare hereditary disease of the kidney tubules, beginning in childhood and resulting in bone changes similar to those of rickets. The renal tubules fail to reabsorb phosphorus, glucose, and amino acids normally, and the increased excretion of phosphorus results in loss of phosphate from the bones. Acidosis may be present. The serum calcium is normal or low, phosphorus low, and alkaline phosphatase increased. Cataracts, congenital glaucoma, and mental retardation may be present. Treatment consists of the administration of calcium, phosphorus, and vitamin D, together with alkalis to counteract the acidosis.

Renal dwarfism (renal rickets, renal osteodystrophy)

Renal dwarfism is a rare disease of childhood characterized by chronic renal insufficiency from impaired glomerular filtration, disturbance of the calcium-phosphorus metabolism, and skeletal changes simulating those of rickets. Decreased urinary excretion of phosphorus leads to a high level of phosphorus in the blood and the excretion of phosphorus in the intestine, where it decreases the absorption of calcium by precipitating as insoluble calcium phosphate. Secondary hypertrophy of the parathyroid glands may occur.

Pathology. The nephritis is evidenced by a low urinary specific gravity, frequent albuminuria, diminished urea clearance, and an increase of the nonprotein nitrogen of the blood. Postmortem examinations show an advanced bilateral interstitial nephritis. The bones may exhibit a replacement of red marrow by fat; microscopically there are excess osteoid and defective ossification at the epiphyseal plates. The roentgenographic changes consist of a widening of the epiphyseal lines and a broadening of the diaphyses, as in rickets, but usually to a lesser extent and without the characteristic rachitic cupping (Fig. 58). The epiphyses are not markedly altered but may appear fragmented. Epiphyseal separation is common.

Clinical picture. The clinical course is marked by gradually developing dwarfism, which is usually not evident until about the fifth year, by thirst and polyuria beginning insidiously during childhood and later accompanied by drowsiness, vomiting, and headaches, and by bone deformities that appear near the age of puberty. The advanced stage of renal dwarfism is marked by development of uremia.

98 *Handbook of orthopaedic surgery*

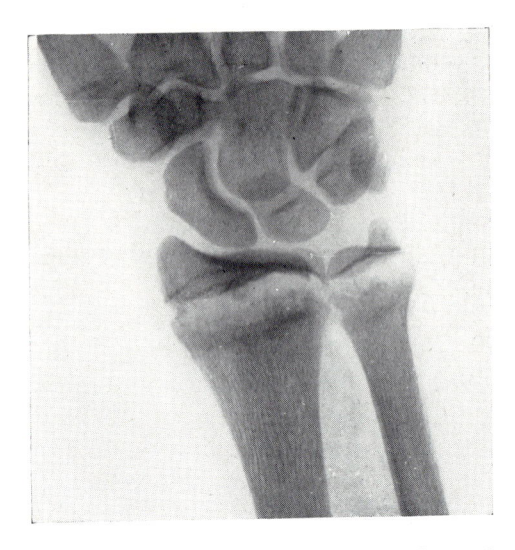

Fig. 58. Roentgenogram of wrist in renal dwarfism. Note wide epiphyseal lines of radius and ulna, normal appearance of epiphyses, and areas of irregular calcification at the metaphyseal margins.

Prognosis and treatment. The disease is almost always fatal, no effective therapy being known. Vitamin D does not help and may do harm. From an orthopaedic point of view the chief importance in recognizing renal dwarfism lies in appreciation of the futility and risk of attempting surgical correction of the deformities. A brace to prevent the increase of deformity is sometimes indicated.

OSTEOMALACIA (ADULT RICKETS)

Osteomalacia is a nutritional disease of adults which corresponds closely with rickets as regards pathogenesis and pathologic changes. It is rarely seen except in northern China, Japan, and northern India. There it occurs typically in women during pregnancy and is ascribed to a combination of high calcium demand, low dietary calcium, and insufficient exposure to sunlight so that little endogenous vitamin D is available.

Etiology. Lack of vitamin D is thought to be the most important cause; it leads to inadequate absorption of calcium and phosphorus from the intestine and as a result the bones are depleted of calcium.

Pathology. The bones may become so soft that they can be cut easily with a knife. The cortex is thinned, the internal structure is greatly altered, and microscopically much of the bone is replaced by osteoid tissue. Characteristic gross deformities of the skeleton are the "heart-shaped pelvis" from pressure at the acetabula, the shortened or "telescoped spine," and marked bowing of the tibiae and femora. As a rule the serum calcium is normal or low, the serum phosphorus low, and the alkaline phosphatase elevated.

Clinical picture. The patient complains of shooting pains referred to the pelvis, back, or hips and on examination shows tenderness in these regions. Severe progressive muscular weakness may be present. The softened spine, pelvis, and long bones develop deformities from muscular and gravitational stresses, and pathologic fractures are common.

Roentgenographic picture. Even in early or mild cases, osteomalacic bones may show transverse lines of rarefaction called *Looser's zones* (Fig. 59). They occur especially in the large long bones and the pelvis, are sometimes bilaterally symmetrical, and probably represent pathologic fatigue fractures with union delayed by lack of mineralization. In later cases of osteomalacia the roentgenograms show a striking loss of calcium and the presence of bony deformities.

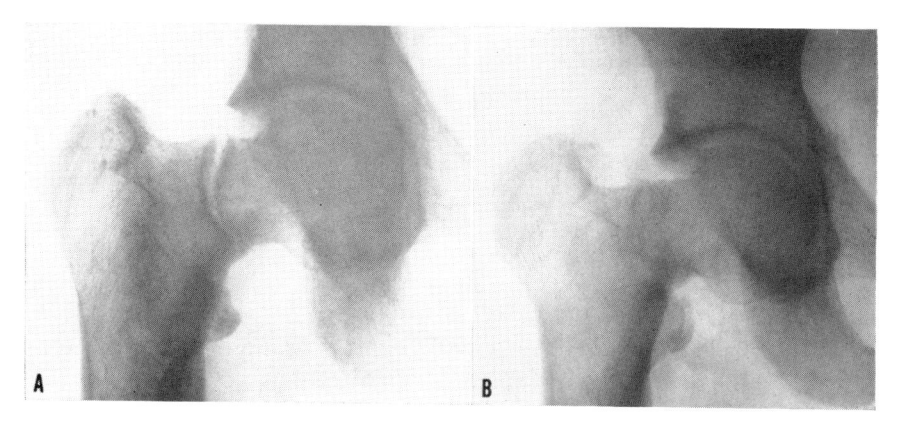

Fig. 59. Looser's zone in the femoral neck of a 40-year-old man with osteomalacia. **A,** Note transcervical pseudofracture line and coxa vara. Hip symptoms had been present for three years. **B,** Note healing of pseudofracture after a year of treatment consisting of the daily administration of 300,000 units of vitamin D. At this time the patient was bearing full weight on the affected limb without hip symptoms.

Diagnosis. In differential diagnosis, osteomalacia secondary to chronic visceral disease should be ruled out. Intestinal disorders with deficient absorption of fats, such as idiopathic steatorrhea and celiac disease, and certain disorders of the kidneys (p. 95), the pancreas, and the biliary system are alike in affecting the availability of calcium, phosphates, and vitamin D and so leading to osteomalacic changes in the bones.

Hyperparathyroidism and occasionally osteogenesis imperfecta, metastatic carcinoma, multiple myeloma, and senile osteoporosis must also be considered.

Treatment. Careful diagnostic studies should be done to rule out underlying visceral disease. Vitamin D concentrate should be given in large doses. Irradiation with ultraviolet light is indicated. A radical change in environment and diet may prove helpful, and an abundance of nutritious foods, calcium, fresh air, and sunshine should be assured. Protective measures to forestall deformity should be combined with careful exercise, adequate to counteract the atrophy of disuse.

RETICULOENDOTHELIOSIS (HISTIOCYTOSIS)

Involvement of the reticuloendothelial system, of unknown cause, is common to the three affections to be described in this group: eosinophilic granuloma, Hand-Schüller-Christian disease, and Letterer-Siwe disease. These diseases are believed to be closely related to one another and possibly variants or phases of the same disorder.

Eosinophilic granuloma

A benign inflammatory lesion of bone, eosinophilic granuloma occurs almost exclusively in children and young adults and is much more common in males than in females. Its etiology is unknown. It involves both long and flat bones and is usually solitary. The lesion is often discovered accidentally by roentgenographic examination or after pathologic fracture. However, its presence may be heralded by local swelling, tenderness, redness, heat, and pain, with some limitation of function.

The usual roentgenographic finding is a circumscribed area of bone destruction from 1 to 4 cm. in diameter with a sharply punched-out appearance (Fig. 60). An involved vertebral body may lose height, becoming greatly thinned. Upon gross pathologic examination the early lesion may have the appearance of soft hemorrhagic granulation tissue; upon microscopic examination there are found numbers of large mononuclear histiocytes, which are phagocytic and contain either droplets of neutral fat or disintegrated cellular material, and collections of eosinophils from which the disease derives its name. Multinuclear giant cells are often present. In the later stages the eosinophils disappear and the histiocytes become foamy. The pathologic tissue is eventually transformed into bone.

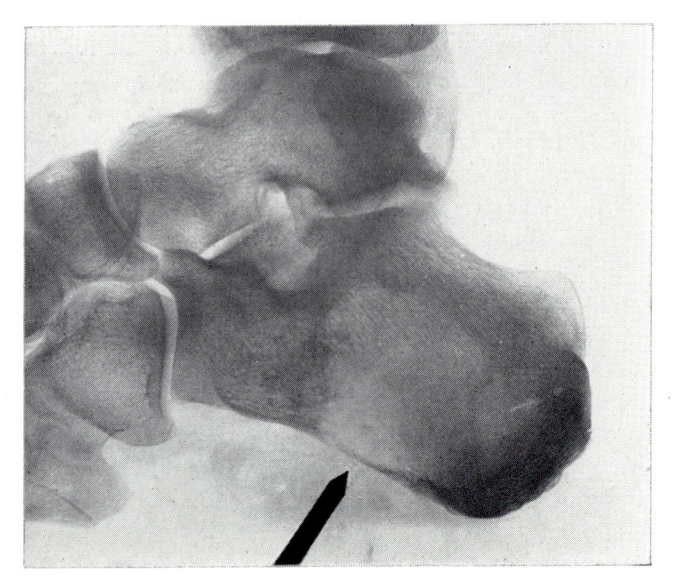

Fig. 60. Roentgenogram of eosinophilic granuloma of calcaneus. Note large circumscribed area of radiolucency.

General affections of the skeleton 101

Differential diagnosis. Eosinophilic granuloma may be confused with osteoid osteoma, osteomyelitis, Ewing's sarcoma, osteogenic sarcoma, multiple myeloma, bone cyst, giant cell tumor, syphilis, tuberculosis, and other conditions.

Treatment and prognosis. Without treatment the lesions may undergo spontaneous healing in from a few months to a year. Excision or curettage, and packing of the cavity with small bone grafts when indicated, usually result in complete cure. Roentgentherapy also may be curative.

Hand-Schüller-Christian disease

The syndrome known as Hand-Schüller-Christian disease is a rare metabolic disorder attended by multiple bone defects that render its differential diagnosis from other bone diseases important. It is characterized by the storage of lipoid substances in bone. These deposits consist microscopically of large numbers of reticuloendothelial cells with a foamlike appearance due to lipoid infiltration. The deposits are most common in the skull but occasionally are found in other bones, giving rise to characteristic defects visible on roentgenographic examination (Fig. 61). They may occur also in the tendons or tendon sheaths and in the viscera. In well-marked cases these changes may be quite extensive.

The disease usually makes its clinical appearance in childhood. Commonly associated factors, dependent upon the localization of the lipoid deposit, are diabetes insipidus, gingivitis, and exophthalmos. Dwarfism and

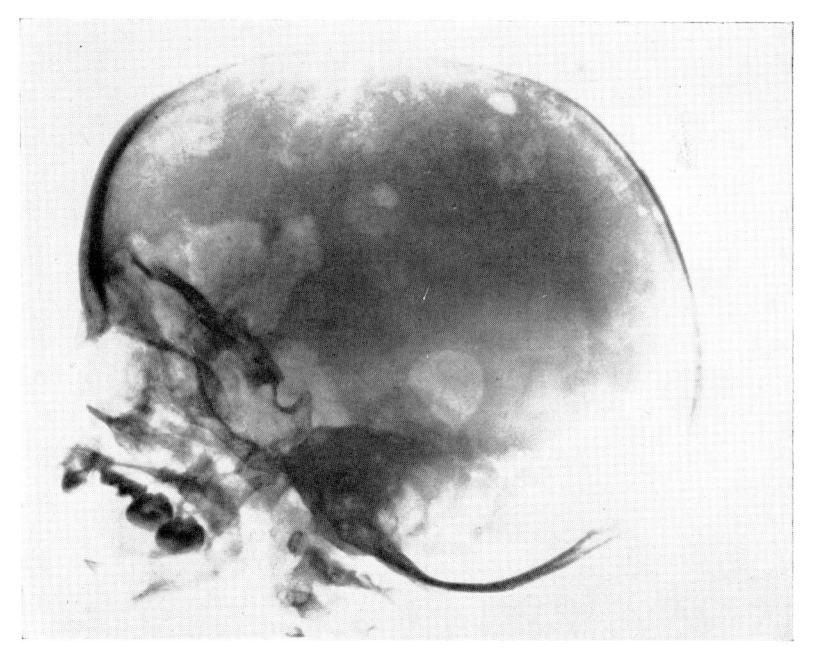

Fig. 61. Roentgenogram of skull in Hand-Schüller-Christian disease. The irregular, punched-out areas contain reticuloendothelial cells infiltrated with lipoid substances.

infantilism are sometimes present, and the patient may be jaundiced. Lipemia is not a constant finding.

Symptomatic improvement may be induced by shrinking the lipoid deposits by means of roentgentherapy. In spite of treatment, cases with extensive involvement of the bones are often fatal.

Letterer-Siwe disease

Letterer-Siwe disease is a rare disorder of infancy, with pathologic changes similar to those of the Hand-Schüller-Christian syndrome, of which it is said to be an acute form because of its rapid, progressive, and fatal course.

The spleen, liver, and lymph nodes are enlarged, and there may be anemia, leukopenia, and thrombocytopenia. Skin manifestations occur early in the disease and include petechial hemorrhages and seborrhea of the trunk and scalp.

Roentgenographic findings consist of multiple rarefied lesions like those of eosinophilic granuloma, especially in the skull. Diagnosis is made by biopsy of the skin lesion or of a lymph node. Treatment is usually ineffective.

GAUCHER'S DISEASE

In Gaucher's disease, histiocytes laden with a lipid known as *kerasin* accumulate in large numbers in the bone marrow, spleen, liver, and other sites. The characteristic cells are called *Gaucher cells*. Their presence in the spleen usually leads to extreme splenomegaly.

A hereditary influence is found in about one third of the cases. Gaucher's disease occurs in an acute infantile and a chronic adult form. The acute infantile cases are characterized by splenomegaly, hepatomegaly, and retarded physical development. Neurologic manifestations including hypertonia and opisthotonos develop, as well as severe pulmonary symptoms. The infant becomes increasingly cachectic and usually does not survive his first year. Niemann-Pick disease is a similar fatal lipoid storage disorder of infancy.

The chronic form is the more common variety of Gaucher's disease. One half of the cases begin in the first decade of life. Abdominal discomfort from enlargement of the spleen is usually the first symptom, but anemia or joint pain secondary to bone involvement may occur initially. Hepatomegaly may develop early or late. Brownish discolorations of the skin, yellow deposits in the conjunctivae, and hemorrhagic manifestations also occur.

The roentgenographic findings are characteristic. Affected bones show reduced density, mottled areas, and radiolucent defects. The lower ends of the femora appear flared, with thin cortex and wide medullary canal. Similar changes may be seen in other bones, such as the vertebrae, pelvis, tibiae, and humeri. Pathologic fractures may result.

Diagnosis is made by demonstration of the characteristic cells in the bone marrow. The treatment is splenectomy to improve the anemia and relieve the abdominal discomfort. Transfusions are indicated for the anemia. The disease progresses slowly to a fatal termination.

CHAPTER 5

General affections of the skeleton—cont'd

Affections caused by congenital developmental abnormalities

ACHONDROPLASIA (CHONDRODYSTROPHIA FOETALIS)

Achondroplasia is a condition of abnormal osteogenesis that produces the typical congenital dwarf of literature and drama. The discovery of a complete achondroplastic skeleton of the early Egyptian period has established this as one of the oldest of known diseases.

Pathology and etiology. Essentials in the pathologic process, which begins early in intrauterine life, are disordered chondrification and ossification of the ends of the long bones. These changes sometimes can be recognized in roentgenograms before birth and sometimes even as early as the third month of pregnancy. Later the epiphyseal plates are abnormally thin. The bones of membranous origin develop normally. Achondroplasia is always congenital and inherited. Its exact etiology has not been established.

Clinical picture. Many achondroplastic infants are stillborn or die in their first year. In children the condition is first noticed usually when the disproportion between length of trunk and of limbs becomes evident. The arms and legs appear short and thickened in contrast to the normally developing torso. The clinical appearance of the achondroplastic dwarf is characteristic and usually permits of ready diagnosis (Fig. 62). The adult height is seldom more than 4 feet. The skull is usually brachycephalic, its anteroposterior diameter being less than normal. The facial expression resulting from high and broad forehead, flattened nose with depressed bridge, and prominent lower jaw is typical. The hands are short and broad with fingers of almost equal length, which tend to spread in a radial manner and have occasioned the term "main en trident." Although growth of the trunk is of essentially normal extent, pathologic anteroposterior and lateral spinal curvatures of secondary nature are common, as is protrusion of the abdomen. Bowing of the femora and tibiae is a frequent finding. Mental development is usually unimpaired, as are the sexual characteristics, although in both respects exceptions occur.

General affections of the skeleton 105

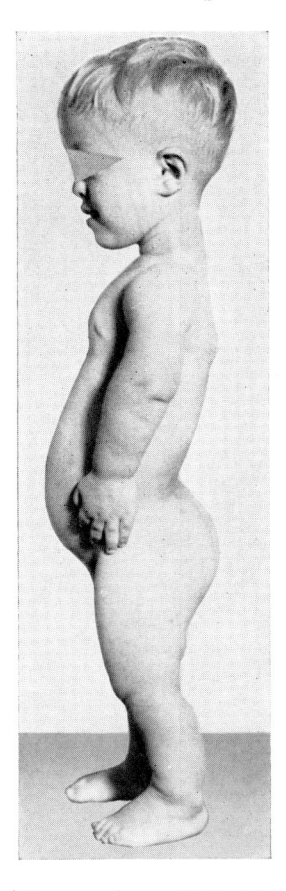

Fig. 62. Achondroplastic dwarf 5 years of age. His height, 32 inches, is 11 inches below average for his age. Note short extremities, long torso, increased lumbar lordosis, protruding abdomen, large head, saddle nose, and short, thick fingers and toes.

Diagnosis. Differential diagnosis is difficult only in infancy, when rickets and cretinism are to be considered. The usual normal mentality of the achondroplastic patient forms an obvious contrast with the impaired mental development of the cretin. The roentgenograms, however, are of greatest value in differentiating sharply the short, broad, normally dense shafts and thinned epiphyseal plates of achondroplasia (Fig. 63) from the poorly ossified bones and epiphyses of rickets, and from the transverse metaphyseal condensations of cretinism.

Treatment. No successful treatment of achondroplasia is known. Occasionally, especial attention is required for the prevention or correction of specific deformities. The prognosis for length of life is good.

DYSCHONDROPLASIA (DIAPHYSEAL OR METAPHYSEAL ACLASIS)

Dyschondroplasia is an infrequent congenital and sometimes inherited skeletal affection of obscure etiology characterized by disorderly carti-

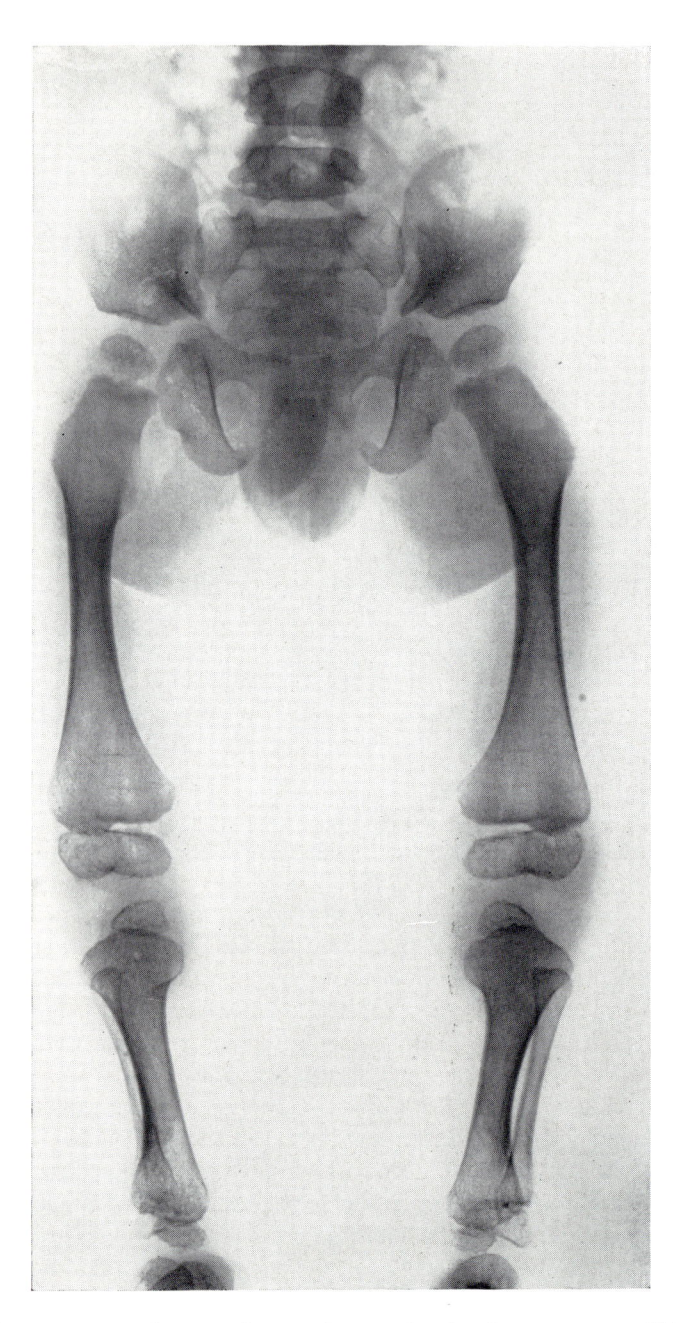

Fig. 63. Roentgenogram showing changes due to achondroplasia in 3-year-old boy. Note the short, thick femora, tibiae, and fibulae, the valgus of the femoral necks, and the slight varus of the knees.

General affections of the skeleton 107

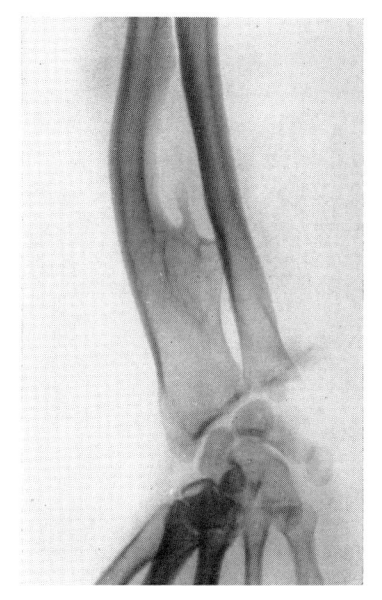

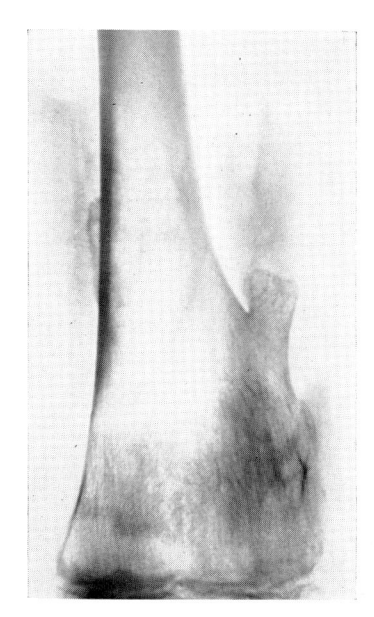

Fig. 64   Fig. 65

Fig. 64. Roentgenogram showing multiple congenital exostoses in a woman 28 years of age. Note the exostosis at the lower end of the radius, which encroaches on the interosseous space, and the lateral bowing of the shaft of the radius.

Fig. 65. Roentgenogram showing multiple congenital exostoses in a 9-year-old boy. Note the broadening of the metaphysis, and the exostosis above the adductor tubercle of the femur. This patient is the son of the patient shown in Fig. 64.

laginous development and irregular ossification at the ends of the long bones (Figs. 64 and 65). Two clinical types of the condition are noteworthy. In one of these, *Ollier's disease*, the deforming overgrowths are of extremely irregular shape and are confined to one extremity or to one side of the body. In the other, *hereditary multiple cartilaginous exostoses*, there are numerous and often roughly symmetrical osteocartilaginous tumors which individually are identical with the benign bone tumor known as osteochondroma. There are various gradations between these two types; in both types, as a rule, secondary bone deformity and dwarfed skeletal growth occur.

Pathology. The site of the pathologic process is the metaphysis, where disorderly overgrowth of cartilage and abnormal and incomplete ossification take place. The bones of purely membranous origin are not usually involved. The changes become most marked where growth in length is greatest, that is, at the shoulders and wrists and about the knees. Multiple tumors often take the form of narrow, elongated pyramids with osseous base at the epiphyseal line and cartilage-covered tip directed obliquely along the shaft. In such cases symmetrical deformities are likely to occur at analogous levels of the limbs. An adventitious bursa may form over the tip of such a tumor, and with maturity the cartilaginous tip may be-

108   *Handbook of orthopaedic surgery*

come completely ossified. Malignant degeneration occasionally takes place.

Clinical picture. Dyschondroplasia is more common in males than in females. The presence of hard painless swellings attached to the ends of the long bones, or to the scapula or pelvis, is usually noticed in early childhood. In less-marked cases such tumors make their appearance only at puberty. Patients with lesions of the more severe type show retarded general skeletal development, associated with which there may be secondary deformities, such as curvature of the bones of the forearm or fusion of the lower end of the tibia and fibula.

Roentgenographic picture. The roentgenograms of dyschondroplasia are, as a rule, pathognomonic, presenting large and irregularly expanded diaphyseal masses with only thin sheets of cortical bone, or multiple bony outgrowths at the metaphyseal regions (Figs. 64 and 65).

Treatment and prognosis. Treatment is chiefly concerned with the surgical removal of discrete tumors that by local pressure on tendon or nerve

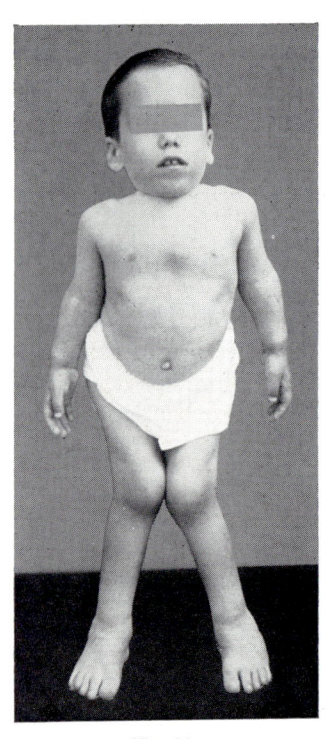

Fig. 66 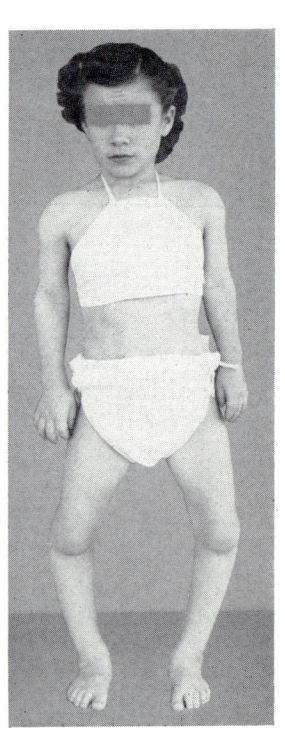   Fig. 67

Fig. 66. Morquio's disease (chondro-osteodystrophy). Boy 8 years old whose height, 36 inches, is 13 inches below average for his age. Note large head, flexion of the hips and knees, bilateral genu valgum, and short extremities.

Fig. 67. Morquio's disease (chondro-osteodystrophy). Girl 13½ years old whose height, 47½ inches, is 14 inches below average for her age. Note large head, bilateral genu varum, and short, stubby fingers and toes.

are causing pain or are interfering with the function of an adjacent joint. After ossification of the epiphyses has taken place, no further increase in deformity is likely to occur, and operative correction of outstanding deformities may be indicated. The prognosis for length of life is excellent.

MORQUIO'S DISEASE (MORQUIO-BRAILSFORD CHONDRO-OSTEODYSTROPHY)

Morquio's disease is a congenital affection characterized by dwarfism, spinal deformity, and widespread changes in the epiphyses (Figs. 66 and 67). In approximately one third of the reported cases there is a familial history. The disease is usually unrecognized until the child begins to walk, at which time a waddling gait is noted. There are characteristic changes in the spine and centers of ossification, especially in the capital femoral epiphyses.

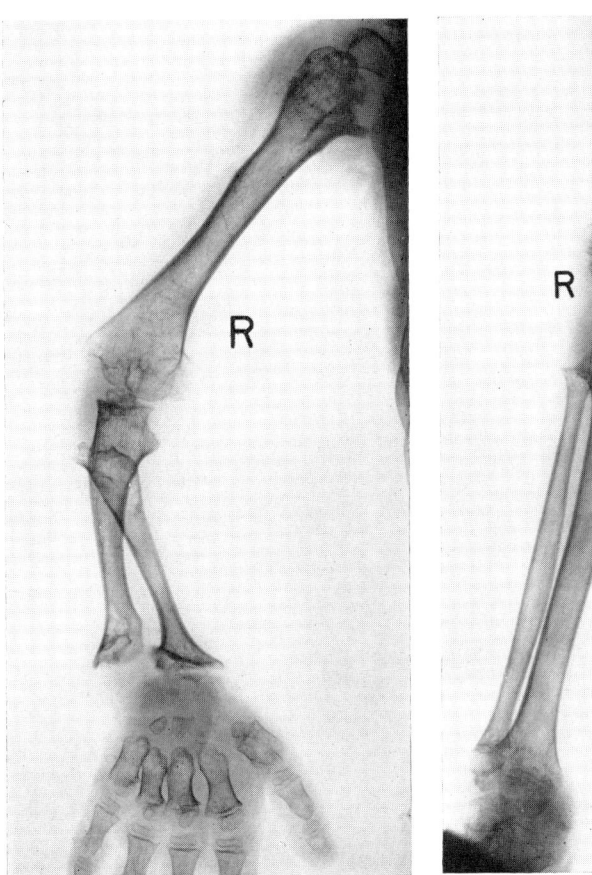

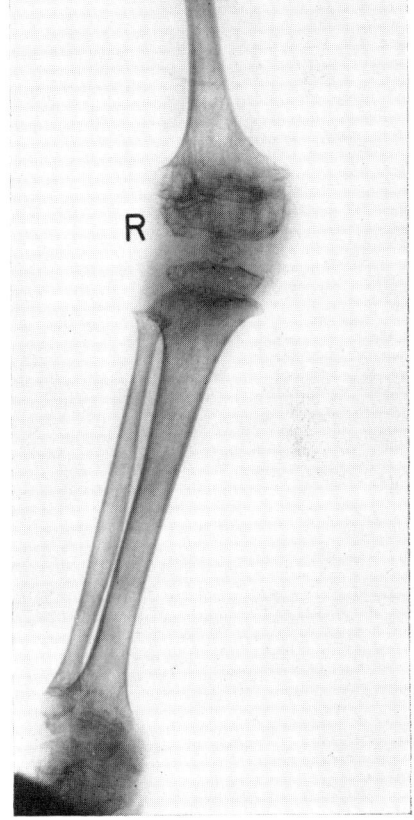

Fig. 68

Fig. 69

Fig. 68. Morquio's disease. Roentgenogram of upper extremity of patient shown in Fig. 66. Note deformities of epiphyses and long bones.

Fig. 69. Morquio's disease. Roentgenogram of lower extremity of patient shown in Fig. 66. Note genu valgum, deformity of epiphyses, and thinning of femoral shaft.

The femoral heads become enlarged and irregular, with resulting limitation of external rotation of the hips. The spine is stiff and usually presents a sharp kyphosis at the dorsolumbar junction, which may be confused with the gibbus of a tuberculous spine. There may be a compensatory lumbar lordosis. There is gross deformity of the vertebral bodies, particularly at the dorsolumbar junction, where the front half of the vertebrae may appear to be missing. The neck and trunk are short in contrast to the limbs. The phalanges and metacarpal bones may be stubby and the ulna and fibula short (Figs. 68 and 69). The intelligence is usually normal.

The only treatment is that which may be indicated to correct deformities.

HURLER'S SYNDROME (GARGOYLISM, LIPOCHONDRO-OSTEODYSTROPHY)

Hurler's syndrome is a deforming congenital and familial disease of children, associated with widespread deposition of lipid or protein in various tissues of the body. It is usually fatal in the second decade of life because

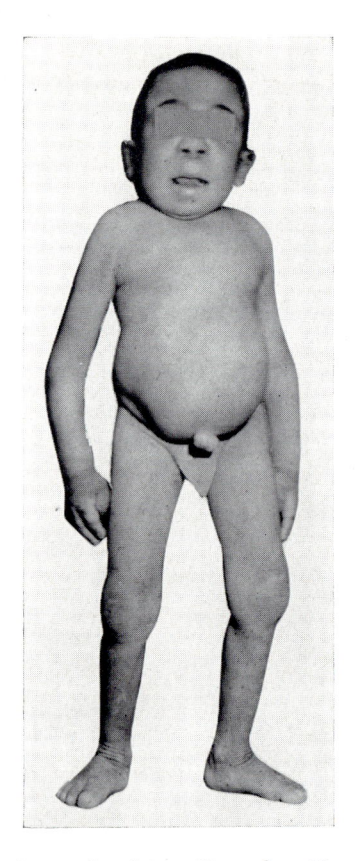

Fig. 70. Hurler's syndrome (gargoylism) in a Negro boy 12 years of age. Note shortness of neck and trunk, protruding abdomen, and characteristic facies. This patient also had an umbilical hernia. He died of congestive heart failure three months after this photograph was made.

of heart failure from lipid infiltration. It is characterized by marked shortening of the trunk and neck (Fig. 70), a dorsal kyphosis, protruding abdomen, and enlargement of the liver and spleen. The facial features are coarse and somewhat repulsive. There are a misshapen, enlarged skull, prominent forehead, widely spaced eyes, prominent supraorbital ridges, "saddle-nose," thick tongue, and prognathism. The corneas are clouded by multiple deep opacities. There are usually short arms, impaired joint mobility, and flexion deformities of the joints, especially of the fingers, which are thickened. Because of cerebral infiltration by the lipid substance, mental deficiency develops. Characteristic roentgenographic changes include abnormalities in development of the cranial bones, abnormal vertebral contours, widening of the medial ends of the clavicles and underdevelopment of their lateral ends, and tapering of the distal phalanges. There is no known treatment.

OSTEOGENESIS IMPERFECTA (FRAGILITAS OSSIUM, IDIOPATHIC OSTEOPSATHYROSIS, BRITTLE BONES)

Osteogenesis imperfecta is a rare congenital and usually inherited skeletal disease in which the occurrence of multiple fractures is rendered inevitable by extreme fragility of the bones. Fractures may be evident in the skeleton of the newborn infant. In roentgenograms the bones often show a generalized thinning of the cortex, osteoporosis, decreased thickness of the shafts, and coarse trabeculations (Fig. 71). The fractures are often undisplaced.

Etiology. The cause of the excessive bone fragility is not known. An endocrine disturbance has never been proved. Abnormal numerical or functional characteristics of the osteoblasts have been postulated, as well as other disturbances leading to an alteration of the process of ossification of the developing bone. The underlying pathologic change appears to be a mesenchymal defect.

Clinical picture. Broad lines may be drawn clinically between certain types of this disease. There is a severe form, to which the term "osteogenesis imperfecta" is restricted by some clinicians, in which the disease is obvious at birth from the occurrence of multiple fractures and definite shortening of the extremities as compared with the trunk. In these infants the prognosis for survival is poor. A less severe form of the disease, to which the term "idiopathic osteopsathyrosis" is sometimes applied, is characterized by the occurrence of fractures only in early or late childhood. It is probable that a third group of cases, patients who show perhaps two or three successive fractures after episodes of only moderate trauma, represent a milder form of the disease.

In many of the patients with osteogenesis imperfecta a very definite China-blue coloration of the sclerae will be noted. This color has been attributed to a decreased opacity of the sclerae, which permits the pigmentatation of the deeper coats to show through. The combination of bone fragility and blue sclerae is an inherited dominant characteristic. Many of these

112   *Handbook of orthopaedic surgery*

patients also show hypermobility of the joints, thinning of the skin, and otosclerosis after 20 years of age; all are of short stature.

Treatment and prognosis. Since the underlying etiology is unknown, treatment is empirical and, in general, unsatisfactory. The diet and vitamin

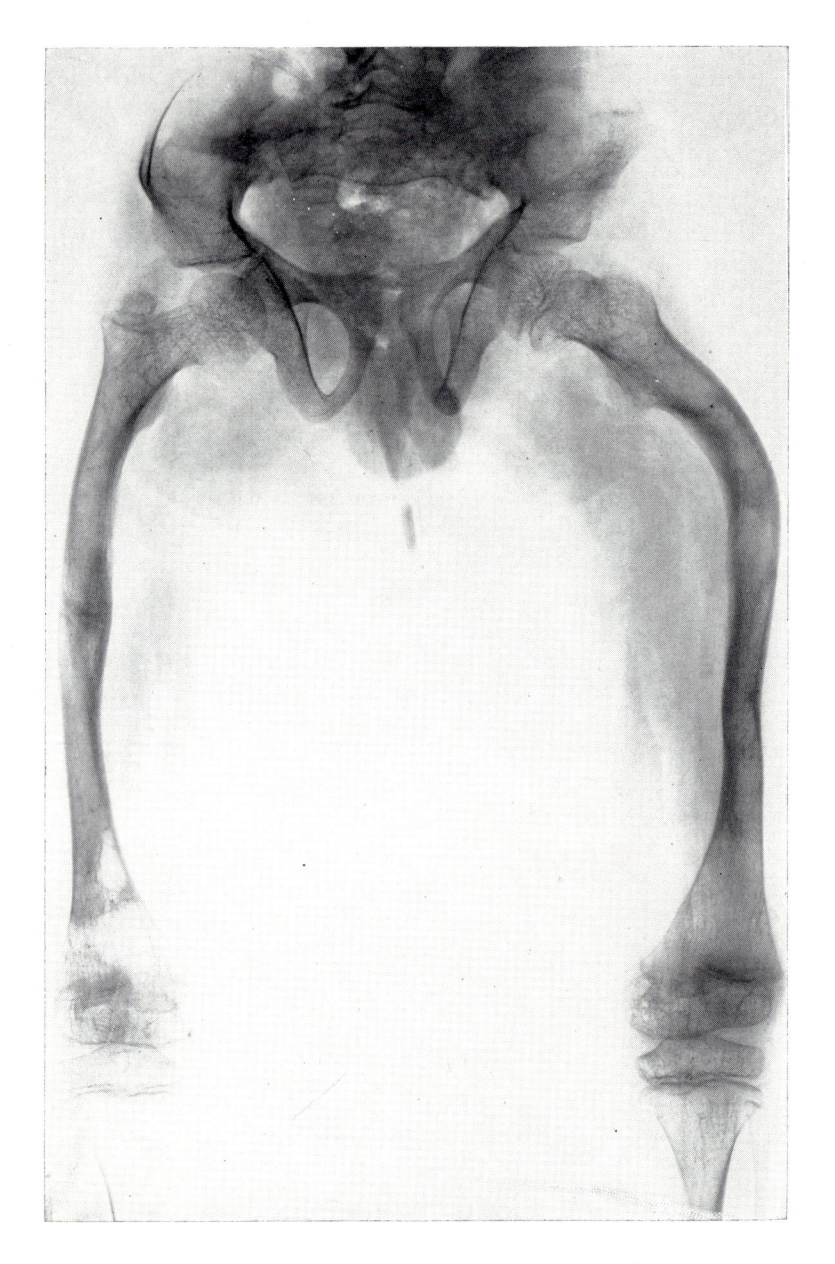

Fig. 71. Roentgenogram showing osteogenesis imperfecta in boy 10 years of age. One femur has been fractured four times and the other twice. Note deformity of femora, uneven density and thinning of cortices, and heart-shaped pelvis.

intake should be adequate. Reduction and immobilization after fracture are carried out as usual. An effort should be made to keep the child as active as possible in order to stimulate bone formation.

The prognosis for union of these fractures is excellent. It is a matter of clinical experience that the fragility of the bone does not entail a loss of its capacity to unite after fracture. Union may be accomplished by exuberant callus formation of tumorlike appearance. With repeated fractures of various bones, it is not surprising that extensive deformities may ultimately develop. In the more severe cases deformities also result from bending of the shafts of the bones because of their plasticity. Corrective osteotomies and intramedullary fixation are occasionally indicated. After the age of puberty has passed, the prognosis for disappearance of the abnormal fragility is good.

FIBROUS DYSPLASIA

Fibrous dysplasia is a chronic bone affection characterized by the presence of one or many skeletal lesions in which bone is replaced by an abnormal proliferation of fibrous tissue. Its etiology is unknown; it is ordinarily considered to be a dysplasia of congenital origin.

Clinically fibrous dysplasia is seen in *polyostotic* form, wherein more than one bone is affected, and in *monostotic* form, in which the lesion involves only one bone. The monostotic type has not been shown to progress to the polyostotic, and the exact relationship between the two remains obscure.

Polyostotic fibrous dysplasia

Polyostotic fibrous dysplasia is somewhat more common in girls than in boys. It is seldom seen in infants but develops usually during the later years of the growth period. The course of the lesions is variable; whereas severely involved cases may progress rapidly in childhood, in many instances the lesions enlarge slowly or not at all after growth has ceased. Unilateral distribution is a common but by no means constant finding. Most frequently involved are the long bones, especially the femur, and the pelvis, ribs, and skull.

The presenting complaint is usually increasing deformity, a limp, pain in the affected area, or disability associated with a pathologic fracture.

Albright's syndrome, seen almost exclusively in girls, is the relatively rare combination of polyostotic fibrous dysplasia, irregularly edged café au lait pigmentation of the skin, and an endocrine disorder evidenced by sexual precocity.

Pathology. Grossly the tissue of the early lesions is gray and of soft, gritty consistency; when more mature it is yellow and firm. Microscopic sections show a fibroblastic matrix embedding scattered bone spicules. Osteoid is present, as well as occasional areas of cartilage, and degenerative changes may be superimposed.

The blood chemistry findings are normal except after a major fracture

114   *Handbook of orthopaedic surgery*

or in the presence of extensive skeletal involvement, when the serum alkaline phosphatase is often elevated.

Roentgenographic picture. The affected bones show radiolucent areas of ground-glass appearance, thin cortices, deformed contours, and fractures. The fractures usually heal well with the exception of those of the upper

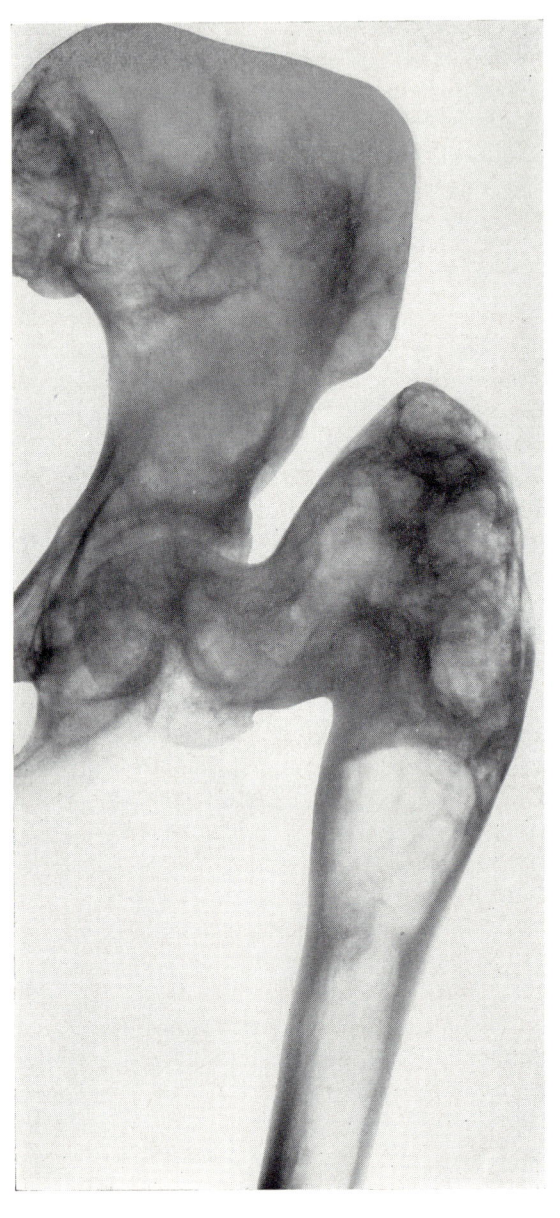

Fig. 72. Roentgenogram of polyostotic fibrous dysplasia in a woman 33 years old. Note the extensive radiolucent areas in femur and pelvis, and shepherd's-crook deformity of upper end of femur. Almost all bones of the body were involved.

third of the femur, which cause some of the most crippling features of the disease. After multiple fractures in the upper third, the femoral deformity may be quite severe (Fig. 72) and has been called a shepherd's crook deformity. The unilateral bone lesions tend to be segmental, leaving normal bone adjacent to the radiolucent areas.

Treatment. The fractures and deformities often need orthopaedic treatment, especially the bowing and pseudarthrosis of the upper femur. The latter may require osteotomy and grafting. There is no treatment for the underlying disease.

Monostotic fibrous dysplasia

In about half of the reported cases of monostotic fibrous dysplasia the lesion has involved a rib, possibly because of the frequency of routine chest roentgenograms. The lesion has been found in many other bones, long and flat, membranous and enchondral, particularly the upper femur, tibia, and mandible. Notably, the bones of the hands and feet seem to escape.

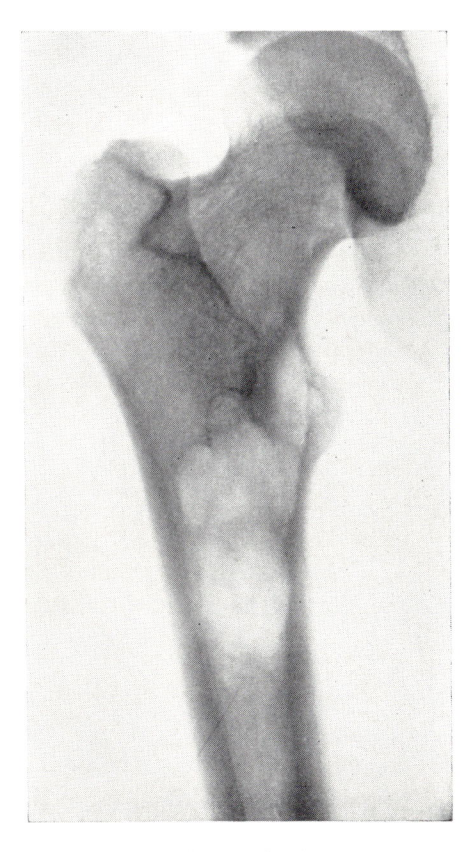

Fig. 73. Roentgenogram of monostotic fibrous dysplasia involving the femur. Note multilocular radiolucency extending from above the lesser trochanter down into the shaft.

Monostotic fibrous dysplasia may be asymptomatic or may present itself by local swelling, pain, tenderness, or pathologic fracture. The lesion may remain static or slowly enlarge. Roentgenograms show a localized area of rarefaction (Fig. 73), which is not pathognomonic. The gross and microscopic appearance of the pathologic tissue is similar to that of the lesions in polyostotic fibrous dysplasia

Treatment. Biopsy is indicated when the diagnosis is in doubt. At the time of biopsy pathologic tissue may be removed by thorough curettement and the resulting cavity may be packed with small grafts of autogenous bone.

OSTEOSCLEROSIS

Under this term may be grouped a number of interesting but rare and little-known skeletal diseases characterized by areas of increased bone density. The affected bones have a typically opaque roentgenographic appearance; in some of them the cortex is greatly thickened and the medullary canal may be obliterated. The bone changes do not as a rule cause symptoms and are often discovered as an incidental finding during roentgenographic examinations. The etiology of these diseases is unknown, although the sporadic association of various factors in individual cases has led to a variety of hypotheses. These affections are sometimes hereditary or familial. Excessive fluorine intake may cause bone changes of this type. Symptomatic treatment is occasionally indicated.

Osteopetrosis (Albers-Schönberg disease, marble bones)

The areas of increased bone density in this disease are widespread, often including pelvis, vertebrae, skull, and extremities. The affection may be manifest in infancy. Transverse pathologic fractures may occur, usually in the long bones; they ordinarily heal without incident. Hydrocephalus, blindness, enlargement of spleen and liver, malnutrition, and progressive myelophthisic anemia may be associated. In severe cases there may be mental retardation. The face may be wrinkled and have a mongoloid appearance.

In roentgenograms the affected bones show greatly increased density and loss of normal architecture. The medullary canal is narrowed or obliterated. The metaphyseal portion of the long bones may have a "celery stalk" appearance with dense longitudinal striations.

Osteopathia striata

Osteopathia striata is a form of osteosclerosis in which there are coarse, longitudinal striations running the entire length of the shaft, especially marked in the metaphyseal areas. After epiphyseal closure the striations extend the entire length of the bone. The skull and clavicles are seldom affected. The bony contour is normal and no symptoms are referable to the disorder. The cause is unknown, but there are strong hereditary and familial factors.

Osteopoikilosis (spotted bones)

In osteopoikilosis the areas of condensation are small and scattered, giving the affected bones a spotted appearance in roentgenograms (Fig. 74). The dense areas consist of thickened trabeculae in the spongiosa. The metaphyseal and epiphyseal regions are most often involved. Symptoms are slight or absent, and discovery of the lesions may be entirely fortuitous.

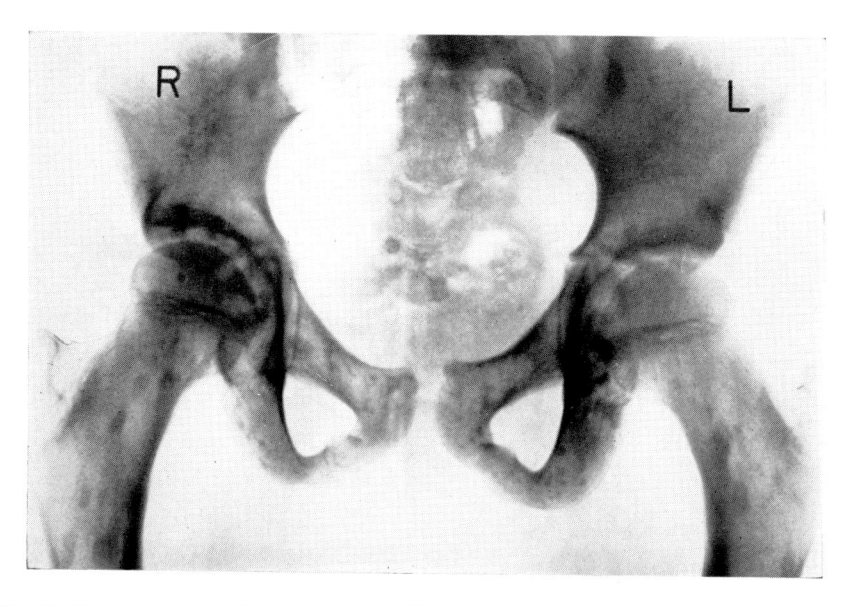

Fig. 74. Roentgenogram showing osteopoikilosis in girl 12 years of age. Note small, dark areas of bone condensation in pelvis and femora.

Melorheostosis

As its name implies, this disease is a "flowing" hyperostosis of the bones of one extremity. It is rare, occurs somewhat more often in males than in females, and begins in childhood but may be found at any age. Pain is the most common complaint and may be transient. Melorheostosis is characterized roentgenographically by an increased density and an enlargement of the cortical bone, both of which are limited to a single side of the bones. The roentgenographic changes have been compared to tallow, or wax, dripping on the side of a burning candle (Fig. 75). In severe cases the skin temperature over the affected bones may be elevated and there may be periarticular bony deposits that cause discomfort and joint stiffness.

PROGRESSIVE DIAPHYSEAL DYSPLASIA (ENGELMANN'S DISEASE)

Progressive diaphyseal dysplasia is a rare affection characterized by a symmetrical expansion and sclerosis of the diaphyses of long bones in young children. The involved bone proliferates by both an endosteal and a perio-

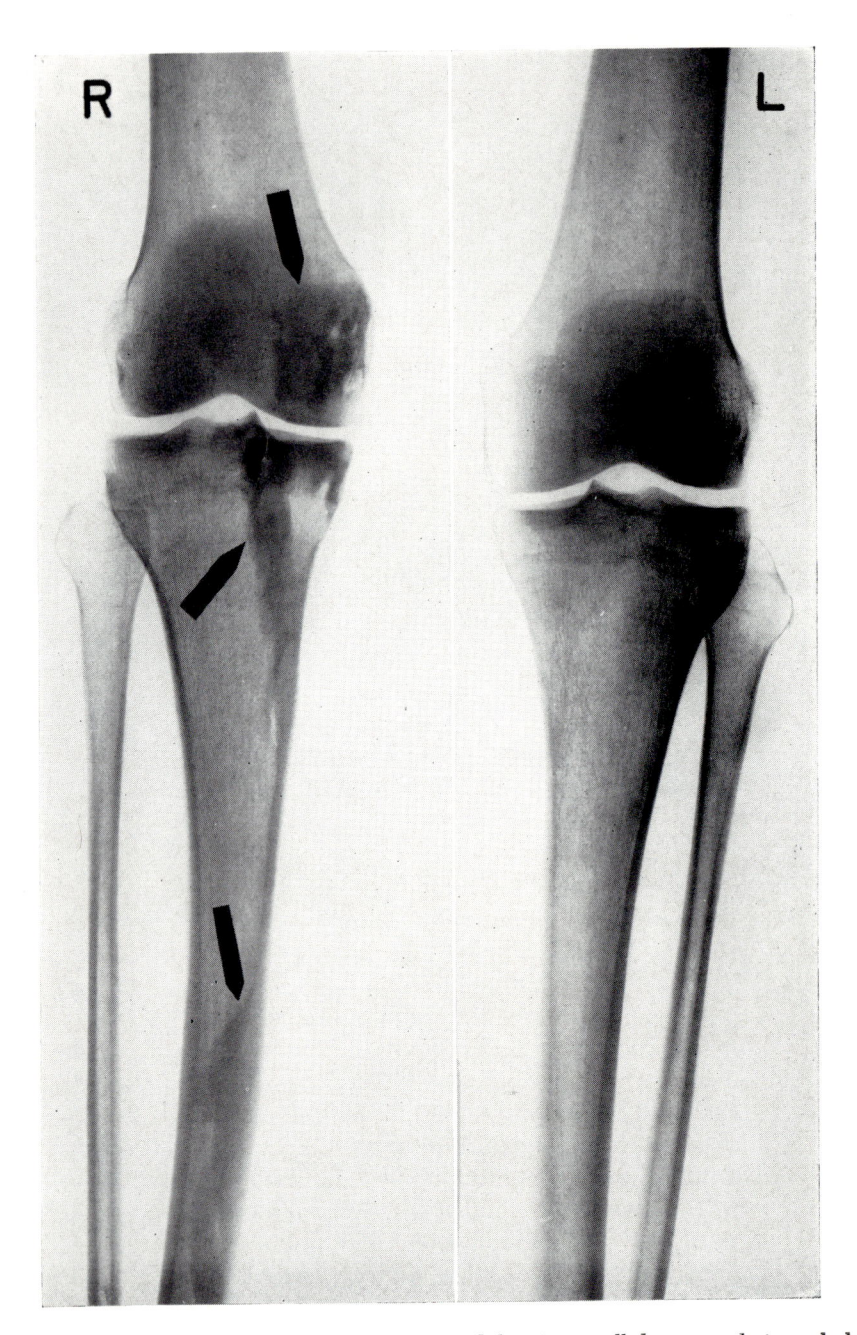

Fig. 75. Roentgenograms of melorheostosis in adult. Note well-demarcated, irregularly shaped areas of increased density in right femur and tibia. This has been described as a dripping candle-wax appearance.

steal reaction, producing a thickened cortex without trabecular pattern. Coxa valga is usually associated. There may be an increase of bone density at the base of the skull.

The patients have increased fatigability, leg pain, abnormalities of gait, and delayed development. No treatment is known, and the ultimate prognosis has not been determined.

PROGRESSIVE MYOSITIS OSSIFICANS

While not primarily a disease of the skeleton, progressive myositis ossificans is conveniently considered here because in its advanced stage it is characterized by a transformation of muscles and fasciae into immobile structures of bony consistency (Fig. 76). The disease is rare, and its cause is unknown. An interesting hypothesis of the pathogenesis is that the mesenchymal cells do not possess the normal property of tissue differentiation, and hence progress ultimately to widespread development of bone. It is four times as common in the male as in the female.

Clinical picture. The disease begins in childhood, sometimes as early as the first year. Malalignment and decrease in size of the great toes are frequently present. As a rule the muscles of the neck or back are first involved by the process of ossification, and although there may be remissions, one group of muscles after another gradually becomes stiffened. Ultimately the patient becomes bedridden, and as a rule death ensues from intercurrent infection.

Diagnosis and treatment. The diagnosis presents difficulty only in the

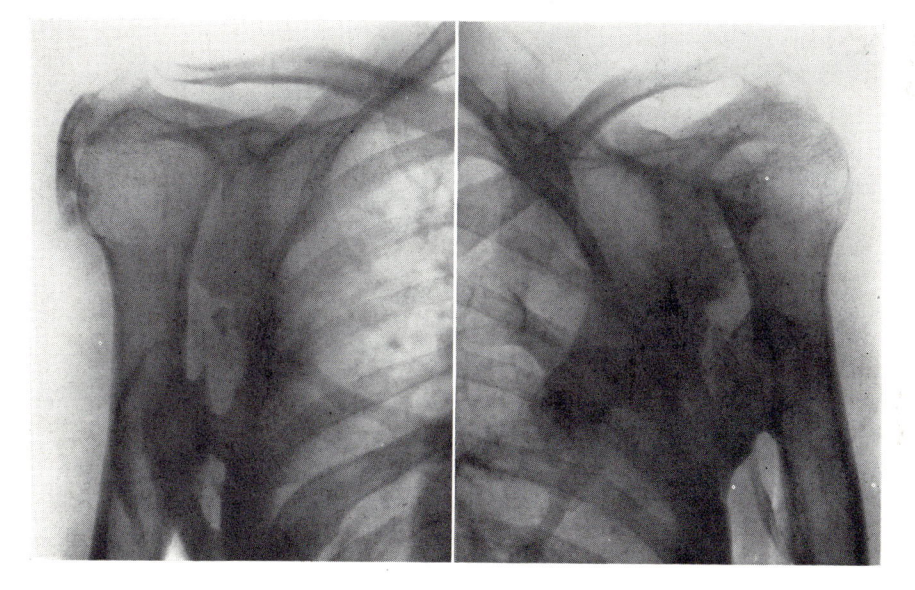

Fig. 76. Progressive myositis ossificans. Roentgenograms of the shoulders of a 32-year-old woman who had had gradual progression of joint stiffness and palpable bony masses in various muscle groups since the age of 4 years.

early stage of the disease. Muscle biopsy may then be helpful. At the present time no effective treatment is known.

Affections caused by endocrine abnormalities
HYPOPITUITARY DWARFISM

Certain congenital anomalies of the anterior part of the pituitary gland or its destruction in early childhood by tumors, syphilis, reticuloendotheliosis, or tuberculosis may result in pituitary dwarfism.

Clinical picture. Growth retardation in the congenital case is noticed within the first few years of life. Irrespective of age, the proportions between head, trunk, and extremities are those of a normal child (Fig. 77). There are two types of pituitary dwarfism: one with normal sexual development and the other with hypogonadism or deficient sexual development. The intelligence of pituitary dwarfs is usually normal.

Roentgenographic examination shows the fontanels to be open beyond

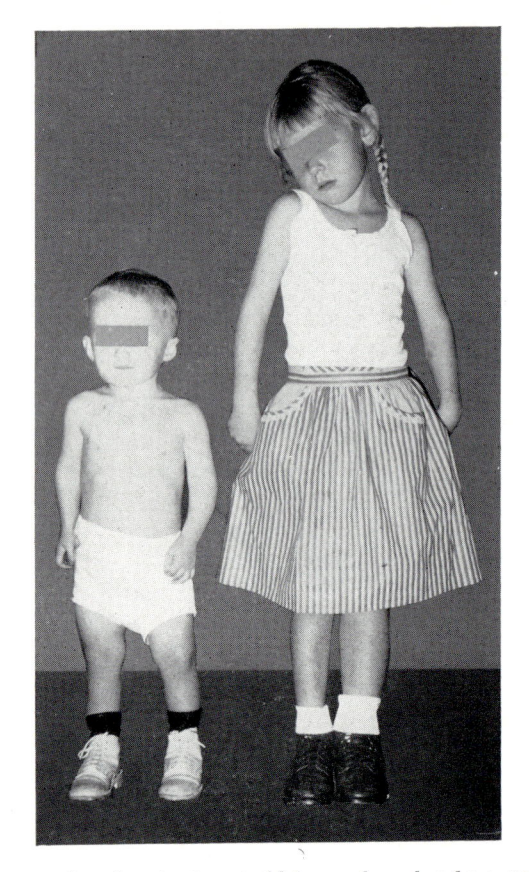

Fig. 77. Hypopituitary dwarfism in 4-year-old boy, whose height is 25 inches. The girl is also 4 years old and has the normal height of 39 inches. The dwarf has a normal facies, as well as head, trunk, and extremities of normal proportions.

the second year, osteoporosis of the skull and long bones, and delay in the appearance of ossification centers and in the closure of epiphyses.

Prognosis. The prognosis depends upon the etiologic factor.

Treatment. Striking improvement has been observed after the daily oral administration of 5 to 15 mg. of methyl testosterone to pituitary dwarfs. Caution against masculinization of females must be taken. During and after adolescence, girls are given, in addition to testosterone, 1 mg. of stilbestrol daily to promote development of secondary female sex characteristics.

HYPERPITUITARISM
Gigantism

Gigantism is a condition in which skeletal overgrowth results from a pathologically increased activity of the anterior portion of the pituitary gland during youth. It is thus of orthopaedic interest in demonstrating clearly a close relationship between skeletal development and endocrine function. Subjective symptoms are slight or absent. Treatment in these cases belongs to the neurologic rather than to the orthopaedic surgeon.

Acromegaly

The bone changes of acromegaly are believed to represent the reaction of the adult skeleton to hyperactivity of the anterior lobe of the pituitary gland. Acromegaly in the adult thus corresponds in etiology to *gigantism* in the youth.

Clinical picture. The characteristic changes of acromegaly usually appear first in early or middle adult life and are slowly progressive. They include a gradual enlargement of the bones of the skull, jaw, spine, hands, and feet, and an associated involvement of the soft tissues. The lower jaw protrudes. The orbital and zygomatic arches are prominent, and the nose, ears, lower lip, and tongue are large. Kyphosis of the thoracic spine is commonly present, the hands and feet become massive, and the fingers and toes may be strikingly thickened (Fig. 78). The costochondral junctions become enlarged, forming the acromegalic rosary, and with advancing ossification the ribs lengthen and the chest thickens. There may be marked rarefaction of the bones, due to nitrogen deficiency or insufficient intake of calcium and phosphorus. The thyroid gland may be enlarged. The urinary excretion of calcium may be doubled.

Diagnosis and treatment. The typical deformities are often associated with other evidences of endocrine disorder and with progressive symptoms, such as disturbances of vision, which are secondary results of the local intracranial changes. These associated symptoms are of diagnostic value, as are roentgenograms of the sella turcica. Myxedema and osteitis deformans are to be excluded. Treatment by surgery, irradiation, or a combination of the two is the prerogative of the neurologic surgeon. The administration of thyroid and sex hormones may be followed by improvement.

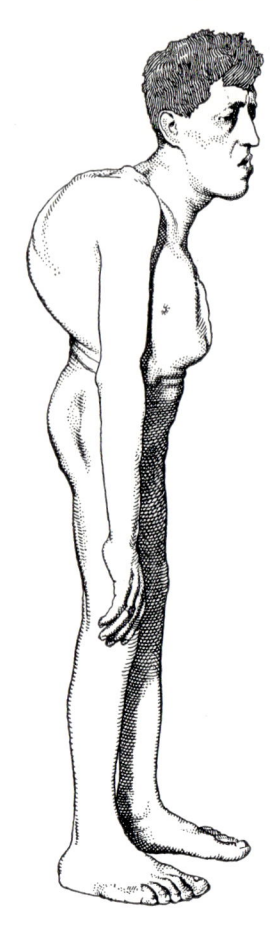

Fig. 78. Acromegaly. Note prominence of supraorbital areas, protuberance of jaw, kyphosis, and enlargement of hands and feet. (From clinical material of Dr. Walter E. Dandy.)

CRETINISM (HYPOTHYROIDISM)

Cretinism is a form of dwarfism caused by hypofunction of the thyroid gland. The condition first manifests itself usually in the second six months of life. The usual cause is a congenital lack of thyroid tissue. Cases of endemic type occur frequently in goitrous regions and may be ascribed to a lack of iodine in the mother. In such instances the fetus may develop as a cretin in utero.

The cretin must be carefully differentiated from the rachitic and the achondroplastic (Fig. 62) dwarfs. Hurler's syndrome (Fig. 70) should also be excluded. The cretin has a large tongue which often protrudes between his thickened lips, a flattened nose with sunken bridge, puffy eyelids, and a dry skin. The facial expression is characteristically stupid and usually the mental development is obviously impaired. Ossification of the epiphyses is irregular and delayed. Since the kidneys are unable to excrete phosphate in normal amounts, it accumulates in the blood serum although the epiphyseal cartilages may remain ununited for twenty or thirty years, growth of the long bones ceases, and the arms and legs remain short and stumpy. The roentgenograms show transverse bony shadows at the ends of the diaphyses.

Cretinism may be treated by the administration of thyroid preparations.

HYPERPARATHYROIDISM (GENERALIZED OSTEITIS FIBROSA CYSTICA, VON RECKLINGHAUSEN'S DISEASE OF BONE)

By secreting excessive amounts of parathormone, a circumscribed parathyroid hyperplasia (or *parathyroid adenoma*) may lead to demineralization of the skeleton, localized areas of bone destruction, characteristic changes in serum calcium and phosphorus levels, nephrolithiasis, and renal insufficiency. The mechanism of parathormone action on bone and kidney is still not completely understood.

Blood chemistry. The serum calcium is consistently increased and the serum phosphorus usually decreased. The alkaline phosphatase level is elevated and always rises further as the osseous changes become more severe; this is thought to be the result of increased osteoblastic activity. The excretion of calcium in the urine is also increased.

Pathology. The essential features are a gradual resorption of bone trabeculae and replacement by fibrous tissue. Macroscopically this tissue presents a picture of disordered arrangement with numerous areas of hemorrhage. Hemorrhagic cysts of irregular size and distribution often occur as the result of local degenerative changes; such cysts may have fibrous walls and may contain a grumous, serosanguineous fluid. Bone destruction is manifested microscopically by thin and disappearing lamellae, about which may be grouped numerous osteoclasts; in some places the appearance may be such as to suggest giant cell tumor. Other areas may show new bone formation with abundant osteoid and osteoblasts. The gradual loss of cortical bone results in decreased strength, which may lead to curvature, compression, or spontaneous fracture.

Secondary changes in the kidneys are sometimes marked. The increased urinary excretion of calcium and phosphorus not infrequently leads to the formation of renal calculi. Chronic nephritis and renal insufficiency may result from the precipitation of calcium phosphate within the parenchyma of the kidney.

Clinical picture. This type of hyperparathyroidism is uncommon, may occur at any age, and is seen mostly in the middle years of life. The symptoms are extremely diverse, depending upon the site of major involvement in the individual case, and a number of more or less well-defined clinical types have been described. General lassitude and muscular hypotonia due directly to the hypercalcemia may be the presenting symptoms. Gastrointestinal complaints and urinary disturbances, such as polyuria, are common. Skeletal involvement may be evidenced first by deep-seated pain and tenderness, the local swelling of an area of bone expansion, or the disability of a spontaneous fracture. Cases developing in late middle life and ushered in by backache, progressive kyphosis, and decrease in stature, form a major group. Deformity of bones other than the vertebrae is usually a late manifestation. In some cases of hyperparathyroidism, particularly those in which renal calculi cause the presenting complaint, skeletal symptoms and bone changes in the roentgenograms may be entirely absent.

Roentgenographic picture. The loss of bone causes a generalized decrease in roentgenographic density, which may be complicated by the secondary changes of deformity, local areas of rarefaction, and fractures. In addition to the generalized radiolucency, roentgenograms of the spine may show cupping, wedging, and crushing of the vertebral bodies, as well as various degrees of kyphosis with a "pigeon breast" deformation of the chest. The skull may have a moth-eaten appearance.

Differential diagnosis. The varied clinical picture leads to simulation of numerous other diseases. Skeletal types of hyperparathyroidism must be differentiated from senile osteoporosis, osteomalacia, osteitis deformans, solitary bone cyst, giant cell tumor, fragilitas ossium, fibrous dysplasia, cystic angioma of bone, myasthenia gravis, multiple myeloma, and metastatic malignancy. The biochemical and roentgenographic examinations are usually of chief differential value.

Treatment. The treatment is parathyroidectomy. After excision of the parathyroid adenoma, marked improvement, both in symptoms and in general nutrition is to be expected; usually regression of the bone changes also occurs. Orthopaedic treatment consists of appropriate measures, such as braces and splints, for the prevention of deformity. Support is especially indicated when the spine is involved. In some cases, after parathyroidectomy has been performed and bony strength has been restored, corrective operations, such as osteotomy, may be indicated.

Affections caused by unknown acquired abnormalities
OSTEITIS DEFORMANS

Osteitis deformans was first described by Sir James Paget in 1876 and is often called *Paget's disease*. It is a chronic skeletal disease of middle and late life, beginning insidiously and characterized by progressive structural changes and typical deformities occurring in the long bones, spine, pelvis, and cranium.

Etiology. The causative agent is unknown. Attempts to establish heredity, infection, or an endocrine defect as the etiologic factor have failed through lack of proof.

Pathology. The initial bone lesion is considered to be destructive (osteolytic), and to be followed by bone proliferation (osteoblastic). The outstanding skeletal changes are a gradually developing thickening and bowing of the shafts of the long bones, particularly the tibiae and the femora, and a generalized thickening of the cranium (Fig. 79). Frequently, osteitis defor-

General affections of the skeleton 125

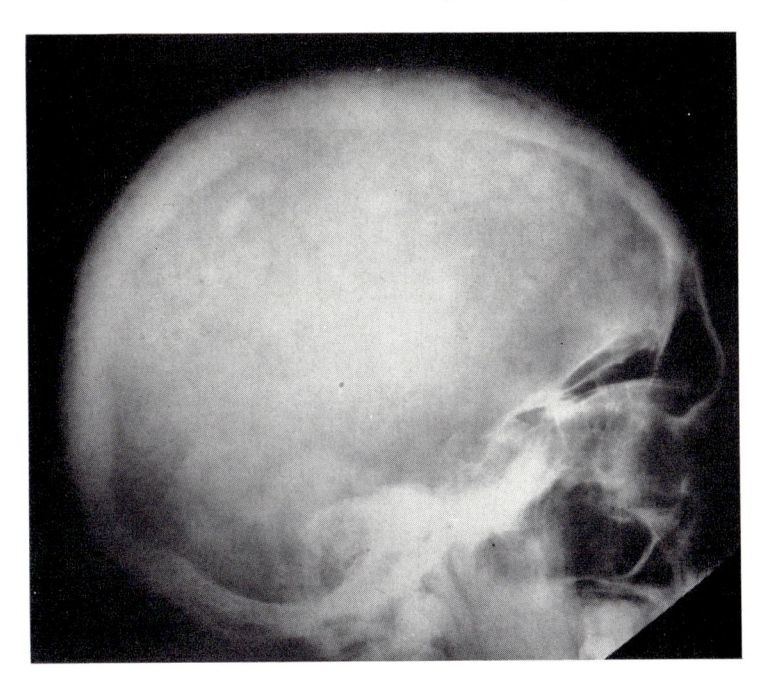

Fig. 79. Lateral roentgenogram of skull in osteitis deformans, showing great thickening of calvarium, irregular bone density, and indistinct peripheral margin.

mans affects only a single bone. In the early stages the bones lose much of their ability to withstand normal stresses, and an increase in their degree of curvature results. In the spine, which is very frequently involved, there is often collapse of one or more of the vertebral bodies, which results in a kyphosis. In later stages more bony matrix is laid down, which calcifies, often producing finally a thick, hard osseous structure. The surface of the involved long bones is of characteristic unevenness and is furrowed by the periosteal vessels. Section discloses a thickened cortical layer which has lost its dense character and sharp outline and encroaches upon the marrow cavity. The marrow cavity may be filled with spongy tissue and may contain small scattered cystic areas filled with gelatinous material. Microscopically the bone marrow may be largely replaced by a vascular fibrous tissue, in which are present irregular areas of osteoid of abnormal, mosaic appearance.

The serum alkaline phosphatase may be greatly increased, particularly in early stages of the disease and in patients with multiple bone involvement, and it usually continues elevated as long as the disease remains active. The serum calcium and phosphorus are usually within normal limits.

Clinical picture. In many instances bones affected by Paget's disease remain asymptomatic throughout the individual's life. Estimates including such cases place the over-all incidence of the disease at approximately 3% of the adult population. According to several statistical studies, osteitis

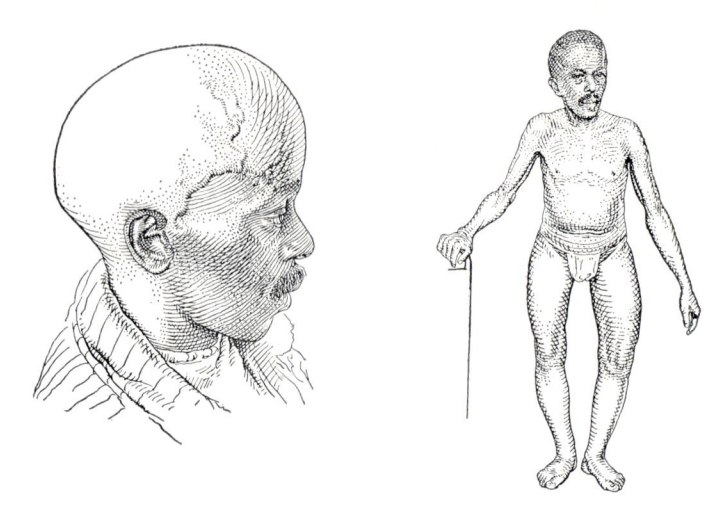

Fig. 80. Osteitis deformans. Note massive cranium with enlargement of superficial veins, bowing of the lower extremities, and decreased height. (From clinical material of Dr. George W. Wagoner.)

deformans affects men more frequently than women, and occasionally it occurs in families.

Most patients are between 40 and 60 years old when the first symptoms develop. The patient may complain of fatigue or aching in the legs, which simulates the discomfort of chronic arthritis; may suffer chiefly from headache and backache; may be affected by stiffness or clumsiness; or may simply have noticed that he is becoming bowlegged, that his back is stooped, or that his head is becoming larger, as evidenced by the tight fit of his hat.

The patient suffering from osteitis deformans in its moderately advanced stage presents a characteristic clinical appearance (Fig. 80). The head appears massive and too large for the body, while the face is relatively small. The head may be dropped forward, and a long dorsal kyphosis may be present. The chest is likely to be barrel-shaped, the lumbar spine flexed, and the legs bowed outward and forward. This posture gives to the arms an exaggerated length, which has been compared to that of an anthropoid ape. There are no mental changes other than those of advancing age. As the disease progresses there may develop a deafness and tinnitus and an impairment of vision from pressure on the cranial nerves. Clinical diagnosis in well-established cases presents little difficulty.

Roentgenographic picture. Roentgenograms are of diagnostic value, as the changes of osteitis deformans are characteristic. The contour of the bone is altered by an increase of its normal curvature. The cortex is enlarged sometimes to as much as four or five times its normal thickness and presents a blurred, fluffy appearance; the medulla is narrowed; there is a loss of the normal definitive line between cortex and medulla; and the pelvic bones often show an abnormally prominent and coarse trabecular pattern. In all cases of suspected osteitis deformans, roentgenograms of the skull should be made, since its appearance is pathognomonic. The bones of the cranium are greatly thickened, with obliteration of the sutures and vascular channels, indistinct outlines, and uneven density that produce a "cotton-wool" appearance.

Diagnosis. The characteristic deformities and roentgenographic changes of osteitis deformans are usually adequate to ensure its recognition. A high serum alkaline phosphatase level supports the diagnosis. In the differential diagnosis, syphilis, hyperparathyroidism, metastatic carcinoma, and osteomalacia must be considered. Diagnosis of the localized form of osteitis deformans, in which only a single bone is involved, sometimes presents difficulty. In such cases biopsy is occasionally desirable in order to exclude primary or metastatic tumor.

Treatment and prognosis. At the present time the treatment of osteitis deformans is of symptomatic type. Salicylates and barbiturates are useful for the relief of pain. In the more active cases braces may be indicated for the prevention of deformity, and rarely a deformity that has become established may be corrected by osteotomy.

The prognosis for length of life is good. Cardiovascular complications are the most common cause of death. Pathologic fracture is the most common complication. It occurs most often in the femur. There is no prolongation of the healing time except in late stages of the disease, and the treatment is that of the uncomplicated fracture. A more serious complication, occurring in from 2 to 15% of the patients in reported series of cases, is the development of malignancy. The commonest type is osteogenic sarcoma. Most of the patients who develop this die within two years of diagnosis. Compression of the spinal cord by the thickened vertebrae is a rare complication.

SENILE OSTEOPOROSIS

Senile osteoporosis, which is found more than twice as often in women as in men, is most commonly manifested as an impairment of the bony strength of the spine. It develops when the bone that is being lost by normal catabolism is not replaced in equal measure by new bone formation. The defect is an insufficient deposition of bone matrix, resulting from decreased osteoblastic activity, and is quite different from the chemical failure of osteoid to calcify, which occurs in osteomalacia.

The cause of the decrease of osteoblastic activity is not known with certainty; however, it may be related to changes in the gonads and adrenals and to the normal inactivity of the aged. Accordingly senile osteoporosis is probably related to postmenopausal osteoporosis, in which there is faulty protein metabolism due to deficiency of estrogen, and to the osteoporosis of disuse, or disuse atrophy (Fig. 49), in which there is an excessive excretion of urinary calcium (hypercalciuria).

Clinical picture. Senile osteoporosis is most often discovered when an elderly person, following lifting or bending, develops sudden pain in the lower dorsal or lumbar region of the back, often accompanied by a snap or crack. Roentgenograms will usually show compression of a vertebral body,

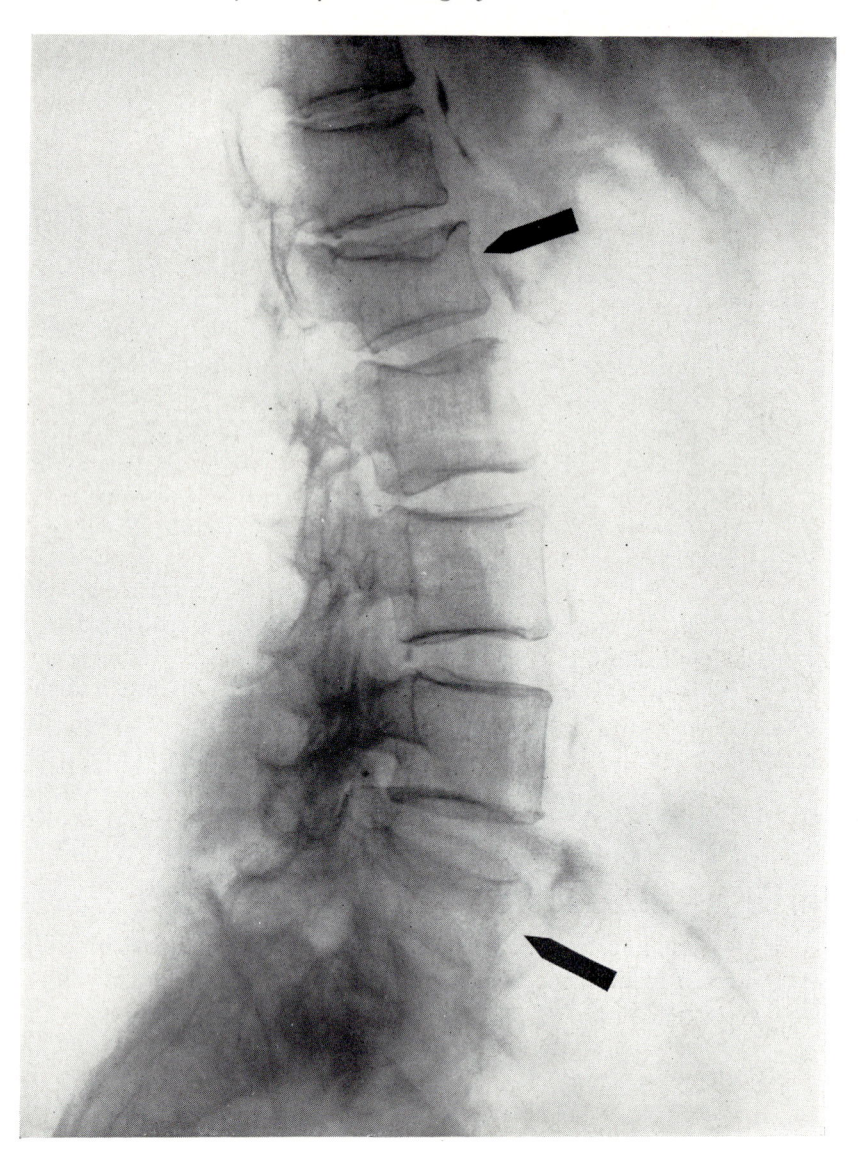

Fig. 81. Roentgenogram of senile osteoporosis in patient 65 years of age. Note greatly decreased density of vertebral bodies while their narrow margins remain distinct. The bodies of the first and fifth lumbar vertebrae (as well as the bodies of three thoracic vertebrae) had sustained compression fractures from minor trauma.

with increased radiolucency of the whole spine (Fig. 81). The vertebrae most often showing collapse are about the lumbodorsal junction. The vertebral bodies often appear biconcave. The remainder of the skeleton also shows some rarefaction but not to the degree present in the spine.

Treatment. The deposition of bone matrix cannot be increased by dietary measures or vitamin medication. The administration of androgens (testosterone) and estrogens (conjugated estrogens and estradiol) relieves the symptoms but has not been proved to result in bone production. Fractures of the spine and other bones should be treated as indicated in the individual case.

SECONDARY HYPERTROPHIC PULMONARY OSTEOARTHROPATHY (BAMBERGER-MARIE DISEASE)

Secondary hypertrophic pulmonary osteoarthropathy, called also *pulmonary osteoarthropathy of Marie* and evidenced clinically by the common clubbed fingers, is always secondary to chronic wasting disease. Pulmonary tuberculosis, empyema, lung abscess, bronchiectasis, and cardiac disease are the common causes; intrathoracic tumors and long-standing infections elsewhere in the body are occasionally responsible. Chronic gastrointestinal disease, cirrhosis of the liver, and amyloid disease may also be causes. The mechanism by which these diseases produce the bone changes is not understood but is probably of either circulatory or toxic nature. The characteristic pathologic process is a thickening of both soft tissues and bone; the bony proliferation is brought about by a very chronic ossifying periostitis.

Clinical picture. The affection is more common in men than in women. The first clinical sign is a generalized, symmetrical, and painless enlargement of the distal portion of the fingers, due to thickening of the soft tissues (Fig. 82). The nails become slightly cyanotic. They may show thickening, ridges, and an increased convexity and may bend down over the ends of the phalanges. They have been called "hippocratic fingers." Analogous changes may appear in the toes and toenails simultaneously. Wrists and ankles also may

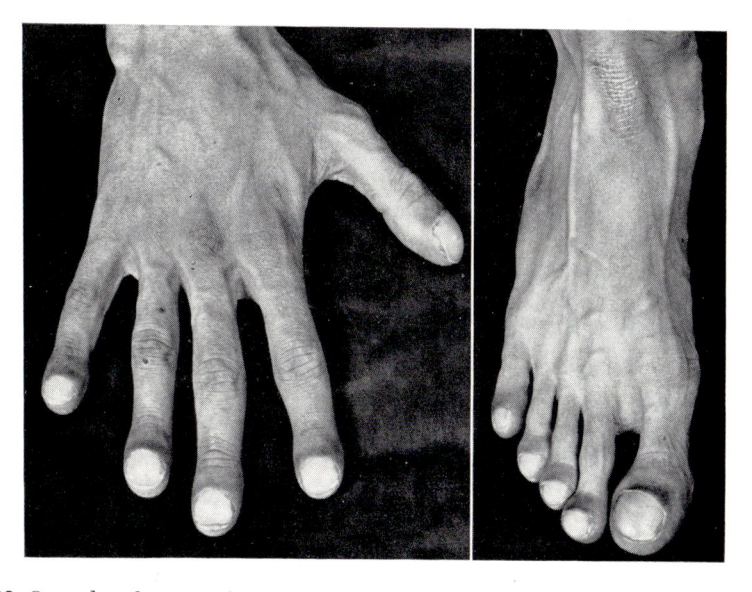

Fig. 82. Secondary hypertrophic pulmonary osteoarthropathy. Note the clubbed appearance of the ends of fingers and toes and the broadening of the nails.

130 Handbook of orthopaedic surgery

become swollen, and the joints may contain increased fluid. The roentgenograms show proliferative bony changes, sometimes with spurring, and in severe cases the shafts of the bones of forearm and leg may be obviously thickened from subperiosteal formation of new bone.

Treatment. The primary visceral disease must be investigated and treated. If this is cured promptly, the clubbing may regress. In the majority of cases, however, the bone lesions when once established either remain unchanged or show a very gradual progression.

INFANTILE CORTICAL HYPEROSTOSIS (CAFFEY'S DISEASE)

Caffey's disease is an affection characterized by subperiosteal new bone formation on the shafts of the long bones and mandible in infants under 6 months of age.

Etiology. The etiology is unknown. Because of the associated fever, leukocytosis, and increased sedimentation rate, many observers believe it to

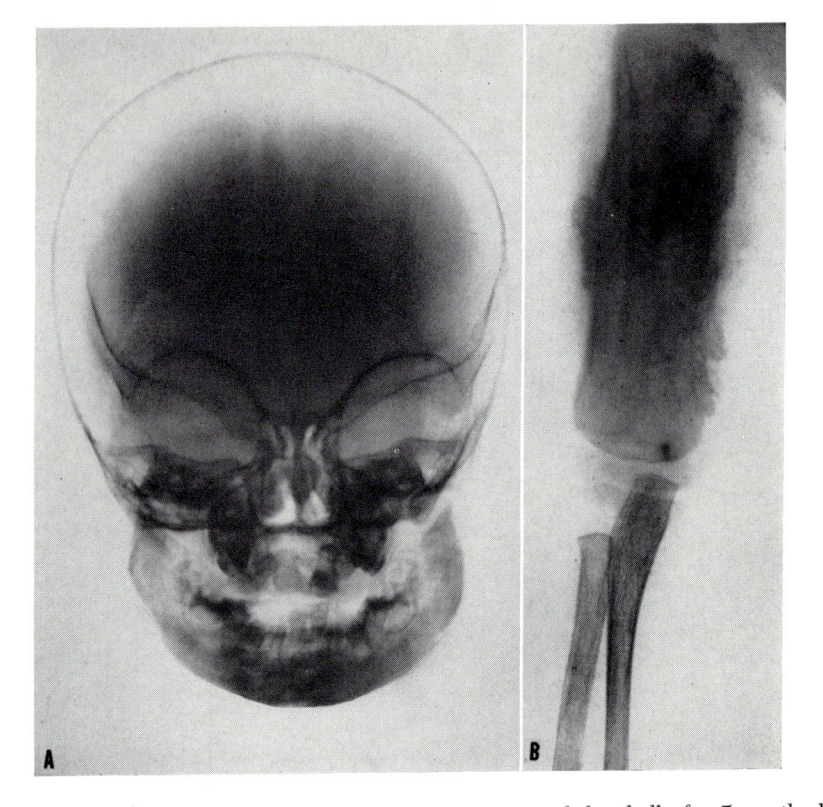

Fig. 83. Infantile cortical hyperostosis. **A,** Roentgenogram of the skull of a 7-month-old infant, showing massive subperiosteal overgrowth of the mandible. **B,** Roentgenogram of the upper limb of a 3-month-old infant, showing massive new bone about the humeral shaft. In this infant the mandible, clavicles, and several ribs showed similar but less extensive involvement.

be an infection, possibly a virus infection. However, all serologic tests and cultures are negative.

Clinical picture. Boys are affected more often than girls. The earliest signs are irritability and swelling of the face, over a clavicle, or in an extremity, in whole or in part. These swellings are sudden in onset, tender, of wooden induration, and appear to be located beneath the subcutaneous fat in the muscular planes; they begin to subside by the time roentgenographic changes appear. The first roentgenographic changes are subperiosteal shadows over the whole or part of the bone. These increase in size and may give the appearance of an enlarged and thickened over-all bone structure (Fig. 83). With healing, the proliferative bone disappears and normal bone structure is restored in from a few months to two years, the average period being eight months.

Diagnosis. Infantile cortical hyperostosis must be differentiated from scurvy, hypervitaminosis A, progressive diaphyseal dysplasia, trauma, osteomyelitis, syphilis, and neoplasm. Hypervitaminosis A, with which it is most often confused, never occurs in the infant under 1 year of age.

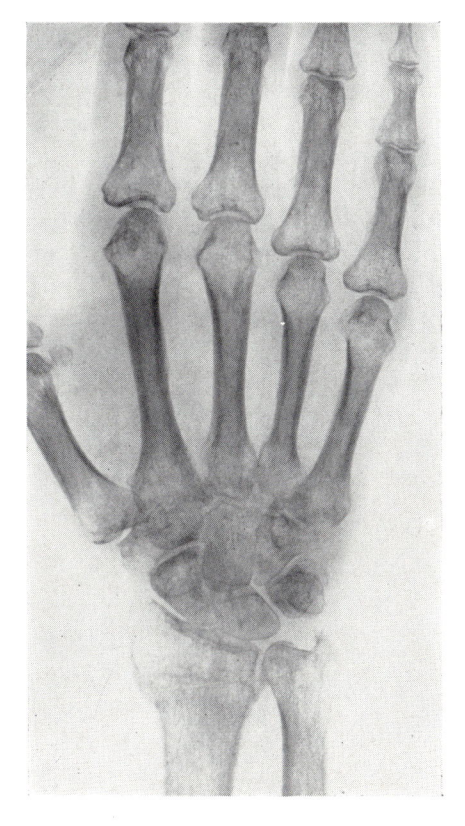

Fig. 84. Roentgenogram of hand in Sudeck's atrophy following a Colles' fracture. Note healed fracture of distal end of radius and marked bone atrophy. The patient's disabling pain gradually subsided with treatment, which included a dorsal sympathectomy.

Treatment. No specific treatment is indicated. The prophylactic use of antibiotics is justifiable until the possibility of an infection has been ruled out. Surgery is contraindicated.

POSTTRAUMATIC PAINFUL OSTEOPOROSIS (SUDECK'S ATROPHY, POSTTRAUMATIC OR REFLEX SYMPATHETIC DYSTROPHY)

Occasionally an injury of an extremity or of a peripheral nerve is followed by prolonged local pain, vasomotor instability, trophic changes in the soft tissues, and diffuse, patchy rarefaction and atrophy of bone. The trauma may be of quite minor nature, and the disturbance of function is always greater than that which would be expected from the injury alone. This condition, termed posttraumatic painful osteoporosis and first described as an entity by Sudeck in 1900, must be distinguished carefully from simple disuse atrophy of bone, with or without malingering, and from causalgia due to a lesion of a peripheral nerve. The bone atrophy may have an irregular and spotted appearance (Fig. 84); it may be band-shaped, subchondral, metaphyseal, or diffuse.

Etiology. The pathogenesis is not well understood. Much of the evidence suggests that disturbed function of the sympathetic nerve supply, due to injury or compression, is the major factor. Accordingly the changes may represent the terminal phase of a neurodystrophic process.

Treatment and prognosis. Although the period of disability is always long, most patients recover spontaneously or with simple treatment, such as immobilization followed by physical therapy and active use of the extremity. In the more intractable cases, sympatholytic drugs, repeated procaine block of the sympathetic ganglia, ganglionectomy, or periarterial sympathectomy may be indicated. Rarely a permanent deformity and disability result despite treatment.

CHAPTER 6

Infections of bones and joints (exclusive of tuberculosis)

BONE INFECTION or *osteomyelitis* and joint infection or *septic arthritis* may be acute or chronic. To a large extent the nature and degree of the inflammatory reaction, whether in bone or in joint, are determined by the characteristics of the invading organism. Types of bone and joint infection warranting description here include those caused (1) by bacteria *(Staphylococcus, Streptococcus,* pneumococcus, gonococcus, *Salmonella,* and *Brucella);* (2) by fungi *(Actinomyces, Blastomyces,* and *Coccidioides);* (3) by the parasite *Echinococcus;* and (4) by the *Treponema pallidum.*

PYOGENIC OR SUPPURATIVE OSTEOMYELITIS

Incidence. Since the advent of antibiotic therapy for primary pyogenic infections, hematogenous osteomyelitis has become uncommon. Its incidence is much higher in children than in adults, and in boys than in girls. Any bone may be involved. Those most commonly affected are the tibia, femur, humerus, and radius.

Routes of infection. In hematogenous osteomyelitis the invading organisms reach the bone by transportation in the blood stream from a distant focus, such as a furuncle, pustule, infected laceration, or the nasopharynx. In other forms of osteomyelitis the bone is infected by spread from a contiguous focus, such as a pyarthrosis, or by direct introduction through a wound, as in open fracture (Fig. 85).

Etiology. In at least 80% of the cases the infecting organism is the *Staphylococcus aureus. Streptococcus haemolyticus* is the next most common organism, being responsible for about 10%. Trauma, causing minute hemorrhage in bone, may play a part in the etiology by providing a locus in which the organisms of a transient bacteremia may lodge, survive, and multiply. Any debilitating disease may be a predisposing factor.

Pathology. In children, hematogenous osteomyelitis usually starts in the

134 *Handbook of orthopaedic surgery*

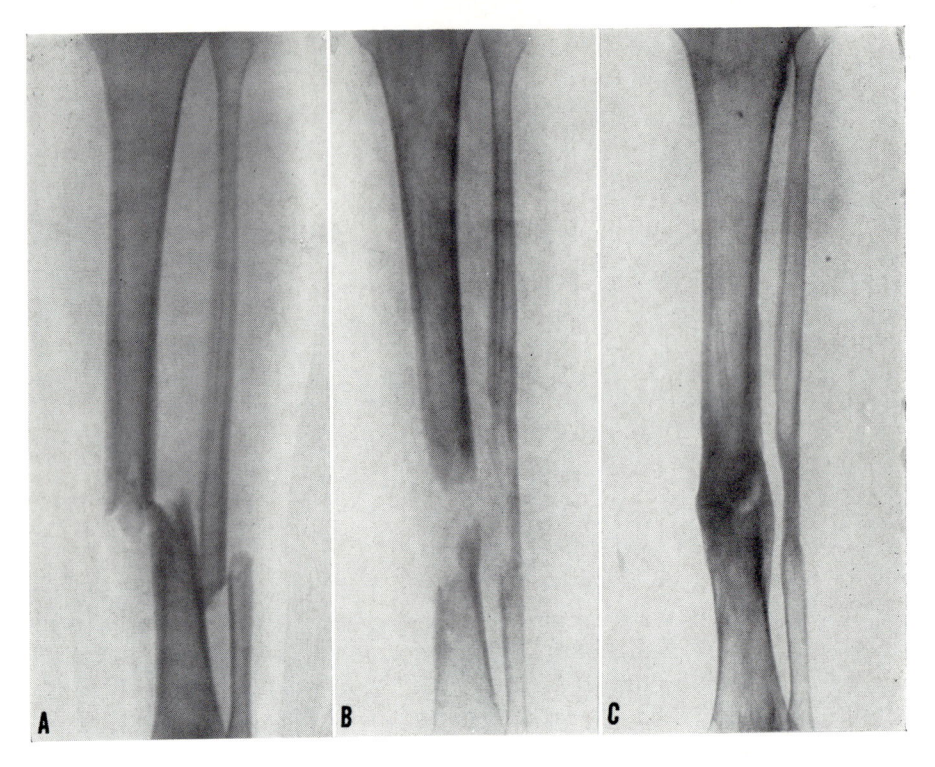

Fig. 85. Osteomyelitis secondary to open (compound) fractures of tibia and fibula in a 19-year-old boy. **A**, Fractures on day of injury: before debridement, reduction, and immobilization. **B**, Ten months after fracture: osteomyelitis has involved all fragments, necessitating sequestrectomy which has produced a wide tibial defect. The limb has remained completely disabled, and there is extensive bone atrophy. **C**, Four years after fracture: bone grafting, performed after all signs of infection had disappeared, has been followed finally by restoration of tibial continuity.

metaphysis, or cancellous end of the diaphysis. The circulation in this region is relatively sluggish, and here are found end arteries in which the bacteria are thought to lodge, causing a septic infarction. Hyperemia, edema, and infiltration of polymorphonuclear leukocytes ensue. Leukocytes destroyed by bacterial toxins liberate a proteolytic enzyme. Further necrosis of ischemic tissue culminates in abscess formation. With increasing tension the septic process spreads in the directions of least resistance (Fig. 86) centrally toward the medullary cavity, and outwardly through haversian and Volkmann's canals, or through erosions of the thin metaphyseal cortex, to form a subperiosteal abscess. The subperiosteal pus may spread for some distance along and around the shaft; it may then re-enter the medullary cavity or may perforate the periosteum and extend into the overlying soft tissues.

In children the epiphyseal cartilage plate acts as a barrier to the infection, preventing or delaying extension into the epiphyseal end of the bone and thence into the joint. When the metaphyseal area is intracapsular, however, infection may spread quickly into the joint. An important example is the hip joint. Osteomyelitis of the neck of the femur may lead very quickly to the serious complication of septic arthritis of the hip. Often the joints develop a secondary synovitis before they become actually infected.

With the accumulation of pus beneath the periosteum, new bone is laid down on its inner surface, forming an *involucrum*. In this new bone numerous openings or *cloacae* for the discharge of pus and bone debris appear. Certain areas of bone may become ischemic from the stripping up of periosteum and the thrombosis of cortical capillaries. These areas become necrotic and separate, forming *sequestra* (Fig. 87). Small sequestra may be extruded through the involucral cloacae into sinuses draining upon the skin surface. It is impossible, however, for the larger sequestra to be extruded, and they may have to be removed surgically. Sequestra may become sur-

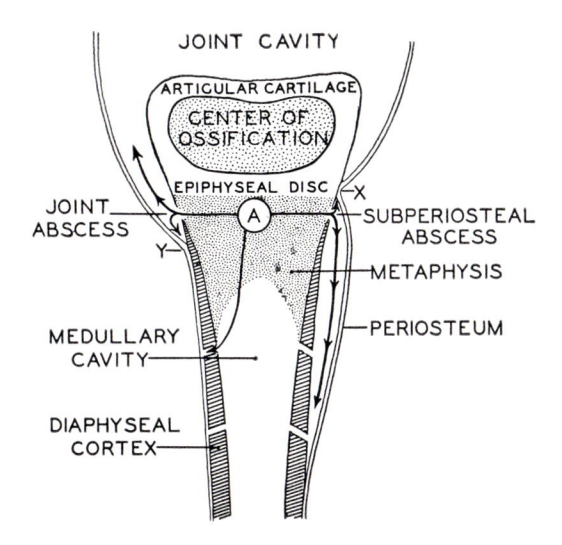

Fig. 86. Diagram showing direction of possible spread of infection from focus **A** in metaphysis. **X** and **Y** mark the junction of synovial membrane and periosteum in subperiosteal abscess and joint abscess, respectively. (After Hart.)

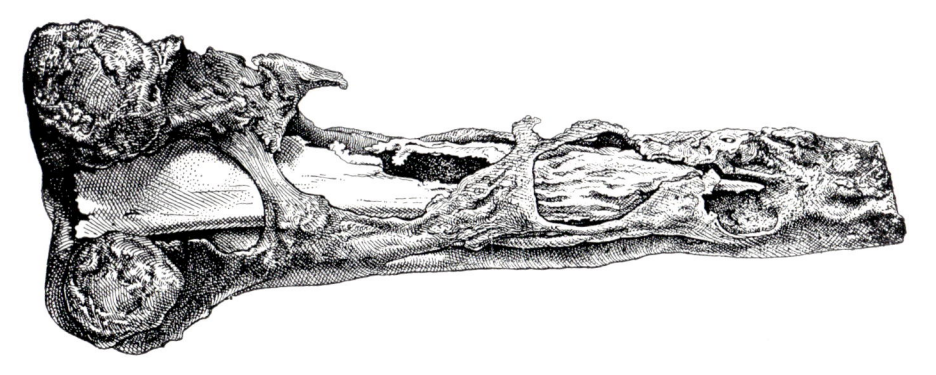

Fig. 87. Chronic osteomyelitis of femur, showing large sequestrum and surrounding involucrum. (Drawing from museum specimen.)

rounded by granulation tissue and gradually disintegrated and absorbed by the action of proteolytic ferments liberated in the purulent exudate.

Accordingly, the microscopic picture of acute osteomyelitis is characterized by masses of polymorphonuclear leukocytes, areas of necrosis, and cell detritus about bone trabeculae. In later stages of the disease microscopic sections show fibrotic bone marrow, many round cells, the dead bone and empty lacunae of sequestra, and the new trabeculae and osteoblasts of involucra.

In extensive osteomyelitic involvement of the shaft of a long bone, pathologic fracture occasionally occurs. This is particularly likely to happen if stress is placed upon the bone before sufficiently mature involucrum has restored its strength.

All pyogenic osteomyelitis is not accompanied by the formation of sequestra. Atypical infections from relatively avirulent organisms are not uncommon. The defenses of the body, especially when supplemented by antibiotics, may early overcome the infection, which then completely subsides. Osteomyelitis in infancy rarely results in gross sequestration.

Osteomyelitis of a long bone in childhood frequently produces a slight overgrowth in length.

Clinical picture. Acute osteomyelitis usually starts with malaise, general weakness, and aching, followed by an elevation of body temperature and intense pain in the affected region. In the early stages, when the infectious process is within a deeply situated bone, there may be no sharply localized tenderness. Nearly always a septicemia is associated with acute osteomyelitis, blood culture is positive, and the patient is extremely ill. A leukocytosis of from 15,000 to 40,000 cells, depending upon the severity of the infection, may be present. Ordinarily there is protective muscle spasm, the joint nearest the disease focus being held in flexion. As the infection advances, there may be localization of the process, with swelling, redness, increased heat, and acute tenderness about the infected area. Rarely, extensive infection of the shaft of a bone may be unaccompanied by evidence of localization. If the resistance of the body, aided by antibiotics, is sufficient to overcome the infection, the acute inflammatory symptoms will subside; if not, they will persist until pus is released by a surgical procedure or liberates itself spontaneously. Afterward the fever gradually decreases, but even in the presence of adequate drainage it may persist for several weeks. The local signs of acute inflammation usually subside slowly after evacuation of the pus.

In infants, acute osteomyelitis may be attended by little or no fever. The chief signs are irritability, loss of function of the affected extremity, tenderness, and swelling. The clinical course is relatively rapid.

After liberation of the pus and subsidence of the acute symptoms, the draining sinus or sinuses of *chronic osteomyelitis* may develop. The drainage will persist as long as there remain infected granulation tissue and dead bone that act as a foreign body. Accumulation of pus from inadequate drainage may cause periodic exacerbations of symptoms. Prolonged disuse of the infected parts leads to muscle atrophy, and if the joints are not properly splinted contractures often develop. There may be at first no general symptoms, but when purulent drainage has continued for a period of years nephritis or amyloid disease may develop. The constant inflammation of epithelial cells at the mouth of such a sinus may lead to a squamous cell carcinoma. Recurrence of infection may take place many years after apparently complete healing of an osteomyelitis. Osteomyelitis of a long bone in childhood may stimulate growth to produce slightly increased length; if the epiphyseal plate is involved, however, growth may cease or occur in asymmetrical manner, leading to deformity.

Roentgenographic picture. Bone changes are seldom visible in the roentgenograms in less than ten days from the time of onset; they appear later in adults than in children, and several weeks may elapse before definite bony abnormality can be demonstrated. Often the first change in the affected bone is an area of haziness or of mottling in the metaphysis, caused by the destruction of trabeculae. This is soon followed by new bone formation under the periosteum. Later there may be destructive areas in the shaft (Fig. 88) and evidences of sequestration. Roentgenographic changes may be atypical or absent when the course of the infection has been modified by early antibiotic treatment.

Differential diagnosis. Acute osteomyelitis must be distinguished from acute rheumatic fever with its migratory polyarthritis. Acute cellulitis must be differentiated. Pyogenic arthritis causes more swelling and spasm than does aseptic synovitis secondary to osteomyelitis and can be identified by aspiration of the joint, smear, and culture. In diagnosing chronic osteomyelitis one should rule out Ewing's sarcoma, osteogenic sarcoma, osteoid-osteoma, fungus infections, tuberculosis, and syphilis. In adults, vertebral osteomyelitis is sometimes a difficult diagnostic problem.

Prognosis. With antibiotic treatment the mortality of hematogenous osteomyelitis has been reduced from more than 20% to perhaps 1% or less. The most serious cases are those in infants and young children with septicemia. The course of the disease depends largely upon the promptness with which effective antibiotic therapy can be started. Frequently the bacteremia disappears quickly and the local infection is controlled before extensive necrosis of bone can take place. Less favorable cases progress to chronic osteomyelitis with its periodic exacerbations. In chronic cases of long standing, nephritis or amyloid disease may prove fatal.

Treatment. The type of treatment depends upon the stage to which the septic process has progressed.

Acute stage. In the acute stage, the patient is suffering not only from a local bone lesion but also from a blood stream infection with severe general reaction. It is most important that he receive systemic antibiotic therapy as promptly as possible, this being preceded, however, by the taking of a blood culture. The usual drug is penicillin; it should be given in large doses, such as 300,000 units or more every six hours. If the organism proves to be resistant to penicillin, as shown by lack of clinical response in about two

138   *Handbook of orthopaedic surgery*

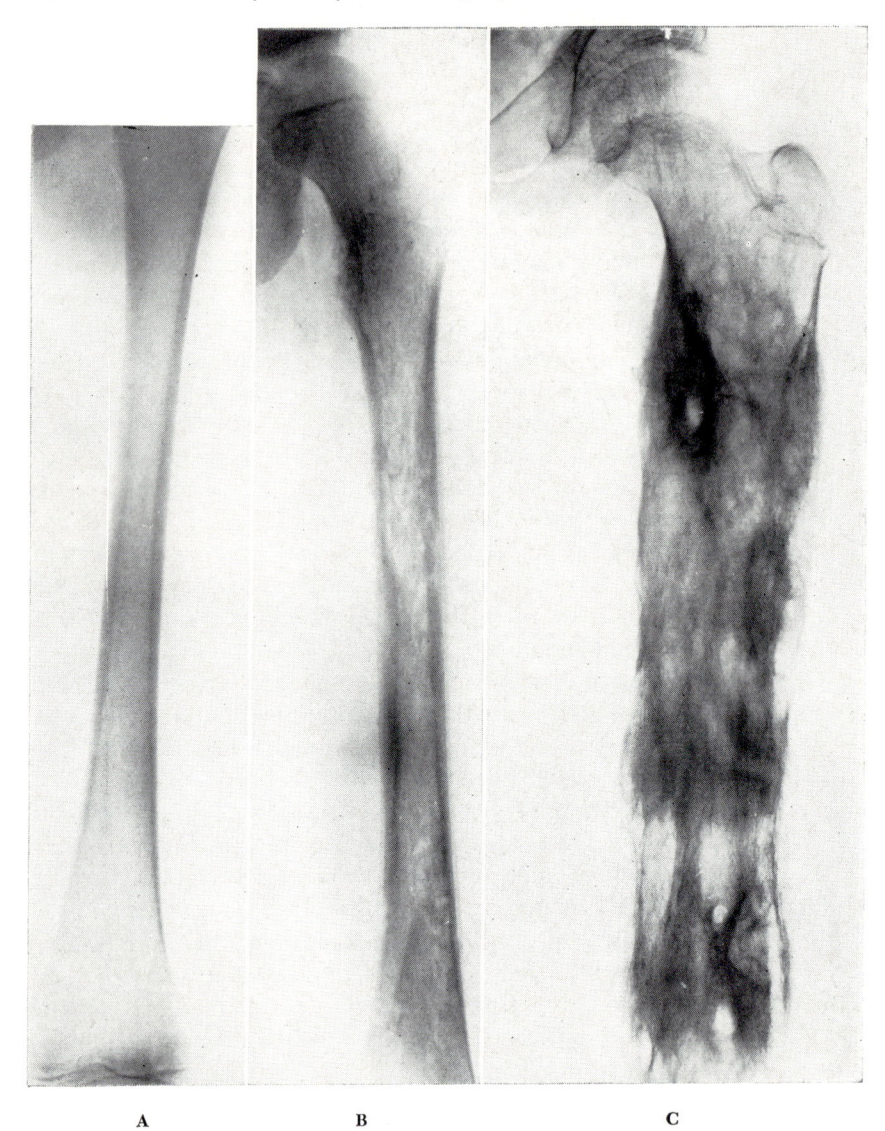

A   B   C

Fig. 88. Osteomyelitis of femur. **A,** Absence of roentgenographic changes three weeks after acute clinical onset in 9-year-old boy. **B,** Three weeks later. Widespread mottling and periosteal elevation. **C,** Three years later. Note shaft thickened by massive involucrum, irregular areas of bone absorption and bone proliferation, and cloacae marking sites of draining sinuses.

days, a different antibiotic should be started. By this time the results of antibiotic sensitivity testing of the organism cultured from the blood or from a subperiosteal abscess may be available. Because of the frequency of toxic reactions, allergic phenomena, and bacterial resistance, selection of the proper antibiotic from the large number of available preparations is often difficult. When penicillin is contraindicated, a member of the erythromycin group is often the best choice. As a rule, antibiotic therapy should be continued for at least three weeks.

The acutely ill patient requires constant bed rest and skilled nursing care. His course should be followed by blood cell counts and blood cultures. Attention to hydration and electrolyte replacement is important.

The affected limb should be put at rest in good functional position by means of traction or the support of a splint or plaster shell. Hot moist dressings may be applied; in some clinics ice bags are preferred.

With early intensive treatment of the patient's general condition, including antibiotic therapy, it is possible to delay surgical operation upon the infected bone and in many cases to avoid it altogether. After the local signs, of which the most useful is fluctuation, indicate that a subperiosteal abscess has formed, it should be aspirated of as much pus as can be obtained. The pus should be examined by Gram stain and cultured. An antibiotic may be instilled directly into the abscess cavity. If the abscess recurs, it may be best to effect surgical drainage. Operation upon the bone itself is inadvisable in the early stage of the disease but later may become necessary. As the acute condition subsides a cast must usually be applied, especially if the destruction of bone has been extensive. The patient must be followed carefully during his convalescence.

Chronic stage. In the chronic stage, the patient is no longer obviously ill but has a local infection of low grade which may be manifested by persistent drainage from one or more cutaneous sinuses and by recurrent episodes of local pain, increased heat, and swelling. Chronic osteomyelitis is still seen frequently despite improved treatment of early hematogenous infections and of compound fractures. Attempt should be made to improve the patient's general condition by giving a high caloric diet and supplementary vitamins, and transfusions may be helpful. The drainage from sinuses should be cultured, the sensitivities of the causative organism and any secondary invaders determined, and appropriate antibiotic treatment started. Antibiotics may be relatively ineffective, however, because of the poor circulation in scarred soft tissues and sclerotic bone. Surgical removal of dead bone, or *sequestrectomy,* is indicated when the patient is in good general condition, the necrotic bone is roentgenographically well separated, and an adequate involucrum has been formed. In the absence of persistent diffuse infectious changes in the affected bone, individual sequestra are best removed through sinuses or small incisions. If roentgenograms show most of the bone to be still involved by chronic infection, however, the much more extensive surgical procedure of *saucerization* may be indicated. It includes removal of all scar tissue, infected granulation tissue, sequestra, sclerotic bone, and overhanging bone edges; it leaves a long flat depression in the bone with a grossly clean and freely bleeding surface. An antibiotic or sulfonamide may be put into the wound. In some cases closure of the soft tissues is practicable, whereas in others it may be necessary to leave the wound open and fill it with petrolatum gauze (the *Orr method*); in either case an ample cast is applied to rest the affected structures and protect the weakened bone. In the Orr method the cast and dressings are changed only at infrequent intervals, when the odor becomes offensive or the cast softened. Later, skin grafting for coverage or even bone grafting for strength may be indicated.

In the chronic stage it is often difficult to obliterate large cavities, especially when they occur in the thick lower end of the femur or upper end of the tibia. Skin grafting may be required before bone surgery can be done. Sometimes it is possible to close these cavities by removing completely the superficial layer of bone lining the cavity, together with all infected soft tissue, and allowing the remaining soft tissue to collapse into the cavity. If this proves unsuccessful, it may be necessary to carry out a "bone-filling" operation of transplanting muscle and fascia or fat into the cavity. Sometimes cancellous bone chips may be packed into the cavity after complete saucerization.

Amputation is occasionally indicated in chronic osteomyelitis. There are a few adult patients in whom chronic infection over a long period of years has responded so poorly to the usual treatment that amputation improves their general health and function.

BRODIE'S ABSCESS

Brodie's abscess is a localized form of chronic osteomyelitis dating back to a recognized or unrecognized bacteremia, which may have preceded the clinical appearance of the abscess by many years. The abscess has a thin wall of fibrous tissue and sclerotic bone; it contains pus that on culture may be sterile or may contain staphylococci of low virulence. The most common site is the lower end of the tibia. These abscesses occur most often in older children and young adults. Clinically the onset is gradual. The chief symp-

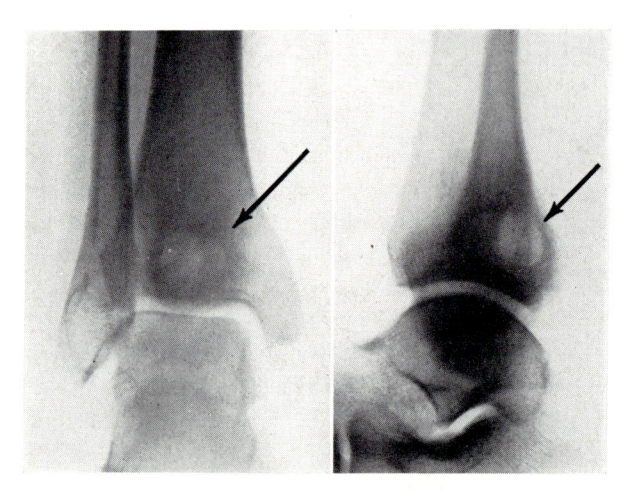

Fig. 89. Roentgenograms showing a Brodie's abscess of the distal end of the tibia in a man 29 years of age. Note circular, well-demarcated area of decreased density, indicating site of the abscess.

tom is local pain, often worse at night, and usually there are slightly increased heat and tenderness over the site of the lesion.

Diagnosis. The roentgenographic appearance of an area of decreased density surrounded by sclerotic bone (Fig. 89) confirms the clinical diagnosis. Brodie's abscess is to be differentiated from osteogenic sarcoma, osteoid-osteoma, eosinophilic granuloma, bone cyst, and fibrous dysplasia.

Treatment. The treatment consists of operation and the local and systemic administration of an antibiotic. The abscess should be thoroughly cleaned out or excised. Usually the wound may be closed, after which a cast is applied.

SCLEROSING OSTEITIS (GARRÉ'S OSTEITIS)

In 1893 Garré described as a form of chronic osteomyelitis a sclerosing osteitis, usually in the shaft of a long bone, which is characterized clinically by local pain and roentgenographically by a fusiform thickening and increased density of the cortex.

Etiology. Hypotheses have incriminated infection of low virulence and local anoxia from impaired circulation. Since the affected bone is usually sterile and its microscopic appearance is not pathognomonic, it may be that etiologically Garré's osteitis is not an entity.

Differential diagnosis. Osteoid-osteoma, Ewing's sarcoma, osteogenic sarcoma, syphilitic periostitis, and localized osteitis deformans should be considered.

Treatment. It has been customary to drill holes through the dense cortical area or to excise a part of it. These measures usually relieve the pain, as well as provide material for culture and biopsy.

OSTEITIS PUBIS

Osteitis pubis is a painful, usually nonsuppurative affection of the pubic symphysis, occurring most often after prostatic operations in older men. A few cases have been reported in young adults after local trauma and in women during or after pregnancy. Urinary tract organisms have been cultured from the diseased area in some cases. However, it is questionable whether osteitis pubis is a low-grade infectious process or a noninfectious sequel of trauma.

Clinical picture. Characteristically, two to eight weeks following prostatic surgery there is sudden onset of pain over one side of the symphysis, with pubic tenderness. The pain rapidly becomes more severe, especially with activity, and is worse on coughing, defecation, and urination. The patient tends to lie in one position, with flexed hips and marked adductor muscle spasm. Recovery is often spontaneous but slow.

Roentgenographic picture. Several weeks after the clinical onset, the margins of the symphysis become irregular and the pubic bodies and rami osteoporotic. Decalcification may extend laterally to the ischium and even to the acetabulum. Early the symphyseal interval may appear widened; much later it may be narrowed or obliterated.

Differential diagnosis. Osteitis pubis must be distinguished from strain of the adductor muscles, from frank osteomyelitis with its more severe local and systemic reactions, and from metastatic malignancy and tuberculosis.

Treatment. The pain is treated by bed rest, appropriate medication, and local application of heat or cold. A short bilateral hip spica cast may afford much relief. An antibiotic should be given if signs of infection are present. Accumulation of pus may require aspiration or incision and drainage.

PYOGENIC OR SUPPURATIVE ARTHRITIS

Incidence. Pyogenic arthritis is more common in children than in adults but is seen frequently in both. Males are affected more commonly than females. The hip and knee are the most frequent sites of infection.

Etiology. Trauma probably influences the localization of the infection. As in osteomyelitis, the *Staphylococcus aureus* and the *Streptococcus haemolyticus* are the common infecting agents. Less commonly, joints are infected by any of a variety of microorganisms including pneumococcus, gonococcus, meningococcus, *Salmonella, Brucella,* colon bacillus, and many others.

Routes of infection. Organisms reach the joint by one of three routes: (1) by vascular transfer from a distant focus, such as an infected abrasion, furuncle, or upper respiratory tract infection; (2) by direct or lymphatic extension from a neighboring infected area, such as an osteomyelitis; or (3) by direct inoculation of infected material through a penetrating wound. Of the last type is infection from a contaminated aspiration or injection, a grave complication that can almost always be prevented by the use of strictest aseptic technic when a needle must be introduced into a joint.

Pathology. Depending upon the numbers and virulence of the organism, the resistance of the patient, and the duration of the infection, three distinct types of synovitis and joint effusion—serous, serofibrinous, and purulent—are to be noted.

Serous effusion. If the infection is mild there may be only synovial edema and moderate increase of synovial fluid. The fluid may, however, become cloudy and show an increased cell count.

Serofibrinous effusion. The second stage of inflammation is more serious. A layer of fibrin forms over the synovial membrane, which is swollen and infiltrated by polymorphonuclear leukocytes. The fibrinous exudate may be replaced by granulation tissue with the formation of intra-articular adhesions.

Purulent effusion. Purulent effusion occurs in the most severe type of inflammatory reaction. All articular structures rapidly become involved. The cartilage becomes eroded, especially at points of pressure, leading to inflammatory changes in the underlying bone and later to frank osteomyelitis. The amount of destruction depends upon the virulence of the organism and the length of time during which the infection has been present. Pathologic dislocation sometimes occurs. Septic joints of this type often progress to a fibrous or bony ankylosis (Figs. 117 and 118).

In addition to the local inflammatory process, the widespread pathologic changes associated with septicemia may be present.

Clinical picture. The symptoms vary with the degree of the joint inflammation. In the serous type of reaction there may be only moderate swelling and slight pain. There is an increase of local heat, and the joint usually becomes flexed because of protective muscle spasm. Palpation of the distended joint capsule yields the sensation of fluctuation, and often the outline of the capsule can be defined. Attempts to move the joint are accompanied by pain. Fever and leukocytosis are present but not of great degree.

In the serofibrinous type of arthritis the joint is much more painful and all of the signs of inflammation are more intense.

In the purulent or suppurative type of inflammation the symptoms are still more severe. There is usually an extreme systemic reaction with a marked elevation of temperature (104° to 105° F., 40° to 41° C.) and leukocytosis. The patient is usually apprehensive. The joint is extremely painful on examination. The infection may spread to the neighboring structures, giving rise to brawny induration and thickening of the periarticular tissues.

Differential diagnosis. To make a definite diagnosis of pyogenic arthritis it is necessary to aspirate the joint fluid, examine a smear microscopically, and culture the fluid. Acute osteomyelitis, periarticular cellulitis, and purulent bursitis are often confused with pyogenic arthritis. Gonococcal arthritis must be remembered. Frequently pyogenic arthritis must be differentiated from acute rheumatic fever. Acute rheumatoid arthritis, gout, tuberculosis, scurvy, hemophilia, and acute poliomyelitis must also be excluded.

Acute appendicitis may cause psoas spasm, resulting in flexion of the right hip which may suggest pyogenic arthritis of the hip. Acute pelvic inflammatory disease may cause symptoms referable to either hip joint.

Treatment. Therapy should be prompt and vigorous. If fluid aspirated from the joint is cloudy, several hundred thousand units of penicillin in saline solution may be instilled immediately into the joint and systemic penicillin treatment started. A different antibiotic should be substituted later if culture and sensitivity tests so indicate.

The inflamed joint structures should be put at rest by means of traction, splint, or bivalved cast.

Aspiration, culture, gentle irrigation, and instillation of antibiotic may be done, at first daily and then at longer intervals as the local and systemic signs of infection subside. If such improvement does not begin promptly and continue, and in particular, if the aspirate remains purulent and the patient febrile, surgical drainage is indicated. Irrigation with an antibiotic may be done at operation and at daily postoperative dressings. A windowed cast may be used to support the joint in its best functional position. After the inflammation has subsided and the cast has been removed, mobility and strength are restored by gradually increasing exercise. When severe damage of intra-articular structures has made ankylosis inevitable, care should be taken that it occur in the position of maximum usefulness (p. 197).

Prognosis. Serous effusions are rapidly absorbed and recovery takes place quickly and completely. If a serofibrinous or purulent exudate is present, however, some limitation of motion usually results and occasionally the final outcome is bony ankylosis. When the pyarthrosis is associated with a septicemia, which happens more frequently in children than in adults, there is danger of a fatal outcome.

PYOGENIC ARTHRITIS OF THE HIP IN INFANTS

This entity warrants individual emphasis because of its difficulty of diagnosis, need of prompt treatment, and serious consequences if inadequately handled.

Pathology. In all probability the infecting organisms usually enter the hip joint from an expanding focus in the intracapsular metaphysis of the femoral neck. In some instances they may lodge first in synovial membrane or bony portion of the capital epiphysis. The epiphysis, which in infancy is wholly or largely cartilaginous, may be severely damaged or destroyed by proteolytic enzymes in the exudate and by impairment of its blood supply resulting from increased intra-articular pressure. Pathologic dislocation is a common sequel.

Diagnosis. The systemic reaction, especially in premature infants, may be deceptively mild, without fever or leukocytosis. Permanent, irreparable joint damage may occur unless the diagnosis is made early. It should be suspected from the local, acute inflammatory signs of swelling and pain on motion and should be confirmed by prompt aspiration.

Treatment. Unless the diagnosis has been made and local and systemic antibiotic treatment has been started as early as a day or two after onset, prompt surgical drainage is usually indicated, followed by rest in a spica cast with the hip in extension, slight internal rotation, and moderate abduction to forestall subluxation.

PNEUMOCOCCAL ARTHRITIS

Pneumococci are occasionally the cause of pyogenic arthritis, in most instances as a complication of pneumonia. As a rule the arthritis affects only a single joint; most commonly involved is the hip. The inflammatory process may be of mild, serous type but may progress to severe suppurative changes. The diagnosis is confirmed by aspiration, smear, and culture; the treatment consists chiefly of antibiotics given systemically and into the joint; the prognosis, as a rule, is excellent.

GONOCOCCAL ARTHRITIS

Gonococcal arthritis, now an uncommon entity, is usually a metastatic sequel of inadequately treated acute gonorrheal urethritis. Males between 20 and 30 years of age are most often affected.

Clinical picture. The joint involvement usually appears two to three weeks after the onset of a urethral or vaginal discharge, but it may occur much later. The arthritis may be polyarticular or monarticular. Fleeting pains are sometimes present in multiple joints for several days before obvious infection becomes localized in a single joint. The knee is affected most commonly, and next the ankle. Periarticular inflammation may involve tendon sheaths and bursae.

In acute cases the joint is extremely painful and tender, with redness, increased heat, swelling, glossy overlying skin, and severe muscle spasm; the systemic reaction includes fever and marked leukocytosis. Cases of more chronic type are often characterized chiefly by pain in several joints, swelling, restricted mobility, and little systemic reaction.

Diagnosis. In acute cases the diagnosis is suggested by the clinical picture and by identification of the organisms in the urethral or vaginal discharge. It is important to exclude *Staphylococcus* and *Streptococcus* infection and acute rheumatic fever. Early diagnostic aspiration of the affected joint and bacteriologic study of the aspirate should be carried out. Within the first ten days of the infection gonococci will often be found in the joint fluid. In chronic or subacute cases there may be some difficulty in finding the organisms and in differentiating the condition from rheumatoid arthritis, Reiter's syndrome, and tuberculosis.

Treatment. Therapy should be directed toward cure of the primary focus, as well as the inflamed joint. Penicillin should be given systemically in large doses. The affected joint may require elevation, heat, support in good functional position, aspiration, gentle lavage, and instillation of penicillin. After the infection has subsided, the joint should be gradually mobilized. Unsuccessfully treated cases may be followed by fibrous or even bony ankylosis.

SALMONELLA OSTEOMYELITIS AND ARTHRITIS

In many countries typhoid osteomyelitis, which is caused by *Salmonella typhi,* is now rare. Infections of bone or joint by other members of the *Salmonella* group are seen occasionally. Their incidence is relatively high in children with sickle cell anemia. Several bones may be involved, with local pain, tenderness, and roentgenographic changes, in the later stages of an enteric fever; a chronic localized osteomyelitis resembling Brodie's abscess may make its clinical appearance years after a *Salmonella* septicemia; or a low-grade pyogenic osteomyelitis or arthritis may occur without recognized primary infection. The diagnosis is made on culture of the organism. The treatment is similar to that of other forms of pyogenic osteomyelitis and arthritis. Chloramphenicol has proved effective in most *Salmonella* infections.

BRUCELLA OSTEOMYELITIS AND ARTHRITIS

Human brucellosis, an uncommon disease in the United States, is seen chiefly as a result of direct contact with cattle or swine or of drinking unpasteurized milk. Its orthopaedic manifestations are of two types: (1) excessive fatigue, aches, and pains without local infectious foci, and (2) localized osteomyelitis, arthritis, and bursitis. Involvement of the spine tends to destroy contiguous vertebral surfaces and disk, ending in bony ankylosis of the bodies. The diagnosis may be suspected from the clinical picture, strengthened by serum agglutination testing, and proved by culture. *Brucella* is cultured more readily from tissue removed at operation than from joint fluid or the drainage from sinuses. The treatment includes use of the tetracycline drugs and streptomycin.

FUNGUS INFECTIONS OF BONES AND JOINTS

Although the fungi which may infect bones and joints are of many varieties, mycotic osteomyelitis and arthritis are uncommon or rare entities. In some instances the disease is systemic, and the organisms reach a bone or joint focus through the blood stream; in others, involvement takes place by direct extension from infected overlying tissues. The lesions, in general, are infectious granulomas; as a rule they are osteolytic, and differentiation from tuberculosis is sometimes difficult. Whereas serologic and skin tests may be helpful, final diagnosis depends upon identification of the organism in smear, culture, or histologic section. Some of these infections respond to specific antibiotic therapy; for some, surgical drainage, extirpation, or amputation is indicated.

Actinomycosis occurs about the jaw in more than half of the cases, involving soft tissue primarily and spreading later to the mandible. Indurated areas and deep abscesses are characteristic. A purulent exudate containing mycotic colonies, the so-called sulfur granules, is often extruded through multiple sinus tracts.

Blastomycosis may be disseminated widely from the lungs via the blood stream, causing a chronic destructive osteomyelitis of vertebrae, ribs, skull, and other bones. Such cases often prove fatal, despite treatment.

Coccidioidomycosis is endemic in the southwestern part of the United States. Primary pulmonary infection may be followed by a systemic phase with multiple bone, joint, and visceral lesions and a grave prognosis.

ECHINOCOCCUS CYST

Occasionally cysts caused by the parasite *Echinococcus granulosus* are formed within bone; in North America such cases are very rare. The lesions involve the pelvic bones most commonly and next in order the spine and the long bones. The embryos are brought by the blood stream to bone, where they produce multiple small intraosseous cysts, rather than the single large cyst seen in the liver or lung. Pain, which begins only in late stages, occurs usually from the leakage of fluid or from pathologic fracture. Eosinophilia is frequently present. Hydatid fluid may be used for complement fixation, precipitation, and intradermal tests to aid in establishing the diagnosis.

Treatment. Complete excision of the cystic areas, when practicable, is the treatment of choice.

SYPHILIS OF BONES AND JOINTS

Involvement of bones and joints occurs in both the congenital and the acquired forms of syphilis and may mimic many other diseases. With early antibiotic treatment, premarital serologic testing, and supervised prenatal care, syphilitic bone and joint infections have become rare in many parts of the world. Often they are of chief interest from the standpoint of differential diagnosis. Several types warrant brief description. Included here are osteochondritis, localized periostitis, diffuse periostitis and osteoperiostitis, symmetrical serous synovitis, and gummatous arthritis.

Osteochondritis

Pathology. In early infancy syphilitic infections may cause characteristic changes in the epiphyses. Radiographically an irregular deposit of lime salts appears along the epiphyseal line. Histologically the cartilage cells are of abnormal appearance; they multiply in a disorderly manner with the production of many immature forms. Areas of necrosis are present. If the disease is unchecked, it may cause suppuration and the development of frank syphilitic osteomyelitis. Occasionally the epiphysis separates from the shaft and extreme distortion results. The neighboring joint may exhibit a synovitis or even a destructive arthritis.

Clinical picture. The lesions of syphilitic osteochondritis are most often of symmetrical distribution and involve, in order of frequency, the lower end of the femur, the lower ends of the tibia and fibula, and the lower ends of the radius and ulna. The joints become swollen and tender, but no local or general febrile reaction is present. Often the infant appears to be partially paralyzed; this condition has been called *pseudoparalysis.*

Prognosis. If proper antisyphilitic therapy is instituted, the prognosis for recovery is good.

Localized periostitis

In a form of syphilitic periostitis called *periostitis ossificans,* bone production in and beneath the thickened periosteum causes the formation of a hard, dense, circumscribed swelling. This swelling is always found on the convex side of the bone. When the tibia is involved, the condition is sometimes spoken of as *saber shin.*

Diffuse periostitis and osteoperiostitis

In the late stage of syphilis a gummatous periostitis and osteitis causing necrosis of bone are sometimes observed. There is little or no pain. The skull, as well as the long bones, may be involved. The process may lead to suppuration and may simulate pyogenic osteomyelitis. There may be diffuse thickening of the bony cortex with the formation of small hyperostoses that present a characteristic appearance. Pathologic fracture may occur.

Symmetrical serous synovitis

A painless hydrarthrosis of the knees, called *Clutton's joints,* may develop in children and subside at about the twentieth year without residuals. Its recognition is important in obviating exploratory operation and in leading to antisyphilitic medication.

Gummatous arthritis

In late syphilis a gumma of subchondral cancellous bone may extend into the contiguous joint and produce a destructive arthritis. Similar gummas sometimes begin in synovial membrane. With adequate antisyphilitic treatment, the prognosis for recovery is good.

CHAPTER 7

Tuberculosis of bones and joints

TUBERCULOSIS OF BONES AND JOINTS is a localized, progressively destructive disease resulting from the activity of *Mycobacterium tuberculosis* in bone or articular structures. It is secondary to tuberculous infection in another part of the body, such as lungs or lymph nodes.

Incidence. In recent decades great improvement in living conditions and better methods of prevention and treatment have reduced the incidence of active tuberculous infections and their complications. Osteoarticular tuberculosis, which constitutes no more than 2 or 3% of tuberculous infections in general, is no longer a common disease in many areas.

Tuberculosis of bones and joints may occur at any age but is most frequent in childhood. It affects males somewhat more often than females and is most common in groups whose living conditions are substandard. Although any bone or joint may be involved, the most frequent sites are, in order, the spine, the hip, and the knee. In many patients more than one joint is affected.

Routes of infection. Tuberculous joints are seen in patients with recognized pulmonary tuberculosis, in whom the mycobacteria have traveled from lung to bone or joint via the blood stream. Trauma and lowered resistance may have some influence on localization and survival of the organisms. In some instances they may spread via lymphatic channels or by direct extension. Bone and joint tuberculosis is seen also in individuals who have no obvious primary lesion. In such cases the initial focus may be a bronchial lymph node that the mycobacteria reach after being inhaled or a mesenteric node they reach after being ingested. In many countries infected cattle and unpasteurized milk are still important sources of tuberculous infection.

Pathology. An outstanding characteristic of tuberculous infection of bone is destruction with little tendency toward the formation of new bone. The process usually begins in subchondral or metaphyseal bone and then by gradual extension along the line of least resistance enters the joint. In some instances it starts in the synovial membrane and involves secondarily the bone beneath the joint surface.

Localization of the mycobacteria in bone leads to the formation of tubercles. Microscopically the typical tubercle contains epithelioid cells and one or more Langhans' giant cells with their peripherally placed nuclei. In the earliest stages polymorphonuclear leukocytes are present. Later, numerous lymphocytes infiltrate the marginal areas. Adjacent tubercles may coalesce to form larger ones, and the expanding lesion gradually destroys and replaces surrounding tissues. Necrosis of ischemic and toxic origin may take place near the center of such a granuloma, progressing slowly to liquefaction, while about the periphery fibroblasts lay down collagen that tends ultimately to wall off the lesion.

As the destructive process near the end of a bone advances, it soon penetrates into the nearest joint along an edge of its articular cartilage. Rapid dissemination of the tuberculous material then takes place over synovial membrane and cartilage. Although relatively resistant to tuberculous destruction, the articular cartilage may be undermined at its synovial margins, gradually separated from the underlying bone, and destroyed. These changes are accompanied by the formation of a purulent, cheesy exudate containing remnants of necrotic tissue. The bone becomes disintegrated and destroyed on its exposed joint surfaces. If the destructive process is unchecked by treatment, the increasing exudate may dissect the surrounding joint structures along the planes of least resistance, enter the soft tissues to form an abscess, and penetrate the overlying skin to produce a chronically draining sinus that soon becomes infected secondarily with pyogenic bacteria.

If the infection is overcome, the exudate is slowly absorbed and replaced by fibrous tissue. Bone about the edges of the lesion is stimulated to proliferate, and gradually the evidences of active infection subside. Tuberculous organisms in the tissues may remain viable for long periods.

Tuberculous abscesses are called "cold abscesses" because of the absence of an acute inflammatory reaction with marked increase in local heat, redness, and pain. As the focus feeding a deep tuberculous abscess subsides with treatment, the pus is slowly absorbed. The abscess wall becomes shrunken and fibrotic; it may become partially calcified.

Except in very early infections, tuberculosis completely within bone and without extension into a joint is unusual. It is seen occasionally in phalanges, metacarpals, metatarsals, or ribs, and rarely in other bones.

Clinical picture. The onset of local symptoms is insidious. Sometimes they are preceded by poor general health, loss of weight, or respiratory infections. As a rule the involvement is monarticular. Spontaneous pain, pain on motion of the affected joint, and restriction of its mobility by spasm (Fig. 90) may be the first evidences of tuberculosis; they are followed quickly by muscle atrophy. In other cases pain may be slight or absent. A painless kyphosis, or even the appearance of a cold abscess, may be the first manifestation of spinal tuberculosis, and a painless limp may be the first sign of involvement in the lower extremity. In superficial joints swelling is an

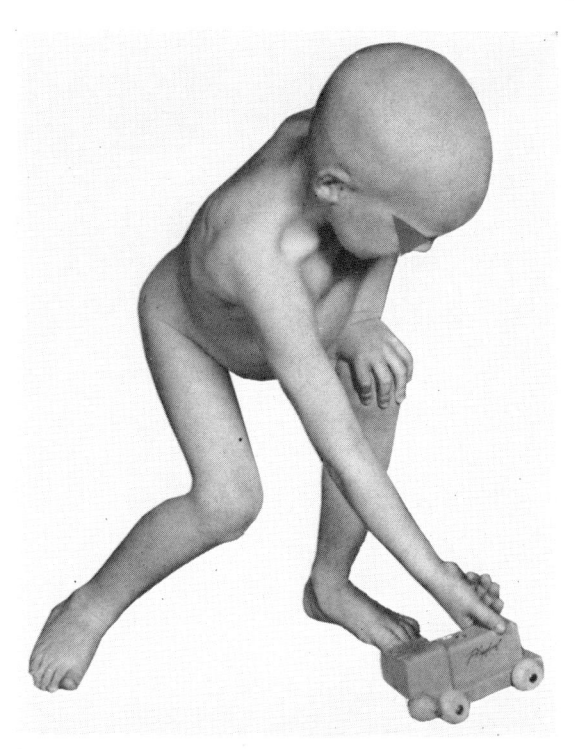

Fig. 90. Tuberculosis of lumbar spine in a 4-year-old boy. Note how, in picking up an object from the floor, the patient protects his spine in extension by flexing hips and knees and propping with his left hand.

early sign; they usually show no redness, little heat, and only slight tenderness. In children night cries and night sweats may occur, and there is usually a slight afternoon elevation of temperature. A mild leukocytosis may be present. In later stages severe deformity may result from contractures and bone destruction.

Roentgenographic picture. Early changes are slight and often not diagnostic. Later the bones show decalcification, faint joint outlines, and irregular notching of the joint surfaces. There is sometimes a circumscribed area of decreased density without surrounding sclerosis. In tuberculosis of the spine (Fig. 91), loss of disk space and erosion and collapse of the vertebral bodies are seen. The most characteristic feature of the roentgenograms, however, is the almost complete lack of bone regeneration in the early cases. In later stages of the infection new bone may be seen and the joint outlines again become sharply defined. In late stages sequestra are occasionally visualized.

Diagnosis. Since early, accurate diagnosis is of the greatest importance, free use should be made of aspiration and biopsy technics. Positive diagnosis depends upon the identification of *Mycobacterium tuberculosis* in smear and culture or the demonstration of tubercles in microscopic sections. Guinea pig inoculation is sometimes helpful.

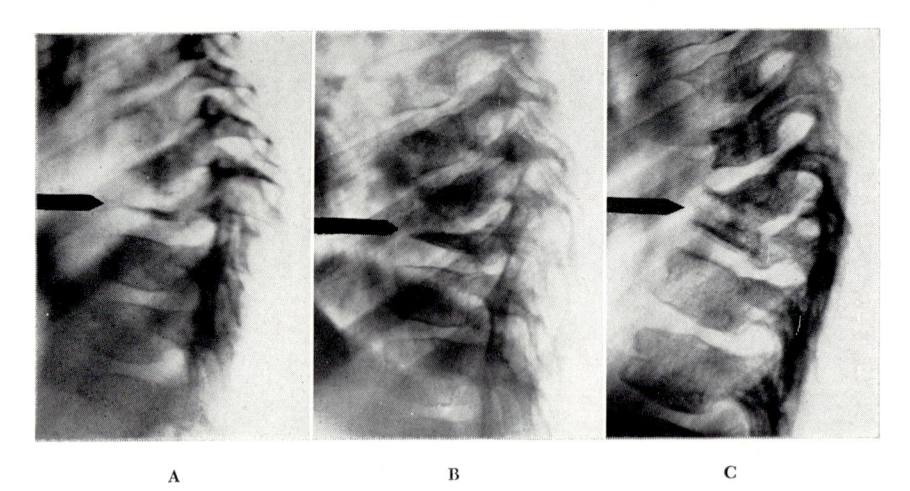

Fig. 91. Lateral roentgenograms of tuberculosis of spine in boy 3 years of age. **A,** Note the destruction of bodies of seventh and eighth thoracic vertebrae and the kyphosis. **B,** In same patient, two years later. Treatment has consisted of rest on Bradford frame and immobilization in plaster body cast. Note sharp, well-demarcated outlines of the diseased vertebral bodies, indicating healing. **C,** In same patient, eighteen months later. Note well-demarcated outlines and fusion of the diseased vertebral bodies. If antituberculous drugs had been available when this patient was treated, his disability period might have been shortened.

The intracutaneous tuberculin test often provides useful information. Especially in children, a positive test is suggestive but not conclusive evidence of tuberculosis somewhere in the body. Rarely is tuberculosis present when the tuberculin skin test is negative and remains so even when repeated with increased concentrations of tuberculin.

Treatment. Until the recent development of antituberculous drugs, the treatment of bone and joint tuberculosis was, as a rule, limited to support of the patient's immunologic defenses by general hygienic measures and to improvement of his joint lesion by putting it at rest with a brace or arthrodesis. Almost invariably the optimal end result was bony ankylosis in good functional position. By their bacteriostatic action, antibiotics have shortened the course of the disease and made it possible occasionally to eradicate the joint lesion without leading necessarily to ankylosis. With chemotherapeutic coverage, surgery can be done earlier and more safely.

The treatment of bone and joint tuberculosis includes general measures, which apply to all cases, and local measures that vary with the site and extent of the tuberculous lesion.

General measures. Prolonged bed rest and nutritious diet are indicated. They are especially beneficial for debilitated patients, patients with concomitant active pulmonary infections, and patients with multiple bone and joint foci.

At present the most useful antituberculous drugs are streptomycin, para-aminosalicylic acid, and isoniazid (isonicotinic acid hydrazide). As a rule their administration should be started early, continued for a year or more, and repeated as needed. Since the effectiveness of an individual drug decreases rapidly through the development of resistant strains, it is customary to prescribe the antibiotics concurrently. At times two are given at the start of treatment while the third is reserved, to be added later at the time of surgical operation.

Streptomycin is given intramuscularly in doses that vary from 1 Gm. twice a week to 2 Gm. daily, depending upon the age of the patient, the nature of the infection, and the imminence of toxic reaction to the drug. Such reactions include vertigo and deafness that is sometimes permanent. *Para-aminosalicylic acid* is given by mouth in doses of 10 to 20 Gm. a day. It may cause gastrointestinal symptoms, such as vomiting and diarrhea, and occasionally produces allergic reactions. *Isoniazid* may be given by mouth or by intramuscular injection. The usual dosage is 200 mg. daily for adults, and 4 mg. per kilogram of body weight for children. For some types of tuberculosis much higher doses have been recommended. The toxic complications of isoniazid, which include mild skin and neurologic changes, are uncommon. For patients receiving large doses, vitamin B_6 (pyridoxine) may be used to forestall peripheral neuritis.

Local measures. The object of the local treatment of bone and joint tuberculosis is to make conditions at the site of the lesion optimal for prompt and permanent healing. This is accomplished by (1) initial immobilization to provide local rest from mechanical stresses such as tension and compression, (2) extirpation of the lesion, when possible, to permit the approximation of healthy tissues, and (3) arthrodesis when destruction of the joint has made permanent support advisable. Specific therapy for the individual case is determined by the extent and location of the lesion and by the nature of the patient's reaction to the infection.

Immobilization of some degree is usually indicated from the time the diagnosis is first suspected to the end of the treatment period. It may be secured simply by rest in bed on fracture board and foam rubber mattress, or by traction, braces, or plaster casts. Rarely a case is seen so early that the small focus of tuberculous infection can be reached readily by antibiotics in the blood and healed spontaneously, requiring only prolonged external immobilization; such a patient may be treated by traction in recumbency for several months, followed by a brace and ambulation for several months, and further followed by re-examination at long intervals to rule out recurrence. Most patients are seen much later, however, when the joint structures have been extensively destroyed, painless movement and stability cannot be regained, and the permanent immobilization of arthrodesis is desirable.

The optimal time for operation is when the patient's resistance is strong (as indicated by apyrexia, a low sedimentation rate, and a high lymphocyte-monocyte ratio) and when the lesion is no longer advancing. Most tuberculous joints require arthrodesis and bone grafting. With the arthrodesis, partial excision of the pathologic tissue can often be combined. Virtually complete excision of early lesions, such as a tuberculous synovitis or a small bone focus, is occasionally possible, and in such cases arthrodesis may not be indicated. Tuberculous sinuses and abscesses that persist despite medical treatment can often be successfully excised after the bone or joint lesion has regressed with immobilization and antibiotics. Abscesses that are causing symptoms but cannot be resected may be evacuated. Amputation is occasionally indicated, most often for extensive, secondarily infected tuberculosis of the ankle and foot of an adult.

Postoperatively the antituberculous chemotherapy should be continued for a year or longer, until mycobacterial activity can be presumed to be no longer present. The affected joint requires appropriate protection by means of a cast or brace until healing is sound and mature. The period of postoperative immobilization may last several months to a year or more. The patient's activity is increased gradually to a normal level. To prevent possible recurrence he should be re-examined at increasing intervals for at least several years.

Prognosis. The prognosis in bone and joint tuberculosis depends much upon early diagnosis and treatment. Most of the patients recover. Retention of joint mobility, however, is unusual; especially is this true in adults.

The outlook is relatively grave when the patient also has active pulmonary tuberculosis or when he has involvement of more than one major joint. Prolonged suppuration may lead to amyloidosis. Tuberculosis of the spine or hip is more serious than that of other joints.

TUBERCULOSIS OF THE SPINE

The spine is the most common site of bone and joint tuberculosis, being involved in approximately half the cases. Children are affected more often than adults. Any level of the spine may be involved; the greatest incidence

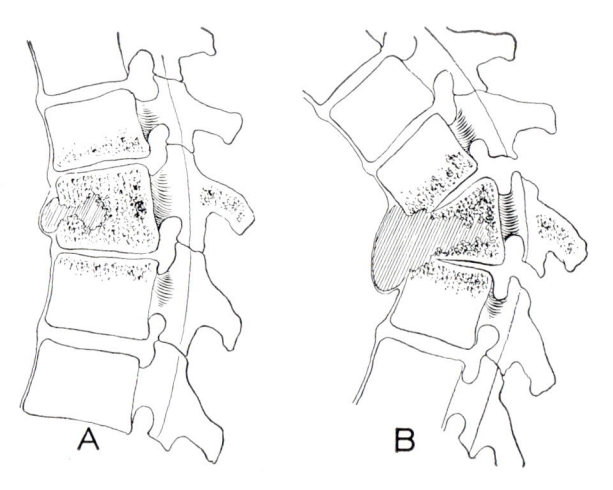

Fig. 92. Tuberculosis of the spine. Stages in the process of bone destruction and abscess formation: **A**, early, and **B**, late. (After Calot.)

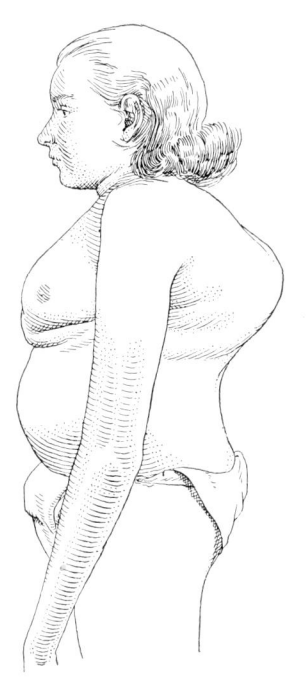

Fig. 93. Severe kyphosis from tuberculosis of dorsal spine. (From clinical material of Dr. G. E. Bennett.)

is in the lower thoracic region. Spinal tuberculosis is sometimes called *Pott's disease* because in 1779 Sir Percivall Pott described a painful deformity of the spine, accompanied by paraplegia, which is thought to have been tuberculous. Because of anatomic differences, tuberculosis of the spine varies considerably in pathology, complications, and treatment from tuberculosis of the joints of the extremities.

Pathology. Tuberculosis of the spine is thought to begin in the cancellous bone of a vertebral body (Fig. 92). Uncommonly it may start in posterior arch, process, or contiguous joint structures. The infection may extend beneath the anterior longitudinal ligament or directly across affected disks to involve several adjacent vertebrae. In some instances multiple foci are separated by uninfected vertebrae. With increasing destruction the strength of the involved vertebral body becomes so impaired that it collapses under continued stress, producing a posterior protrusion of the spine, or *kyphosis* (Fig. 93). This deformity is greater when it involves the thoracic level of the spine, which normally has a moderate posterior convexity. In the cervical and lumbar portions of the spine, where the convexity is normally anterior, kyphosis following collapse of the vertebral bodies may not become noticeable until the disease is far advanced. Healing takes place by gradual fibrosis and by new bone formation with resulting bony ankylosis of the collapsed vertebrae.

Abscesses. Some degree of abscess formation doubtless occurs in every

156   *Handbook of orthopaedic surgery*

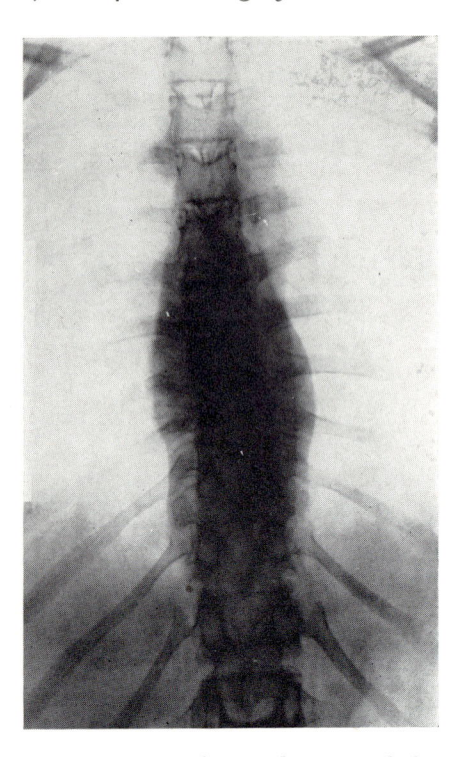

Fig. 94. Anteroposterior roentgenogram showing large spinal abscess in 33-year-old man who had tuberculosis of the mid-thoracic vertebrae.

case of vertebral tuberculosis. When treatment of the bony focus is delayed or ineffective, the abscess may become quite large. It may appear in anteroposterior roentgenograms as a fusiform or flask-shaped shadow encircling the spine at and just below the level of the involved vertebrae (Fig. 94). These abscesses tend to gravitate along fascial planes and to present themselves in characteristic locations. Cervical abscesses may appear in a retropharyngeal position or in the deep muscles on either side of the neck. Thoracic abscesses may point in the posterior mediastinum, rupture into the pleura or lung, or reach the chest wall. The typical lumbar abscess descends along the psoas fascial sheath; it may point posteriorly, laterally, or in the groin or upper, inner thigh as a *psoas abscess*. Untreated, such abscesses may rupture through the skin, producing sinuses that become secondarily infected.

Paraplegia. Paralysis of the lower extremities has in the past complicated from 6 to 24% of reported cases of tuberculosis of the spine. With earlier diagnosis and more effective treatment, it is much less common. It is seen mostly in tuberculosis of the upper or middle thoracic vertebrae, where the spinal cord is relatively large in diameter, the spinal canal narrow, and the spine slightly kyphotic.

The spinal cord may be compressed by an abscess, a caseating or granulating mass, or an edge of bone or disk that protrudes posteriorly as the kyphosis increases. Edema of the cord and thrombosis of local vessels may play a part.

The first symptom may be a gait disturbance from inability to control the legs and feet. The paraplegia is usually of spastic type with hyperactive deep reflexes. The sphincters are sometimes involved; sensory changes are usually slight.

Treatment. The general antituberculous treatment, outlined previously (p. 152), is essential. The local treatment often consists of three phases: preoperative recumbency, surgical treatment, and postoperative immobilization.

Preoperative recumbency. Rest on a foam rubber mattress over a fracture board may be adequate to relieve stresses on the diseased vertebrae. More efficient support of the spine may be obtained by having the patient lie on a Bradford frame, which is a pipe frame across which canvas is tightly stretched. Body casts provide excellent immobilization. In some orthopaedic institutions full-length posterior plaster shells are used. Lesions of the cervical spine are often treated by recumbency with head traction or with a brace incorporating the head, neck, and trunk. Nonoperative treatment is ordinarily continued for at least several months and often much longer (Fig. 95.) The patient is usually considered ready for operation when he has no fever, his erythrocyte sedimentation rate is low, and serial roentgenograms suggest slowing of the destructive process.

Surgical treatment. Arthrodesis, or surgical fusion, of the spine is usually indicated to provide relatively prompt internal splinting and permanent rest of the affected vertebrae. The surgical technic used most frequently is the posterior arthrodesis devised in 1912 by Hibbs. It consists of splitting the spinous processes into small fragments, chipping up the outer surfaces of the laminal arches, removing the cartilage from the articular facets, and

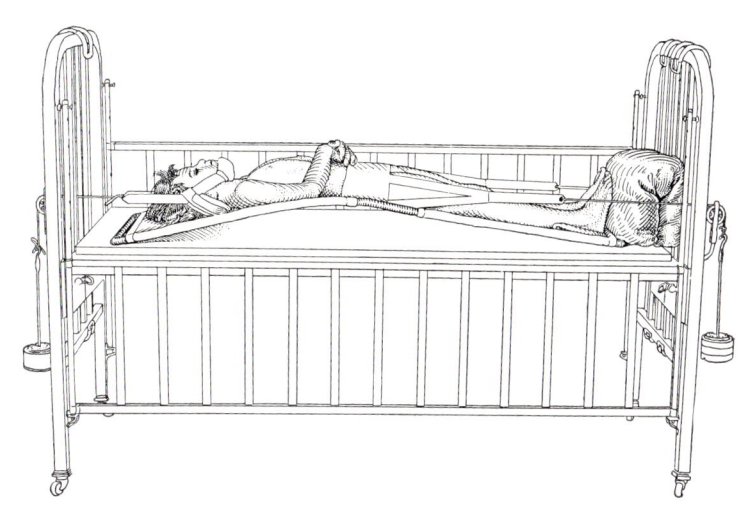

Fig. 95. Whitman frame with head and pelvic traction for treatment of tuberculosis of the lumbar spine. Note fracture board in place of mattress.

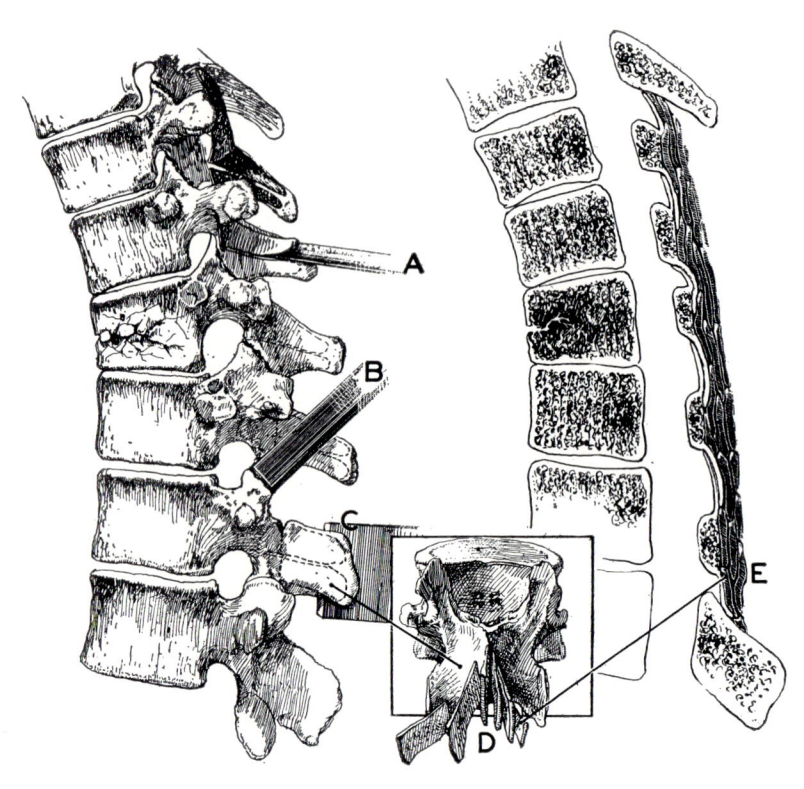

Fig. 96. Hibbs method of stabilization of the spine. **A,** Gouge splitting off and turning down chips from spinous processes and laminae; **B,** chisel removing cartilage from articular facets; **C,** splitting of spinous processes; **D,** posterior view showing splitting of spinous processes; **E,** sagittal section of spine showing continuous layer of small grafts posterior to the denuded laminae.

placing the bone chips as bridges across the denuded bone of the posterior surfaces of the vertebral arches (Fig. 96). It is often advisable, especially in adults, to reinforce this bridge of bone chips with additional autogenous bone from the iliac crest or the tibia or with bone from a bone bank. The Albee method of spinal arthrodesis, now seldom used, comprises longitudinal splitting of the spinous processes and inserting a long cortical bone graft from the tibia between their two halves.

Very early cases of spinal tuberculosis may respond favorably to evacuation of the pus, necrotic soft tissue, and sequestra. After thorough removal of the diseased tissue, bone grafts may be inserted. Occasionally a costotransversectomy, lateral rhachotomy, or laminectomy is indicated when paraplegia secondary to spinal tuberculosis fails to respond to nonoperative treatment.

Postoperative immobilization. Recumbency and antibiotic therapy are continued as healing of the spine takes place. A period of three to six months in bed is often advisable, after which the patient is allowed to be up with a plaster body jacket (Figs. 97 and 98) or a brace (Fig. 99) for perhaps

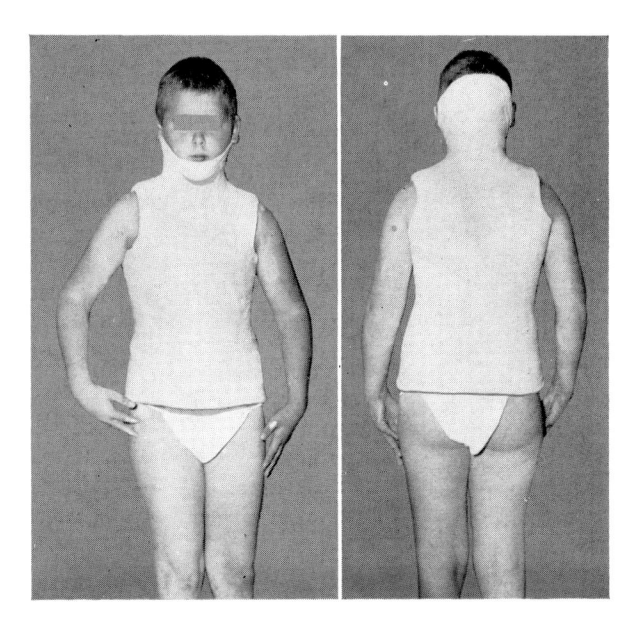

Fig. 97. Modified Calot jacket (sometimes called Minerva jacket) for immobilization of upper dorsal or lower cervical spine.

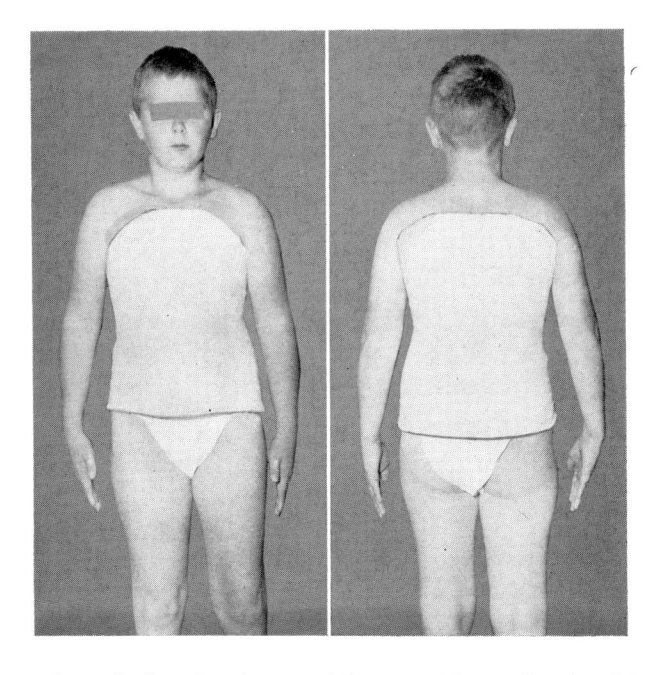

Fig. 98. Sayre plaster body jacket for immobilization of lower dorsal and lumbar spine.

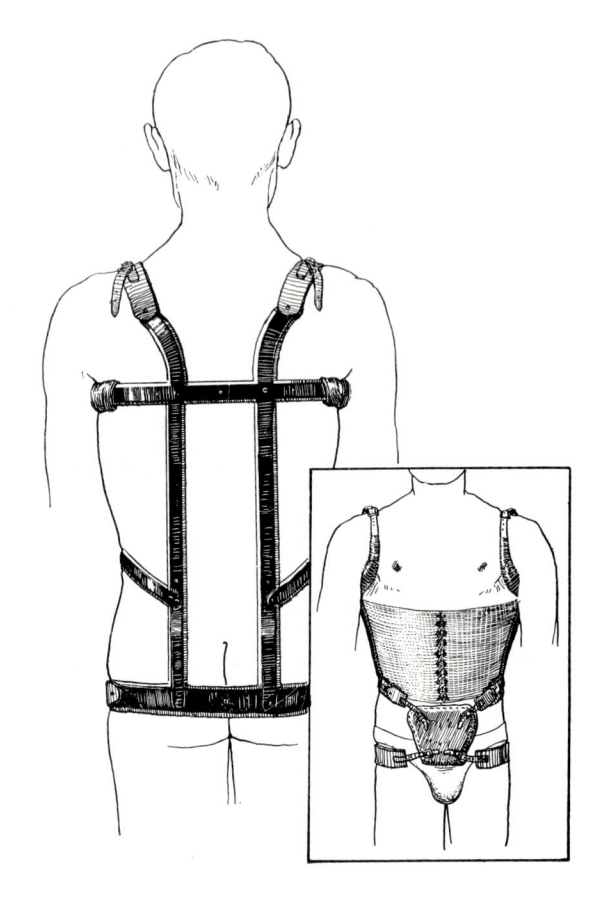

Fig. 99. Large spinal brace for treatment of tuberculosis of lower dorsal or upper lumbar spine (modification of Taylor and Bennett braces).

another six months, the support being discarded when roentgenograms show mature bony fusion.

Subsequently the patient should be re-examined at regular intervals for several years in order that any reactivation of tuberculous infection may be recognized and treated early.

TUBERCULOSIS OF THE SACROILIAC JOINT

Sacroiliac tuberculosis is uncommon, chiefly affects young adults, and may be associated with tuberculous foci in lungs or spine.

Clinical picture. The first symptom may be dull low back pain, often with hip or sciatic radiation. There may be a limp. In such cases differentiation from more common low back entities, such as disk lesions or Strümpell-Marie arthritis, is important and sometimes difficult. Roentgenograms showing distortion of the sacroiliac joint margins by irregular erosive changes support the diagnosis of tuberculosis. Abscess formation usually becomes obvious in late cases; occasionally it is the first evidence of disease.

Treatment. General measures include antituberculous drugs and rest. The affected joint may be immobilized by a short double spica cast extending from chest to knees. The surgical treatment, often done early, usually includes extirpation of the diseased tissue and arthrodesis of the joint. After a period of postoperative immobilization to allow bony fusion, activity is gradually resumed.

TUBERCULOSIS OF THE HIP

Of the joints of the extremities, the hip is most frequently involved by tuberculosis (Figs. 100 to 103). The clinical picture and the treatment vary greatly with the promptness with which the lesion has been recognized; they exemplify principles that apply also in tuberculosis of the other joints of the extremities.

Clinical picture. In the *early case*, with a small tuberculous focus which is intraosseous or intrasynovial, there may be no symptoms except a limp and slight discomfort in the hip or referred to the knee. The only physical signs may be slight restriction of passive mobility by spasm and possibly some tenderness over the hip. When a case is diagnosed and treated at this early stage, the patient has a good prognosis for retaining hip function.

In the *later case*, with tuberculous destruction of the joint surfaces, there may be severe muscle spasm, deformity, swelling of the joint, atrophy of the muscles, and some shortening of the extremity. An abscess may appear, and the disability is severe.

Treatment. In the *early case*, in which intra-articular changes are mini-

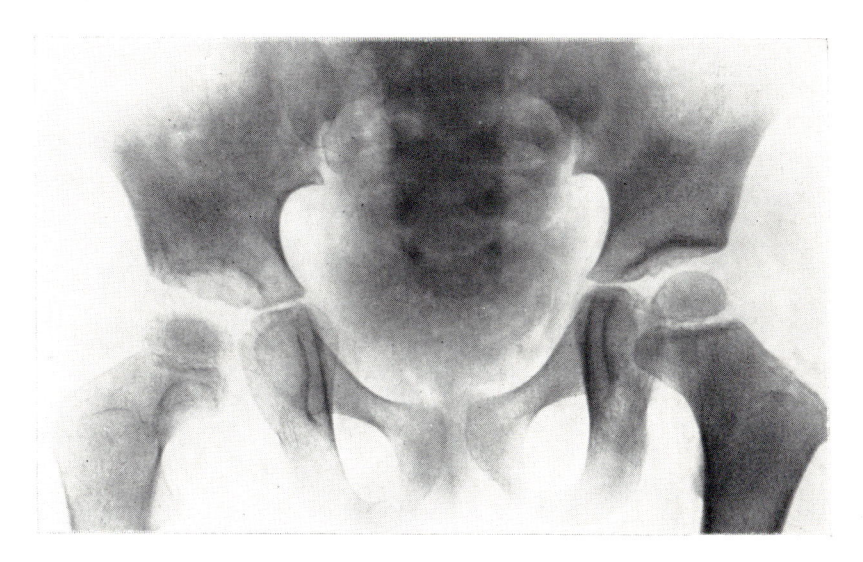

Fig. 100. Roentgenogram of tuberculosis of right hip in boy 3½ years old. Note changes in inferior portion of femoral neck, osteoporosis of upper end of femur and acetabulum, flattening of capital epiphysis, and lateral displacement of femoral head with relation to acetabulum.

162   *Handbook of orthopaedic surgery*

mal, healing without loss of joint mobility is the goal of treatment. Antituberculous drugs are given for many months, and the joint is put at rest by means of traction or cast (Figs. 104 and 105). Early operation may be indicated to eradicate necrotic tissue and pus about or in the joint. After the lesion has healed, weight bearing is cautiously resumed.

In the *late case* and in cases which have responded poorly to early treatment, extensive intra-articular destruction has usually occurred, painless mobility cannot be regained, and a fused hip becomes the therapeutic goal.

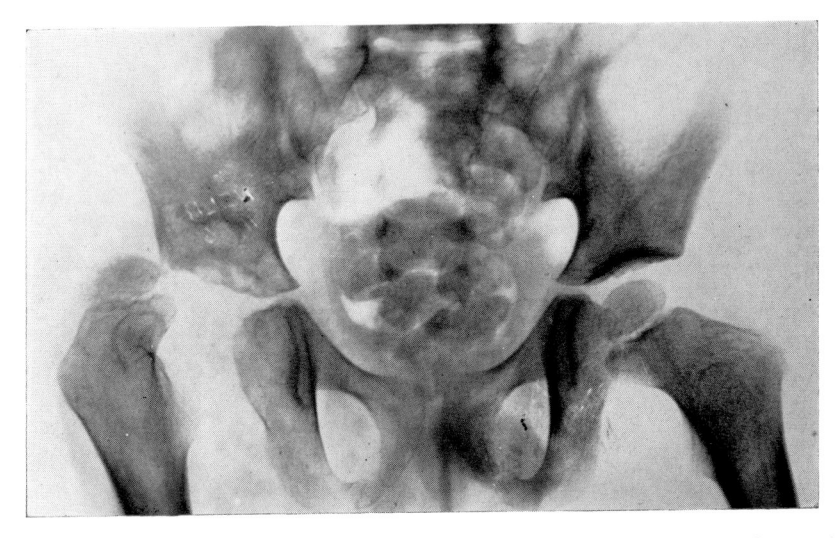

Fig. 101. Roentgenogram of same patient as shown in Fig. 100, one month later. This pathologic dislocation of his tuberculous right hip occurred when skin traction was removed.

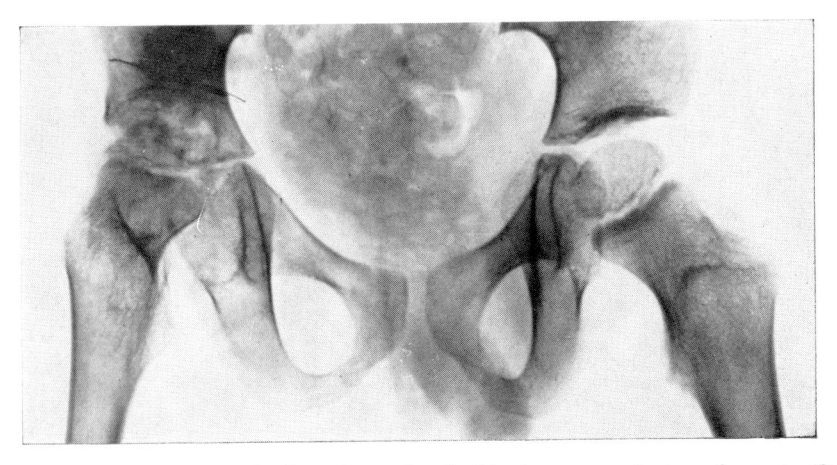

Fig. 102. Roentgenogram of tuberculosis of right hip in same patient as shown in Fig. 100, after two years of immobilization in plaster casts. Antituberculous drugs had not yet been made available. Note erosion of acetabulum, density changes in capital epiphysis, and upward displacement of femur.

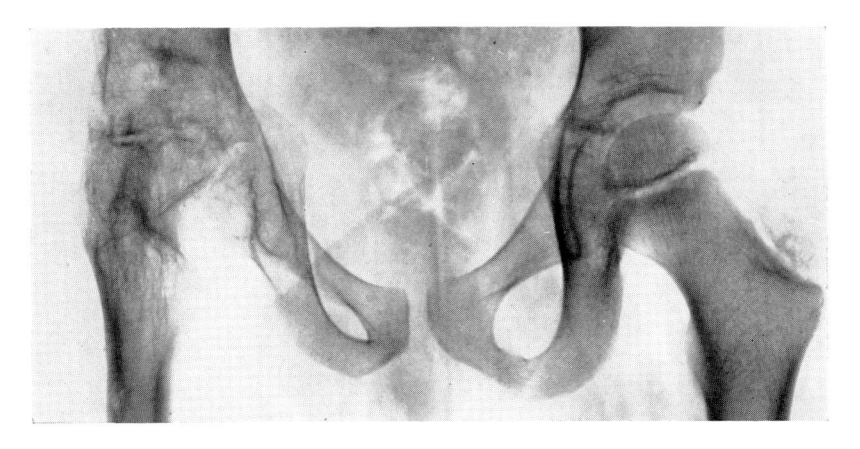

Fig. 103. Roentgenogram of tuberculosis of right hip in same patient as shown in Fig. 100, four and one half years later. Arthrodesis had been done two and one half years previously. Note continuous bony structure from pelvis to upper end of femur, upward displacement of femur, and marked atrophy of femoral shaft.

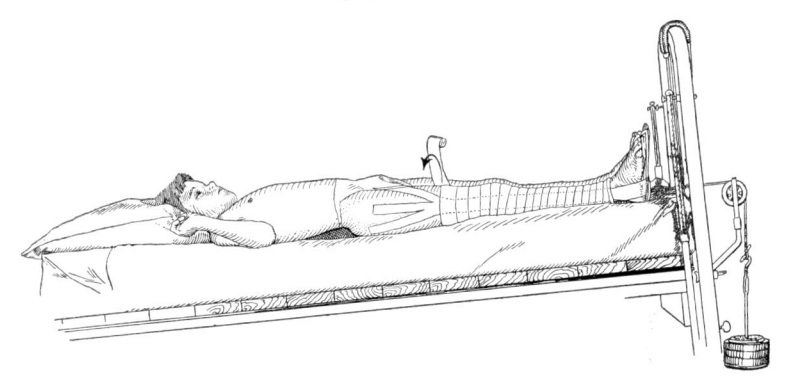

Fig. 104. Skin traction used in treating tuberculosis of right hip. Longitudinal strips of cloth lined by foam rubber or an adhesive are held in place by an elastic cotton bandage. For countertraction the foot of the bed has been elevated.

A hip solidly ankylosed in good functional position is permanently strong, painless, and unlikely to develop reinfection. As a rule the optimal position (p. 198) consists of about 5 degrees of abduction, 5 degrees of external rotation, and 10 to 25 degrees of flexion. When intra-articular structures have been destroyed by tuberculosis, arthrodesis is usually advised as soon as the patient's general condition will permit. Tuberculous tissue is cleaned out of the joint, the cancellous bone of the femoral head is placed in contact with that of the acetabulum, and an iliac graft is fixed from ilium to femur. Subtrochanteric osteotomy may be done to relieve stress at the hip joint line. The operation must be followed by an ample and closely fitting bilateral spica cast for at least six to nine months, or until roentgenograms show strong bony union, after which a gradual return to weight bearing under supervision is allowed.

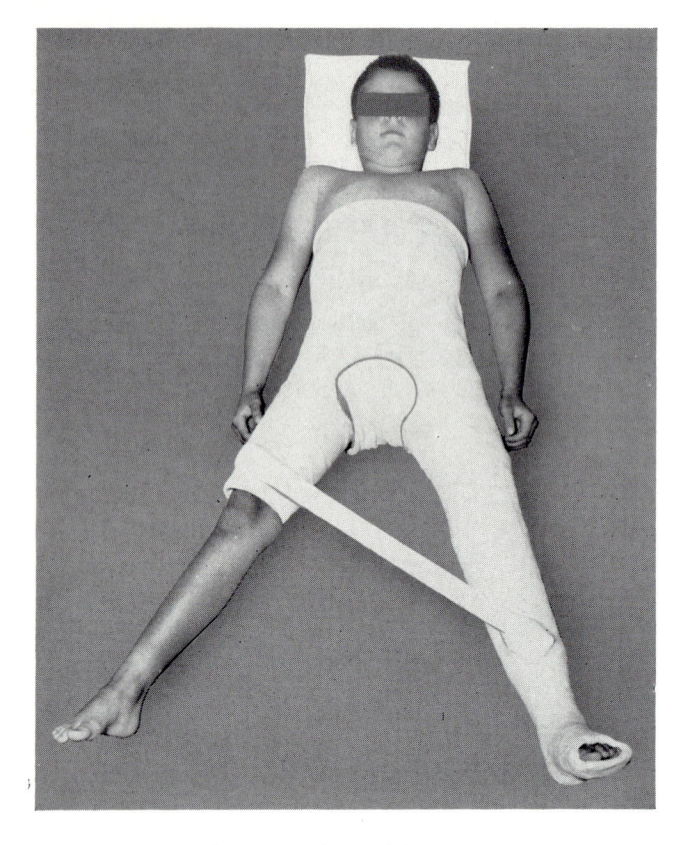

Fig. 105. Bilateral spica cast for immobilizing left hip. This type of cast is useful in acute and chronic infections, injuries, and postoperative treatment.

A method of fusing the upper portion of the femoral shaft to the ischium by osteotomy and bone graft has been described by Trumble and modified by Brittain. Direct femoro-ischial transplantation has been described by Bosworth. These operations have the advantage of permanently relieving the diseased hip joint of the pressure of weight bearing. They are particularly useful in late cases when there has been extensive destruction of the ilium or the upper end of the femur

TUBERCULOSIS OF OTHER JOINTS

Although the spine and, next, the hip are most commonly involved by tuberculosis, any joint of the body may on occasion be affected. Third in frequency is the knee. Tuberculosis of the ankle or foot is more common in adolescents and adults than in young children, tends to respond poorly to treatment, and ends occasionally in amputation. Tuberculosis of the upper extremity, according to Steindler, is only one seventh as common as that of the lower extremity. In the upper extremity the elbow is most frequently involved, next the shoulder, and then the wrist; all are seen more often in adults than in children. Relatively frequent in children, however, is tuberculous dactylitis, which may involve the metacarpals, metatarsals, or phalanges.

The diagnosis and treatment of tuberculosis in these locations follow the principles previously outlined.

CHAPTER 8

Chronic arthritis

THE most important cause of pains and aches in the joints is *chronic arthritis*, which in this context includes *rheumatoid arthritis, osteoarthritis,* and several related, less common forms of chronic joint disease.

In individual cases the disability caused by chronic arthritis varies from trivial and temporary to complete and permanent. In the aggregate, disability from chronic arthritis is enormous because of its high incidence in adult years and its chronicity. Statistical studies have indicated that in the United States 4,500,000 persons have chronic arthritis and that of this number 800,000 are partially disabled and 200,000 totally disabled.

The causes of chronic arthritis have not been established. In recent years investigation of this and related problems has been greatly accelerated. In the United States this research has in large part been guided and financed by a number of scientific, lay, and governmental organizations dedicated to clearer understanding of arthritis and to better treatment of arthritic patients.

Most general practitioners and many specialists are concerned with evaluating and treating the patient who has chronic arthritis. To his therapy orthopaedics can frequently make a number of helpful contributions. In many early cases pain can be relieved and deformity prevented by the use of appropriate physical therapy, braces, and casts. In late cases major improvement of deformity and disability can often be accomplished by carefully chosen surgical procedures and postoperative orthopaedic rehabilitation.

Until more accurate knowledge of the causes and interrelationships of its subvarieties becomes available, no completely satisfactory classification of chronic arthritis can be devised. Two major types which can be clearly differentiated, however, and which warrant detailed consideration are *rheumatoid arthritis* and *osteoarthritis (degenerative joint disease).*

This chapter is adapted from the *Primer on the rheumatic diseases* prepared by the American Rheumatism Association and published by the American Medical Association in 1959.

RHEUMATOID ARTHRITIS
(ATROPHIC ARTHRITIS, PROLIFERATIVE ARTHRITIS)

Rheumatoid arthritis is a connective tissue disease characterized by chronic inflammatory changes in the synovial membranes and other structures, by migratory swelling and stiffness of the joints in its early stage, and by more or less deformity, ankylosis, and invalidism in its late stage.

Incidence. Rheumatoid arthritis occurs throughout the world but is most frequent in temperate climates. Women are affected three times as often as men; 80% of the cases begin in persons between 25 and 50 years of age; the highest incidence is found between 35 and 40 years.

Etiology. The cause of rheumatoid arthritis has not been determined. A slight familial tendency has been proved. Hypotheses of the etiology have included infection, abnormality of the peripheral circulation, endocrine imbalance, metabolic disturbance, allergic phenomenon, faulty adaptation to physical or psychic stress, and many other concepts. Despite the tremendous amount of data provided by recent laboratory and clinical investigation, no hypothesis is as yet supported by enough evidence to be accepted as the true or major explanation of the disease.

Rheumatoid arthritis is currently regarded as belonging to a group of connective tissue diseases that exhibit somewhat similar clinical and pathologic changes. Other members of the group are systemic lupus erythematosus, polyarteritis nodosa, dermatomyositis, scleroderma, and rheumatic fever. Fundamental relationship between these diseases, however, is questionable.

Pathology. Of the pathologic changes which may be found in many parts of the body in rheumatoid arthritis, the most constant and most characteristic affect the joints.

The earliest change is inflammation of the synovial membrane. It becomes congested and edematous, is infiltrated by leukocytes and chronic inflammatory cells, and is further thickened by the proliferation of synovial cells and villous hypertrophy. Peripheral portions of the articular cartilage are involved in the inflammatory reaction, undergo lysis, and are replaced by granulation tissue. Similar inflammatory changes take place in the subchondral marrow spaces, and there is resorption of bony trabeculae. A thin layer of granulation tissue, called a *pannus,* spreads from the synovial lining over parts of the articular cartilage, covering and eroding its surface. Adhesions of granulation tissue may undergo fibrosis and restrict joint mobility. The synovial fluid tends to be cloudy; its white cell content is increased. In later stages the discolored and thinned articular cartilage becomes eroded, exposing areas of cancellous bone. Maturing granulation tissue between the bone ends may lead to fibrous ankylosis or, with ossification, to solid bony ankylosis. Unless preventive measures have been taken, the position of ankylosis may be one of deformity and severe disability.

Many patients with rheumatoid arthritis show more or less typical pathologic changes in extra-articular tissues. The most characteristic histologic lesion is a granuloma-like nodule of chronically inflamed connective tissue, which has been found in the subcutaneous tissues in 15 to 20% of the cases. In the skeletal muscles, focal infiltrations of lymphocytes are a common finding, together with atrophy and fibrosis. Cardiac changes including pericarditis, myocarditis, coronary arteritis, and granulomatous inflammation of the valves, rarely of sufficient magnitude to cause symptoms, have been demonstrated frequently at necropsy.

Symptoms. The type of onset and the progression of rheumatoid arthritis vary widely. In 75% of the cases the onset is insidious. The joint symptoms may be preceded by periods of fatigue, lassitude, and muscular stiffness, associated with loss of weight. At first there may be fleeting pains in one or more joints. These are followed by joint symptoms of more persistent type, consisting first of constant pain, swelling, and stiffness. Additional joints may become involved. Later severe muscle atrophy develops. The joints may become deformed and ankylosed. The proximal interphalangeal and metacarpophalangeal joints of the hands are often affected first, and next the knees. The pain is usually not limited to the joint but may be felt in adjacent muscles, tendons, and ligaments. The symptoms tend to be worse with bad weather, overexercise, and fatigue.

About one fourth of the cases begin more acutely, with an abrupt onset of pain, swelling, and tenderness in one or several joints. These changes may progress rapidly to produce severe deformities within a few weeks, or they may subside to a less acute phase.

The constitutional symptoms frequently include weakness and fatigue. Malaise and fever are common during periods of acute joint inflammation. The disease often seems to be influenced by emotional and psychologic factors.

Physical signs. Periarticular swelling is usually the earliest local sign. It is most characteristically found in the smaller joints of the hands and feet, especially in the middle joints of the fingers, where it produces a spindle-

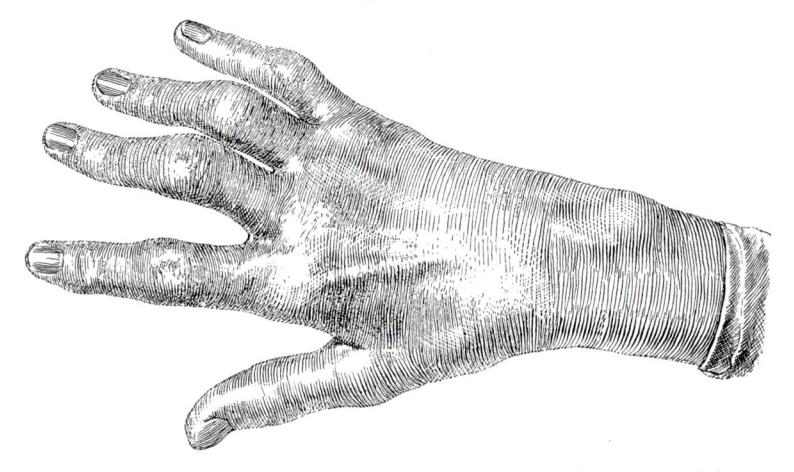

Fig. 106. Rheumatoid arthritis of the hand, early stage. Note enlargement of the proximal interphalangeal joints. (After Duncan.)

Chronic arthritis 169

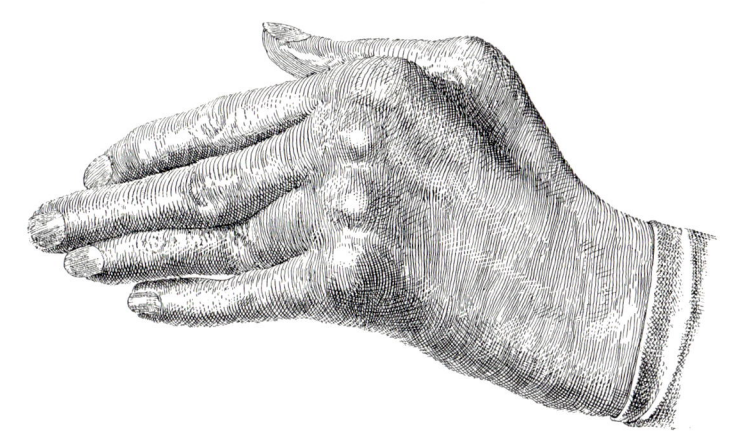

Fig. 107. Rheumatoid arthritis of the hand, late stage. Note enlargement and flexion contracture of metacarpophalangeal joints, ulnar deviation of the fingers, subluxation of proximal interphalangeal joint of ring finger, and atrophy of the hand. (After Duncan.)

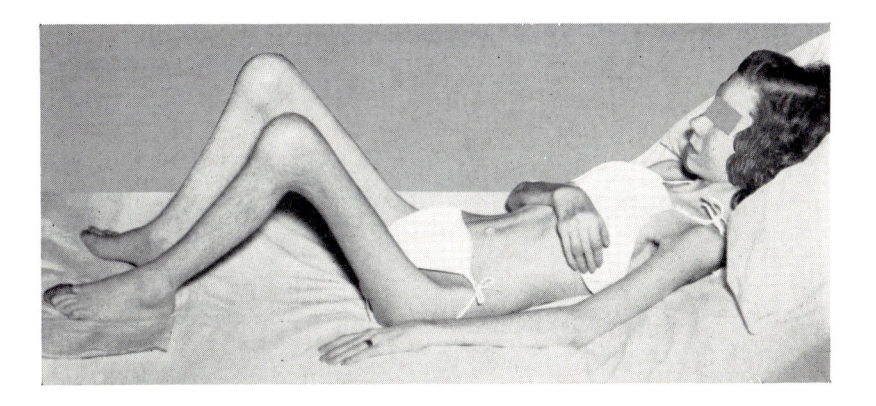

Fig. 108. Rheumatoid arthritis (Still's disease) in 16-year-old girl. Note enlargement of knees and ankles, flexion contractures of hips and knees, equinous contractures, and severe muscle atrophy in right hand, thighs, and legs.

shaped appearance (Fig. 106). Any joint of the body may be involved. In early stages the joints may be acutely tender; later they become less sensitive. The tenderness may extend into the adjoining muscles and tendon sheaths. There is slight increase of surface temperature over the joints, but redness is unusual. Muscular weakness and atrophy are quite characteristic (Fig. 107). Flexion deformity may result from positions that are assumed in an effort to relieve pain.

In the extremities the skin may become thin and glossy. The fingers are often cool and moist. In 15 to 20% of the patients fibrous nodules occur in the subcutaneous tissue, especially about the elbows and the phalangeal joints. Generalized lymphadenopathy of moderate degree is a common finding.

There are many phases and *variants* of rheumatoid arthritis, as well as

possibly unrelated diseases which closely simulate it. Among them are the following:
1. *Still's disease,* or *juvenile rheumatoid arthritis* (Fig. 108), an uncommon, crippling disease of childhood, with which is associated enlargement of the lymph nodes and spleen.
2. *Felty's syndrome,* a severe arthritis associated with leukopenia and splenomegaly.
3. *Reiter's syndrome,* an ill-defined disease occurring chiefly in adult males and characterized by the triad of arthritis, nongonorrheal urethritis, and conjunctivitis.
4. *Psoriatic arthritis,* the intimate association of rheumatoid arthritis and psoriasis. In these patients exacerbations and remissions of the two diseases coincide, the distal interphalangeal joints are involved, and resorption of bone occurs at the articular margins.
5. *Palindromic rheumatism,* characterized by repeated, brief episodes of acute arthritis without residual joint damage. This may be an atypical or prodromal form of rheumatoid arthritis.
6. *Intermittent hydrarthrosis,* a recurring joint effusion usually in the knee and possibly representing a phase of rheumatoid arthritis. It is accompanied by characteristic local symptoms and signs (p. 410).

Clinical course. Many patients improve spontaneously, but their recovery may be hastened by treatment. When the disease is of short duration, there may be no objective joint changes. A long course, marked by exacerbations and remissions, is frequently seen. In about half of the cases the disease is progressive, with severe joint involvement and permanent changes in the joint tissues. Deformity may develop because the joint is held in the position of greatest comfort; thus the knees, for example, are likely to develop a flexion deformity. Maintenance of the flexed position may be followed by capsular contractures and destructive changes within the joint; later the development of adhesions and of partial or complete ankylosis causes a permanent deformity. However, at any stage the disease may become quiescent, in which event gradual improvement of the general health follows.

Roentgenographic picture. Swelling of the tissues about the affected joint is usually visible in the roentgenogram. In early stages the joint cavity may be distended by increased synovial fluid. Bone atrophy, evidenced by rarefaction and most marked in the epiphyseal areas, gradually becomes conspicuous. The contour of the articular surfaces is not necessarily altered. The cartilage space later becomes narrowed, however, and small areas of bone absorption, referred to as punched-out areas, may be seen; the edges still remain distinct. In advanced stages the articular margins may show bony spurs, ridges, and prominences. These hypertrophic features of the late case resemble the changes of osteoarthritis and tend to obscure the true atrophic character of the bone lesions. In late stages the articular surfaces may become ankylosed. There also may be subluxation or dislocation.

Laboratory findings. During active phases of the disease the erythrocyte sedimentation rate is usually elevated, the C-reactive protein test commonly positive, and a slight leukocytosis occasionally present. In these patients there is usually a normocytic, hypochromic anemia refractory to iron.

The serum globulin is increased in relation to the albumin. In most cases the serum, apparently because of the presence of abnormal macroglobulins sometimes called the "rheumatoid factor," will agglutinate or flocculate suspended particles such as hemolytic streptococci, sheep erythrocytes sensitized with amboceptor, and latex or bentonite particles sensitized with human gamma globulin. Several tests based on this property of the serum in rheumatoid arthritis have a diagnostic specificity as high as 85%. Their results may not be positive, however, in the first weeks or months of the disease. As a rule they are negative in juvenile rheumatoid arthritis, ankylosing spondylitis, and psoriatic arthritis.

The synovial fluid may appear cloudy and may clot spontaneously in vitro. Its viscosity is decreased. Its white cell count is high, varying with the severity of the arthritis. During acute attacks polymorphonuclear leukocytes are most numerous; in chronic stages most of the cells are lymphocytes.

Differential diagnosis. As a rule, late rheumatoid arthritis is easily recognizable; in early cases, the diagnosis may be obscure. Affections requiring differentiation include acute rheumatic fever, osteoarthritis, pyogenic arthritis, gonococcal arthritis, tuberculosis, gout, systemic lupus erythematosus, and syphilitic arthritis.

Rheumatic fever in its acute inflammatory stage may present a migratory polyarthritis simulating that of early rheumatoid arthritis. The patient with acute rheumatic fever is more likely to have had a streptococcic throat infection and to have electrocardiographic changes and a high fever. Serologic tests may aid in the differentiation. After the acute phase of rheumatic fever the joints recover completely, contrasting with their usual course in rheumatoid arthritis.

Osteoarthritis, or degenerative joint disease, may be confused with rheumatoid arthritis, especially in the aged. The following are the most significant points in differentiation: (1) rheumatoid arthritis is a systemic disease and the patients are sick, whereas in osteoarthritis they are not sick, (2) acute inflammatory signs and cutaneous changes are more commonly associated with rheumatoid arthritis, (3) weight-bearing joints are more often involved in osteoarthritis, (4) in the fingers, the proximal interphalangeal joints are more often involved in rheumatoid arthritis and the distal interphalangeal joints in osteoarthritis (Heberden's nodes, Fig. 109), (5) subcutaneous nodules are not seen in osteoarthritis, and (6) osteoporosis and bony ankylosis are uncommon in osteoarthritis. Erythrocyte sedimentation and serologic tests aid in differentiation.

In pyogenic arthritis, as a rule, a single large joint is involved. High fever and leukocytosis may distinguish the early case from rheumatoid arthritis, and destructive changes in the roentgenograms the late case. Aspiration of the joint may yield pus, and a positive culture confirms the diagnosis.

Gonococcal arthritis may simulate rheumatoid arthritis. Careful questioning and thorough examination of the patient are important. Frequently in acute gonorrheal arthritis the gonococcus can be demonstrated in the joint fluid.

Joint tuberculosis in its early stages may be confused with rheumatoid arthritis; however, tuberculosis is more often monarticular, is more insidious in its onset, and is likely to show more bone destruction roentgenographically. Culture of the joint exudate, inoculation of a guinea pig with it, or biopsy of the synovial membrane may be necessary to establish the diagnosis.

Gout must frequently be considered in the diagnosis. Its high blood uric acid is characteristic, especially in the absence of an increase of the nonprotein or urea nitrogen. In gout the joint quickly loses its tenderness between attacks, and the great toe is often the first part of the body to be affected (Fig. 110). Chronic gout is more often confused with rheumatoid arthritis than is acute gout. Roentgenographically the punched-out areas in bone characteristic of gout may be found also in rheumatoid arthritis. Biopsy of synovial membrane or suspected tophi may be indicated.

Systemic lupus erythematosus may be difficult to distinguish from rheumatoid arthritis. The exact relationship between these two diseases of connective tissue is unknown. In lupus erythematosus the patient usually shows minimal joint changes, severe systemic symptoms, and the characteristic L.E. cell phenomenon.

Syphilis can cause multiple joint involvement similar to that of rheumatoid arthritis. A positive complement fixation reaction in the blood, and sometimes also in the synovial fluid, is helpful in the differentiation.

Treatment. The treatment of rheumatoid arthritis must be suited to the individual patient after a careful survey of the various factors in his particular case. The most important elements in the treatment are general measures, drug therapy, local treatment of joints, prevention of deformity, and correction of deformity.

General measures. Rheumatoid arthritis is a systemic disease requiring treatment of the individual as a whole as well as treatment of his affected joints. Among general measures, rest is of first importance. During acute stages of the disease, complete bed rest may be indicated. With it should be combined a program of selected exercises, including deep breathing, to improve general muscular tone and minimize atrophy. Massages are beneficial. As the patient improves he is allowed to do more, but not to the point of fatigue. His day should be planned to include periods of therapy, exercises, recreation, and rest.

The diet should be well balanced, and undernutrition or obesity should be corrected. Anemia, if present, should be treated. Care should be taken to prevent exposure to cold or dampness. Any infectious process that appears to be impairing the patient's general health should be treated. Anxiety and worry, which hinder recovery, should be mitigated. The physician's attitude toward the patient should demonstrate sympathetic and reassuring interest.

Drug therapy. As yet no specific, curative drug for rheumatoid arthritis has been found. Among preparations in current use are salicylates, phenylbutazone, antimalarials, gold salts, and steroids.

The salicylates are most helpful for the alleviation of pain. Plain, coated, or buffered aspirin is the most commonly used drug. It may be given in dosage of one to three 325 mg. (5-grain) tablets two to six times a day, depending upon the severity of the arthritis and the patient's tolerance.

Phenylbutazone will sometimes produce dramatic relief of arthritic symptoms, but it is in no way curative. It may be given in an initial dosage of 600 mg. a day and gradually reduced to 100 to 200 mg. daily. If the toxic effects of a drug rash, thrombocytopenia, or leukopenia appear, use of the drug should be promptly discontinued. Many rheumatologists consider phenylbutazone too dangerous to be given over a long period of time.

Antimalarial compounds, such as chloroquine phosphate, often seem to exert a slow but long-lasting suppressive effect in rheumatoid arthritis. They may produce toxic reactions, however, which necessitate discontinuance of the drug.

Treatment with soluble gold salts, or chrysotherapy, may suppress or even arrest the active rheumatoid process and so induce lengthy remission. Chrysotherapy is especially effective in early cases. Its mode of action is not well understood. Gold salts are given by intramuscular injection in small doses over a long period of time. The usefulness of gold therapy is distinctly limited by its occasionally dangerous toxic effects on kidneys, intestines, and skin; toxic effects appear in from 10 to 20% of the treated patients. Nevertheless, some observers consider chrysotherapy the best form of treatment for all early rheumatoid arthritis and report good results in 50 to 60% of the patients so treated.

The steroid drugs, cortisone and the new synthetic hormones, have an important but limited place in the treatment of active rheumatoid arthritis. They are potent anti-inflammatory agents which may produce dramatic alleviation of symptoms and signs, reduction of fever, reversal of abnormal laboratory findings, and psychologic improvement. However, they do not alter the fundamental pathologic process of rheumatoid arthritis. Their suppressive action is temporary, whereas their prolonged administration may lead to adverse changes like those of adrenocortical hyperfunction in Cushing's syndrome. The long list of these undesirable effects includes such formidable complications as skeletal demineralization, pathologic fracture, peptic ulcer, edema from sodium and water retention, hypopotassemia and muscle weakness, depressive psychosis, reactivation of infections such as tuberculosis, and atrophy of the adrenal cortex. Continued investigation may discover a steroid derivative less prone to cause these complications. Currently, steroid therapy should be reserved for the management of patients whose active disease remains resistant to other forms of treatment.

Local treatment of joints. Physical therapy is helpful in all stages of rheumatoid arthritis. Local applications of heat by means of warm moist compresses or packs, infrared radiation, whirlpool baths, or diathermy usually alleviate the acute pain. Paraffin baths are most helpful for arthritic hands and feet. Heat should be followed by gentle massage of the muscles above and below the affected joints. Liniments rubbed lightly on the joints will often ease the discomfort. To minimize joint stiffness and muscle atrophy, active exercise of the affected joints, without weight bearing, should be carried out several times a day. In these exercises the joints should be put through their full range of voluntary motion. Pain and fatigue must be avoided. The amount of exercise may be increased gradually if there is no unfavorable reaction. After the acute stage of the disease has passed, most patients can be helped by occupational therapy. Posture exercises are often indicated.

In acute arthritis the pain is sometimes so severe that it is advisable to provide rest for the joint by immobilizing it in a light splint or plaster cast. Immobilization should be continued no longer than is necessary to relieve the pain, and as soon as possible the joint should be taken out of the splint at least once a day and be put actively through its full range of motion or through as much motion as the pain will allow. Aspiration of synovial fluid will sometimes relieve the pain of an acutely distended joint capsule. Intra-articular injection of an anti-inflammatory steroid such as hydrocortisone may be helpful. Despite all technical precautions, multiple or repeated injections entail risk of infection.

Prevention of deformity. The prevention of deformity in rheumatoid arthritis is of the utmost importance because of the frequency of fibrous and bony ankylosis. The most important preventive measure is to alternate periods of splinting in good functional position with periods of active range-of-motion exercises. When an ankylosis cannot be averted, however, care should be taken that the joint become stiff in the best position for function (p. 197). This can be accomplished by fixing the joint in its optimal position by means of traction, a plaster splint, or a brace.

Correction of deformity. Most deformities from rheumatoid arthritis can be either greatly improved or corrected by orthopaedic means without resort to surgery. A common example is flexion contracture of the knee, a disfiguring and disabling deformity making it impossible for the patient to stand or walk in anything approaching normal fashion. Often the knee flexion can be gradually overcome by skin traction without too much discomfort and with care to prevent posterior subluxation of the upper end of the tibia. An alternative treatment is the use of a long leg cast, which is cut transversely back of the knee and wedged at intervals of a few days into increasing extension or which is straightened gradually with turnbuckles. Such casts must be well padded and used with caution to avoid causing pressure sores. Forceful manipulation to correct the deformity, with or without anesthesia, is usually best avoided because of the likelihood of causing additional injury to already damaged and weakened joint structures. To prevent recurrence of the flexion deformity, the goal of treatment must be complete extension, and it should usually be maintained for at least several months by means of a long leg brace.

Arthritic deformities that fail to respond to closed methods can often be corrected readily by surgical means. Such operations must be chosen with great regard for the qualifications and needs of the individual patient. A resistant knee flexion contracture may be treated by *capsulotomy*, or surgical release of the constricted or adherent joint capsule. Secondary contracture of an overlying tendon may require *tenotomy* and lengthening. A knee joint chronically enlarged by arthritic thickening of its lining membrane may be improved by *synovectomy*. The crippling deformity of bony ankylosis in flexion is correctible by *osteotomy*.

In some joints the stiffness that follows rheumatoid arthritis can be treated successfully by *arthroplasty* (p. 200). As a rule the hip and elbow are the joints most favorable for arthroplasty. To mobilize the stiffened hip the orthopaedist must decide whether to advise a cup arthroplasty, replacement of the femoral head with a metal prosthesis, an osteotomy, or other type of reconstructive operation. Mobility can be restored to an ankylosed jaw by resecting the condyle of the mandible. Surgical fusion, or *arthrodesis* (p. 197), may be indicated for an arthritic joint when maximum stability and freedom from pain are desired.

A spine partially ankylosed in a position of kyphosis can sometimes be improved by mobilization with exercises and recumbency in hyperextension; a strong back brace is then applied to maintain the corrected position. Bony ankylosis in severe kyphosis may be improved by vertebral osteotomy; the operation must be done with great care to prevent injury of the spinal cord. For the wrists and fingers, intermittent support in functional position and elastic or spring tension splinting to overcome contractures are of the greatest value. Late arthritic disabilities of the hand can often be helped by carefully selected surgical procedures.

The patient who has been severely disabled by arthritis is usually most grateful for any improvement of joint position or motion, although it be only the ability to put one hand behind the head to comb the hair. When a deformity is permanent, even its partial correction may be extremely helpful.

Prognosis. When rheumatoid arthritis is recognized early as a systemic disease and is treated with vigor and persistence, reasonably good results can usually be obtained. Patients with slight changes in the joints may recover spontaneously; in late cases, long remissions may occur. With proper orthopaedic therapy, the serious consequences of the disease can usually be prevented or greatly ameliorated.

OSTEOARTHRITIS (DEGENERATIVE JOINT DISEASE)

Osteoarthritis is a form of chronic arthritis found commonly in middle-aged and elderly people, affecting especially the weight-bearing joints, and characterized by degenerative changes in articular cartilage and bony overgrowth at the joint margins.

Etiology. The cause of osteoarthritis is obscure; it seems to include mechanical, dystrophic, and genetic factors. Degenerative changes in articular cartilage are more common and more severe with advancing age, in the weight-bearing joints, and in joints which have become incongruent or have been used abnormally. The fact that osteoarthritic changes are often localized to only part of a single joint suggests that there are causative factors other than age and attrition. Mechanical injury, which may consist of a single major trauma or of repeated minor traumas, may cause intra-articular changes that act as a predisposing or aggravating cause. In people over 45 years of age whose parents have suffered from arthritis late in life there is a greater susceptibility than in those who have no family history of arthritis. Although no clear-cut relationship between endocrine abnormalities and osteoarthritis has been established, degenerative joint changes occurring in women at the menopause have sometimes been spoken of as *climacteric* or *menopausal arthritis.*

Pathology. In osteoarthritis, in contradistinction to rheumatoid arthritis, characteristic early changes appear in articular cartilage rather than in the synovial membrane. The cartilage seems to lose some of its ability to withstand mechanical stresses. A number of microscopic degenerative changes have been described, such as swelling of the chondrocytes and chondromucoid softening of the matrix. Grossly the cartilage undergoes splitting, fibrillation, gradual thinning, and widespread degeneration. In late stages the underlying bone may become denuded. About the cartilaginous edges, reactive chondro-osseous spicules or *osteophytes* form quite early. These appear in roentgenograms as spurs and lipping. Occasionally the osteophytes become detached and form loose bodies within the joint. As degeneration of the cartilage progresses, the underlying bone usually becomes eburnated and deformed. In osteoarthritis, atrophy of the bone trabeculae occurs quite late and is thought to be partly the result of a decrease in physical activity. There are often marked changes of shape in the end of the bone, increased bony deposits in and about the areas of cartilaginous degeneration, and erosion of bone beneath the destroyed cartilage. The synovial membrane and periarticular tissues usually show little change but may become considerably thickened. The amount of synovial fluid remains essentially normal.

Symptoms and signs. In the early stages of osteoarthritis the patient usually complains of stiffness of one or more joints, associated with an aching pain in or about the affected joint. The involvement is more often monarticular than polyarticular. This stiffness tends to become less noticeable after moderate use of the joint. Continued use is followed, however, by marked discomfort, which may be relieved by rest, support, and heat. The patient tires easily on exertion. His symptoms are worse in cold, wet weather. In this stage there is slight enlargement of the affected joints, which may be slightly tender about their margins; these changes are usually most noticeable in the fingers and knees. Bony enlargement of the distal interphalangeal joints (*Heberden's nodes*) is one of the commonest signs (Fig. 109).

Later in the course of the disease there are marked limitation of joint motion and considerable disability, especially in the larger joints. There may be referred pain from pressure upon nerve roots. Pain may then be present while the joint is resting, as well as when it is in motion. Malalignment of the joint is a frequent result of the irregular degeneration and loss of articu-

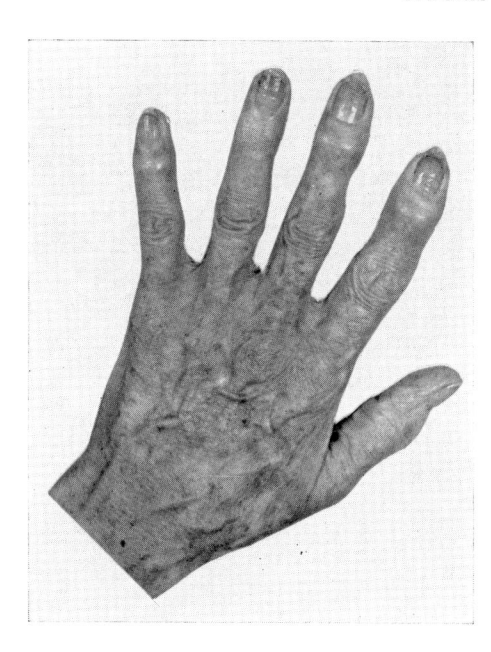

Fig. 109. Osteoarthritis of the hand. Note enlargement of distal joints of the index, middle, and little fingers (Heberden's nodes).

lar cartilage. Crepitation may be frequently noticed, and loose intra-articular fragments may produce transient locking. Examination at this stage reveals moderate swelling and puffiness and a loss of the normal joint contour.

A tendency to early fatigue is characteristic of osteoarthritis. Many of the patients are obese. There may be a disturbance of body mechanics with a sagging, protuberant abdomen, a flat chest, and abnormal weight-bearing lines in the feet, knees, and hips, resulting in chronic strain of these joints. Generalized arteriosclerosis is often associated.

Clinical course. Osteoarthritis usually exhibits a slowly progressive and often intermittent course. Periods of improvement are frequent, especially under proper treatment. Trauma may intensify and prolong the symptoms. More disability follows involvement of the spine and lower extremities than that of the upper extremities. As the condition progresses in the spine, there may be a limitation of the normal range of motion, localized pain from impingement of the sensitive bony overgrowths, and radiating pain from impingement of bony overgrowths on nerve roots. Osteoarthritis may progress to the point of causing an extreme disability of one or more joints but, unlike rheumatoid arthritis, seldom results in bony ankylosis except in the spine.

Roentgenographic picture. Roentgenographic signs of osteoarthritis may antedate the symptoms, or the reverse may occur. Thinning of the degenerated cartilage appears as narrowing of the cartilage space. Proliferation of bone produces sharpening of intra-articular prominences, spurs, lipping, bridging between adjacent vertebral bodies, and condensation of articular margins. At the same time cystlike spaces frequently appear in the subjacent cancellous bone. Bone atrophy may be noticeable.

Laboratory findings. There are no diagnostic laboratory findings. The blood picture, including the sedimentation rate, is usually normal. No characteristic changes are found in the synovial fluid.

Diagnosis. The diagnosis can usually be made after careful analysis of the history, and of the joint changes as shown by physical and roentgenographic examination. Osteoarthritis is sometimes difficult to distinguish from rheumatoid arthritis, and the two may coexist. Osteoarthritis may be simulated also by gouty, tuberculous, syphilitic, or neuropathic joint disease. Osteitis deformans should be excluded. Occasionally neoplasms must be considered in the diagnosis. In doubtful cases biopsy may be indicated.

Treatment. Treatment includes general measures, drug therapy, local treatment of joints, prevention of deformity, and surgical measures.

General measures. It is important to relieve the patient's apprehension and secure his constructive attitude toward treatment by explanation and reassurance. Usually he may be told that, although his joint structures cannot be restored to normal, the osteoarthritic process is essentially benign and will not shorten his life or cause complete joint stiffness and that ordinarily the symptoms can be satisfactorily controlled by appropriate treatment.

Adequate rest is important. Afternoon rest periods may be helpful. The patient must be taught to adjust his physical activity to a level which his affected joint or joints will tolerate. He should steer a middle course, not allowing himself to become either fatigued from overexercise or weak from inactivity. In some instances a change of occupation is required.

The patient should also be instructed in a simple program of brief range-of-motion, nonweight-bearing exercises. Such exercises, done once or twice daily, will do much to maintain joint mobility, ward off symptoms, and improve body mechanics.

Since obesity is often an aggravating factor when the weight-bearing joints are affected, gradual reduction of weight by dieting is frequently indicated.

Drug therapy. There is no medication specific for osteoarthritis. Salicylates, as in other joint diseases, relieve pain. Aspirin may be given in doses of 0.6 to 0.9 Gm. three to five times daily. Phenylbutazone may be used but because of its potential toxicity must be carefully controlled. Steroid hormones have proved to be of no permanent value but may at times be used to relieve acute symptoms.

Local treatment of joints. Some degree of rest of the involved joint is nearly always beneficial. For weight-bearing joints, either a restriction of standing and walking or the temporary use of crutches or cane may be indicated. Local rest may be facilitated by means of a splint or brace, but no joint should be completely fixed for long periods. Usually physical therapy proves helpful in relieving the symptoms. Heat in the form of baking, hot packs, whirlpool or paraffin baths, or diathermy is indicated. Massage of the muscles above and below the affected joints may make the patient more comfortable. Active, nonweight-bearing exercises are usually helpful but should not be continued to the point of fatigue.

Injections of hydrocortisone into painful joints sometimes give temporary relief; such injections may be repeated several times. The greatest care must be taken not to introduce infection.

Prevention of deformity. The danger of developing fixed deformity is much less in osteoarthritis than in rheumatoid arthritis. Most of the deformity is caused by changes in the shape of the articular ends of the bones. At times, however, the hips may become flexed and adducted, the knees flexed, or the feet pronated; selected exercises and splinting will do much to prevent such deformities.

Surgical measures. In osteoarthritis, surgical treatment is often indicated if the joint changes have become so advanced that nonoperative measures no longer control the symptoms effectively. Operations are used primarily to relieve pain on motion and secondarily to correct deformity, restore mobility, or provide stability.

Loose bodies, which occasionally appear in osteoarthritic joints and cause pain and locking, should be removed. Synovectomy may be indicated if the lining membrane is chronically thickened and joint movement is painful. Denervation of a joint by section of its sensory nerves is sometimes helpful but cannot be relied upon for complete or permanent relief. Arthrodesis is ordinarily followed by permanent freedom from pain. Arthroplasty may improve the pain without producing stiffness; it is especially useful for one major joint when the involvement is bilateral. Careful selection must be made among these and other useful procedures in the surgical treatment of the osteoarthritic hip (p. 191) and the osteoarthritic knee (p. 193).

Prognosis. The prognosis for relief of the symptoms and control of the arthritic process is better in osteoarthritis than in rheumatoid arthritis. The damaged joints can be made less disabling and less painful by well-advised treatment. Despite roentgenographic evidence of advanced changes, the patient will experience remarkably little pain when a suitable therapeutic regime is prescribed and diligently followed.

GOUT

Gout is a familial metabolic disease characterized by an abnormality of purine metabolism in which uric acid, the normal end product, is involved. Its cause is unknown. Approximately 95% of the patients are males; they are usually past the age of 30 years. Rarely is gout observed in Negroes.

Clinical picture. Early stages of gout are marked by recurring attacks of acute monarticular pain and inflammation, and the later stages by chronic deforming articular changes. The attacks are precipitated by excessive intake of meats and other foods high in protein, fatigue, overindulgence in alcohol, and occasionally by trauma or surgery of the involved joint. Between attacks the patient is symptom-free unless permanent joint damage has taken place.

The joints most often involved are those of the foot (classically the first

180 Handbook of orthopaedic surgery

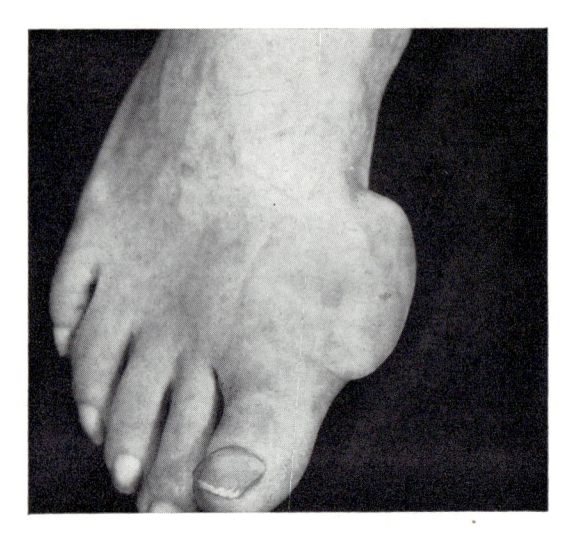

Fig. 110. Gout. Note mass at base of great toe, resulting from urate deposits. This case is of long duration.

metatarsophalangeal joint, Fig. 110), hand, wrist, knee, and elbow. Seldom is the hip, shoulder, or spine affected. In acute attacks the involved joint is usually red, swollen, warm, tender, and extremely painful on motion; veins in the overlying skin may be distended.

Pathology. The joint lesions consist of creamy or chalky deposits of sodium urate surrounded by foreign-body inflammatory reaction; they occur in synovium, capsule, articular cartilage, and periarticular bone. Such urate deposits, known as *tophi*, are sometimes found in the lobes of the ears. They may occur also in subcutaneous tissue, fascia, kidneys, heart, and other viscera.

Roentgenographic picture. In early gout, roentgenograms may show no bone changes. In later cases, typical small punched-out areas appear near the ends of the bones at the affected joint.

Laboratory findings. The blood uric acid is usually elevated (5 to 15 mg. per 100 ml.) during the acute episode. However, the acute attack is not caused by the high uric acid level in the blood, either clinically or experimentally.

Treatment. Although no cure for gout is known, certain drugs provide dramatic relief of the pain and swelling. Colchicine is most useful; it may be given hourly in doses of 0.5 mg. until the pain subsides or until toxic gastrointestinal upsets supervene. Phenylbutazone often relieves the symptoms within forty-eight hours or less. If taken for a longer period it may cause toxic effects such as edema, nausea, and granulocytopenia which must be watched for and prevented, the drug being discontinued if they appear. In acute attacks, corticotropin may be effective and intra-articular injection of hydrocortisone very helpful.

In chronic gout, disabilities from tophaceous deposits can be prevented and to some degree reversed through the prolonged use of a uricosuric agent such as probenecid. The patient should follow a low-purine diet and avoid excessive alcohol and trauma. In late cases, large tophi may require surgical extirpation. As a rule gout does not alter life expectancy.

CHAPTER 9

Chronic arthritis of individual joints—ankylosis and arthroplasty

CHRONIC ARTHRITIS of the spine, hip, and knee present individual problems that can best be considered separately. The classification into rheumatoid arthritis and osteoarthritis has again been followed.

CHRONIC ARTHRITIS OF THE SPINE
Rheumatoid arthritis

Incidence. Rheumatoid arthritis of the spine often accompanies rheumatoid arthritis of the joints of the extremities but may occur independently. It affects both sexes and is seen most frequently in the early decades of adult life, between the ages of 25 and 45 years. Occasionally it occurs in children, in association with multiple joint involvement, splenomegaly, and generalized lymphadenopathy *(Still's disease)*.

Pathology. The pathologic findings are essentially the same as those described for rheumatoid arthritis elsewhere in the body. The initial change is thought to be a synovitis of the facet joints. The vertebrae and cartilages become atrophic. In the later stages of rheumatoid arthritis the spine is more likely to develop fibrous ankylosis than bony ankylosis. The subcutaneous nodules of rheumatoid arthritis may also be present.

Clinical picture. Back pain and stiffness usually begin insidiously and increase slowly. The discomfort is especially marked upon bending over and lifting and is relieved but does not subside completely with recumbency. The symptoms often begin in the cervical or upper dorsal region; in other patients the lower dorsal or upper lumbar level may be first affected. At times the pain may radiate to the front of the chest and abdomen or down the legs. Coughing and sneezing often cause sharp pain in the back. It is not uncommon for the symptoms to appear in recurrent attacks which may follow minor infections, excessive exercise, or slight trauma. As the condition progresses, muscle spasm and contractures may lead to dorsal kyphosis and secondary postural changes in the cervical and lumbar regions. The stiffness becomes gradually more marked but usually does not progress to bony ankylosis. As a rule, rheumatoid arthritis of the spine is accompanied by rheumatoid arthritis in several joints of the extremities; often the smaller joints are so involved.

Diagnosis. The diagnosis is based upon the character of the onset, the findings on clinical examination, the roentgenographic evidence, and the frequent association with rheumatoid involvement of other joints.

Differential diagnosis. Rheumatoid arthritis of the spine must be differentiated from other causes of pain and stiffness in the back. Most important of these are Strümpell-Marie arthritis, osteoarthritis, tuberculosis, malignancy, intervertebral disk lesions, vertebral epiphysitis, fracture, sprain, and visceral disease with referred pain.

Treatment. The treatment is discussed at the end of this section, p. 188.

Strümpell-Marie arthritis (ankylosing spondylitis)

Strümpell-Marie arthritis, although commonly described under rheumatoid arthritis, has a number of characteristics that distinguish it as a sepa-

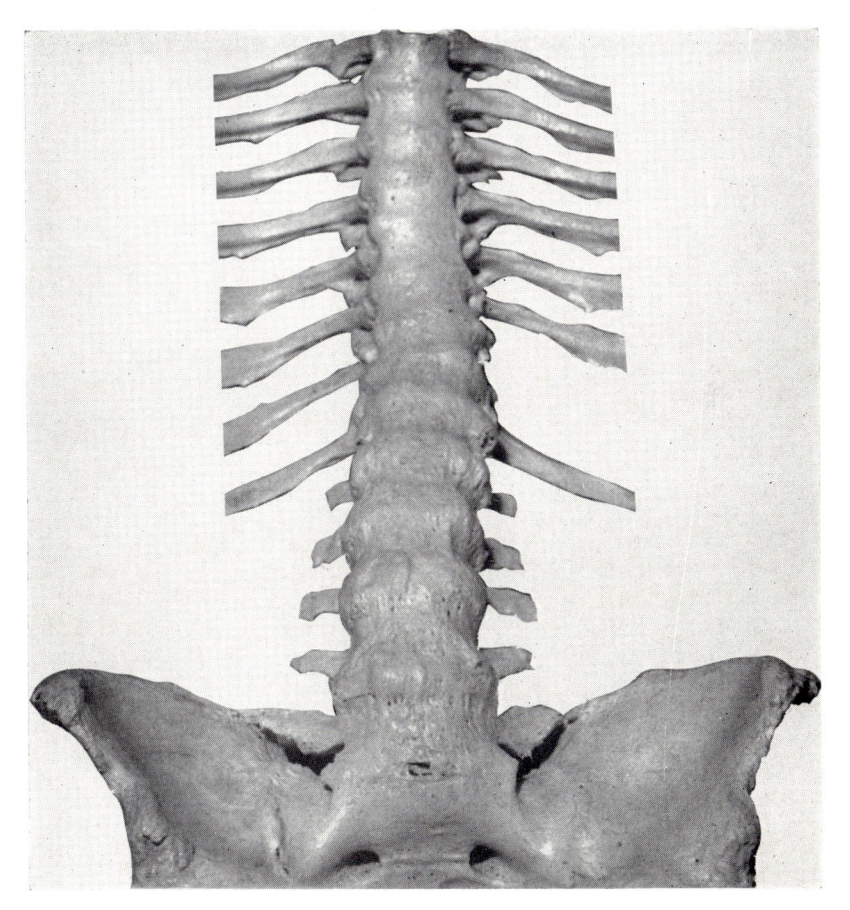

Fig. 111. Specimen of advanced Strümpell-Marie arthritis, showing bony ankylosis of vertebrae and sacroiliac joints.

rate entity. It was first described clinically in 1884 by Strümpell in Germany and in 1898 by Marie in France. It is characterized by ossification of the ligaments of the spine and by involvement also of the hips and shoulders. The sacroiliac joints are affected early in its course. Its cause is unknown. Infection and trauma have been considered contributing influences, but without proof. Factors related to sex and age may play a part, since Strümpell-Marie arthritis is ten times as common in men as in women and usually begins between the ages of 20 and 40 years.

Pathology. The pathologic changes begin like those of rheumatoid arthritis and proceed gradually to an extensive bony ankylosis. Progressive ossification occurs in the capsular and other intervertebral ligaments, fusing the lower and often in later stages the entire spine into a single mass. The costovertebral joints may become ankylosed. In the intervertebral disks, peripheral ossification takes place much earlier than does central ossification. The vertebral bodies tend to become osteoporotic; their contour changes little except in the dorsal spine, where they often become wedge-shaped.

There may be irregular spur formation and lipping of the vertebrae. The typical gross specimen has an appearance suggesting that liquid bone

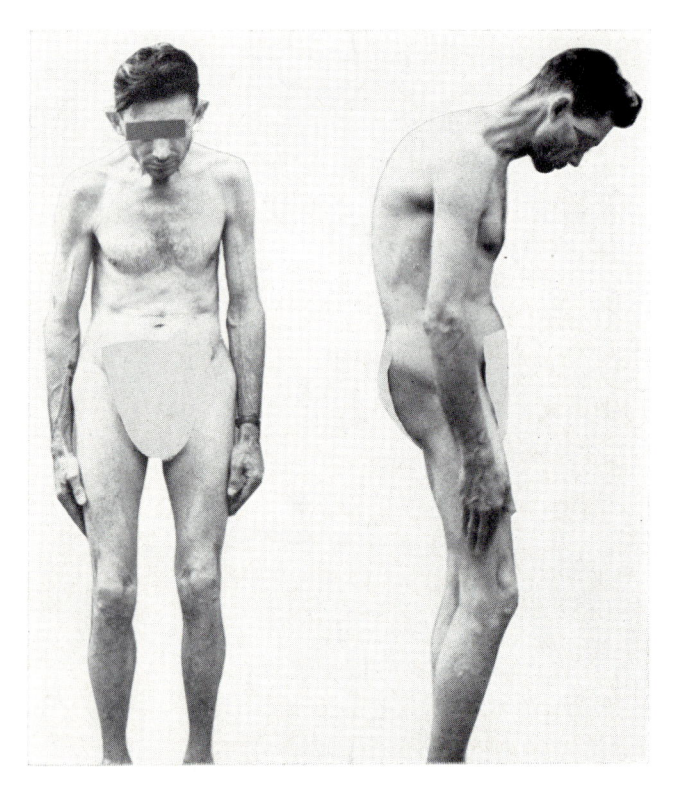

Fig. 112. Strümpell-Marie arthritis in a 46-year-old man with ankylosis of entire spine in faulty position.

Chronic arthritis of individual joints 185

has been poured upon the anterior surface of the vertebral column and has congealed as it flowed down (Fig. 111).

Clinical picture. The onset may be associated with acute pain but, on the contrary, stiffness without pain is sometimes the first symptom. The pain first appears in the hips, buttocks, or lumbosacral region. Low back pain that comes on while the patient is recumbent in early morning hours suggests the diagnosis. Decreased spinal mobility and diminished chest expansion are characteristic signs. As the disease progresses, kyphosis and flatten-

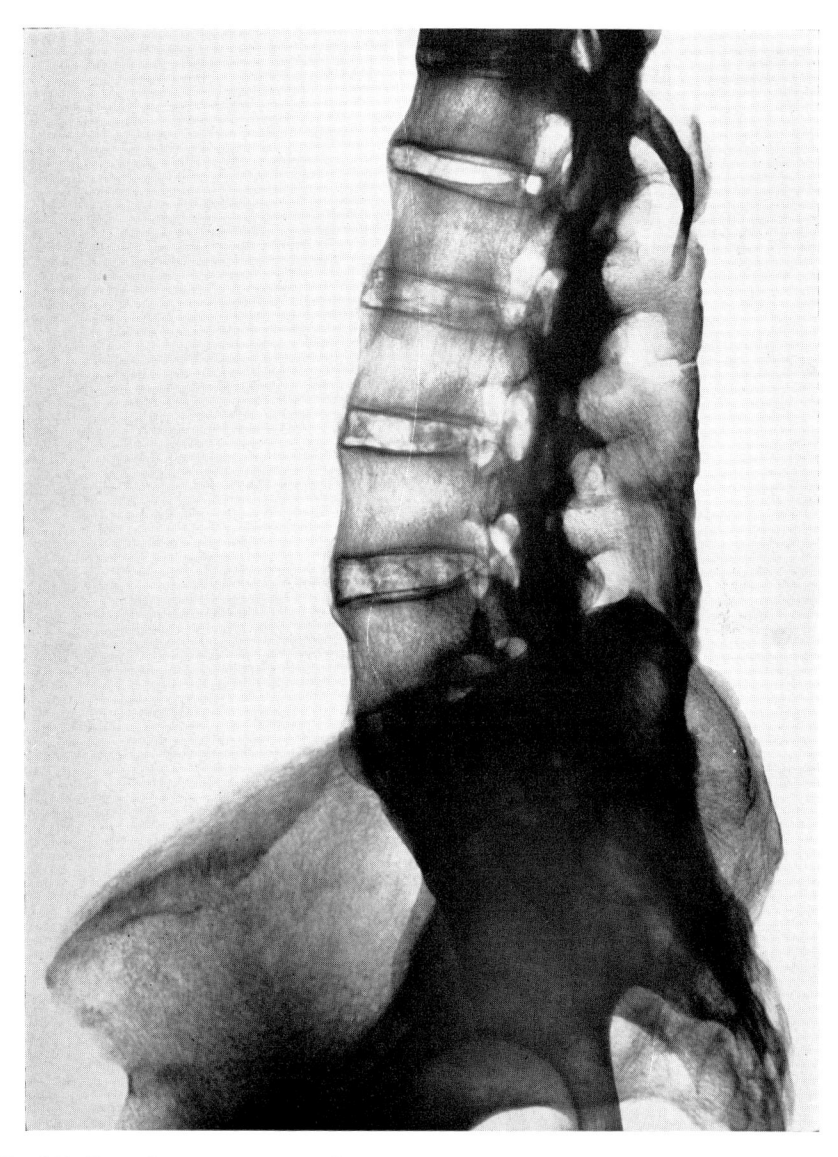

Fig. 113. Lateral roentgenogram of specimen in Fig. 111, showing ossification between vertebrae anteriorly and posteriorly as well as in the intervertebral disks.

ing of the chest frequently develop unless preventive measures are taken. The pain, followed by stiffening, may progress very slowly from the low back farther and farther upward until finally the entire spine becomes ankylosed (Fig. 112). The pain tends to lessen as the stiffness increases. The arthritic process may extend to involve the hips and shoulders. If the hips become stiff, a characteristic gait develops in which the pelvis is rotated from side to side to compensate for the lack of hip motion. In typical cases there is no involvement of the smaller joints.

Roentgenographic picture. Roentgenographic changes may not appear until many months after the onset of symptoms. As a rule the earliest findings are changes in density along the margins of the sacroiliac joints. As the disease progresses, small erosions and narrowing appear in the apophyseal joints. Late changes include obliteration of the sacroiliac and apophyseal joint spaces, ossification of the periphery of the annulus fibrosus (giving the appearance sometimes called "bamboo spine"), and bony bridging of the laminae and spinous processes (Fig. 113).

Diagnosis. The diagnostic criteria are similar to those of rheumatoid arthritis of the spine. Characteristic features, however, are the high incidence in young men, the onset of symptoms and signs in the low back and their slow proximal progression, the roentgenographic changes in the sacroiliac joints, and the absence of arthritis in the smaller joints of the extremities.

Differential diagnosis. The differential diagnosis is similar to that of rheumatoid arthritis.

Treatment. The treatment is discussed at the end of the section, p. 188.

Osteoarthritis

Incidence and etiology. Osteoarthritis of the spine is seen most often in stocky and obese persons over 40 years of age and is more frequent in males than in females. It is much more common than rheumatoid arthritis of the spine or Strümpell-Marie arthritis. It is most often observed in the lumbar spine. The repeated minor traumas of constant use of the back probably constitute an important causative factor. Faulty body mechanics probably play a part by putting added strain upon localized areas of the spine.

Pathology. The pathologic changes of osteoarthritis described previously (p. 176) take place in the spinal diarthroses, or intervertebral joints. Although the articular cartilage becomes frayed and thinned, these joints do not undergo bony ankylosis. Marked eburnation of bone may occur about the articular facets.

Thinning of the intervertebral disks, and lipping and spur formation at the anterolateral margins of the vertebral bodies result from disk degeneration and reactive bone production; although these changes, often termed *spondylosis* or *spondylophytosis*, usually accompany osteoarthritis of the spinal diarthroses, they probably constitute a related but distinct degenerative process. In later stages the vertebral bodies become flattened, and much new bone may develop about their margins, producing so-called bridging and leaf formation. Such changes, demonstrable in roentgenograms, are present to some degree in a high percentage of older people who have never had back pain; this is especially true of heavy individuals.

Clinical picture. Following slight trauma or strain there may be complaint of pain in the lower part of the back, with considerable stiffness and lameness. Stiffness may be most noticeable on first getting up in the morning. Pain that radiates around toward the chest or abdomen or down the legs or arms is often present; such pain may be a result of compression of nerve roots, caused by small outgrowths of bone near the intervertebral foramina. Radiating pain is particularly common in involvement of the lumbosacral and sacroiliac joints and of the intervertebral foramina of the cervical spine. Examination of the patient's back is likely to show muscle spasm, restricted mobility, pain at the extremes of motion, and very little tenderness. Deformity of the lumbar spine, often consisting of lateral curvature and a decrease of the normal lordosis, may develop. Ankylosis of some

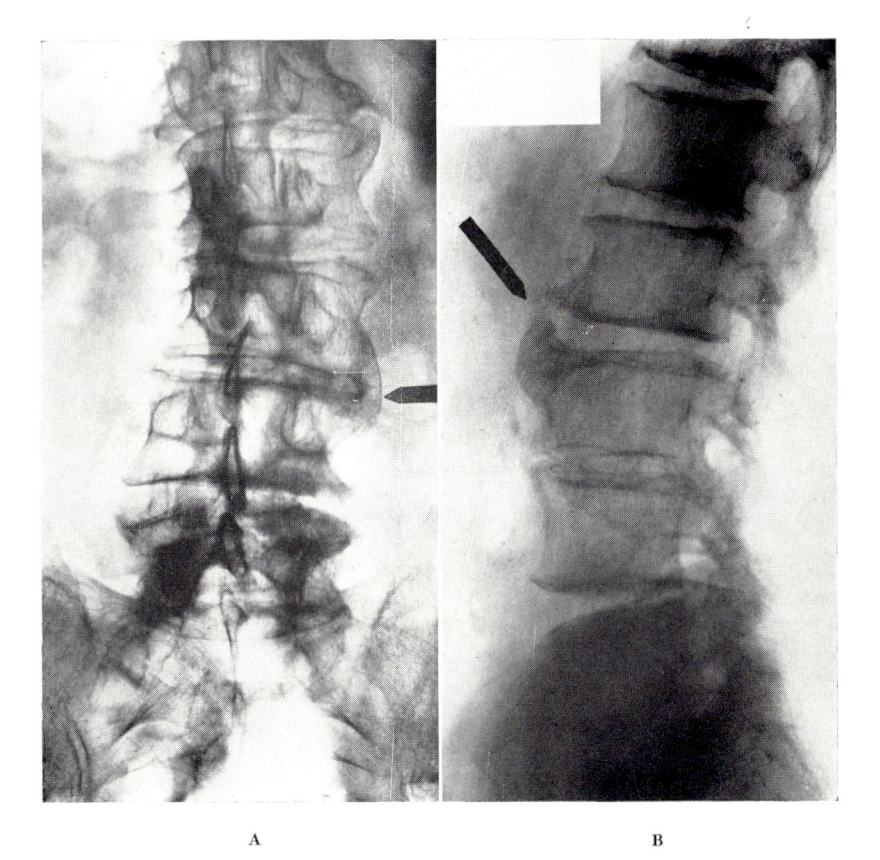

Fig. 114. Osteoarthritis of the lumbar spine in a man 70 years of age. **A,** Anteroposterior roentgenogram showing deformity of spine with spur formation and large bridge of new bone. **B,** Lateral roentgenogram showing spur formation, almost complete anterior bridging between second and third lumbar vertebrae, and narrowing of third lumbar interspace.

areas of the spine may follow. The lumbar and lower dorsal spine is more often involved than higher levels of the back and frequently is the first to become stiffened.

Diagnosis. The diagnosis is made from the history, the physical findings, and the associated roentgenographic changes of lipping, spurs, and irregular bone formation about the vertebral margins (Fig. 114).

Differential diagnosis. The differential diagnosis is similar to that of rheumatoid arthritis of the spine. Osteoarthritis must also be differentiated from neurogenic arthropathy and from osteitis deformans. It should also be differentiated from the localized vertebral lipping associated with collapse or fibrosis of an intervertebral disk called spondylosis, and from the traction spurs that may follow localized injury of an intervertebral articulation.

Treatment of chronic arthritis of the spine

The treatment of chronic arthritis of the spine includes general measures, local measures, roentgentherapy, and surgical treatment.

General measures. General measures include ample rest and a well-balanced diet. The caloric intake should be regulated to correct any obesity or undernutrition. A chronic infectious process that is impairing the patient's general health may require treatment. Back pain and aching can usually be relieved effectively and safely by aspirin. Phenylbutazone may be used with proper regard for its toxicity.

Local measures. Local measures are indicated for the relief of pain and the prevention and correction of deformity. Throughout the acutely painful stage of any form of chronic arthritis of the spine the patient should be kept in bed. If there is a tendency for kyphosis to develop, hyperextension exercises should be given and the position of hyperextension should be maintained. Hyperextension in recumbency can be obtained conveniently by using a hinged fracture board on a reversed Gatch bed. In some instances the support provided by a Whitman frame or a posterior plaster shell may be advisable. When the patient begins to stand, the back should be supported by a strong belt, surgical corset, brace, or plaster jacket. For Strümpell-Marie arthritis the Baker or the Jewett three-point brace is particularly useful, as it tends constantly to correct flexion. Massage and postural exercises, preceded by hot packs or other form of heat, may be given daily. Particular attention should be paid to preserving and increasing the chest expansion by means of deep breathing exercises. In arthritis of the cervical spine it may be necessary to use head traction to correct a flexion deformity of the neck, after which a Thomas collar or a Schanz cotton collar may be applied.

Roentgentherapy. The use of roentgentherapy will often relieve the pain and may check the progress of Strümpell-Marie arthritis but usually is best avoided because of the danger of causing sterilization in young women or of leading to the development of leukemia. Roentgentherapy has not proved successful in the treatment of other forms of chronic arthritis.

Surgical treatment. Spinal operations are seldom indicated. When there is localized pain with roentgenographic evidence of bone changes over a small segment of the spine and when nonsurgical treatment has failed to produce a satisfactory result, an arthrodesis may be indicated for permanent relief of the discomfort. Such instances are uncommon. To correct severe flexion deformity of the back in late rheumatoid or Strümpell-Marie arthritis, an osteotomy of the spine may occasionally be indicated. The results are best when the osteotomy can be done at the dorsolumbar junction.

CHRONIC ARTHRITIS OF THE HIP

The hip joint may be involved primarily in either rheumatoid arthritis or osteoarthritis. In either type the hip affection is often a part of a widespread arthritic process. Osteoarthritis virtually limited to the hip, however, is a common and disabling affection of degenerative nature in middle and late adult years. It has been termed *malum coxae senilis*.

Malum coxae senilis

Etiology. Although the cause of malum coxae senilis is not thoroughly understood, trauma associated with incongruity of the joint surfaces is thought to be the most important factor in many cases. Osteoarthritis may not follow immediately after a major injury or repeated minor injuries of the hip, but may develop insidiously years later. It is often a late sequel of congenital dysplasia of the hip, a congenital subluxation, a reduced congenital dislocation, or a congenital coxa vara. It often appears many years after an epiphyseal disturbance such as coxa plana or slipping of the capital femoral epiphysis. Ischemic necrosis of the femoral head, of whatever origin, is likely to result in distortion of the articular surface, leading sooner or later to osteoarthritis of the hip.

Pathology. The initial changes, which have been shown to begin in areas of the femoral head not subject to weight-bearing pressure, are fibrillation, erosion, and thinning of the articular cartilage. The cartilage becomes irregularly worn away over the head and in the acetabulum and is replaced by hard, eburnated bone. Proliferation of new bone around the head may take place, in the form of a collar. New bone is formed also around the margin of the acetabulum. The acetabulum grows larger as the head of the femur flattens. The femoral neck may become short and broad. In addition to spurring and gross changes of contour, roentgenograms show irregular areas of increased bone density, mottling of the head and neck, and numerous small cystlike areas near the articular surfaces (Fig. 115). The synovial membrane usually becomes thick and fibrous. It may be completely replaced by fibrous connective tissue.

Clinical picture. Often both hips are involved; when this is the case, the changes are usually more advanced on one side than the other.

The onset is insidious. Although stiffness without pain may be the first symptom, most patients complain initially of aching in the hip region, together with slight stiffness or pain down the thigh to the knee, following excessive exercise, which is completely relieved with rest. After standing or

190 *Handbook of orthopaedic surgery*

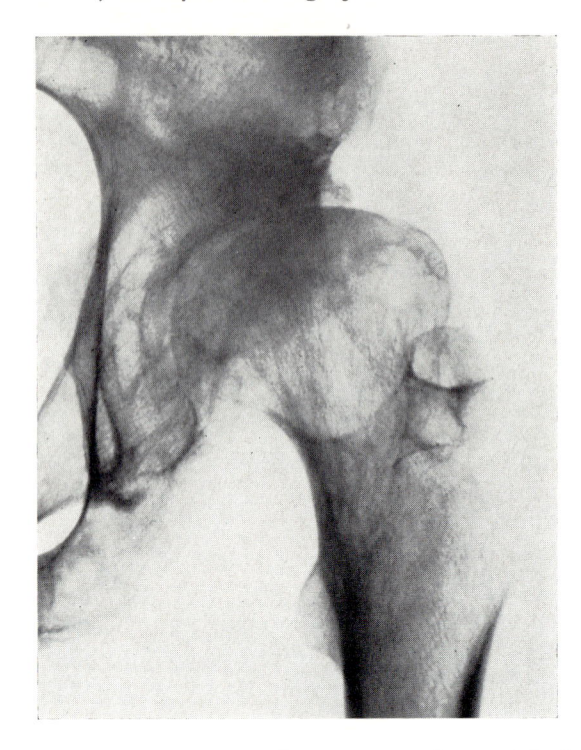

Fig. 115. Anteroposterior roentgenogram showing osteoarthritis of the hip in a 57-year-old man. Note narrowing of articular cartilage space, flattening and widening of femoral head, bony proliferation about the acetabular margin, and areas of rarefaction and of sclerosis in the head and about the acetabulum.

sitting there may be a slight catching sensation and pain in the hip on starting to walk. As the condition progresses, these symptoms appear most often in the morning and wear off during the day. After activity, however, the symptoms recur with increasing regularity. Gradually muscle spasm develops, causing flexion and adduction of the hip. Associated with the limitation of motion, there is usually discomfort upon pressure about the joint. Later, slight shortening of the leg and a limp become noticeable. Creaking and grating may develop in the joint with motion, and the muscles atrophy. Later there is considerable pain on weight bearing. Radiating pain often extends down the front of the thigh to the knee but is sometimes more marked on the posterior aspect. The extremity gradually becomes externally rotated, and the prominence of the greater trochanter increases. Abduction is impaired early, and internal rotation, as well as all other motions, becomes decreased in range. As the deformity of the hip increases, the added stress which is put upon the low back may cause troublesome symptoms. Arthritic changes may develop in the lumbar spine as a result of strain. Recurrent, protracted periods of severe pain and disability are characteristic of the later stages.

Diagnosis. As a rule, the diagnosis is not difficult. The roentgenographic findings, as well as the history and clinical signs are quite characteristic.

Differential diagnosis. Ischemic necrosis of the femoral head, tuberculosis, neuropathic joint disease, rheumatoid arthritis, and subacute or late forms of pyogenic arthritis may simulate malum coxae senilis.

Prognosis. There is little possibility of complete restoration of function. If treatment is started early and is continued faithfully, however, the pain may be relieved. The hip usually becomes quite restricted in motion, and the limitation may progress to complete stiffness. When a flexion and adduction deformity develops, the disability is severe because of shortening of the leg.

Treatment. The treatment includes both general and local measures.

General treatment. General measures include weight reduction by low-calorie diet, when the patient is obese, and regulation of physical activity to ensure adequate rest from prolonged weight bearing.

Local treatment. In early cases the relatively mild hip pain can often be relieved for long periods by *conservative* forms of local treatment. Heat and massage are often helpful. Active, nonweight-bearing exercises of the hip should be carried out daily in an effort to preserve its range of motion. If the extremity has become shortened, a heel raise may be tried. Weight-bearing stresses on the affected hip can be lessened by using a cane in the opposite hand; for short periods crutches are sometimes indicated. As a rule ischial-weight-bearing braces are difficult for the middle-aged patient to wear effectively and comfortably. For temporary relief during an acutely painful episode, intra-articular injection of hydrocortisone may be helpful; repeated injections are contraindicated by the danger of introducing infection. For hip pain that persists despite these measures, a period of several weeks of recumbency with traction on the affected lower extremity and daily physical therapy may be most helpful. On returning to activity the patient can continue to use the traction at night. Occasionally, when the disease is not too far advanced, cautious manipulation under anesthesia may bring about relief of pain and increase of mobility, but usually such improvement is only temporary.

In the later stages of osteoarthritis of the hip, the only effective treatment is *surgical.* Operation is indicated if the patient's pain is intolerable despite thorough trial of other forms of treatment and if his general condition is good enough to withstand major surgery. Of the many operations devised for the osteoarthritic hip, none completely abolishes the symptoms. Selection of the procedure best suited to the needs of the individual patient requires experience and judgment.

Since the primary object of treatment is to relieve hip pain, *neurectomy,* or section of the sensory nerves to the hip joint, is sometimes done when more strenuous surgery or long convalescence is contraindicated. The results of sensory neurectomy, however, have been undependable and often disappointing.

The most useful types of surgical treatment are arthroplasty, arthrodesis, and osteotomy.

By *arthroplasty* both the pain and the stiffness of malum coxae senilis can often be satisfactorily reduced. Arthroplasty is used more freely in older than in younger individuals because its early good results sometimes deteriorate in later years. The *cup* or *mold* arthroplasty (p. 201), pioneered by Smith-Petersen, includes placing a metal cup between the reshaped acetabulum and remodeled head. In the *replacement arthroplasty* the femoral head is excised and replaced by a metal prosthesis with a long stem that traverses the medullary canal of lower neck and upper shaft.

Since *arthrodesis* provides complete and permanent relief of hip pain, it is usually the operation of choice for young and active individuals despite the drawbacks of long postoperative convalescence, hip stiffness, and possible later discomfort in the low back. The procedure usually includes complete removal of articular cartilage from the acetabulum and femoral head, bridging from ilium to femur with massive bone grafts, metallic internal fixation, and the application of a hip spica cast.

The pain of malum coxae senilis can often be relieved by a subtrochanteric *osteotomy,* which presumably redistributes to some extent the weight-bearing stresses in and about the joint. McMurray's operation of osteotomy at the level of the lesser trochanter and medial displacement of the femoral shaft, followed by internal fixation or a hip spica cast or both, is frequently used.

CHRONIC ARTHRITIS OF THE KNEE

The knee joint may be affected in both types of chronic arthritis. Usually both knees are involved. The etiologic factors and pathologic changes are essentially the same as those discussed in the preceding chapter. The knee is the most frequent large joint to be involved by osteoarthritis. Most of the affected individuals are heavy, and the increased weight is probably an important predisposing factor.

Clinical picture. Chronic arthritis of the knee often starts with slight stiffness in the joint after sitting, or a tightness in the back of the knee associated with creaking. It becomes difficult to walk up stairs. Tenderness may be accompanied by swelling and increase of joint fluid, which together with muscle atrophy give the knee a spindle-shaped contour. Attempts to straighten the knee may cause pain, and a flexion contracture may develop. Occasionally in chronic cases the tibia may become subluxated backward; this occurs more often in rheumatoid arthritis than in osteoarthritis. In osteoarthritis, the roentgenographic appearance of the knee (Fig. 116) is typical, with spurs and lipping appearing about the margins of the femur and tibia as well as around the articular surface of the patella. Within the joint are often found loose bodies that have broken off from the small marginal projections of bone.

Diagnosis. The diagnosis is made from the clinical findings and the roentgenograms. The picture is typical and is not often confused with that of other conditions. In the differential diagnosis, synovitis of other types, tuberculosis, and neuropathic joint disease must be considered.

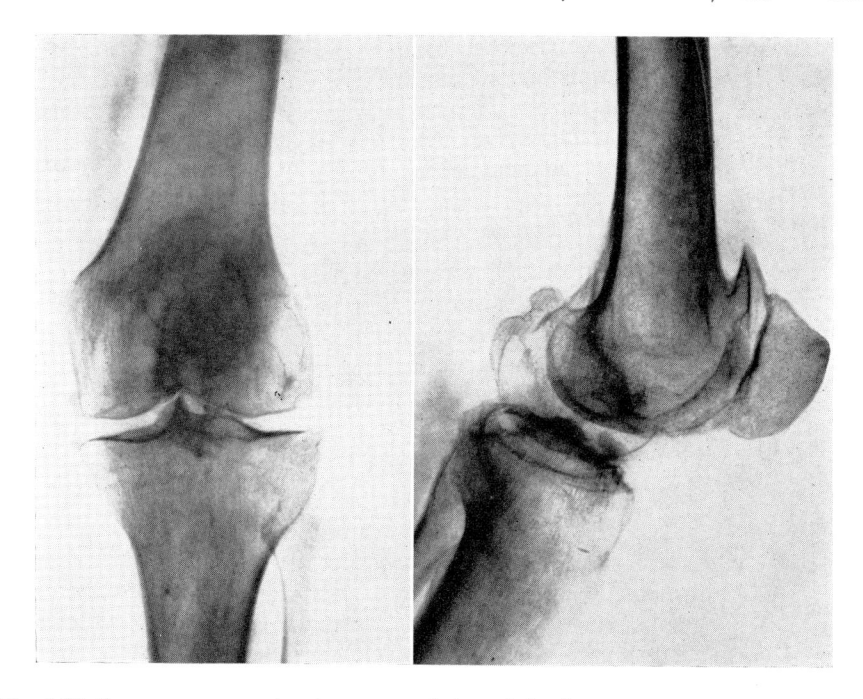

Fig. 116. Roentgenograms showing osteoarthritis of the knee in a woman 65 years of age. Note spurs about the margins of the femoral and tibial condyles, the tibial spine, and the upper and lower poles of the patella, as well as a possible loose body in the intercondylar fossa.

Prognosis. In advanced rheumatoid arthritis of the knee the outlook for recovery of function is poor. In early osteoarthritis the symptoms can be relieved, although slow progression of the degenerative changes usually continues.

Treatment. The general treatment has been outlined in the preceding chapter. Locally, rest is important: the strain of weight bearing should be relieved at once. The knee should be protected with an elastic support, brace, or cast, and crutches may be advisable. Hot applications may relieve the pain. Regulated exercise of quadriceps and hamstring muscles will increase the circulation, maintain muscle tone, and assist in preventing flexion contracture.

Knee flexion contracture in rheumatoid arthritis may be very difficult to correct. Traction or wedged casts may be used, followed by a brace to maintain extension. Posterior *capsulotomy* may be necessary. If the knee has retained mobility in flexion, supracondylar *osteotomy* of the femur will allow correction of the unsightly flexion deformity and preserve the range of motion. Bony ankylosis in flexion is also correctible by osteotomy.

In rheumatoid arthritis, *synovectomy*, or excision of the synovial membrane, is indicated when the arthritic process has become quiescent throughout the body but has left persistent pain, thickening of the synovium, and limitation of motion in the knee. Advanced arthritic changes with roentgenographic evidence of destruction of the joint surfaces are often indications for *arthrodesis,* or surgical fusion. Complete ankylosis of the knee in a young person with good musculature and no active arthritis elsewhere in the body may warrant *arthroplasty,* but as a rule a painless ankylosis in good position is preferable to a postarthroplasty knee which may sooner or later develop pain or instability or both.

In osteoarthritis with pain and crepitation limited to the anterior aspect of the knee and unrelieved by nonoperative treatment, *patellectomy* is often indicated. In selected cases it may be advisable to combine patellectomy, synovectomy, and excision of degenerated cartilages and bony spurs; after so extensive an operation, several weeks of traction and physical therapy are essential.

ANKYLOSIS

Ankylosis is a restriction of the normal range of motion by tissue changes within or without the joint cavity. Ankylosis may occur with the joint in a position favorable for function or in an attitude of deformity.

Etiology. Ankylosis is often a result of the incomplete healing or restoration of joint structures damaged by chronic arthritis, infection, or trauma. A severe burn about a joint sometimes results in ankylosis. Ankylosis is of two kinds: (1) fibrous, partial, or false (when connective tissue adhesions between the articular surfaces or extra-articular tissues are not accompanied by actual bony union) and (2) bony, complete, or true (when solid new bone has been formed between the articular surfaces). Fibrous ankylosis may follow joint inflammations, intra-articular fractures, repeated intra-articular hemorrhages, or extra-articular changes resulting from infection, trauma, or prolonged immobilization. Bony ankylosis is often the end result of a more severe infection or a more advanced rheumatoid arthritis, which has destroyed the cartilaginous surfaces and allowed the apposition of denuded bone.

Clinical picture. In fibrous ankylosis a small amount of motion may be present and pain may be experienced when the joint is manipulated. In bony ankylosis (Fig. 117) no joint motion is possible. Often it is difficult to determine whether the ankylosis is true or false. Roentgenograms of the joint should always be examined but at times they are deceptive. The films may appear to show a solid bony fusion when definite joint motion can be elicited clinically or can be demonstrated later at operation. The most reliable roentgenographic criterion of bony ankylosis is the presence of fine bony trabeculae which can be traced directly across the region of the former joint space (Fig. 118).

Treatment. In the early stages of joint involvement the best assurance against the development of ankylosis is proper treatment of the original disease or injury. In pyogenic arthritis it is often necessary to place the joint absolutely at rest in order to avoid injury of the articular surfaces. In rheumatoid arthritis the joint may be best treated by alternating periods of

Chronic arthritis of individual joints 195

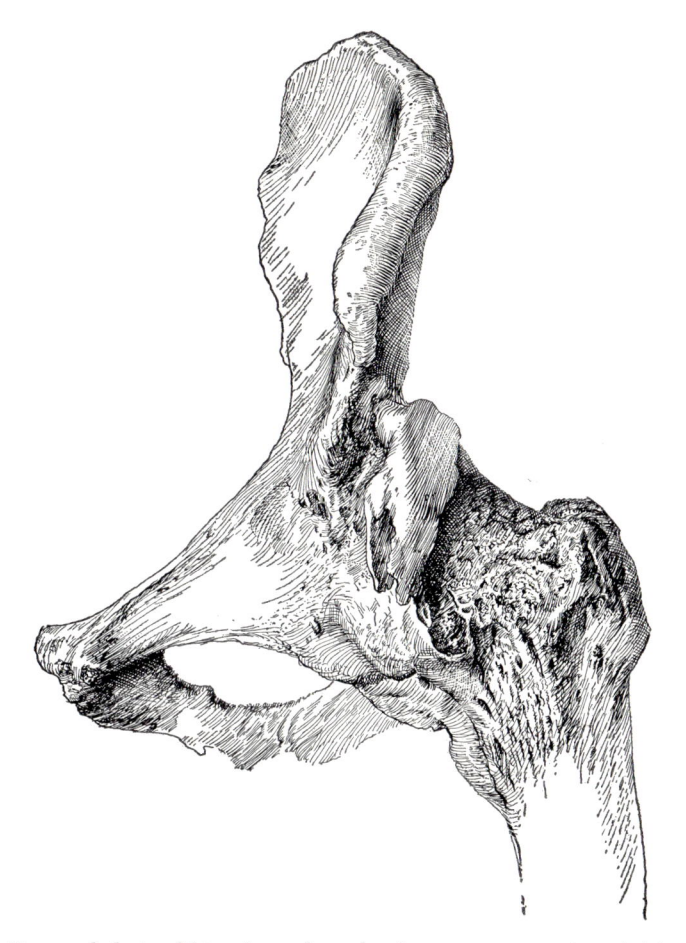

Fig. 117. Bony ankylosis of hip, the end result of a severe pyogenic arthritis. (Drawing from museum specimen.)

splinting and of regulated exercise. When the knee or the hip is involved, traction applied below the joint and designed to lessen the pressure of the apposed articular surfaces is often an effective aid in preventing joint destruction and ankylosis. In order to minimize the danger of ankylosis, casts used in the treatment of fractures should immobilize no joint without good reason, should be discarded as soon as early union will permit, and should be followed by active exercise of all affected joints.

If fibrous ankylosis has taken place, it may be possible by means of physical therapy to preserve or increase a useful range of motion in the joint. Vigorous active exercise is essential; preliminary heat and massage may be of some help. Passive motion should never be forced if the movement is accompanied by pain, since additional damage and stiffening may result and since the discomfort may serve to discourage further endeavors. Electrical stimulation of muscles about the joint and insistence on active contraction of these muscles will often help. A joint which by gentle physical

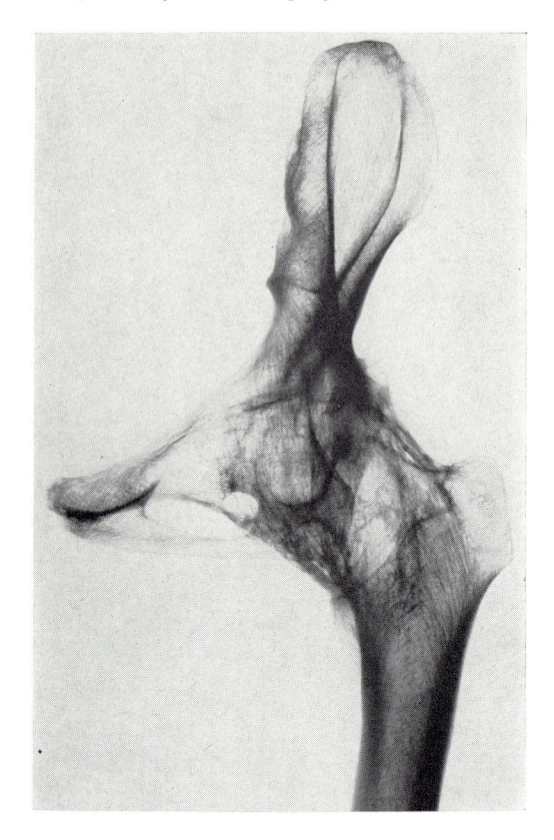

Fig. 118. Bony ankylosis of hip. Roentgenogram of specimen illustrated in Fig. 117, showing bony trabeculae extending from pelvis to femur.

therapy can be restored even partially to motion will usually preserve its regained function.

If forcible mobilization of a partially ankylosed joint becomes necessary, the manipulation should be done gently under anesthesia. In an occasional case it may be desirable to perform repeated manipulations. If the adhesions and contractures can be overcome with a minimum of effort, the prognosis for improved joint function is good, provided that muscle tone and strength are adequate, but if considerable force is used the outcome is at best doubtful. The bones about these partially ankylosed and little-used joints are very atrophic and weak. Care should therefore be taken not to exert too much force, as the bones fracture easily. The smaller joints do not respond well to manipulation. Of great importance is the patient's cooperation in a program of vigorous active exercise after the manipulation.

If an ankylosis has occurred with the joint in good position, arthroplasty, or other operation for mobilization, may be indicated. When the ankylosis has occurred in a faulty position, however, operations for improvement of the deformity, as well as those for restoration of joint motion, must be kept under consideration. In a partial extension ankylosis of the knee such as sometimes occurs following a fracture of the lower half of the femur, with contracture of the quadriceps muscle, a lengthening of the quadriceps tendon (Bennett operation) or a resection of the scar tissue about the quadriceps tendon and muscle fibers (Thompson operation) may be followed by a useful increase of the range of flexion.

OPTIMUM POSITIONS OF JOINT FIXATION

In many patients with joint disease it becomes impossible to prevent ankylosis. Should ankylosis become inevitable, the position most suitable for future function of the extremity must be determined early, and efforts must be made to prevent ankylosis from occurring in any less favorable position. This is a vital factor in the preservation of function, as well as in the prevention of disfigurement. Many orthopaedic operations are made necessary only because ankylosis in poor functional position has been allowed to take place.

The therapeutic procedure of producing a bony ankylosis by surgery is called *arthrodesis*. Arthrodesis may be indicated (1) to eradicate an intra-articular disease, as in tuberculosis; (2) to abolish intractable pain on motion, as in chronic arthritis with severe intra-articular damage; or (3) to provide permanent stability for a joint rendered flail by paralysis.

In arthrodesis, care must be taken that the ankylosis occur with the joint in the position most favorable for function.

The best positions for ankylosis, subject to slight modifications depending upon the individual patient's occupation and habits, are indicated below for the spine, shoulders, elbow, wrist, hip, knee, and ankle, respectively.

Spine. The vertebral column should be so supported that its antero-posterior curves remain relatively normal. Ankylosis should never be al-

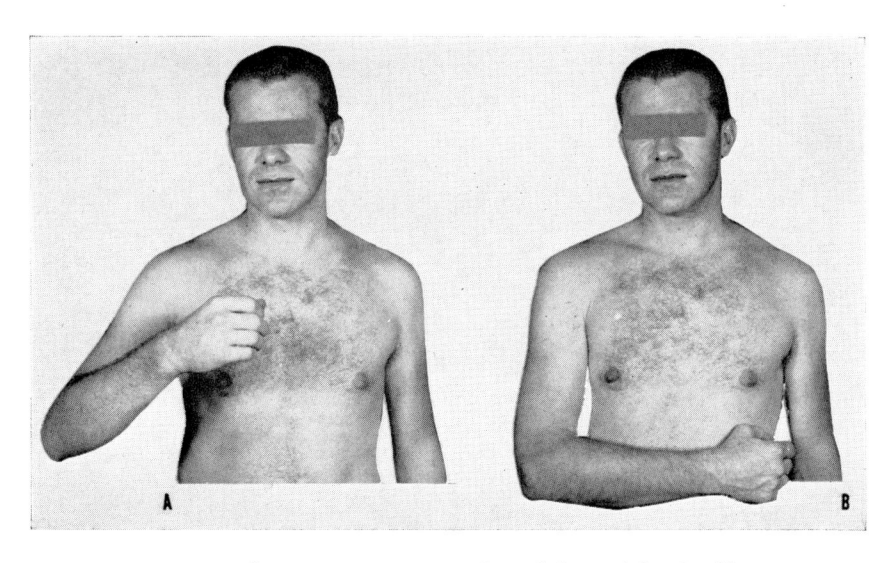

Fig. 119. Correct, **A**, and incorrect, **B**, positions for ankylosis of the shoulder.

198   *Handbook of orthopaedic surgery*

lowed to take place with the spine in a flexed or laterally deviated position.

Shoulder. In children the shoulder should be allowed to ankylose in from 50 to 75 degrees of abduction; in adults abduction of 50 degrees is preferable. The arm should also be brought forward 45 degrees from its resting position at the side of the body and should be so rotated that the hand approaches the face when the elbow is flexed (Fig. 119).

Elbow. The elbow should be allowed to ankylose at a right angle (Fig. 120) with the forearm in a position midway between supination and pronation. When both elbows are affected, one should be allowed to ankylose at about 100 degrees of flexion and the other at 80 degrees of flexion.

Wrist. The wrist should be allowed to ankylose in from 15 to 35 degrees of dorsiflexion (Fig. 121). This is most important, as ankylosis in flexion severely limits the usefulness of the hand.

Hip. The hip is ankylosed preferably in about 5 degrees of abduction, 5 degrees of external rotation, and 10 to 25 degrees of flexion. The most suitable degree of flexion depends largely upon the habits of the individual. If the patient's occupation is sedentary, ankylosis of the hip in full extension would obviously be undesirable (Fig. 122).

Knee. The knee may be ankylosed in full extension, but in women and in men of sedentary occupation flexion of from 20 to 30 degrees forms a less

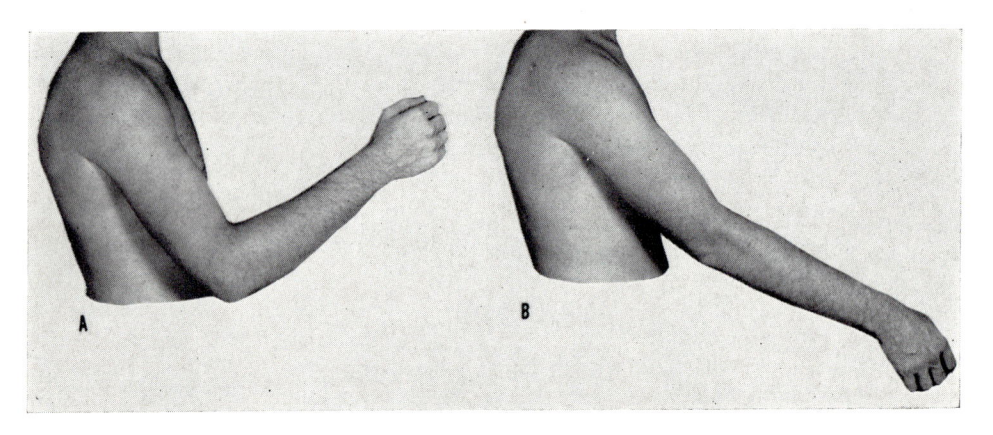

Fig. 120. Correct, **A**, and incorrect, **B**, positions for ankylosis of the elbow.

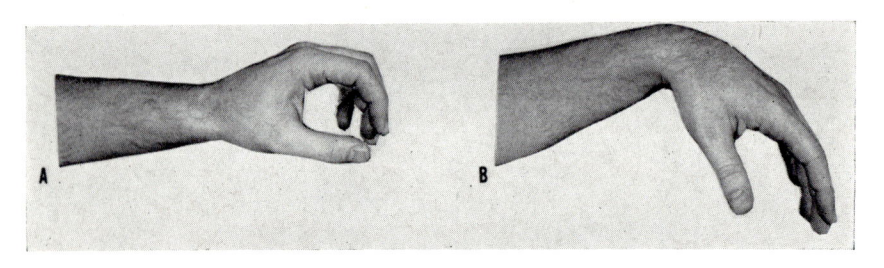

Fig. 121. Correct, **A**, and incorrect, **B**, positions for ankylosis of the wrist.

Chronic arthritis of individual joints 199

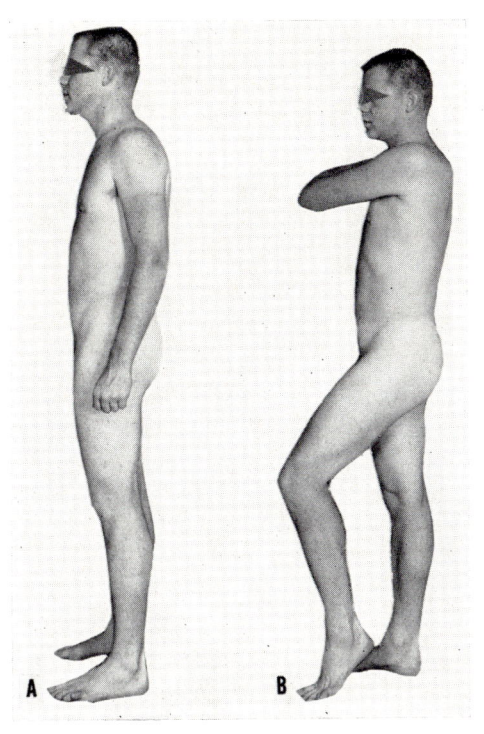

Fig. 122. Neutral, **A**, and incorrect, **B**, positions for ankylosis of the hip.

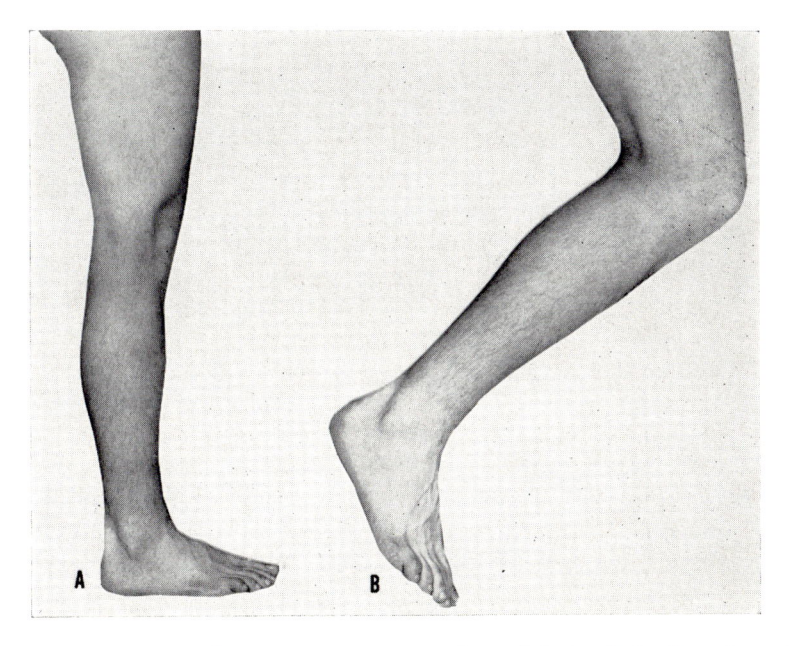

Fig. 123. Correct, **A**, and incorrect, **B**, positions for ankylosis of the knee in a child. In adults slight flexion is often preferable to the neutral or fully extended position.

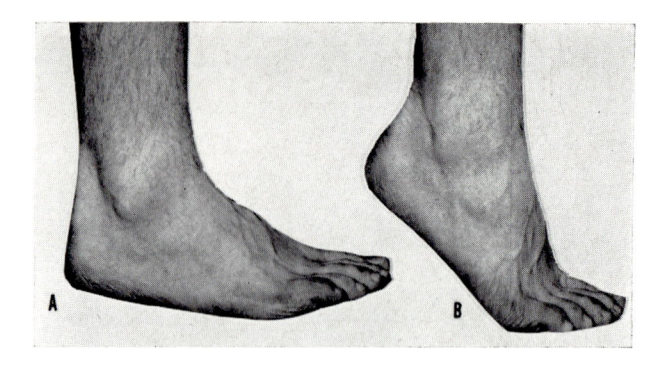

Fig. 124. Correct, **A**, and incorrect, **B**, positions for ankylosis of the ankle. Slight equinus is usually desirable to allow for the height of the shoe heel and to facilitate push-off in walking.

awkward position. In children full extension is essential, because with growth an increase of flexion is likely to occur (Fig. 123).

Ankle. The ankle should be allowed to ankylose in neutral zero position with the foot at a right angle to the leg, or in slight equinus to allow for the height of the shoe heel (Fig. 124). If the affected leg is shortened, slight equinus provides a more serviceable extremity. Care should be taken to avoid rotation deformity, by aligning the foot with the ankle. When the ankle, knee, or hip undergoes ankylosis, the position should be such that a line drawn from the anterior superior iliac spine to the middle of the patella and projected to the foot passes either through or close to the second toe.

ARTHROPLASTY

Arthroplasty is a surgical procedure for restoring motion to a stiffened joint. At the same time the necessary stability of the joint and its freedom from pain must be preserved. In properly selected cases the results of arthroplasty are often satisfactory. The best results are obtained in the hip, elbow, and jaw. Of the many arthroplastic technics that have been described, few attempt to restore the detailed anatomy of the joint.

Arthroplasty is most likely to be successful when the ankylosis has resulted from trauma or osteoarthritis. In joints ankylosed from rheumatoid arthritis there is often a tendency for some degree of stiffness to recur gradually after arthroplasty. In many rheumatoid patients, however, the ankylosis is bilateral and even a partial restoration of mobility is most helpful. Ankylosis following pyogenic or tuberculous arthritis is relatively unfavorable for arthroplasty because of the danger of reactivating the infection. In selected cases arthroplasty may be done after the infection has remained quiescent for at least a year and with care to provide appropriate antibiotic coverage.

The most favorable patient for arthroplasty is a well-motivated young adult with ankylosis of only one joint and good musculature above and below it. Arthroplasty is most likely to be successful when the joint has become ankylosed in a relatively normal position and when little bony overgrowth has developed about it. Arthroplasty is contraindicated in children before the epiphyses have united and is usually inadvisable for any weight-bearing joint of a person whose occupation requires heavy manual labor.

In arthroplasty sufficient bone must be removed to permit free movement in the desired directions. The bone ends should often be separated ½ inch or more; they are shaped, smoothed, and usually covered with some type of interposing material. Fascia lata was for many years the most popular interposing material. In arthroplasty of the hip, Smith-Petersen's technic of inserting a cup of inert metal over the head of the femur (Fig. 125) has given good results. Postoperatively, traction is helpful. Early mobilization is essential and should be encouraged by an extended program of physical therapy with emphasis upon active exercise. Improvement of mobility and strength after arthroplasty may continue for several years, during which the patient should be kept under periodic observation.

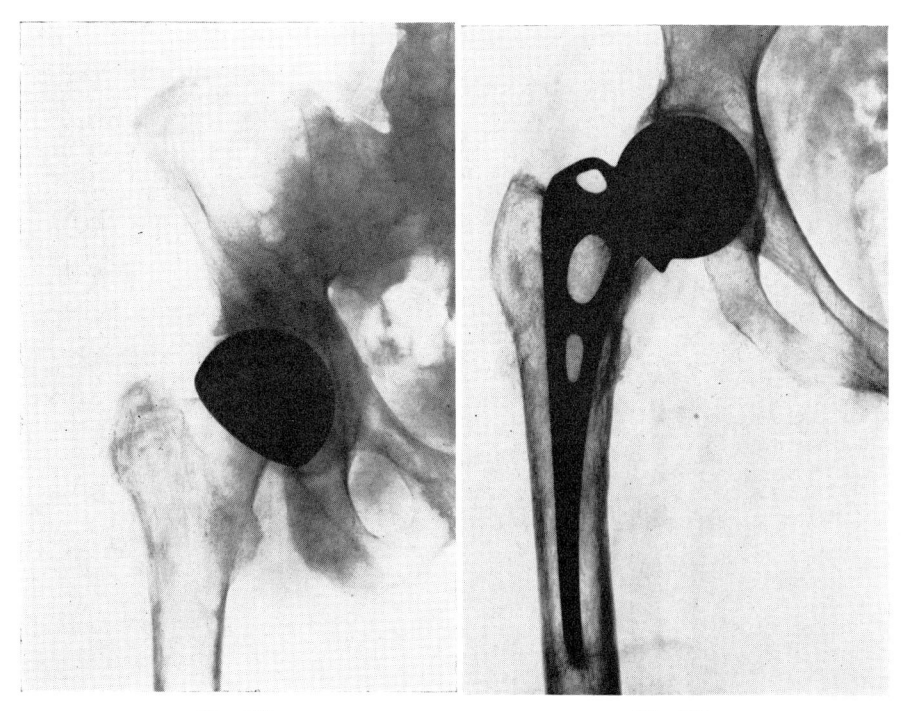

Fig. 125   Fig. 126

Fig. 125. Roentgenogram of hip following Smith-Petersen cup arthroplasty, in a 41-year-old man who had had pain and partial ankylosis of the hip from Strümpell-Marie arthritis.

Fig. 126. Roentgenogram of hip following replacement arthroplasty with Austin Moore prosthesis, in a 75-year-old woman who had had nonunion of a femoral neck fracture and ischemic necrosis of the femoral head.

In recent years replacement arthroplasty of the hip has been much used as a treatment for chronic arthritis, ischemic necrosis of the femoral head, and high, vertical fractures of the femoral neck in elderly persons. In this technic the femoral head is replaced by a metal endo-prosthesis with a stem extending distally through the neck and down into the medullary canal of the upper part of the shaft (Fig. 126). When done on proper indication by a well-trained surgeon, replacement arthroplasty usually produces satisfactory early relief of disabling hip symptoms. Some of these hips become painful several years after operation, however, and it is too early for accurate evaluation of the long-term results.

CHAPTER 10

Neuromuscular disabilities—poliomyelitis

POLIOMYELITIS, OR INFANTILE PARALYSIS, is an acute infectious disease caused by a group of filtrable viruses that attack the nervous system and have an especial tendency to affect the anterior horns of the gray matter of the spinal cord; hence the disease is often called *anterior poliomyelitis*. The infection is often accompanied by a paralysis, which is entirely incidental and not essential to the diagnosis. The disease occurs most often in infancy and in early childhood during epidemics; hence the term "infantile"; yet it is seen also in adults, especially young adults. The incidence is higher in boys than in girls, but among adults it is relatively high in pregnant women. With the use of recently developed vaccines the incidence has decreased tremendously in the past few years.

Poliomyelitis may appear in either sporadic or epidemic form. The greatest number of cases occurs in midsummer and early fall. It has been reported that in an epidemic 6% of all exposed persons will acquire the disease, but only a very small percentage of this number will develop paralysis.

Etiology. Poliovirus, of which there are three types, is a member of the Enterovirus group, which includes the Coxsackie and ECHO viruses. It has recently been demonstrated that certain other viruses of this group can produce diseases, paralytic as well as nonparalytic, which are clinically and pathologically indistinguishable from poliomyelitis. Poliovirus isolated from human cases has been proved to be the infecting agent of poliomyelitis by the results of inoculating monkeys. Poliomyelitis develops in the inoculated animal and can be transmitted to others. Poliovirus and many other members of the Enterovirus group can be propagated in tissue cultures of human and simian cells.

Poliovirus can be isolated from the feces of patients and of persons in contact with them. It is frequently isolated from the oral secretion. During epidemics it has also been isolated from flies. The alimentary tract, particularly its upper portion, the mouth, pharynx, and esophagus, is considered to be the chief pathway for entry of the virus and spread of the disease. From the intestinal tract the virus enters the blood. It has been found in muscle and heart tissue as well as in the nerves. The susceptibility of different individuals varies and is thought to be increased by recent tonsillectomy, inoculations, and pregnancy. It has been shown that one attack confers absolute immunity against only one type of the virus.

Pathology. In the acute stage of the disease the virus has been found chiefly in parts of the central nervous system and in the alimentary tract. It is thought to spread from the alimentary tract by way of the peripheral nerve trunks or blood stream to the central nervous system. The virus has a peculiar affinity for neuronal tissue, especially the motor portion, rather than for the supporting glial tissue. After entering the central nervous system the virus diffuses in all directions, usually traversing the short chain motor pathways. By the time the disease is manifest clinically, evidence of widespread focal involvement of the brain, the spinal cord, and sometimes the meninges may be noted. The clinical findings are never an accurate index of the extent to which the central nervous system has been involved.

The greatest changes appear in the anterior horn cells of the gray matter, especially those in the lumbar enlargement of the cord. These changes result in a motor paralysis. Occasionally the posterior horn cells or root ganglia or the higher sensory centers may be involved in the acute stage with the production of sensory disturbances. The cell bodies of these areas show evidence of atrophy and disintegration and may be replaced by scar tissue. The damaging effects upon the nerve cells may come (1) from direct toxic action by the virus; (2) from anemia through the constriction of local blood vessels; or (3) from direct pressure as the result of hemorrhage, exudate, or edema. There are also changes within the lymphatic system, such as swollen mesenteric glands, congested Peyer's patches, and enlargement of the spleen. In the chronic stage, when the motor cells have been replaced by scar tissue, degeneration of the peripheral nerves occurs and is accompanied by disuse atrophy of muscle, tendon, and bone. In the chronic stage, microscopic examination of affected muscles shows areas of atrophy, fatty or fibrous replacement, and hypertrophy of the undamaged fibers.

Clinical picture. Clinically, the disease may be abortive (without involvement of the central nervous system); it may be nonparalytic (without gross evidence of flaccid paralysis); or it may be paralytic (with varying degrees of muscle weakness or paralysis). The abortive type is of little clinical concern; the nonparalytic type is characterized early by muscle tightness, particularly of the neck, back, and hamstring muscle groups. The paralytic type forms the chief discussion of this chapter. It may be (1) ataxic, in which there are pathologic changes in Clarke's columns, the cerebellum, or the basal ganglia with an accompanying nystagmus; (2) cortical, in which the lesion is in the upper motor neuron with resulting spastic paralysis and hyperactive reflexes; or (3) spinal or subcortical, in which the lesion is in the lower motor neuron and results in flaccid paralysis. The last type is by far the most common. Upper spinal involvement is usually termed bulbar poliomyelitis.

The average incubation period is from seven to fourteen days, although it may be as long as thirty-five days. After the onset of the disease there are three distinct stages: (1) the acute stage or stage of onset, which lasts from one to four weeks; (2) the stage of convalescence and recovery, which lasts from six months to two years; and (3) the residual stage, during which little or no spontaneous improvement occurs.

Acute stage. The symptoms during the acute stage may be divided into three groups: systemic, meningitic, and paralytic.

The most characteristic *systemic* symptom is fever, which may reach from 100° to 104° F. (38° to 40° C.), lasts from one to six days, and then subsides either by lysis or crisis. In this stage intense headaches, rapid pulse, and marked gastrointestinal symptoms, such as vomiting, constipation, and abdominal distress, are often observed. There may be associated upper respiratory symptoms, as well as drowsiness and irritability when the patient is aroused. Urinary retention occurs frequently. The cervical lymph nodes may be enlarged. Pain may be present spontaneously in the muscles or may be felt only when they are subjected to pressure.

The *meningitic* symptoms may consist of hyperactive reflexes and muscular twitchings or convulsions. Stiffness of the back and neck, with inability to touch the chin to the knees, is usually present, and is a valuable diagnostic sign. Kernig's sign, or resistance to extending the knee when the hip is flexed, is usually positive but not so constantly as in bacterial meningitis. The spinal fluid is clear with a moderate increase in cells, polymorphonuclear in the early stages and later mostly lymphocytic, and there may be slight increase of its globulin and albumin content.

The *paralytic* symptoms appear usually on the second or third day and seldom after the eighth day. Resistance to muscle-stretching movements is the most common early sign. With the development of flaccid paralysis the reflexes become hypoactive or absent, the first affected being the abdominal and cremasterics. In the occasional instances of cortical involvement the paralysis may be spastic in type with hyperactive reflexes. Paralytic symptoms are much more common in the lower extremities than in the upper; asymmetrical involvement is usual. Partial paralysis of a muscle is much more common than total paralysis. The return of muscle power begins usually in the first two weeks but may not become obvious until later. The most serious cases, which constitute the bulbar type, are those with paralysis of the diaphragm and of other respiratory muscles. Often the bulbar symptoms quickly follow paralysis of the upper extremity and particularly paralysis about the shoulder girdle.

Great care should be taken to recognize paralysis of the abdominal and spinal muscles, since such paralysis may later lead to curvature of the spine. After weakening or paralysis of any muscles becomes evident, it is most important to determine which groups are involved, since the affected muscles need immediate rest. Tenderness of the muscles may be slight or extreme;

it is a most characteristic symptom and has been known to persist for as long as sixteen weeks, although the average duration is six weeks. Gentle active exercise tends to decrease muscle tenderness.

In an epidemic there may be patients who show all the neurologic, febrile, upper respiratory, and gastrointestinal symptoms but without evidence of paralysis. Such patients are said to have the nonparalytic type of the disease. In a recent large epidemic, one fourth of the patients diagnosed as having poliomyelitis were in this group; however, the percentage varies a great deal in different epidemics. On the other hand, many patients with no apparent evidence of paralysis and diagnosed initially in an epidemic as having nonparalytic poliomyelitis may later show a mild paralysis of some muscle groups.

Convalescent or recovery stage. In the convalescent stage the muscle tenderness has subsided and there may be a progressive increase of muscle power. The improvement in muscle strength may continue for a period of from eighteen months to two years.

Periodic examinations of the different muscle groups should be made in order to follow the degree of muscle improvement. Much important information can be gained from careful observation of the gait. The so-called *steppage* or *foot-drop gait,* in which the anterior portion of the foot strikes the floor first with each step, is an indication of paralysis of the anterior muscles of the leg. This paralysis is often associated with equinus deformity, and there may be accompanying genu recurvatum, especially when the flexors of the knee are paralyzed. In paralysis of the quadriceps the patient often inclines his body forward and places his hand on the front of the thigh. This braces or stabilizes the knee in extension and prevents sudden flexion on weight bearing. In paralysis of the gluteus maximus muscle the trunk sways backward in walking to prevent a sudden flexion of the body on weight bearing. In paralysis of the gluteus medius muscle the body sways toward the affected side to maintain balance.

Weakness of the abdominal muscles is considered by many to be the most common cause of scoliosis and lordosis after poliomyelitis. In paralytic scoliosis of moderate to severe degree, the patient usually cannot raise his trunk from a supine to a sitting position without the aid of his arms.

Residual stage. The paralytic symptoms and signs in this stage are stationary or very slowly regressive. Deformities may have begun to appear or may already be fully developed (Figs. 127 to 129). They will be described under the treatment of established deformity.

Diagnosis. Except during epidemics the diagnosis is frequently not made until after the paralysis appears. It is usually based upon the history of slight systemic upset, the stiffness of the neck, the muscle tenderness, the paralysis, and the findings on examination of the spinal fluid. It may be verified by isolation of the virus from fecal specimens or pharyngeal swabbings.

Differential diagnosis. In the *acute stage* poliomyelitis is to be differentiated from (1) acute febrile affections usually not accompanied by paralysis, such as acute rheumatic fever, fever associated with upper respiratory

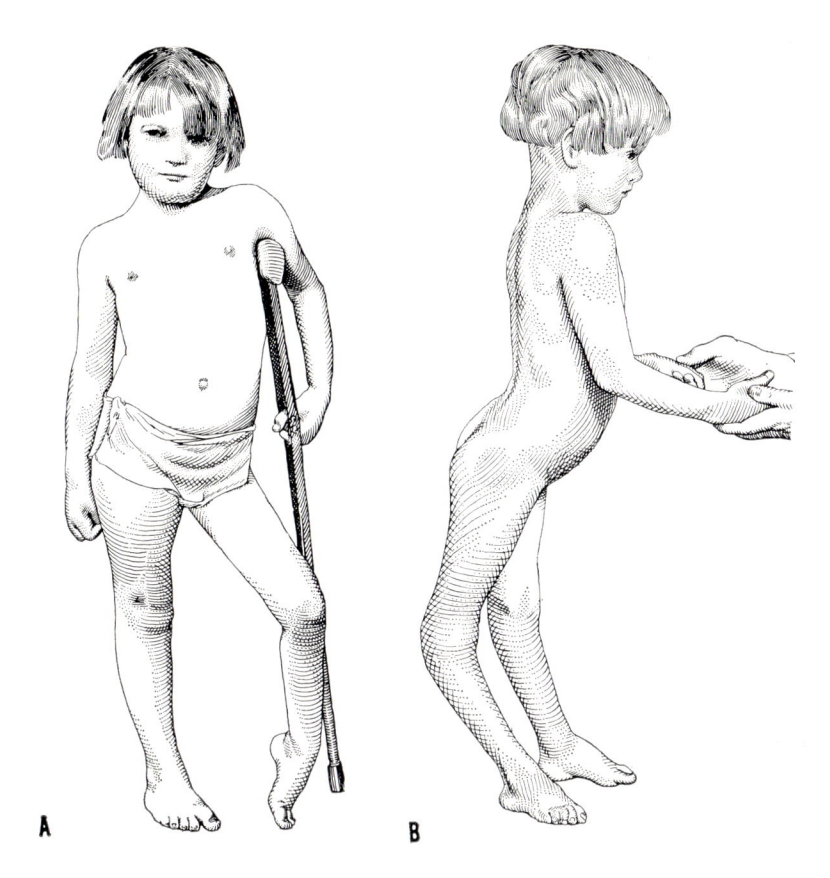

Fig. 127. Deformities in poliomyelitis. A, Note flexion contracture of left hip and knee and equinovarus deformity of left foot. B, Note increased lumbar lordosis and bilateral hip flexion contracture, genu recurvatum (back-knee), and equinus. (A, After Ombredanne and Mathieu.)

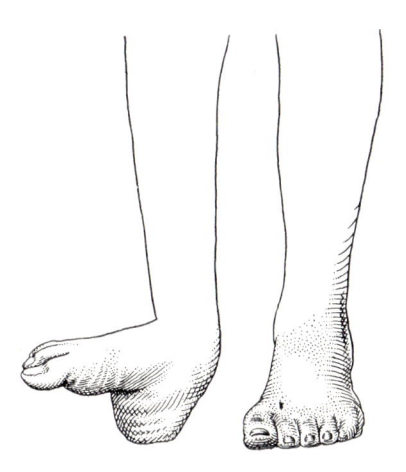

Fig. 128. Deformities in poliomyelitis. Note marked calcaneocavus of right foot.

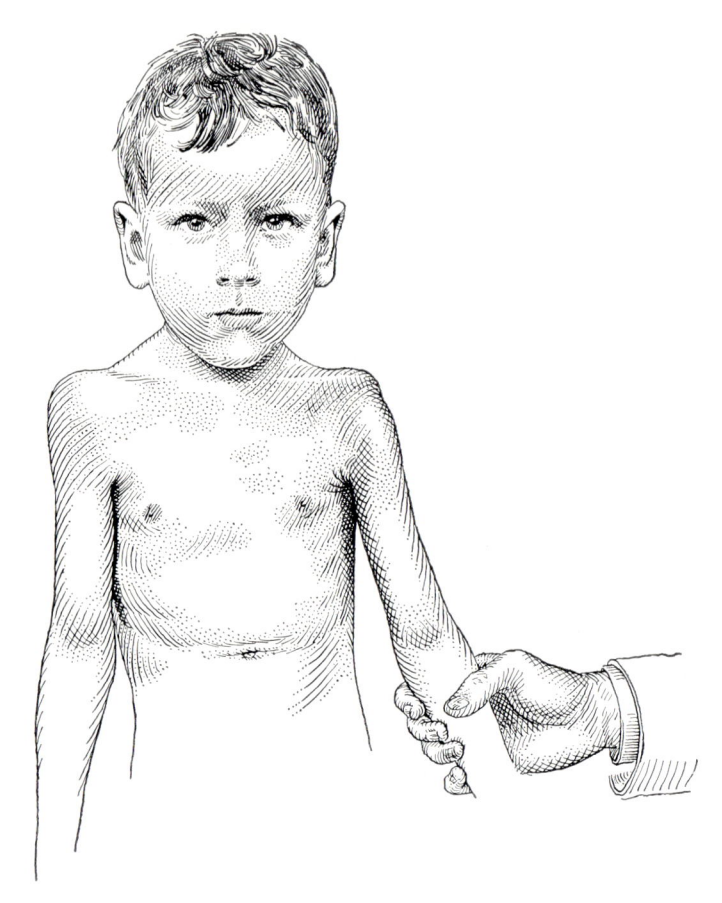

Fig. 129. Deformities in poliomyelitis. Note atrophy and subluxation of left shoulder from paralysis of the deltoid muscle.

infection, pyogenic arthritis, and osteomyelitis, and (2) febrile affections that may be associated with paralysis, such as other enterovirus infections, diphtheria, the Guillain-Barré syndrome, and other forms of polyneuritis. In the *chronic stage* it is to be differentiated from (1) primary affections of the central nervous system, such as alcoholic polyneuritis, encephalitis, meningitis, brain tumor, cerebral palsy, transverse myelitis, lead poisoning, and infantile spinal muscular atrophy; (2) diseases accompanied by pseudoparalysis or spasm, such as pseudohypertrophic muscular dystrophy, syphilis, hypervitaminosis A, infantile cortical hyperostosis, scurvy, and rickets; (3) other conditions that present deformity and loss of function, such as congenital clubfoot and congenital dislocation of the hip; and (4) peripheral nerve injuries, including obstetric paralysis.

Prognosis. The mortality rate is from 3 to 20% during epidemics and increases with age. Ordinarily it is greater in males than in females; however, pregnant women have the highest mortality rate. In bulbar cases the mortality is very high, usually 50% or more. Death is often caused by hypoxia from partial paralysis of the respiratory muscles, with pooling of secretions in the throat, or from involvement of the respiratory or the circulatory center in the medulla.

The prognosis as to function is extremely uncertain. The extent of recovery of muscle power depends wholly upon the survival of the affected nerve cells. No method of determining the amount of power that will return to the paralyzed muscles is known. The prognosis is very favorable if there is a rapid return of power after the initial paralysis, and it is usually better for the upper extremities than for the lower. The prognosis is unfavorable in patients in whom muscle tenderness has been persistent. It is poor when the muscles have remained paralyzed for as long as three months without evidence of return of power. If sufficient rest and support can be given the paralyzed muscles during the acute and convalescent stages, the prognosis is relatively favorable. Spontaneous improvement, if it occurs, starts within a few weeks after the onset of the paralysis and is most rapid during the first six months. Complete recovery after extensive paralysis is uncommon, but after moderate paralysis it is quite common. An extremely high percentage of paralyzed patients in poliomyelitis epidemics either recover completely or are left with a very slight residual paralysis. In a careful two-year follow-up of 673 individuals with paralysis in two Maryland epidemics there were found to be 55% with complete recoveries, and 81% with good recoveries. Retardation of the growth of the affected extremity may occur as a result of disuse.

Treatment. The treatment will be discussed in relation to prophylaxis and to the acute, convalescent, and residual stages, respectively.

Prophylactic measures. Great care should be taken in isolating the patient, especially as regards contact with the nasal secretions and disposal of the feces. Such isolation should be maintained from the onset to forty-eight hours after the temperature becomes normal. During epidemics it is advisable that children avoid fatigue, crowds, swimming pools, and contact with other children. Every effort should be made to exterminate flies, as it has been shown that they are sometimes carriers of the virus.

The Salk vaccine is a most valuable preventive agent. Its efficacy in protecting against paralysis has been estimated to range from 80 to 90% or higher. It is recommended that it be given in three doses to everyone under 45 years of age, and especially to children between 2 and 8 years of age and to pregnant women. It has no effect in decreasing the severity of poliomyelitis if given after the disease has begun. The recently developed Sabin vaccine of living, attenuated virus, which is administered by mouth, shows great promise of eradicating poliomyelitis but currently is recommended only for community-wide use.

Acute stage. In the acute stage constant rest in bed with the joints supported in a neutral position is essential. It relieves the pain and prevents contractures. During this time the patient should not be allowed to become constipated. Inflammation of the nose and throat should be treated symptomatically. Lumbar puncture and intravenous injections of hypertonic glucose during the acute stage reduce the cerebrospinal fluid pressure and are of value in treating meningismus. Hot moist packs may be helpful in relieving pain. In some clinics good results in relieving sustained muscle contraction by the use of muscle-relaxant drugs have been reported. The weakened muscles should be maintained in an attitude free from strain, and any affected joints should be held in the position of maximum functional utility. This part of the treatment is most important in preventing the development of deformity. If a choice of the muscles to be protected in order to prevent deformity is necessary, groups that maintain the erect position—i.e., the hip extensors, the knee extensors, the abdominals and erector spinae, and the dorsiflexors of the ankle—should be given first consideration. Next in importance are the abductors of the shoulder, the dorsiflexors of the wrist, and the adductors of the thumb.

When, in bulbar cases, the respiratory muscles become involved, the patient should be kept quiet with his head down. The administration of oxygen is essential if the patient is hypoxic. Keeping the airway open may require frequent suction. If respiration becomes difficult, from paralysis of the primary respiratory muscles, the patient should be placed in a respirator until recovery of muscle power is sufficient to permit maintenance of normal respiration. He should not be left in the respirator longer than is necessary. If the pharyngeal muscles are paralyzed, care should be taken to forestall choking attacks and the aspiration of mucus. Occasionally tracheotomy becomes necessary. The patient should be fed parenterally and kept at complete rest.

Convalescent stage. The convalescent stage, extending from the subsidence of muscle tenderness to slowing of the process of recovery of muscle power, may last for two years or longer. To prevent joint contracture in this stage it is usually advisable to move the joints passively through their painless range of motion each day. How long the muscles should be kept at rest is a debatable point. Partial immobilization should be continued until an end stage in the return of muscle power has become apparent. Gentle active exercises should be started early in the convalescent stage and gradually increased. Muscles should never be exercised, however, to the point of pain or fatigue. Exercises that do not involve weight bearing will improve the strength of the weakened muscles; however, if too much strain is put upon them, as in weight bearing, their recovery will be definitely retarded. Resistive exercises may be of great value at this stage. In hydrotherapy the support of the water allows muscles to be moved more effectively and provides a pleasant way of carrying out the exercises. The water has no intrinsic therapeutic value. Muscle fatigue, which is to be carefully avoided, can appear with less warning in underwater exercises than in exercises given out of water.

The exercises may be preceded by heat and massage. Selected exercises establish better coordination between partially paralyzed and normal groups. As the patient returns to walking, gait instruction and training should be provided. Great care should be taken to prevent the development of de-

Neuromuscular disabilities—poliomyelitis 211

formities, by proper positioning of the joints and early active corrective exercises. If preventive measures are not taken, permanent bone deformities may later develop as the result of malpositions that have remained uncorrected for a long period of time.

In the convalescent stage, braces and other supportive devices (Fig. 130) are often necessary (1) to enable the patient to stand and walk, (2) to prevent deformity and malposition, and (3) to help in stretching certain groups of muscles that have become contracted. In general, however, bracing is undesirable and should be used only when necessary. A back brace (Fig. 99), removable plaster jacket, or orthopaedic corset may be used for paralysis of the back and abdominal muscles. An abduction arm splint may be used for paralysis of the deltoid muscle. A cock-up splint is used for paralysis of the extensor muscles of the wrist. A walking caliper brace with or without a lock joint at the knee is indicated in paralysis involving the thigh muscles (Fig. 131), and the same type of brace with a waistband and a lock joint at the hip may be used for paralysis of the extensors of the hip. An ankle brace with a right-angle stop joint may be used for paralysis of the dorsiflexor muscles of the ankle (Fig. 132). In paralysis of the gastrocnemius and soleus muscles either an ankle brace with a reversed right-angle stop joint or a

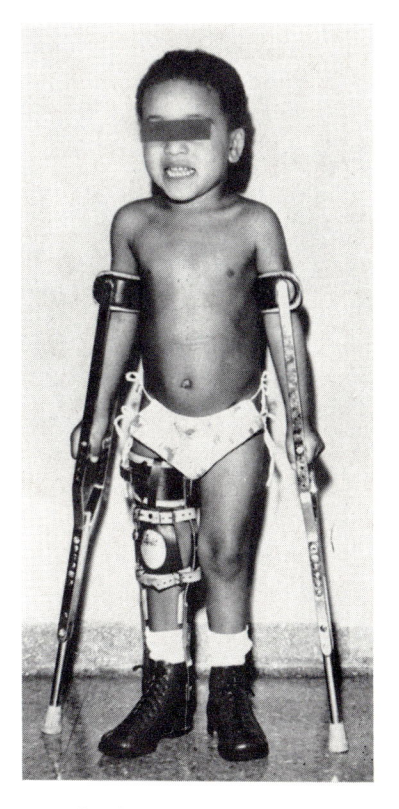

Fig. 130. Convalescent stage of poliomyelitis. Weakened right lower limb is protected by use of a long leg brace and crutches of adjustable length.

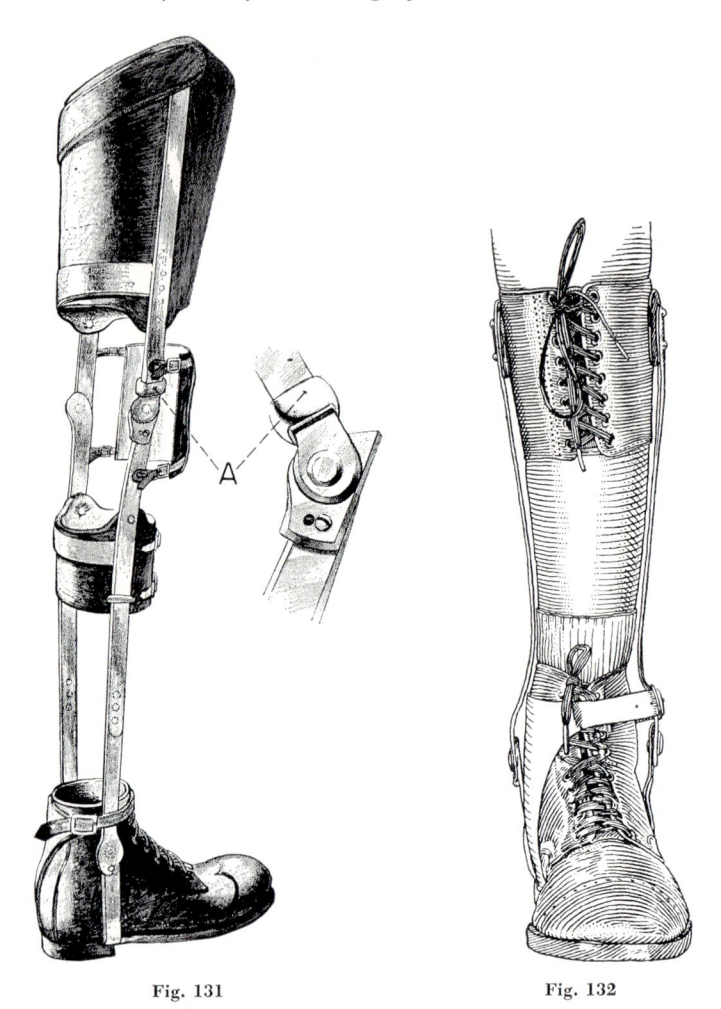

Fig. 131. Long leg brace, with lock joint at knee, **A,** and right-angle stop joint and pull-over **T** strap at ankle. This type of brace is used for the weak lower extremity with paralysis of muscles of the thigh and leg and little or no stability of the knee.

Fig. 132. Ankle brace with **T** strap, for paralysis of muscles of the leg. The **T** strap is used to prevent a deviation of the ankle toward the medial side.

shoe with a raised heel and stiff tongue may be used. In paralysis of the invertors or evertors of the foot a lateral or medial single-bar type of brace with a **T** strap attached to the shoe may be used.

Residual stage. In the residual stage operations are performed to correct deformity, to improve muscle balance, and to secure the stability of joints. In general, procedures of the last two types should not be done until a period of from eighteen months to two years has elapsed from the time of onset of the disease, and procedures of the last type should not be used until the age of 10 years has been reached in the normally developing child or the age of 12 years when the child is underdeveloped.

Surgical treatment. The surgical correction of deformities and disabilities of the joints following poliomyelitis still forms a considerable part of the surgical work on crippled children's services. The procedures, when selected on the basis of sound indications, performed correctly, and followed by adequate aftercare, are productive of most gratifying results. By operation many patients are enabled for the first time to walk, and others who have been in braces and on crutches are enabled to discard these supports. Great care must always be taken, however, that the operation do no harm. In every clinic, individual modifications of accepted surgical procedures have been adopted. No other condition in orthopaedic surgery requires more mature judgment for selection of the most beneficial procedures. Poor results are usually the consequence either of decisions made hastily, on patients who have not been adequately studied or observed, or of operations not followed by sufficient aftercare and observation. Often more information can be gained, and the treatment can be more wisely selected, by watching the patient handle himself and walk than by performing tests of individual muscle function. Too much emphasis cannot be placed upon the necessity of waiting until the child is of adequate age, size, and bony development before proceeding with operations on bony structures, which might later prove futile because of growth changes. Every operation for the correction of deformity or disability resulting from poliomyelitis should be followed by a long period of careful observation.

1. *Operations for the correction of deformities of long standing:*

It often happens that the orthopaedic surgeon does not see the patient until months or years after the onset of the disease and that by this time the deformity has become firmly fixed. Such deformity may involve any one or combination of the following: hip, knee, ankle, upper extremity, and spine.

THE HIP. It is not uncommon to observe a pathologic dislocation of the hip, following paralysis of the gluteus muscles, and flexion-adduction deformity due to persistence of the function of hip flexors and adductors. A snapping sensation on motion of the hip may be associated with an incomplete dislocation. In the treatment of such a dislocation a two-stage shelf operation (Fig. 46) with reefing of the hip joint capsule may be performed. At the first operation the dislocation is reduced, the posterior portion of the capsule is plicated, and the leg is immobilized in a slightly abducted and hyperextended position. At the second operation an exaggerated acetabular shelf is created. Frequently, however, paralytic dislocation of the hip is best treated by arthrodesis.

Hip flexion contracture usually results from allowing the patient to sit up for too long periods during the convalescent stage and can be prevented by keeping the patient in the prone position for a few hours each day during this period. Hip flexion deformity is caused by a contracture of the tensor fasciae latae, iliopsoas, sartorius, and rectus femoris muscles together with weakness of the gluteus maximus muscle. The contracture may at times be gradually reduced by repeated stretching or by the wedging of a bilateral hip spica cast. Occasionally it may be necessary to carry out open division of the tensor fasciae latae muscle at the hip together with manipulation and stretching. A flexion deformity of the hip can usually be relieved by transverse section of the iliotibial band just above the knee *(Yount operation)*, combined with section of the tensor fasciae latae just below the level of the greater trochanter and followed by skeletal traction and plaster fixation. This procedure has been popularized by Irwin. The operation of choice in more severe cases may consist of stripping the fascia lata and associated flexors of the hip subperiosteally from the anterior superior spine and crest of the ilium for a distance of about 1½ inches and of allowing them to slip down the side of the pelvis to become reattached at a more distal site *(Soutter operation)*. This operation is followed by immobilization in a plaster cast for six to eight weeks with the hip in hyperextension. In the most severe cases the anterior superior spine and anterior portion of the crest of the ilium may be detached along with their muscle insertions, slipped down the side of the pelvis, and transplanted *en masse* into the bone at a lower level *(Campbell operation)*. The hip is then immobilized in hyperextension in a plaster cast for eight weeks.

THE KNEE. Flexion deformity of the knee is common. It results from the contraction of strong hamstring and gastrocnemius muscles that are ineffectively opposed by a weakened quadriceps group. It is possible at times to reduce the deformity by applying traction to the leg. Wedged or turnbuckle plaster casts often serve very satisfactorily. Occasionally it may be necessary to lengthen the tendons behind the knee or to perform a *capsuloplasty* in which the posterior attachment of the joint capsule to the femur is released. It is often advisable to combine transference of the tendon of the biceps femoris to the patella with capsuloplasty. For persistent flexion contracture, a supracondylar osteotomy is sometimes indicated.

When a knock-knee deformity develops from quadriceps paralysis with a strong biceps femoris and a tight iliotibial band, it may be necessary to section the band, perform a supracondylar osteotomy of the femur, correct the deformity, and immobilize the extremity in a plaster cast for eight weeks.

When genu recurvatum has developed as a result of weakness of the hamstrings, or walking with an equinus contracture, a caliper brace with a posterior knee strap may stabilize the joint sufficiently to facilitate walking. In more marked cases the patella may be implanted into the upper end of the tibia to act as a bone block and prevent the knee from undergoing hyperextension *(Campbell operation)* or a strong check ligament may be constructed posteriorly from the periosteum of the femur and the fascia lata *(Gill operation)*. A wedge osteotomy of the upper 2 inches of the tibia with its base directed posteriorly and an osteotomy of the fibula, as described by Irwin, are sometimes preferable.

Occasionally posterior subluxation and external rotation of the tibia may develop as a result of weakness of the quadriceps muscle while the hamstrings remain strong. For this deformity it is often advisable to carry out an arthrodesis of the knee; if this is not done, an accurately fitting brace should be applied.

THE ANKLE. An equinus deformity or foot drop may develop as a result of the persistent action of normal gastrocnemius and soleus muscles in opposition to weakened dorsiflexors of the foot. This is by far the commonest paralytic deformity of the ankle. An open lengthening of the Achilles tendon, sometimes accompanied by posterior capsulotomy of the ankle joint, followed by overcorrection in a plaster cast for six weeks, may be indicated. An ankle brace with a right-angle stop (Fig. 132) may then be necessary to prevent recurrence of the equinus. At times it is possible to overcome the contracture with wedged casts or a constant-tension brace. When there is an external rotation deformity of the foot and lower part of the leg due to tibial torsion, correction may be effected by a rotation osteotomy of the tibia.

THE UPPER EXTREMITY. Contracture of the shoulder may develop as a result of paralysis of the abductors and persistence of the adductors. The deformity is one of adduction and internal rotation. It may be possible to overcome the contracture by manipulation. Otherwise the contracted structures should be exposed by open operation and incised. Early cases of deltoid paralysis may be treated with an *abduction brace,* or a *suspension splint* as described by Irwin, to forestall the development of adduction contracture.

Occasionally there may be a luxation of the head of the humerus due to stretching of the joint capsule following paralysis of the deltoid, triceps, and biceps muscles (Fig. 129). When extreme relaxation is present in the chronic stage and is interfering with function, arthrodesis of the shoulder may be advisable (Fig. 137).

Deformities of the elbow, wrist, and hand, resulting from unbalanced muscular pull and the effects of gravity, may be of varied type. Surgical correction of the deformity is occasionally indicated.

THE SPINE. Great care should be taken to prevent the development of lateral curvature. When weakness of the muscles of the back or abdomen becomes evident, recumbency on a firmly supported mattress, corrective exercises, and prolonged use of a back brace may be indicated. Incipient lateral curvature may be treated by recumbency with traction applied to the head and to the pelvis (Fig. 95). Correction of the curvature can usually be accomplished if treatment is started before secondary bone changes develop. In order to prevent the deformity from increasing, it is often necessary to stabilize the spine by surgical fusion of the vertebrae (Fig. 96). Established scoliosis may require forcible correction of the curvature by special cast or brace technics (p. 335) prior to arthrodesis.

Fascia lata transplants are occasionally used to reinforce partially paralyzed abdominal muscles *(Lowman operation),* but on the whole their results in the hands of most orthopaedic surgeons have been disappointing.

2. *Muscle and tendon transplantations:*

In selected cases, improvement in muscle balance may be obtained by muscle and tendon transplantations, or transferences. In tendon transference it is important (1) that any deformity of the joint should have been previously corrected; (2) that the tendon used should arise from a muscle with good power, preferably equal to that of the paralyzed muscle; (3) that the tendon should pass to its new insertion in a straight line through subcutaneous fat or through a tendon sheath; (4) that the tendon should be inserted under slight tension directly into bone; and (5) that, after the period of postoperative immobilization, supervised exercises should be carried out for the patient to learn optimum use of the transferred muscle-tendon unit. Occasionally a portion of another tendon or a transplant of fascia lata is used to supplement the transferred tendon when its length is insufficient. Tendon transference may be indicated in the treatment of hip, knee, foot, shoulder, elbow, or hand disabilities.

THE HIP. The unsightly gait caused by paralysis of the gluteus maximus or of the gluteus medius may often be improved by one of the following operations.

For paralysis of the gluteus maximus muscle two useful surgical procedures have been devised. In one the erector spinae muscles are freed from their lower attachments and a long strip of fascia lata is removed and sutured to them, passed over the paralyzed gluteus maximus muscle, and fixed into the femur at the insertion of the gluteus maximus *(Ober operation)*. In the other, the origin of the tensor fasciae latae muscle with its bony attachment is transplanted into either the posterior superior spine or the adjacent posterior portion of the iliac crest *(Dickson operation)*. After either of these operations a plaster spica cast applied with the hip in full abduction and extension is to be worn for a period of from six to eight weeks.

For paralysis of the gluteus medius muscle the origin of the tensor fasciae latae may be transplanted posteriorly on the crest of the ilium to a point directly above the greater trochanter *(Legg operation)*. This procedure tends to diminish the lateral sway of the body which is characteristic of abductor limp. Similarly, the insertion of the external oblique or of the iliopsoas muscle may be transferred to the greater trochanter.

THE KNEE. Tendon transplantations about the knee frequently result in improvement of its function and stability. For quadriceps paralysis the most satisfactory operation, in the presence of strong hamstring muscles, is transplantation of the biceps femoris tendon, the iliotibial band, and one medial hamstring into the patella. If the hamstrings as well as the quadriceps are weak, the sartorius muscle and the iliotibial band may be transplanted into the patella.

THE FOOT. Tendon transplantations combined with stabilizing operations on the joints often give very satisfactory results. For varus deformity the tibialis anterior muscle may be transplanted into the cuboid bone or into the base of the third or fourth metatarsal bone. For valgus deformity one of the peroneal tendons may be transplanted either into the navicular bone or into the base of the first metatarsal bone; however, these procedures are not so successful as the transplantations for varus deformity. For a calcaneus foot, transplantation of one or both peroneal tendons and the posterior tibial tendon into the calcaneus may prove beneficial, but this procedure is successful only if some power is present in the calf muscles. For a plantar flexion deformity, or foot drop, the tendon of the extensor hallucis longus or one or both of the peroneal tendons may be transplanted to the navicular; these transplants, however, are not too successful. For a depression of the first metatarsal head and dorsiflexion of the great toe the tendon of the extensor hallucis longus may be transplanted to the neck of the first metatarsal; this should be combined with a fusion of the interphalangeal joint. In many clinics this is the most common transfer, and its results are usually satisfactory. On many occasions these transplantations are combined with joint stabilization operations; although the transplanted tendon may not function as intended, the deforming force is removed by the transfer and the result may be very satisfactory. The treatment of clawfoot deformity resulting from poliomyelitis is discussed on p. 422.

THE SHOULDER. For paralysis of the deltoid muscle the acromial portion of the trapezius muscle may be transplanted into the upper part of the humerus *(Mayer operation)*, or the long head of the triceps and the short head of the biceps may be transplanted into the acromion *(Ober operation)*. The arm is then held in an abduction spica cast for several weeks. Frequently the results of these operations are not so satisfactory as those usually obtained after tendon transplantations in the lower extremities.

THE ELBOW. For incomplete paralysis of the flexors of the elbow the origin of the common flexor tendon, together with its bony attachment at the medial epicondyle, may be transplanted into the shaft of the humerus at a point about 2 inches proximal to its original site *(Steindler operation)*. This procedure often results in considerable improvement of the power of elbow flexion; it may even restore active flexion after this movement has been almost completely lost, but it is most effective when some power remains in the biceps and brachialis muscles. Flexor power has also been restored to the elbow by transplanting the insertion of the triceps tendon into the biceps tendon at the radial tuberosity.

THE HAND. The indications for tendon transference in the hand are numerous, and many operations have been described. The most important mechanism in the hand is opposition of the thumb to the forefinger; operations to improve this function are performed most frequently. For paralysis of the opponens pollicis the palmaris longus or the flexor carpi ulnaris may be used as a motor, the tendon being transplanted into the extensor pollicis brevis tendon after having been looped to the ulnar side of the wrist *(Bunnell operation)*. An alternative procedure is to detach the tendon of the flexor sublimis of the fourth finger, loop it about the flexor carpi ulnaris, and fasten it into the base of the first phalanx of the thumb. When no tendon is available for transfer, a bone graft placed between the first and second metacarpal bones will often make opposition of the thumb and fingers possible.

A most important part of tendon and muscle transplantation is the aftercare. Exercise should be started early in order to lessen the likelihood of adhesions. Physical therapy should be continued as long as progressive improvement is demonstrable.

3. *Operations to increase the stability of joints:*

The most useful procedures in the surgical treatment of poliomyelitis are operations that restore stability to flail joints. Arthrodesis is the most important of these surgical procedures. Bone block is an auxiliary measure which often results in marked improvement of function.

Arthrodesis. Arthrodesis may be indicated for the hip, knee, ankle, foot, shoulder, elbow, or wrist.

THE HIP. Arthrodesis of the hip after poliomyelitis is rarely indicated. Postoperative immobilization must be continued until firm union has taken place; this usually requires from twelve to twenty weeks. The return to activity must be gradual.

THE KNEE. Arthrodesis of the knee is indicated only in selected cases. A well-fitting brace with an adjustable lock at the knee is usually preferable to arthrodesis, but for adults or older children who wish to be free from the inconvenience of apparatus, arthrodesis may be advisable.

THE ANKLE. Arthrodesis of the ankle is occasionally indicated. When arthrodesis is performed, the articular cartilage is usually removed through an anterior incision. As a rule, it is wise to fuse the subtalar and mediotarsal joints at the same time; this operation is called a *pantalar arthrodesis.*

THE FOOT. Arthrodesis of the subtalar and mediotarsal joints is the most commonly performed operation in the surgical treatment of disability follow-

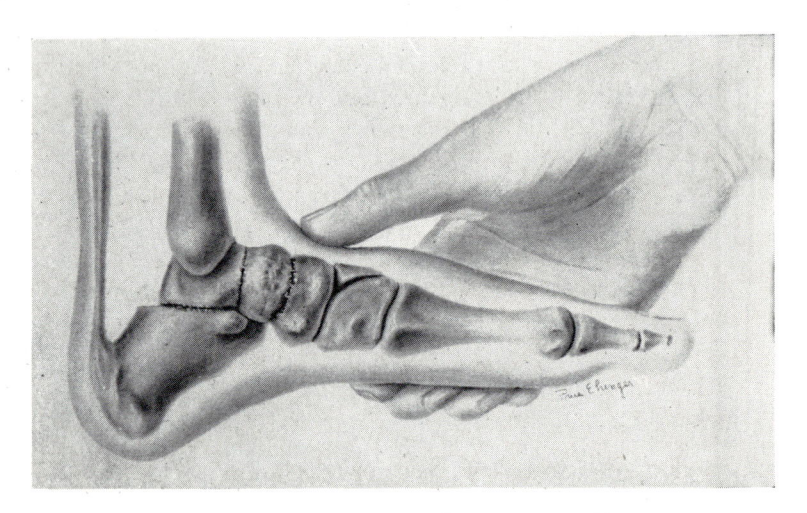

Fig. 133. Hoke operation for stabilizing the foot in poliomyelitis (medial view). Head of the talus has been removed, reshaped, and replaced; articular surfaces have been removed from the talocalcaneal and the talonavicular joints, and foot has been displaced backward on the talus. (Hoke's original drawing.)

ing poliomyelitis. The great value of stabilizing these joints was first shown by G. G. Davis in 1913.

In America the *Hoke operation* (Fig. 133) or one of its modifications is the most popular type of arthrodesis. It may be used for varus, valgus, calcaneus, or equinus deformity. In this operation the head and the neck of the talus are taken out; the subtalar joint surfaces are excised; the cartilage is removed from the posterior surface of the navicular bone; the denuded head of the talus is replaced between the navicular and the body of the talus; and the foot is displaced backward upon the talus. Usually the calcaneocuboid joint surfaces are also removed. When this is done, the combined operation is sometimes known as a *triple arthrodesis* (Fig. 134); this procedure was popularized by Hibbs and Ryerson.

In England the *Dunn operation* or one of its modifications is more popular than the Hoke. In this procedure the navicular bone is completely removed, the subtalar and calcaneocuboid joint surfaces are excised, and the

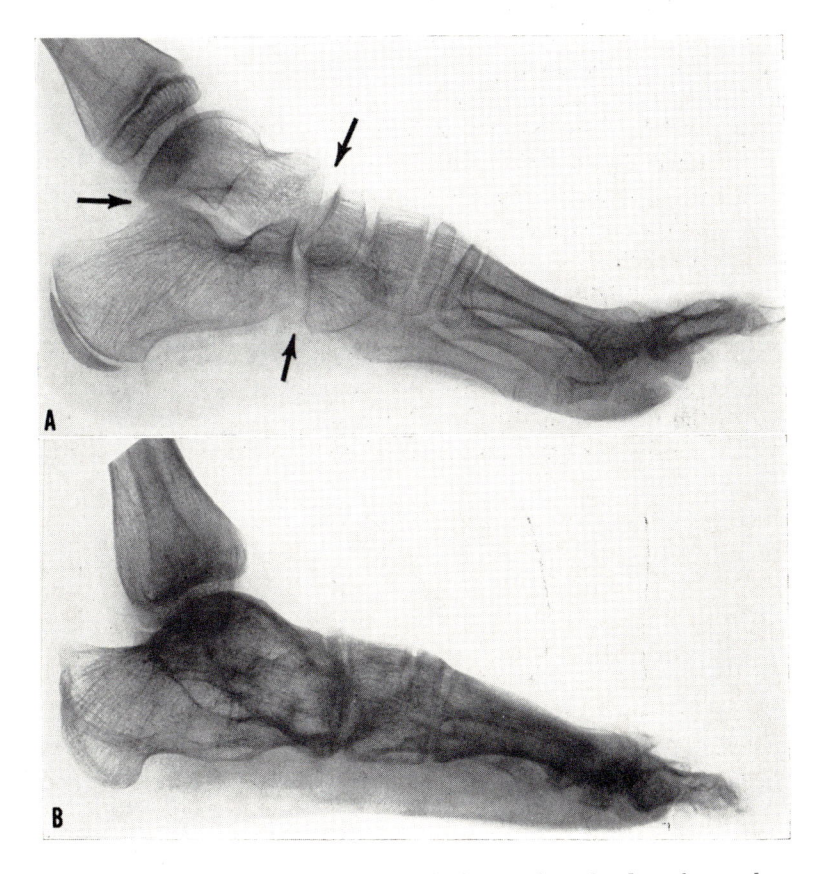

Fig. 134. Roentgenograms of foot before and after triple arthrodesis for weakness and instability from poliomyelitis. **A,** Arrows show the three joints that are to be fused. **B,** Seven years after arthrodesis. Note that the talus, calcaneus, navicular, and cuboid now form a single bony mass providing stability for the foot.

head of the talus and the posterior surface of the cuneiform bones are denuded of cartilage and approximated. Occasionally an arthrodesis of the ankle is performed at the same time. The Hoke and the Dunn operations are most used for the varus or valgus foot. The *Lambrinudi operation* is sometimes used for stabilizing the foot in the presence of weak dorsiflexors of the ankle and fairly strong plantar flexors. The operation consists of (1) removing the whole undersurface of the talus obliquely and the upper surface of the calcaneus, (2) placing the talus in full plantar flexion, and (3) bringing up the forefoot at the mediotarsal joint so that the remainder of the head of the talus lies beneath a prepared bed in the undersurface of the navicular, while the talus and calcaneus are approximated.

For the calcaneus foot (Fig. 135), many orthopaedic surgeons perform a modified triple arthrodesis and in some instances combine with it a fusion of the ankle joint. In combination with triple arthrodesis, the tendons of the peroneals, flexor digitorum longus, and flexor hallucis longus may be transferred into the Achilles tendon and calcaneus. The Whitman astragalectomy has often been used in the past but is seldom done at this time. If an astragalectomy is performed, it is essential that the foot be displaced well backward upon the tibia.

The usual period of immobilization in plaster after arthrodesis of the tarsus is from eight to twelve weeks. It is frequently advisable to change the cast three weeks after operation; at this time, when necessary, manipulation under anesthesia can be carried out to improve the final position of the foot.

Paralytic valgus deformity in young children can be improved or completely corrected by inserting bone grafts into the sinus tarsi to effect extra-articular arthrodesis of the subtalar joint *(Grice operation,* Fig. 136).

THE SHOULDER. Arthrodesis of the shoulder is not to be considered unless the muscles of the shoulder girdle are strong enough to permit shrugging the shoulder and unless useful function of the hand has been retained. Sat-

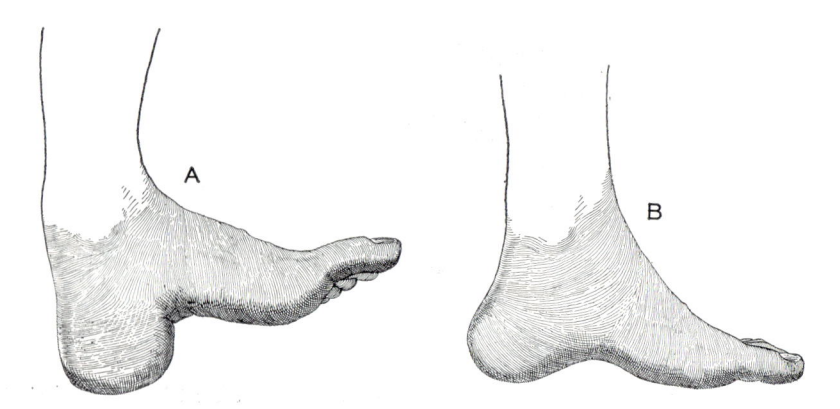

Fig. 135. Calcaneocavus deformity in poliomyelitis (medial view). **A,** Before operation. **B,** After operative stabilization. Note posterior displacement of the foot and correction of the deformity.

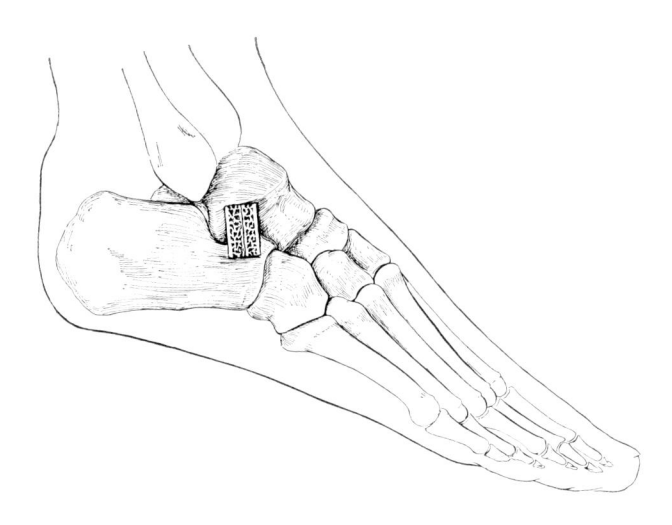

Fig. 136. Grice extra-articular arthrodesis of the subtalar joint for paralytic flatfoot in childhood. Note bone grafts in the sinus tarsi. (Redrawn from Grice, D. S.: J. Bone & Joint Surg. **37-A**:246, 1955.)

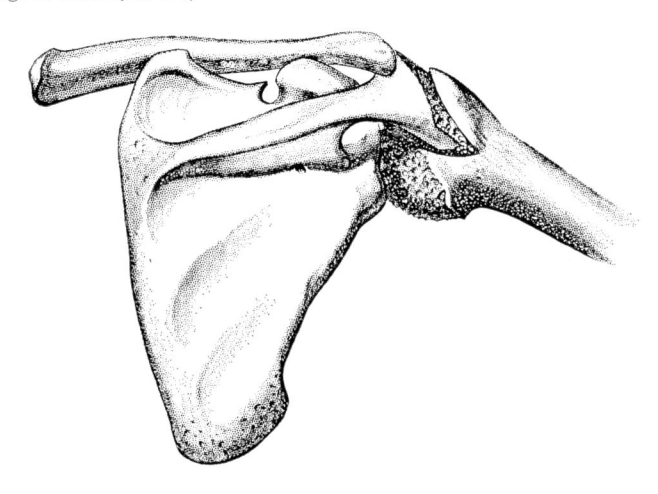

Fig. 137. Arthrodesis of shoulder (Gill). The cartilage has been removed from glenoid and humeral head, and the acromion has been denuded of periosteum, beveled on its flat surfaces, and inserted into a slot in the greater tuberosity of the humerus.

isfactory use of the fused shoulder is dependent upon power in the upper part of the trapezius, the upper two thirds of the serratus anterior, and the pectoralis major muscle. A satisfactory method of arthrodesis is to denude the joint surfaces of cartilage, bevel the upper and lower flat surfaces of the acromion, and then insert this beveled end into a prepared slot in the head of the humerus *(Gill operation,* Fig. 137). Another method of obtaining fusion is to insert a massive bone graft into a hole drilled through the humeral head and into the scapula.

THE ELBOW. Arthrodesis of the elbow is seldom necessary after poliomyelitis.

THE WRIST. Arthrodesis of the wrist is occasionally indicated. It may allow remaining flexors or extensors of the wrist to be transferred for use as motors of the fingers. The cartilaginous surfaces between the carpus and the lower end of the radius should be removed and the wrist immobilized in slight dorsiflexion. A popular technic for arthrodesis of the wrist is to use a cortical bone graft extending from the radius across the denuded dorsum of the carpal bones to the proximal end of the third metacarpal bone. If adequate power is present in the muscles of the fingers, the function of the hand is likely to be improved

Extra-articular check operations about the ankle. It is sometimes useful to abolish undesired ankle motion by creating surgically a bony block. This type of operation is often used to check plantar flexion in paralysis of the dorsiflexor muscles and occasionally to limit dorsiflexion when the plantar flexors are paralyzed. In either case the bone check operation is often preceded by a subtalar arthrodesis.

To check the disabling equinus deformity of paralytic drop foot, either of two procedures may be used. The posterior superior surface of the calcaneus may be denuded and bone chips placed on the raw surface beneath the Achilles tendon. The mass of bone chips should extend up to the lower end of the tibia. When this transplanted bone becomes solid, there is a firm structure behind the ankle which prevents the foot from dropping beyond a right angle *(Campbell bone block operation)*. In the alternative procedure the posterior superior surface of the talus is split, elevated, and held in its new position by the insertion of a small wedge of bone *(Gill operation)*. Gill has also shown that the excessive dorsiflexion of paralytic calcaneus deformity can be limited by creating a bone block anteriorly; the anterosuperior surface of the body of the talus is elevated by an analogous technic. Ryerson and Putti have described similar operations.

4. *Leg equalization operations:*

Frequently after poliomyelitis considerable shortening of the affected leg is produced by the retardation of bone growth. The shortening is proportional to the extent of the paralysis. Slight shortening should be treated by a heel raise. Greater disproportion may indicate surgical equalization of the length of the legs. The indication is sometimes provided by other causes of lateral asymmetry, such as developmental hemihypertrophy or retarded growth following epiphyseal injury. Equalization of leg length may be effected either by lengthening the shorter extremity or by shortening the longer one. Either the tibia and fibula or the femur may be lengthened, rarely as much as three inches, but the end results are often unsatisfactory. The procedure is a gradual stretching of the soft tissues and lengthening of the bone after an osteotomy of special type. After operation the fragments must be maintained in satisfactory apposition and alignment during the lengthening process, and for this purpose many types of apparatus have been devised. Great care and judgment are necessary in the selection of cases suitable for lengthening operations.

In most cases equalization of the length of the legs can be accomplished more satisfactorily by shortening the longer leg, since this is less painful, less hazardous, and less likely to result in inadequate muscular control. The shortening may be accomplished by performing a simple oblique osteotomy of the femur and allowing the fragments to override, or by removing a measured segment of the femur. In either case care must be taken to secure effective internal fixation of the fragments. When a measured segment of the femoral shaft is removed, fixation of the fragments can be satisfactorily maintained with an intramedullary nail.

Gross inequality of leg length in children may often be treated satisfactorily by an operation to retard the growth of the longer leg. Local growth in length may be arrested permanently by fusing the epiphysis to the diaphysis. This operation, called epiphysiodesis, should not be done until the patient is at least 10 years old. In the selection of cases, a careful estimate of the relative rates of growth of the two legs and of the duration of further growth must be made. Since two thirds of the growth in length of the leg occurs about the knee, the usual surgical procedure is fusion of the lower femoral epiphysis or the upper tibial and fibular epiphyses, or all three, to the respective diaphyses. The operative technic must be careful and thorough to prevent later deformity of the knee from incomplete, asymmetrical arrest of growth. An alternative procedure, developed by Blount, is to insert strong metal staples across the epiphyseal plate into epiphysis and diaphysis. Later, if resumption of growth is desired, the staples may be removed. The surgical technic of stapling must be meticulous. Many complications have been reported, caused usually by poor judgment or improper technic.

In recent years, largely through the work of Trueta, there has been a revival of interest in attempts to stimulate epiphyseal growth in the short leg. As yet, however, no reliable method for producing an adequate acceleration of length growth has been devised.

CHAPTER 11

Neuromuscular disabilities (exclusive of poliomyelitis)—involvement of the brain and spinal cord

IN ADDITION TO POLIOMYELITIS, which has been described in the preceding chapter, the disease entities that may give rise to disability of the neuromuscular system are numerous and of diverse etiologic and clinical nature. They are perhaps most conveniently grouped according to the location of the basic pathologic changes. Entities characterized by involvement of the brain and spinal cord will be considered in the present chapter, and in the following one disorders of the peripheral nerves and of the muscles will be described.

Involvement of the brain
CEREBRAL PALSY

Definition. Cerebral palsy is a common and extremely disabling affection seen most frequently in infants and children and characterized clinically by disturbance of voluntary motor function. It includes a variety of neurologic entities; the essential pathologic change is destruction or congenital absence of upper motor neurons. Mental impairment may be present. Involvement of a single extremity is termed *monoplegia;* involvement of both extremities of the same side of the body is called *hemiplegia* (Fig. 138); involvement of both lower extremities, *paraplegia;* and involvement of the four extremities, *quadriplegia* (Fig. 139). Statistics from a large series of cases showed quadriplegia in about 60%, hemiplegia in 20%, and paraplegia in 10%. The incidence of cerebral palsy in reported series is given as 1 to 5 in every thousand live births; the incidence does not vary with sex.

Etiology. The causes of cerebral palsy may be classified chronologically into three groups:

1. *Antenatal,* consisting of congenital defects resulting from an arrested

Neuromuscular disabilities—brain and spinal cord

development of the cerebrum and pyramidal tracts in utero, certain maternal infectious diseases, excessive irradiation, and incompatibilities of the Rh factors when an Rh-negative mother gives birth to an Rh-positive child in her second or third pregnancy.

2. *Natal,* the most frequent type, consisting of nerve cell injury following cerebral hemorrhage due to trauma at birth, or anoxia or hypoxia following winding of the umbilical cord around the baby's neck, too heavy sedation of the mother, or aspiration of mucus by the child.

3. *Postnatal,* consisting of infectious, vascular, or traumatic lesions, such as those of encephalitis, meningitis, syphilis, and vascular accidents.

The antenatal type is common in premature babies. Among children with cerebral palsy, the number of premature births is definitely above the normal expectancy; in one series it was reported to be three times as great. There are an unusually high percentage of complications of pregnancy and a high percentage of previous abortions. Many of the patients of postnatal type are affected before the age of 3 years; in 20% of these children an infectious disease is the etiologic factor.

Pathology. Although direct contusion and laceration of cortical tissue may be present, the factor of intracranial hemorrhage is believed to play

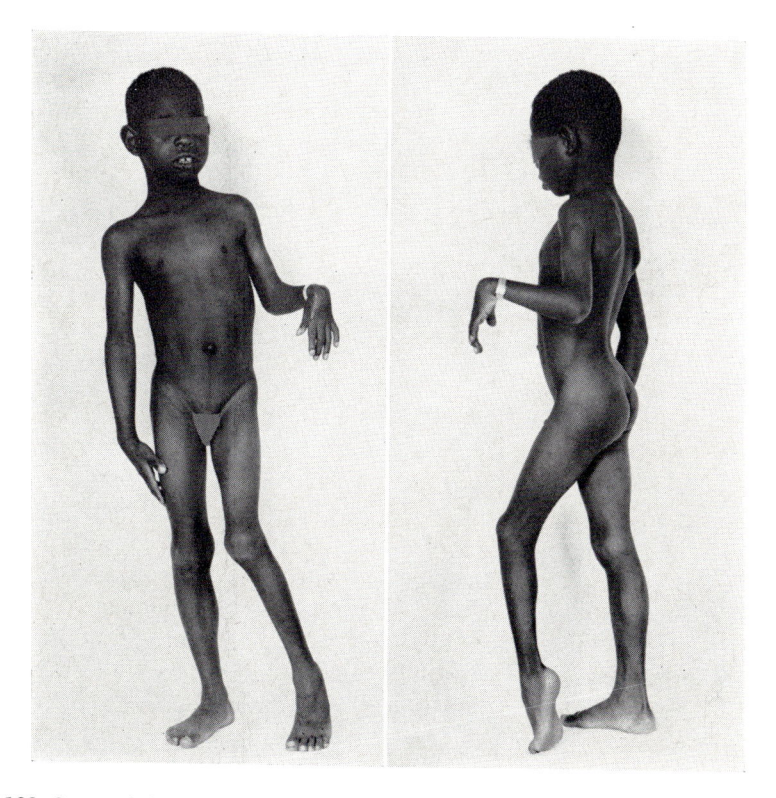

Fig. 138. Spastic left hemiplegia in cerebral palsy. Note abnormal positioning and generalized underdevelopment of left limbs as compared with the right.

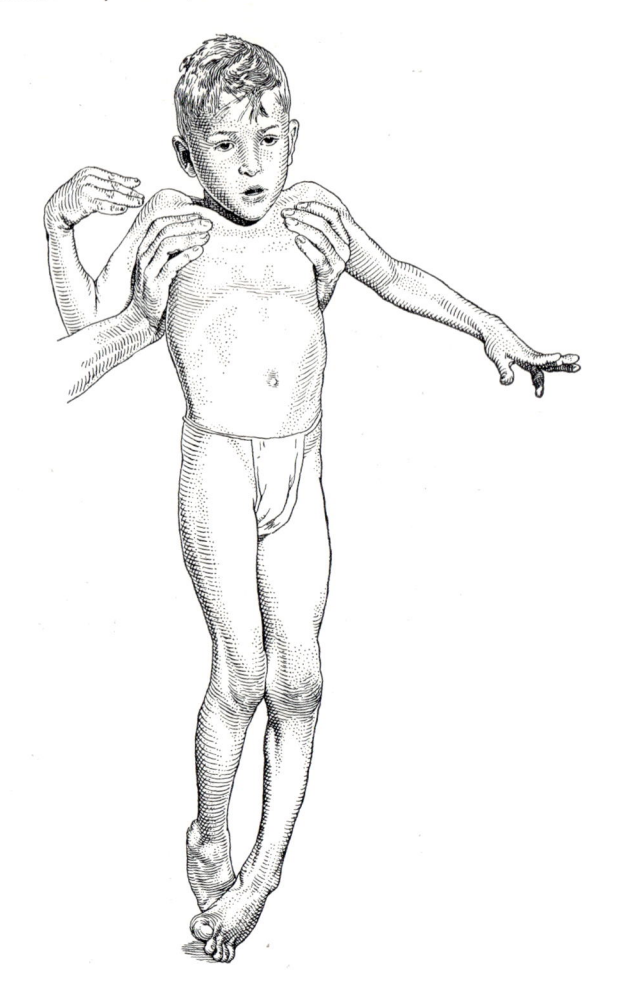

Fig. 139. Spastic quadriplegia in cerebral palsy.

a major role in the pathologic process in most cases. The hemorrhage may occur directly from a vessel ruptured when the dura mater is torn, or it may be of widespread petechial type resulting from increased tension when the venous circulation is temporarily obstructed. Degeneration of the injured nerve cells and fibers ensues and is followed by sclerosis. Grossly the affected areas may show atrophy and softening. The lesions may be more severe either in the cerebral cortex or in the basal ganglia. Degeneration of corresponding tracts in the spinal cord is a constant finding. A severe diffuse injury resulting in multiple hemorrhages through all parts of the brain may produce rigidity with mental retardation. A single hemorrhage or infarct involving the motor cortex may cause spastic hemiplegia or quadriplegia. Jaundice of the newborn, or *kernicterus*, due to incompatible Rh factors, affects the basal ganglia and produces athetosis. Injury of the cerebellum produces ataxia.

Pathologic changes may occur in the spinal cord as the result of injury below the level of the brain. Traction applied during delivery is believed to be an occasional cause of such injuries. The clinical picture is in many respects similar to that of birth injury of the cerebrum or basal ganglia, and it is therefore convenient to consider cases of primary cord involvement together with those resulting from intracranial lesions.

Clinical picture. Intracranial hemorrhage in the newborn infant may be evidenced by severe asphyxia, bulging fontanels, refusal to nurse, spasticity or flaccidity, and convulsions. Lumbar puncture shows the spinal fluid to be bloody and under increased pressure. Many of the infants die shortly after birth. In milder cases the child may be considered normal until unusual delay in holding up the head, sitting, or standing becomes obvious.

Cases of cerebral palsy in older infants and children may be divided into several major groups, according to the location of the lesion within the central nervous system. These groups are characterized by outstanding clinical manifestations, of which the most important are spasticity, athetosis, and ataxia. In many cases the lesions are widespread, however, and the symptoms are of mixed type. Other forms of motor disturbance may also be present. Outstanding among these are *tension*, or widespread muscular hypertonicity or rigidity; *tremor*, or rhythmic involuntary contractions limited to certain muscle groups; and *overflow*, of which an example is involuntary motion of the facial muscles during voluntary movement of the arm.

Spasticity. Approximately 50 to 65% of the cases of cerebral palsy fall into this group. Of the patients with spasticity, nearly one half are hemiplegic. In spasticity the lesion is cortical and the pyramidal tracts are involved. The evidences of spasticity are characteristic. The involved muscles are hyperirritable and contract on the slightest stimulation. The tendon reflexes are hyperactive, the Babinski reflex is positive, and clonus usually is easily elicited. Antagonistic muscle groups, hypersensitive to the stimulus of stretching, contract simultaneously with the protagonists; this results in difficult and inaccurate voluntary movements and in increased muscular resistance to passive manipulation. The involuntary contraction of a spastic muscle when it is suddenly stretched is a useful diagnostic sign; it is called the *stretch reflex*.

An equinus limp is a frequent finding. The equinus deformity may be due not to weakness of the dorsiflexors but to simultaneous contraction of the normally more powerful plantar flexors and to the effect of gravity. In hemiplegia the patient can usually walk, but the affected lower extremity trails and may be of little use.

In paraplegia and quadriplegia occurs the so-called *scissors gait* or *cross-legged progression,* characterized by disabling adduction of the hips resulting from the greater strength of the adductors over the abductor groups and augmented by the force of gravity.

Characteristic deformities develop as a result of the continued contraction of antagonistic muscles of unequal power. The hips may become flexed, adducted, and internally rotated. The knees are flexed. The feet usually assume an equinus or equinovarus position. The shoulders tend to become internally rotated and adducted and the elbows flexed. The forearm is pronated, while the wrist and fingers become flexed and the thumb adducted. When the patient attempts to sit erect, unsightly bowing of the spine and forward protrusion of the head may take place.

Muscle atrophy is usually not conspicuous. Asymmetry of the extremities sometimes becomes marked, however, from retardation of growth of the affected limb due to trophic disturbances. Sensory defects may also be present.

Athetosis. Athetoid patients make up approximately 25 to 40% of the cases of cerebral palsy and according to Phelps can be grouped into twelve types. The lesion is subcortical, the basal ganglia and extrapyramidal tracts being affected. Athetosis is a more or less constant involuntary contraction of successive muscles. These arrhythmic, purposeless contractions become superimposed upon voluntary movements and result in marked incoordination. The reflexes are normal, and the stretch reflex is absent. In athetosis due to an Rh factor incompatibility, there are a hearing loss and a limitation of vertical eye motion; intelligence may be average, and the child can become a good lip reader.

Ataxia. Cases of ataxia, or primary incoordination, are much less numerous than those of spasticity or of athetosis. The lesion is subcortical, and probably cerebellar in most instances. Characteristic clinical manifestations are incoordinated movements, impaired balance, and nystagmus. The reflexes are normal.

Mental status. Some degree of mental impairment, which may be either true deficiency or simply retardation, is usually present. Statistics have shown that the mentality of from 30 to 50% of all cerebral palsy patients is either seriously retarded or otherwise defective, and that approximately 75% have a mentality below average. Some observers, however, believe these figures for mental impairment are too high. Cerebral palsy with spasticity and mental deficiency, of which the ill-tempered, feebleminded, drooling child with scissors gait is the classical example, was described by Little in 1843 and is sometimes called *Little's disease.* Mental deficiency is most marked in the spastic group and more so in quadriplegic and paraplegic patients than in hemiplegic ones. Some patients present obvious idiocy, with characteristically stupid facies and thick, unintelligible speech. In other cases, however, the appearance of subnormal mental endowment is unquestionably exaggerated by inability to control the facial or speech musculature, or by the deficient education that has resulted from absence of the normal locomotor activities of the growing child. Estimation of the mental capacity in the individual case is essential, since it is of primary importance in determining prognosis and treatment.

Diagnosis. Accurate diagnosis is important in order to rule out certain progressive diseases in which the prognosis is unfavorable and treatment is futile. History of difficult, prolonged, or instrumental delivery or of a definite episode of infectious disease during early childhood, although often not obtainable, may be useful auxiliary evidence. The spinal fluid should be examined when congenital syphilis is suspected. Developmental arrest of the central nervous system, hydrocephalus, brain tumor, atypical forms of poliomyelitis, and degenerative diseases of the central nervous system should be considered and excluded. Observation over a period of several months is often useful in ruling out the possibility of a disease process of progressive nature. For proper planning of treatment for the individual patient, an accurate differentiation of the type of cerebral palsy also is necessary.

Prognosis. In untreated cases slow spontaneous improvement in the use of the extremities often takes place as motor experience and better control are acquired during the years of childhood. Well-ordered treatment always results, however, in more rapid and more extensive improvement. Since the ability to cooperate and to learn is essential to effective treatment, the degree of improvement will depend to a large extent upon the mental capacity of the individual patient. Thus patients with paraplegia due to spinal lesions without cerebral involvement may regain considerable muscle function under treatment, whereas patients exhibiting marked mental deficiency improve little, form difficult nursing problems, and often succumb early to intercurrent infection. The prognosis of the patient with frequent convulsive seizures is unfavorable unless the seizures can be controlled with drug therapy.

Treatment. A first step in treatment, which has both nonsurgical and surgical aspects, is the formulation of a realistic goal based on appraisal of the potentialities of the individual patient. Affected children with adequate mental capacity may require a comprehensive program designed to achieve physical capability and social competence. The treatment program should develop speech, self-help, locomotion, psychological adjustment, and appropriate education. The orthopaedic treatment is essentially a process of habilitation and, of necessity, embraces a long program of motor training during which resort to operation is made only as an auxiliary measure. Treatment should begin as soon as the diagnosis has been made, and should start and continue at home as long as possible. Subsequent therapy is governed largely by the patient's response. When the necessary discipline, good hygiene, and freedom from excitement and worry cannot be obtained at home, the therapy can be given more successfully in an institution.

Nonsurgical treatment. Motor education is the most important part of the treatment of most cases of cerebral palsy. The first step is to teach the child how to relax voluntarily; this is particularly important for the athetoid patient. When muscular relaxation can be initiated at will and maintained for as long as several minutes, training in the performance of simple movements is begun. In infants and in older patients with severe involvement attention is concentrated first upon learning to sit or stand. A Thomas collar is sometimes provided to afford helpful support and prevent stretching of the neck muscles. A light corset is sometimes indicated. Braces and plaster shells, worn a part of each day or during the night, are often helpful in the treatment of mild spastic deformities. Daily massage is sometimes of benefit for weakened muscle groups. The most important element of the treatment, however, is a program of exercises selected for the individual patient and carried out daily over a long period of time. Simple reciprocal motions of the extremities are started, at first passive and later active, and finally the patient is taught gradually to combine these simple movements into composite ones such as those of walking. Many aids to activity have been devised, such as ski shoes that allow the patient to stand and shuffle along without fear of falling. In many cases, daily speech training is important.

Many drugs have been tried in the treatment of cerebral palsy. Anticonvulsant medications have been extremely helpful in patients with seizures. Drugs to control muscle tone in spastic and athetoid patients have been less successful. Curare-like drugs relax muscle but are dangerous because of the narrow margin between therapeutic and toxic dosages. Tranquilizing drugs have had limited usefulness and are effective in a small percentage of cerebral palsy patients.

During the long period of training, the details of treatment must be adjusted to the needs of the individual patient; experience, judgment, and patience on the part of the specially trained physical therapist are of the utmost importance. Occupational therapy forms an important part of the treatment of older patients, especially in motor re-education of the upper extremity.

Surgical treatment. As a rule, orthopaedic operations for cerebral palsy are applicable chiefly to cases characterized by spasticity. In many such cases surgical measures serve as a useful adjunct to motor re-education. Operation cannot be regarded as adequate treatment unless accompanied by conservative measures, however, and is unquestionably contraindicated when the disorder is a rapidly progressive one or when the patient possesses too little mental capacity to cooperate in the necessary postoperative training.

The object of surgical treatment in cerebral palsy is to diminish muscle spasm, equalize the power of opposing muscles, stabilize poorly controlled joints, and correct deformity. Of the great variety of procedures that have been devised and employed, many have proved with further experience to be unsatisfactory. In a series of approximately 2,500 surgically treated cases from many different clinics, there were 50% successful results and 50% failures. In this series practically all of the operations upon athetoid patients were failures; however, other clinics have reported favorable results in carefully selected cases. The procedures now in common use may be classified as (1) operations upon motor nerves, (2) operations upon muscles and tendons, and (3) operations upon bone. The operations upon bone are followed by the most uniformly successful results.

1. *Operations upon motor nerves (neurectomy, Stöffel operation):* Division or partial excision of the motor nerves of spastic muscles is a valuable and commonly used procedure. Attempt is made not to paralyze a muscle group and so abolish its entire function, but to produce in the

stronger muscles a loss of power sufficient to result in improved balance and hence increased capability for muscle training. This type of operation has produced better results in treatment of the lower extremity than of the upper. It has proved particularly suitable when applied to the branches of the obturator nerve for adductor spasm and to the branches of the tibial nerve for spasm of the plantar flexors. In selected cases of spastic pronation of the forearm and flexion of the wrist, section of appropriate branches of the median nerve is a helpful procedure.

2. *Operations upon muscles and tendons:* Procedures of this type include tendon transplantation, tendon lengthening, tenotomy, and myotomy. They are often combined advantageously with section of motor nerves to the spastic muscle group. In each case adequate preliminary correction of the deformity must be carried out, care being taken in the release of fibrous contractures of all involved periarticular structures. After operation the immobilization in corrected position and the subsequent physical therapy must be meticulously carried out.

The type of operation must be carefully chosen with regard to the nature and location of the deformity in the individual case. Among the more commonly used procedures are those described below.

AT THE HIP. In cases of severe adduction deformity, tenotomy of a portion of the adductor muscles, followed by immobilization of the thighs for a period of about six weeks in wide abduction, often results in gratifying improvement of the gait.

AT THE KNEE. A number of procedures have been devised to correct incomplete active extension of the knee on standing. Occasionally it is sufficient to lengthen one or more of the hamstring tendons. If the patellar ligament has become elongated, it may be shortened by plication or the tibial tubercle may be transplanted distally *(Chandler operation).* Good results have also followed section of the patellar retinacula and transplantation of the hamstring insertions into the femoral condyles *(Eggers operation).*

AT THE FOOT. Transplantation of the anterior tibial tendon to the lateral side of the dorsum of the foot may be used to improve spastic varus deformity. Lengthening of the Achilles tendon for talipes equinus is indicated only when there is unquestionable structural shortening, since spastic equinus would be all too easily converted into the more disabling deformity of calcaneus type. However, when actual shortening is present, Achilles lengthening is one of the most frequently used and successful operations in the treatment of cerebral palsy. After lengthening of the Achilles tendon, the ankle should be immobilized in a plaster cast in 90 degrees of dorsiflexion.

AT THE SHOULDER. For severe adduction and internal rotation deformity, the tendons of the pectoralis major and subscapularis muscles may be sectioned or lengthened.

AT THE FOREARM. Pronation contracture of spastic origin may be relieved by suitable transplantation of the tendon of the pronator teres muscle.

AT THE WRIST AND HAND. Tenotomy, tenodesis, and tendon transplantation may be helpful in carefully selected cases. Rarely are complicated tendon transplantations successful in cerebral palsy.

3. *Operations upon bone:* Only in carefully selected cases are bone operations indicated. In persistent varus or valgus deformity of the foot, subtalar arthrodesis greatly improves stability and gait. When the wrist is flexed and cannot be held voluntarily in a neutral position, radiocarpal arthrodesis in a position of 35 degrees of hyperextension improves the appearance and in some cases the function of the hand.

NEUROMUSCULAR DISABILITIES OF PSYCHIATRIC ORIGIN (HYSTERICAL PARALYSIS)

Cases of orthopaedic disability due partially or entirely to psychosomatic or psychogenic causes are encountered with considerable frequency. They are especially common in the Armed Forces during wartime. Often a part in the causation is played by the element of financial compensation or the desire to be relieved of some unpleasant duty. Insurance and liability claims are involved in many of these cases. Functional or hysterical paralysis and deformity may simulate a variety of primary osteoarticular or neuromuscular diseases. Hence these disorders, although primarily of psychiatric interest, are of importance in the differential diagnosis of orthopaedic affections.

Clinical picture. Hysterical paralysis may occur in either sex and at any age. The history is likely to include discrepancies that suggest the diagnosis. The joint symptoms are varied, may be out of all proportion to the inciting trauma, and may change unnaturally from day to day. The physical findings also are inconsistent. Spasm and tenderness may be excessive while heat, redness, and swelling are completely absent, and the signs may change as soon as the patient's attention is diverted.

Diagnosis. In diagnosis it must be remembered that organic and functional elements sometimes coexist and that in late hysterical cases a secondary structural element of circulatory changes and of contractures is almost always present. Examination under an anesthetic and roentgenographic visualization of the structures involved are of help. The diagnosis of hysteria should never be made until every effort to establish the presence of an organic lesion has been exhausted. The patient should be kept under observation for a considerable period, and repeated diagnostic examinations should be made.

Treatment. The treatment of functional paralysis and deformity should be largely psychiatric. It is of fundamental importance that the confidence and active interest of the patient be secured. After this has been done it is usually advisable to place the patient upon a regime of gradually increasing corrective physical therapy. Emphasis should be placed upon active motion and active correction. Occupational therapy will often prove of value. When the element of compensation or disability insurance is present, termination of the payments and closure of the case are often followed quickly by relief of the disability.

Involvement of the spinal cord

PROGRESSIVE MUSCULAR ATROPHY (ARAN-DUCHENNE TYPE)

Progressive muscular atrophy is a primary disease of the spinal cord, characterized by a slow degeneration of the anterior horn cells, which produces muscular wasting without sensory losses. It is found most often in adults between 25 and 45 years of age.

Clinical picture. The first evidence of the disorder is usually atrophy of the intrinsic muscles of the hand. The thenar eminence becomes flattened, the interosseous areas deepen, and with progression of the disease a claw-hand develops. Gradually the paralysis extends to the muscles of the arms, shoulders, back, hips, and thighs. Other cases may first show atrophy and weakness in the shoulders, and rarely the legs are first involved. As the condition progresses, the deep reflexes may become hypoactive or absent. Fibrillation of the muscles is a frequent finding and is of diagnostic importance.

When the disease has partially destroyed the pyramidal tracts, as evidenced by spasticity of the legs, hyperactive reflexes, and a positive Babinski sign, it is called *amyotrophic lateral sclerosis.*

Treatment. The orthopaedic treatment is usually conservative, consisting of massage, exercises, and braces. However, if the disease becomes nonprogressive, stabilization of a joint to improve function may be considered.

INFANTILE SPINAL MUSCULAR ATROPHY (AMYOTONIA CONGENITA)

Infantile spinal muscular atrophy is characterized by extreme muscular weakness and hypotonia secondary to gradual degeneration or a developmental defect of the anterior horn cells of the spinal cord. When fully developed at birth it has usually been called amyotonia congenita or *Oppenheim's disease,* whereas it is often called *Werdnig-Hoffmann disease* when the onset follows several weeks or months of normal or nearly normal development. Deep tendon reflexes are absent or gradually lost. These infants will almost never learn to walk. There is inadequate muscle strength to prevent sagging of the head and legs when such an infant is lifted under the back (Fig. 140). Postural deformities, including a severe scoliosis, may develop.

Infantile spinal muscular atrophy should be differentiated from *benign congenital hypotonia,* a syndrome in which there are also marked muscle weakness and hypotonia in infancy, with moderate to marked retardation of sitting and walking. In these patients deep tendon reflexes are at least weakly present, and by the fourth to sixth year these youngsters have usually developed normal strength and appearance. The cause of benign congenital hypotonia is unknown; it may be a retardation of muscle maturation.

Treatment. Massage and exercises may be of some benefit. Braces are sometimes indicated for support of the spine and legs.

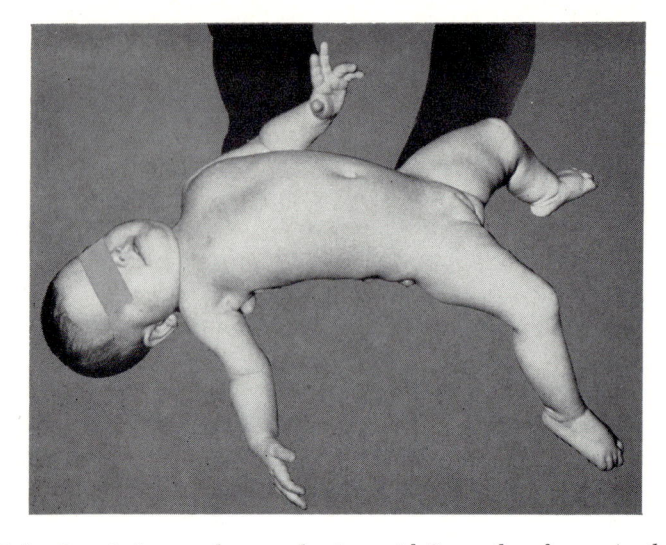

Fig. 140. Infantile spinal muscular atrophy in a girl 6 months of age. As the infant is picked up with support under the shoulders and hips, the head and lower extremities fall backward. Because of muscular weakness, the infant cannot hold her head and lower extremities straight.

FRIEDREICH'S ATAXIA

Friedreich's ataxia is a progressive disease, usually hereditary or familial, which often affects several children of the same family. It develops in early childhood, about 90% of the cases appearing before the fifteenth year. The essential pathologic change is an extensive degeneration or sclerosis of the nerve fibers in the dorsal and lateral tracts of the spinal cord.

Clinical picture. The affection is characterized by weakness of the legs, ataxia, and a swaying, irregular gait with the feet placed widely apart. Nystagmus is characteristically present. The speech is usually thick. Equinovarus deformity of the feet is almost always present, and lateral curvature of the spine is often associated. Early in the disorder the deep reflexes are decreased, but the Babinski sign is present. Later there is often a loss of position and vibratory sensations in the lower limbs, and disturbances of other types of sensation are sometimes observed.

Treatment. At the present time no curative treatment is known. Muscle re-education and massage may help. Braces are sometimes indicated. Occasionally, when the disease is no longer progressive, surgical stabilization of the feet is useful to improve the gait.

SUBACUTE COMBINED SCLEROSIS

In pernicious anemia and deficiency diseases such as pellagra, the development of numbness and tingling in the hands and feet may be followed by the gradual onset of weakness. Later a well-marked flaccid or spastic paralysis of the legs may be present, and secondary deformities are likely to appear.

Treatment. Deformities secondary to the paralysis may respond to physical therapy, and braces may be of benefit. Rarely is lengthening of the Achilles tendons or stabilization of the feet indicated in an effort to improve the gait. Vitamin B_{12} is indicated when the primary disease is pernicious anemia, niacin when it is pellagra.

NEUROPATHIC DISEASE OF BONES AND JOINTS

Etiology. Chronic disease of the spinal cord may cause extensive trophic changes in the bones and joints. Such osteoarticular lesions are seen typically in association with the spinal cord involvement of *tabes dorsalis* and of *syringomyelia*. Statistics show that joint symptoms occur in from 3 to 4% of patients with tabes and in from 10 to 40% of those with syringomyelia. The smaller joints of the foot are frequently involved in patients with diabetic neuropathy. Similar joint changes occur less commonly with other affections of the spinal cord, including traumatic conditions, congenital malformations such as spina bifida with myelomeningocele, tumor, tuberculosis, acute myelitis, poliomyelitis, and progressive muscular atrophy. They have been reported after involvement of the peripheral nerves by trauma, toxic neuritis, or leprosy, and in association with the cerebral changes of dementia paralytica or of cerebral hemorrhage with hemiplegia. Although more than one factor is probably involved, repeated minor trauma of the anesthetic joint seems to be most important in the pathogenesis. The patient, unable to appreciate painful stimuli arising in the joint, fails to protect it, voluntarily or involuntarily, from harmful forces.

Pathology. The changes in neuropathic osteopathy include a thinning of the cortical bone and a diminution in lime salts, which may lead to spontaneous, painless fracture. Healing of such fractures occasionally takes place with the formation of an enormous amount of callus, which may show degenerative changes leading to a second fracture.

The neuropathic arthropathies, often called *Charcot's joints* because they were first described by Jean Martin Charcot in 1866, are most frequently encountered in tabes. The articular cartilages and adjacent bone surfaces become worn away while at the same time hypertrophic, sclerotic changes take place at the joint edges, and loose bodies of irregular shape and size appear. Marked deformity and instability result from mushrooming of the bone, relaxation of the ligaments, and accumulation of intra-articular fluid. The roentgenographic picture of fully developed cases is striking (Fig. 141). Both atrophic and hypertrophic bone changes are present. The joint surfaces appear extensively eroded and deformed. The bone margins are jagged, blurred, and sclerotic, and there may be many irregular pieces of detached bone.

Clinical picture. In neuropathic arthropathy the early signs are insecurity, false motion, and swelling of the affected joint. These may increase rapidly or slowly, but pain is notably absent. Examination shows a tense or boggy nontender swelling, not uniform but containing indurated masses. As a rule the range of joint motion is increased. Although most frequently only a

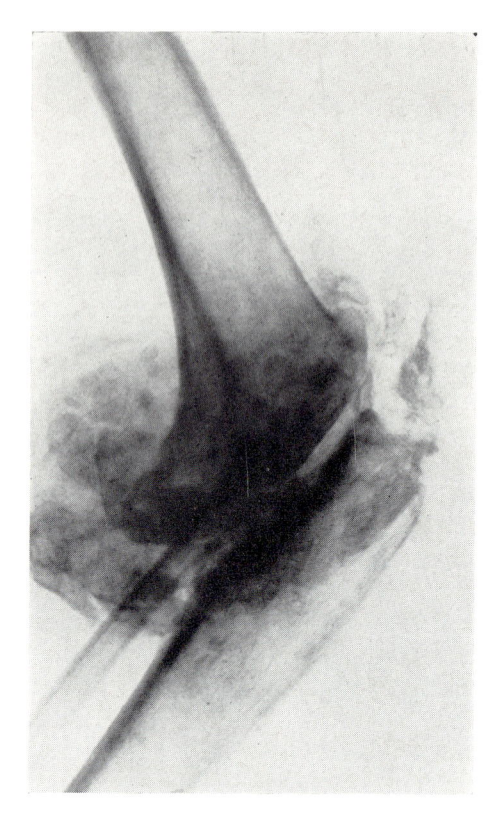

Fig. 141. Roentgenogram of advanced neuropathic disease of the knee (Charcot joint). Note erosion of articular ends of femur and tibia, subluxation, and multiple loose fragments of bone.

single joint is involved, bilateral symmetrical lesions are occasionally seen and rarely a large number of joints may be affected, especially in syringomyelia. The knee, hip, shoulder, tarsus, elbow, wrist, and ankle are most frequently involved, in this order. Lesions of the spine are also encountered. Seventy-five per cent of the tabetic arthropathies occur in the lower extremity, whereas 80% of the joints involved in syringomyelia are those of the upper extremity.

Diagnosis. In advanced cases the diagnosis is often obvious, but in the early stages it may be difficult. In neuropathic arthropathy the local triad of swelling, instability, and absence of severe pain should always suggest the diagnosis, and the roentgenographic evidence is most helpful. The findings of the general history and physical examination are of confirmatory value. In the case of tabes, the Argyll Robertson pupil, absent knee or ankle jerk, and diminished position and vibratory sensations are important findings. Suggestive of syringomyelia are loss of pain and temperature sensations and atrophy of the small muscles of the hand.

Treatment. In tabes, antisyphilitic treatment is a major consideration although it may be too late to have any effect on the disintegrated joint. In neuropathic arthropathy protection for the affected joint is afforded by means of a brace, such as a walking caliper splint for the knee. Crutches may be necessary. With conservative treatment the progress of the disease may sometimes be retarded to a gratifying degree. Arthrodesis of the affected joint is not always successful but in some cases has given excellent results, particularly at the knee. Rarely, in extreme involvement of the knee or ankle, the impossibility of securing adequate stability either by apparatus or by arthrodesis may make amputation the procedure of choice.

SPINA BIFIDA

Spina bifida is a congenital anomaly consisting of a developmental gap or defect in one or more of the vertebral arches (Fig. 142), through which the contents of the spinal canal may protrude and with which partial or complete paralysis of the legs may be associated. Spina bifida sufficiently marked to produce clinical deformity is present in about 1 in 1,000 births. Of these infants, 80% die within the first year. The projecting meningeal sac usually extends posteriorly (Fig. 143) but occasionally extends anteriorly

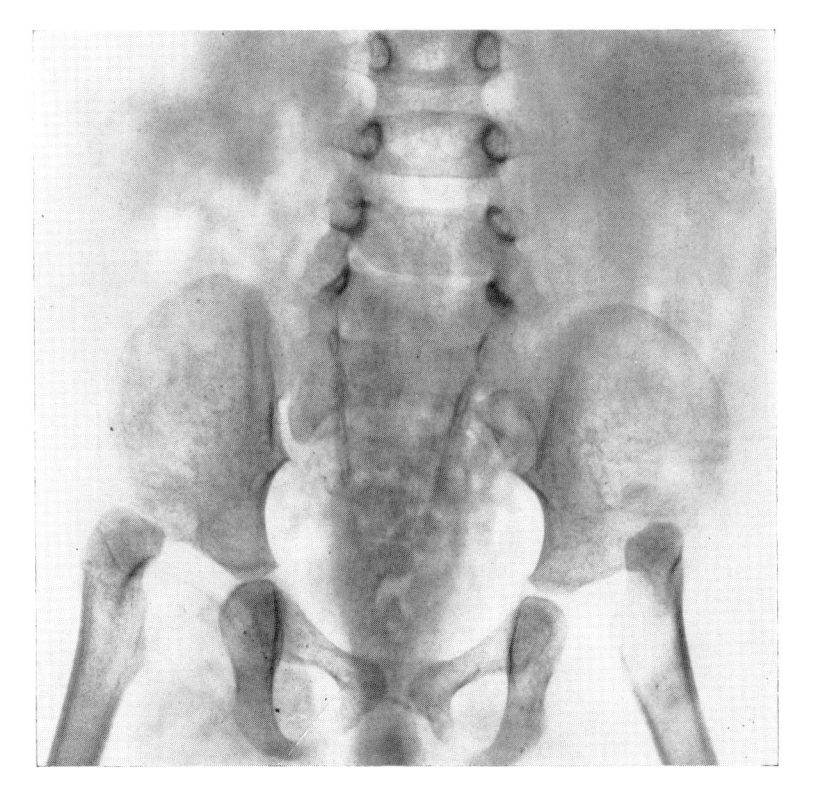

Fig. 142. Spina bifida in boy 3 years of age. Note wide defect in laminal arches of lower three lumbar vertebrae and sacrum, and bilateral dislocation of hips. This patient had had a myelomeningocele removed at 1 month of age.

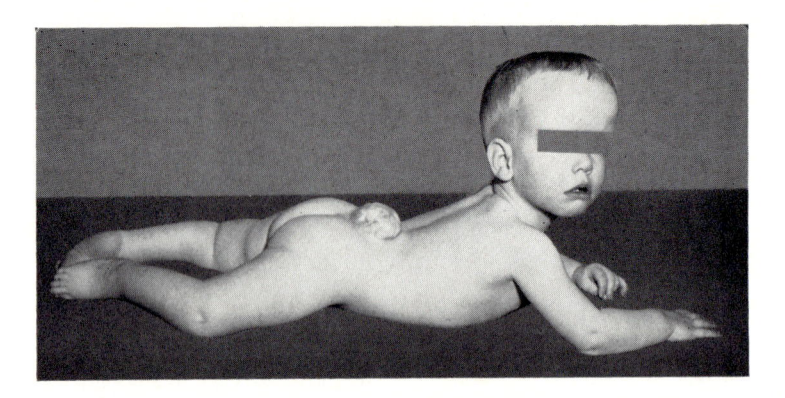

Fig. 143. Spina bifida with myelomeningocele and hydrocephalus in boy 2½ years of age. There were associated contractures of the knees and clubfeet.

into the pelvis, abdomen, or thorax; the condition is then called an *anterior spina bifida*.

Pathology. The essential pathologic characteristic of spina bifida is incomplete development of the roof of the neural arch due to failure of complete fusion of the embryonic neural canal.

Each vertebra has three centers of ossification: one for the body and one for each half of the neural arch. The neural arch is formed by the posterior, midline fusion of the two laminae arising from their separate centers of ossification. Union of the laminae begins in the thoracic region and extends in both directions along the length of the developing spine. The lumbosacral and cervical regions are the last to unite, and it is in these two areas, particularly the former, that faulty closure, resulting in spina bifida, is seen most frequently.

In the normal human embryo the entire neural tube is closed at the end of the third week, and by the eleventh week the partially ossified neural arches of the vertebrae are closed from the first cervical to the third or fourth sacral segments. The spinal cord and the vertebral column are of equal length until the twelfth week. With further growth of the fetus, however, the vertebral canal becomes proportionately longer, so that in the adult the conus is at the level of the twelfth thoracic or first lumbar vertebra. When the nerve roots or the spinal cord is involved in a spina bifida, the upward migration of the cord is prevented. This may be associated with the *Arnold-Chiari malformation*, an elongation of the brain stem and portions of the cerebellum downward through the foramen magnum. Spina bifida may also be associated with *diastematomyelia*, in which a segment of the spinal cord is divided longitudinally by a midline bony spur or fibrous band. Diastematomyelia also secures the dura and prevents migration of the spinal cord.

The defect of spina bifida may be large enough to allow the meninges or the spinal cord to form a protruding soft tissue tumor. According to the extent of the pathologic changes spina bifida has been classified into five types: spina bifida occulta and spina bifida with, respectively, meningocele, myelomeningocele, syringomyelocele, and myelocele.

Spina bifida occulta. A defect is present in the spinous process and laminae of one or more vertebrae (Figs. 203 and 205), but there is no obvious swelling or protrusion. The skin may remain attached to the membranes, nerve roots, or cord by fibrous tissue called the *membrana reuniens*. These subjacent anatomic changes may be suggested by alterations of the skin such as indentations, pigmentations, telangiectases, or hairy patches (hypertrichoses). There may also be associated tumors inside or outside the vertebral canal; among them are lipomas, angiomas, and dermoid cysts. As the growth of the spinal column later exceeds that of the spinal cord, adherence of the overlying structures to the cord may impede its normal ascent. In this manner, as well as through compression of the nerve roots by soft tissue at the site of the laminal defect, paralysis of gradual onset and incomplete type may result at a later age, particularly at a time of rapid growth. In the vast majority of cases, however, spina bifida occulta is discovered as an incidental finding in routine roentgenograms of the low back. In such situations it is usually of no clinical significance.

Spina bifida with meningocele. Through the defect of the incompletely closed arch of one or more vertebrae the meninges herniate and are covered by only a thin, parchment-like layer of skin. The hernial sac contains only cerebrospinal fluid; transillumination will reveal no nerve tissue.

Spina bifida with myelomeningocele. With the bony defect is associated a hernial sac that contains, in addition to cerebrospinal fluid, the spinal cord, nerve roots, or both, either free or attached to the walls of the sac. As compared with meningocele, myelomeningocele is usually much greater in extent, more subject to ulceration if untreated, associated with more neurologic deficit in the lower extremities, as well as bowel and bladder incontinence, and associated more frequently with hydrocephalus.

Spina bifida with syringomyelocele. Syringomyelocele is a severe type of myelomeningocele in which the herniated spinal cord contains a central canal greatly dilated and distended with cerebrospinal fluid.

Spina bifida with myelocele. Also known as *rachischisis,* this condition includes the most severe forms of spina bifida. As a result of the absence of laminae and pedicles, the wide bone defect forms an open groove, partially lined by imperfectly formed spinal cord tissue through which cerebrospinal fluid drains. As a consequence, infection quickly takes place and the infant succumbs early.

Of these five types, the last four are characterized by the presence of a soft tissue tumor due to herniation of the meninges and have been called *spina bifida manifesta*. The involvement of nerve tissue in these cases makes them primarily of neurosurgical interest, but the prevention and correction of secondary paralytic deformities of the lower extremities is of orthopaedic concern.

Clinical picture. The clinical picture is characterized by any or all of three features: (1) the tumor, or protruding soft tissue mass, (2) the neurologic manifestations, and (3) the associated deformities.

The hernial protrusion is located in the midline, most commonly in the lumbar or lumbosacral region. It may vary greatly in size and may increase with violent expiration as in crying. It is usually translucent on transillumination. A defect in the underlying bony structure is apparent on roentgenographic examination.

The neurologic manifestations may be absent in a spina bifida occulta and absent or minimal in a meningocele. In myelomeningocele they may consist of severe motor involvement or complete paraplegia with bowel and bladder incontinence, together with extensive sensory disturbance resulting in trophic ulcerations. The motor involvement is usually a flaccid paralysis and occasionally may be a spastic paralysis.

The most frequently associated deformities are clawfoot, clubfoot, contractures of the knees, malformations of the spine with varying degrees of scoliosis, kyphosis, or lordosis, dislocation of one or of both hips, and hydrocephalus (Fig. 143).

Diagnosis. The diagnosis is obvious in cases with a protruding hernial mass in the lumbar region. Among conditions to be excluded are lipomas and neurofibromas. Spina bifida of the occult type may be diagnosed as an incidental finding in roentgenograms made for other purposes; however, palpation of the area will sometimes demonstrate changes as compared with the normal findings at higher levels of the spine.

Treatment. Neurosurgical exploration and excision of the hernial mass are usually indicated. Drainage of cerebrospinal fluid, ulceration, paraplegia, absence of the anal reflex, constant dribbling of urine, poor general health, or an already existing hydrocephalus may contraindicate operation.

Spina bifida occulta may require operation in later childhood if neurologic signs secondary to involvement of the spinal cord by traction or compression develop. Surgery then consists of careful excision of the membrana reuniens and of any tumor that may be present. The prognosis following this procedure is usually good.

The paralysis and frequent deformity of the lower extremities may require extensive orthopaedic treatment with casts, braces, or operations. These procedures should be carried out in a manner similar to that described in Chapter 10 for corresponding deformities and disabilities following poliomyelitis. Dislocation of the hip with severe weakness of the hip musculature, which is common in severe spina bifida, may be left unreduced, since it is usually impossible to maintain the reduction.

Care must be taken to avoid pressure ulcers. Training the severely involved patient to walk with the aid of crutches and braces and with a three- or four-point gait in the manner of a traumatic or poliomyelitic paraplegic may greatly facilitate his treatment and decrease his invalidism.

CHAPTER 12

Neuromuscular disabilities (exclusive of poliomyelitis)—involvement of peripheral nerves and of muscles

NEUROMUSCULAR DISABILITIES caused by the involvement of peripheral nerves or of muscles include peripheral nerve injuries and certain forms of neuritis, progressive muscular atrophy, and progressive muscular dystrophy.

Involvement of peripheral nerves

PERIPHERAL NERVE INJURIES

Injury of the peripheral nerves is a frequent and serious complication of traumatic lesions of the bones and joints. Every injured extremity must be examined for the possibility of nerve damage, and in a considerable proportion of cases the neurologic lesion will prove of far greater significance than the osteoarticular. It is essential, therefore, that the orthopaedic surgeon become acquainted with that portion of neurology which deals with injuries of the peripheral nerves. The present description can include only a brief introduction; for detailed information reference to the bibliography is suggested.

A short review of the structure of peripheral nerves and their reactions to injury forms a convenient preliminary to consideration of lesions of the individual nerves.

Anatomy. A peripheral nerve is composed of a tremendous number of fibers enclosed in a connective tissue covering. The individual fibers are separated by a loose fibrous tissue termed the *endoneurium*. Fibers are grouped into bundles enclosed by the *perineurium*. The entire peripheral nerve is enclosed by the collagenous *epineurium*, which also sends connective tissue septa between the nerve bundles. The central portion of the individual nerve fiber or *axon* is the axis cylinder; its protoplasm, which is a

241

prolongation of the cytoplasm of the nerve cell, extends the entire length of the nerve. Its extremely thin membrane is continuous with the nerve cell membrane. Surrounding the axis cylinder is a layer of myelin of variable thickness. The axon and myelin in turn are enveloped by the thin Schwann cell membrane. Nerve fibers vary in size. The largest, heavily myelinated axons are motor fibers. Next in size are fibers concerned with proprioception and cutaneous sensation. Fibers conducting pain sensation follow, and the smallest fibers are those of the autonomic system and another type of pain fiber. There is a definite relationship between fiber size and extent of myelination on the one hand and electrical properties on the other; the large, heavily myelinated fibers conduct impulses at a much more rapid rate than do the small, thinly myelinated fibers.

Mechanism of injury. Traumatization of an extremity may involve the nerves in any of several types of injury. These may be classified according to the time of their occurrence with relation to that of the original injury.

At the time of the original injury. The nerves may be directly bruised, lacerated, or completely severed by the rough edge of a fractured bone or by a sharp object from without, such as the blade of a knife or a piece of glass. A portion of the nerve may be torn away; this happens not infrequently in severe gunshot wounds. An additional type of immediate injury is the severe stretch, tear, or even complete rupture of the nerve from strong traction upon the extremity; this type of injury occurs, for instance, in *obstetric paralysis.*

Several hours following the original injury. Temporary loss of nerve function may be occasioned by compression of the nerve from edema or hemorrhage of gradual development.

At the time of treatment of the original injury. Nerve damage is sometimes a result of excessive traumatization during the transportation of the patient when a splint has not been applied or during the reduction of a dislocation or fracture.

Several weeks or more following the original injury. The nerve may undergo gradual compression from cicatricial fibrous tissue or rarely from bony callus.

Several months or more following the original injury. Friction or stretching of the nerve is sometimes the result of a deformity caused by the original injury, as in late traumatic ulnar neuritis.

Gross pathology of the injured nerve. Following an old injury the damaged nerve is often recognizable only with difficulty, because of extensive scarring of its sheath and the adjacent connective tissue. In infected wounds the adhesions are often particularly extensive, and in the proximal segment an ascending neuritis sometimes develops, causing widespread degenerative changes that are followed later by fibrosis. The appearance of the injured nerve varies especially with the degree of completeness of the tear. After complete division the nerve ends retract; a *neuroma,* or small bulblike growth of nerve fibers and connective tissue, forms at the end of the proximal segment; and the end of the distal segment may become narrowed and atrophic or may enlarge to form a *pseudoneuroma,* which is composed of connective tissue only. After incomplete laceration the injured nerve may show a fusiform enlargement, formed by the proliferation of axons, Schwann cells, and fibrous tissue and termed a nerve spindle or *neuroma in continuity.* In some cases there will be found a markedly thin segment which may suggest an incomplete division but which represents essentially a complete one, since all nerve fibers have ruptured and degenerated while only connective tissue sheaths remain intact. In other cases long segments of the nerve fibers may degenerate from friction or stretching while no macroscopic changes of any kind are apparent.

Degeneration and regeneration of nerves after section. The broad outlines of this fundamental and complex subject may be sketched briefly. The distal segment of a peripheral nerve fiber that has been severed undergoes characteristic changes referred to as wallerian degeneration. In the first three days following nerve section no microscopic changes are noted and the distal segment will still conduct if artificially stimulated. From the third day until the end of the first week there is degeneration of the axoplasm and the myelin, which gathers into small globules. Schwann cells begin to proliferate, and an invasion of macrophages occurs. The fiber will no longer conduct, and enzymes associated with acetylcholine metabolism disappear. In the following weeks, the formation of Schwann cell tubules continues, awaiting regenerating axons from the proximal segment.

In the process of regeneration the axis cylinder of the proximal segment, still under the trophic influence of the nerve cell, gradually grows across the gap, enters the empty neurilemmal sheath, and continues to grow distally toward the end-organ while gradual restoration of the myelin sheath takes place. The rate of growth of the axis cylinder, under favorable circumstances, is said to be from 1 to 2 mm. per day.

Since anatomic and functional recovery of the injured nerve is directly dependent upon re-establishment of the pathway from nerve cell to end-organ by means of the regenerating axis cylinder, it is evident that the degree of recovery after any nerve injury will depend largely upon the ability of the axis cylinders to traverse the gap successfully and to find suitable waiting neurilemmas. Hence recovery will not take place if the defect is too extensive or if too much scar tissue is present.

Classification of nerve injuries. Three types of peripheral nerve injury have been described by Seddon: neurapraxia, axonotmesis, and neurotmesis.

Neurapraxia. In neurapraxia there is nerve contusion or compression resulting in segmental damage but leaving the axon structurally intact. Since large fibers are especially vulnerable to this type of injury, motor paralysis in the milder cases may be more prominent than loss of pain sensation. Nerve conductivity is impaired and there may be localized demyelination, but recovery is rapid and always complete. Examples of neurapraxia include crutch palsy, and radial nerve paralysis from sleeping with an arm hanging over the back of a chair.

Axonotmesis. Axonotmesis is an interruption of the axons without damage of the nerve sheath. This type of lesion results from more severe or prolonged compression than that which causes neurapraxia. Since the axons are damaged, recovery must be preceded by wallerian degeneration of the distal segment. In the electromyogram, fibrillation is noted two to three weeks after the injury. Since the epineurium and perineurium are intact, however, the regenerating Schwann cell sheaths are properly oriented and allow the new axons to find their way into correct channels. Recovery is usually satisfactory; the time required for recovery is related to the distance of the lesion from the end-organ.

Neurotmesis. Neurotmesis, in which there is complete interruption of nerve fibers and their connective tissue coverings, is the most severe form of nerve injury in Seddon's classification. There is total paralysis of the involved muscles, and after two weeks their response to faradic stimulation is lost. Electromyographic findings and strength-duration curves show changes typical of degeneration. Cutaneous sensation is lost over the *autonomous zone,* which is the area supplied exclusively by the injured nerve. Examples of neurotmesis are nerve transections in knife and bullet wounds. The prognosis is much poorer than in the milder nerve injuries and depends largely upon the accuracy of surgical repair.

Recovery phase. The recovery of larger, more heavily myelinated fibers is poorer than that of smaller ones. Accordingly the return of motor function is often less complete than that of pain sensation, and touch and proprioception occupy an intermediate position. In axonotmesis and especially in neurotmesis faulty reinnervation may occur, the developing fibers entering inappropriate axon sheaths. Regenerating fibers are often of smaller diameter than the original fibers. Accordingly, incomplete or inappropriate motor innervation may result and sensory function may be disturbed in several ways. In some instances severe pain and burning sensations, occurring spontaneously or provoked by minimal stimuli, result in the disabling condition known as *causalgia.*

As the regenerating axons extend distally, there develops a hypersensitivity that is manifested by a tingling sensation when the regenerating portion of the nerve is tapped. This is called Tinel's sign; usually it appears at the site of the lesion a few weeks after injury and extends distally with nerve regeneration. In favorable cases the return of sensation is followed by motor recovery of variable degree.

Treatment of peripheral nerve injuries. The treatment of nerve injuries is either nonsurgical or surgical, and every case involves a decision as to whether spontaneous recovery can reasonably be expected or whether surgical exploration is the wiser course. A detailed history of the injury and a thorough neurologic examination are essential. Of all the factors involved in the therapy of these cases, perhaps the most important are (1) surgical judgment in deciding when operation is indicated and (2) surgical technic in carrying out the procedure with a minimum of trauma and hemorrhage. The value of physical therapy in nonsurgical treatment and in postoperative care is not to be underestimated.

Nonsurgical treatment. Treatment without operation is always indicated when there is evidence of progressive spontaneous improvement of nerve function, and it is to be employed tentatively when such improvement may be expected following a probably incomplete division of a nerve. It should be explained to the patient at the outset that the course of treatment may be prolonged.

The essentials of nonsurgical treatment are two: (1) support of the paralyzed muscles and (2) physical therapy. The affected muscles must be kept in a position of relaxation; they should not be stretched by normal opponents. To this end, light retentive apparatus suited to the particular case is to be worn most of the time. *Cock-up splints* in radial paralysis and *foot drop braces* in peroneal paralysis are common examples. After a short initial period of rest, physical therapy should be used daily in an attempt to preserve muscle nutrition until regeneration occurs and to prevent the development of adhesions and contractures. It consists at first of heat and massage, passive exercises, and electrical stimulation; later, as recovery begins, muscle re-education and active exercises are added. The progressive recovery of power in paralyzed muscles usually observed in these cases is a source of gratification that makes the extended course of treatment well worth while.

Surgical treatment. Operations for exploration or repair of a damaged nerve may be (1) *primary*, that is, performed immediately after a lacerating injury, or (2) *secondary*, performed after the original wound has healed or when progress in the gradual recovery of nerve function has been unsatisfactory.

It is sometimes possible at the primary operation, as in the repair of a clean laceration, to suture the ends of the sectioned nerve. This is usually inadvisable in the presence of open fractures or bullet wounds. In such cases a secondary nerve suture should be performed after the wound has become perfectly healed and free of infection and after scarring at the severed nerve ends has matured. The interval from nerve injury to nerve suture may vary from several weeks to several months. During this interval the muscles and joints should be kept in as good condition as possible by means of daily physical therapy.

A nerve graft or transplant may be used to replace a defective or missing segment of a nerve trunk. Successful results have been reported in using nerve grafts from nerve banks. Some surgeons use a portion of the sural nerve as a nerve transplant. Sural transplants are more often successful than are grafts from a nerve bank.

The indications for exploratory or secondary operation vary within certain recognized limits. When complete nerve division is suggested by the history and by extensive and persistent sensory and motor losses, exploration should be performed within the first month. If separation, or neurotmesis, has occurred, satisfactory regeneration will not take place without approximation of the nerve ends by suture. The time of appearance of the nerve signs with relation to the time of injury is sometimes of value in differentiating actual rupture from a temporary interruption of function by edema or hemorrhage. When the signs of incomplete interruption are present, nonsurgical treatment should be adopted tentatively, but exploration should usually be carried out if definite improvement has not been shown after three or four months.

In operations upon peripheral nerves, scrupulous precautions to preserve asepsis and hemostasis and to avoid traumatization are essential. *Neurolysis,* or freeing of the nerve from cicatricial adhesions and constrictions, is a common and often very beneficial procedure. It is sometimes necessary to compensate for the shortening of a divided nerve by fixing the adjacent joint temporarily in a suitable position or by transplanting the nerve to a shorter course. Postoperatively braces and physical therapy are used just as in the nonsurgical treatment. Postoperative recovery of nerve function is slow and, as a rule, never quite complete, depending upon many factors, such as the duration of the paralysis, the age of the patient, the type of nerve involved, the level at which it is injured, and the degree of secondary change in muscles, tendons, and joints. Often with careful protection and physical therapy, however, progressive improvement can be expected to continue for as long as two or three years.

INJURIES OF INDIVIDUAL NERVES

Theoretically, every peripheral nerve is susceptible to mechanical injury. Practically, however, and particularly in civil life, the frequent and important lesions are limited to a few of the major trunks. Nerve injury occurs far more commonly in the upper extremity than in the lower. In the upper extremity, lesions of the radial, ulnar, and median nerves are of major significance, and in the lower extremity injuries of the sciatic and peroneal nerves are most important. Lesions of other nerves occur less frequently but are of great interest in the individual case.

Accessory nerve (eleventh cranial nerve)

Etiology. The accessory nerve is sometimes divided by lacerating or perforating wounds of the neck or during neck dissections for tumor of the lymph nodes, cervical rib, or tuberculous lymphadenitis.

Clinical picture. If the nerve is divided in the posterior triangle after emerging from the sternocleidomastoid, only the trapezius muscle is paralyzed. This produces an unsightly deformity consisting of change in the contour of the neck, drooping of the shoulder, and occasionally slight winging of the scapula. Abduction of the arm is at first impaired but later may be partially restored by the action of other muscles of the shoulder girdle. If the nerve is divided in the anterior triangle of the neck, the sternocleidomastoid muscle also is paralyzed, which results in little loss of power but in a noticeable asymmetry.

Treatment. Unless primary suture can be accomplished, the nerve lesion is as a rule irreparable. If winging of the scapula is conspicuous, the deformity may be lessened by surgical measures to limit its displacement.

Brachial plexus

Etiology. The nerves of the brachial plexus are subject to the following types of injury: (1) traction lesions; (2) friction, contusion, or compression lesions; and (3) penetrating lesions.

Traction lesions. If the head is laterally flexed while the opposite shoulder is fixed, or if the shoulder is violently depressed while the head is fixed, the trunks of the brachial plexus become taut and, if the force increases, may be stretched, torn, or even completely ruptured. Such injury occurring during birth causes the common and important *obstetric paralysis* or *birth palsy*. Similar lesions in adults may result from severe stretching of the brachial plexus incident to the trauma of falls or heavy blows upon the shoulder.

Friction, contusion, or compression lesions. Nerve injuries of this type are of particular interest in connection with two clinical entities: (1) *cervical rib* or spasm of the scalenus anterior muscle, which may cause chronic friction or compression (p. 445); and (2) *dislocations or fractures at the shoulder joint*, including displaced fractures of the clavicle, in which the nerves may be injured by the original trauma, by secondary edema or hemorrhage following the original trauma, or by manipulation during reduction of the displacement.

Penetrating lesions. Gunshot wounds form the commonest cause of this type of nerve injury. In the early treatment of these cases hemorrhage from associated injury of the great vessels is often an important factor.

Clinical picture. The symptoms and signs of lesions of the brachial plexus vary widely with the type of trauma and the part of the plexus which is injured. It is therefore convenient to consider the more important clinical entities separately.

Obstetric paralysis

Obstetric paralysis, or *birth palsy*, is a paralysis of the muscles of the upper extremity resulting from mechanical injury of the nerve roots of the brachial plexus during birth and is most commonly seen in infants born after a prolonged and difficult labor. The nerve injury may vary from slight stretching (neurapraxia or axonotmesis) to complete rupture (neurotmesis) of one or more of the nerve trunks. Edema and hemorrhage follow, and later cicatricial fibrosis occurs. In some instances the plexus injury is accompanied by a fracture of the upper end of the humerus or by soft tissue injury of the shoulder. Clinically the newborn infant may present, in addition to paralysis of the arm, transient spasticity of the other arm and the legs as a result of the hematomyelia accompanying avulsion of the nerve roots. Inequality of the pupils may be present from stretching or tearing of the cervical sympathetic nerves. Three main types of paralysis are encountered, depending upon the location of the injury: (1) Erb-Duchenne or upper arm paralysis, (2) Klumpke or lower arm paralysis, and (3) paralysis of the entire arm.

Erb-Duchenne or upper arm paralysis. Upper arm paralysis is by far the

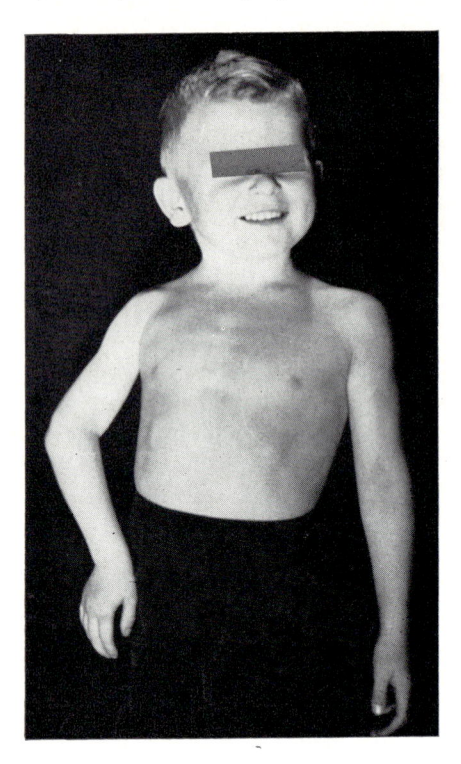

Fig. 144. Right obstetric paralysis in boy 5 years of age. Note atrophy and internal rotation of the shoulder. Extension of the elbow and supination of the forearm were restricted.

most common of these types and is due to injury of the fifth and sixth cervical roots. Because of the distribution of the paralysis, the extremity occupies a typical position, with the shoulder internally rotated and adducted and the forearm pronated (Fig. 144). Movements of the wrist and of the fingers are not affected. There may be slight sensory changes, which in the infant are difficult to evaluate.

Klumpke or lower arm paralysis. Paralysis of the lower arm is much less common; it is due to injury of the eighth cervical and the first dorsal roots. The intrinsic muscles of the hand and sometimes the long flexors of the fingers are paralyzed. The upper arm is not affected. A homolateral *Horner's syndrome* is often present because of involvement of the cervical sympathetic fibers in the first dorsal root; it is characterized by slight ptosis of the eyelid, enophthalmos, and miosis.

Paralysis of the entire arm. In this type of obstetric paralysis, which in frequency occupies a position between the other two varieties, the limb is often completely flaccid and powerless. Extensive sensory losses occur, which in the infant are difficult to demonstrate.

Differential diagnosis. It must be remembered that at birth any of several injuries about the shoulder can cause a flail arm. Separation of the upper humeral epiphysis, fracture of the humerus, and fracture of the clavicle are of fairly common occurrence. Dislocation of the shoulder may be a true congenital luxation or a traumatic displacement due to injury during birth; each is extremely rare. In the infant, cerebral palsy must also be excluded, and in older patients it is necessary to consider the possibility of an old, unrecognized poliomyelitis.

Prognosis. Improvement usually takes place during the months following birth; however, the prognosis varies with the type of paralysis, and perfect recovery is exceptional. In the upper arm paralysis, considerable return of power is to be expected; the lower arm type with paralysis of the intrinsic muscles of the hand has a relatively poor prognosis, and a claw deformity may develop; the palsy of the whole arm is especially likely to show only incomplete recovery. The paralysis is followed by the development of contractures. The typical deformity of internal rotation of the arm is maintained by firm fibrous contractures of the muscles about the shoulder. In extensive late cases the entire arm and shoulder girdle are underdeveloped, and secondary growth changes, such as abnormal prolongation of the acromion and of the coracoid process, take place. In such cases the functional loss is great.

Treatment. The early treatment of obstetric paralysis is conservative. The extremity may be supported by means of a brace in a position combining abduction and external rotation of the shoulder, flexion of the elbow, supination of the forearm, and slight dorsiflexion of the wrist so that the palm of the hand is turned toward the face (Fig. 145). The brace should be removed for care of the infant's skin and after the first few days for gentle massage and manipulation to prevent the development of contractures. While the brace is not being used, the general position of correction should be maintained. When recovery of muscle power has taken place, the brace may be gradually removed. Active and passive corrective exercises should be continued for a long while, and the child should be kept under periodic observation for signs of developing contractures.

Surgical repair of the brachial plexus for birth palsy is rarely indicated. In patients who do not recover spontaneously, intraneural fibrosis is usually so extensive that surgical resection and anastomosis are impossible. In the infant, contractures may be treated by gentle stretching; in older patients, open release is preferable. The procedure described by Sever, comprising section of the contracted pectoralis major and subscapularis muscles near their insertion into the humerus, is often useful. It may be necessary also to section the coracobrachialis and short head of the biceps. If the elongated acromion is limiting abduction, it should be osteotomized at its base and bent upward. Late cases of internal rotation deformity may be treated by rotation osteotomy of the humerus or by tendon transferences favoring external rotation. These operations, although producing no increase of muscle power, may make motion of the arm less awkward. Occasionally in late cases with pronation deformity, tendon transference in the forearm or rotation osteotomy of the radius may be indicated. After any of these

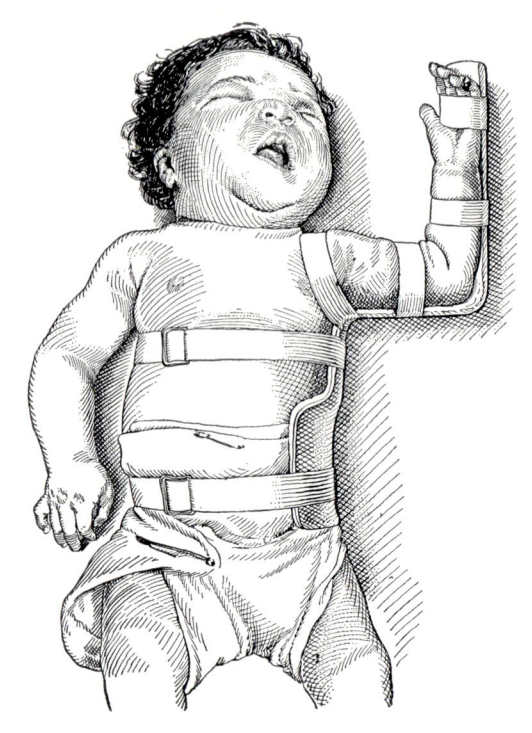

Fig. 145. Left obstetric paralysis in infant, with brace for maintaining abduction and external rotation of shoulder, flexion of elbow, and supination of forearm.

surgical procedures the arm must be adequately supported in the appropriate position, and physical therapy must be careful and prolonged.

Paralysis following dislocation of the shoulder

Paralyses complicating shoulder dislocations are fairly common and fall into two major groups: (1) *supraclavicular traction injuries of the plexus*, produced by the original trauma and independent of the dislocation, and (2) *infraclavicular nerve lesions* resulting from displacement of the humeral head at the time of the original trauma or during its manipulative reposition. Supraclavicular traction injuries are treated by measures similar to those used for the analogous obstetric paralysis. It is advisable, however, to resort to exploratory operation somewhat more often than in birth palsy.

Infraclavicular nerve lesions complicating dislocation may involve chiefly the *axillary nerve*, causing deltoid paralysis and hypesthesia on the lateral aspect of the shoulder and upper arm; the *axillary and the radial nerves*, causing in addition a widespread extensor paralysis; the *medial cord* with paralysis of the intrinsic muscles of the hand and anesthesia in the ulnar distribution; or the *lateral cord* with paralysis of the biceps, coracobrachialis, and the flexors of the fingers supplied by the median nerve. The extent of the paralysis depends in large degree upon the length of time during which the humeral head is allowed to remain displaced and in late cases may be extreme. The treatment of these cases is immediate reduction of the shoulder dislocation, which can usually be accomplished by a closed procedure, followed within a few days by splinting of the shoulder in moderate abduction and flexion and of the wrist in dorsiflexion. Daily physical therapy, including electrical stimulation of the muscles and motion of the involved joints, is helpful. Recovery is sometimes very slow and may continue for many months. Open operation for reduction of a late, untreated dislocation or for exploration of the nerves is occasionally indicated.

Axillary nerve

Etiology. The usual cause of injury is subcoracoid dislocation of the head of the humerus, but rarely the paralysis may follow fracture of the surgical neck of the humerus, the incorrect use of an axillary crutch, or traction injuries of the neck and shoulder.

Clinical picture. The deltoid muscle is paralyzed, causing a loss of true abduction of the shoulder and subsequently an unsightly muscle atrophy, prominence of the acromion, and instability of the shoulder joint. The paralysis of the teres minor muscle is unimportant. There is a variable degree of sensory loss over the lateral aspect of the shoulder and upper arm.

Treatment. Nonsurgical treatment is usually adequate. Surgical repair is difficult because of the short course of the nerve. After irreparable injury a muscle transplantation to provide abduction of the arm is sometimes done (p. 217), or the shoulder may be arthrodesed in 50 to 75 degrees of abduction.

Long thoracic nerve

Etiology. The long thoracic nerve, supplying the serratus anterior muscle, may be injured by (1) the carrying of excessively heavy burdens upon the shoulder or (2) accidental division at operation.

Clinical picture. Paralysis of the serratus anterior muscle results in an inability to raise the arm above the shoulder level in front of the body, loss of forward pushing movements of the shoulder, and winging of the scapula. The deformity and disability are sometimes severe.

Treatment. Rest of the shoulder in an abduction brace and physical therapy are indicated. If recovery does not occur, excessive mobility of the scapula may be corrected by any of several surgical methods involving anchorage of its lower angle to the wall of the thorax.

Radial nerve

Etiology. The radial nerve with its long and exposed course about the humeral shaft is one of the most frequently injured nerves in the body. It is particularly liable to two types of mechanical injury: (1) laceration by the sharp edge of a bone fragment, in fractures of the humeral shaft or in supracondylar fractures, or involvement secondarily in a fibrous scar or in callus; and (2) compression from external objects, as in *crutch palsy*, or

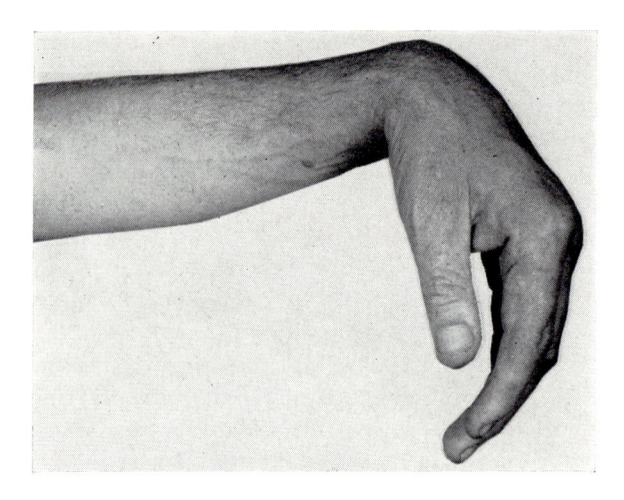

Fig. 146. Wrist drop in complete paralysis of radial nerve.

when the arm is allowed to hang for a long time against an object causing local pressure. Even trivial injuries result usually in a complete rather than a partial motor paralysis.

Clinical picture. Radial palsy involves the extensors of the elbow, wrist, and fingers and causes the characteristic sign of *wrist drop* (Fig. 146). If the lesion is in or below the middle third of the upper arm, paralysis of the triceps is absent as its nerve supply is separated from the main trunk at a higher level. The sensory loss is not so extensive as the wide distribution of the radial nerve would suggest; it consists usually of a small zone of anesthesia on the dorsal surface of the thumb and the adjoining portion of the hand. The posterior interosseous branch of the radial nerve is occasionally injured in wounds of the elbow, with resulting paralysis of the extensor carpi ulnaris and the extensors of the fingers and the thumb.

Treatment. Nonsurgical treatment of radial paralysis consists in the use of cock-up splints and of prolonged physical therapy. Surgical procedures upon the nerve itself—of which neurolysis, end-to-end suture, and transplantation to the anterior aspect of the arm are the most common—are often successful, since the radial nerve is peculiarly capable of functional recovery. When the lesion is irreparable, however, tendon transplantations about the wrist to supplement the weakened muscles can do much to relieve the disability.

Ulnar nerve

Etiology. The ulnar nerve is frequently divided in lacerating wounds and may be injured by fractures in the region of the medial condyle and epicondyle, by dislocation of the elbow, and by secondary inclusion in scar tissue after elbow injury. It may be affected by postural pressure during a prolonged anesthesia. Lesions of the deep motor branch in the hand may result from prolonged use of certain vibrating tools. In addition the ulnar nerve is subject to *late traumatic neuritis* from stretching or from friction against the posterior surface of the medial humeral condyle in valgus deformity of the elbow secondary to old fracture.

Clinical picture. Lesions in the upper arm cause paralysis of the flexor carpi ulnaris, the medial half of the flexor digitorum profundus, the hypothenar muscles, interossei, two medial lumbricals, adductors of the thumb, and the deep head of the flexor pollicis brevis. In cases of long duration the flattening of the hypothenar eminence, interosseous atrophy, and clawhand deformity are characteristic (Fig. 147). A dry and atrophied appearance of the skin and nails due to vasomotor disturbances may be present. Sensory loss is usually marked, even in incomplete division of the nerve, and is located over the ulnar border of the hand, the entire little finger, and the ulnar half of the ring finger. Lesions in the forearm cause motor and sensory losses in the hand, but power in the flexor carpi ulnaris and the flexor digitorum profundus is retained. Lesions at the wrist, below the origin of the large dorsal cutaneous branch, cause the usual motor changes in the hand, with little sensory impairment.

Late traumatic ulnar neuritis or delayed ulnar palsy may be seen in association with (1) recurrent dislocation of the nerve at the postcondylar groove, and (2) old fracture of the lateral condyle with a cubitus valgus deformity. Various degrees of hypermobility of the nerve may occur developmentally or as the result of trauma, and occasionally there is slipping of the nerve trunk anterior to the medial epicondyle with each flexion of the elbow, which produces a typical friction neuritis. The nerve injury after old fractures of the lateral condyle is a result of stretching or friction due to the development of cubitus valgus (Fig. 176A). Pain in the ulnar distribution is likely to be severe, and there may be sensory changes and atrophy of the interosseous muscles.

Treatment. Nonsurgical treatment consists in the use of splints and of

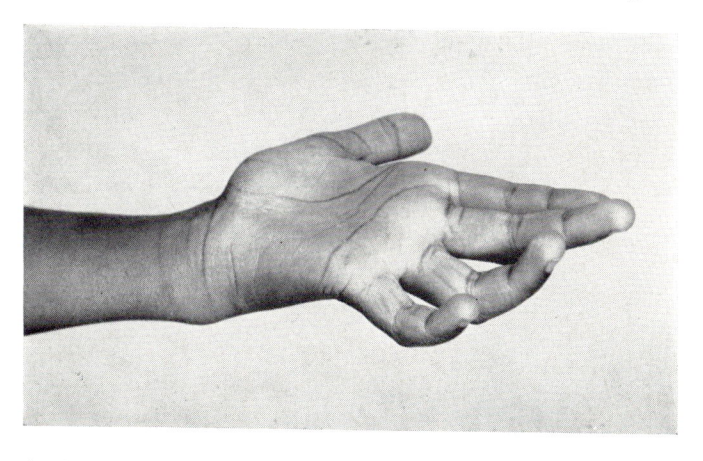

Fig. 147. Clawhand in paralysis of ulnar nerve. Active extension of the interphalangeal joints of ring finger and little finger is impossible because of paralysis of the two medial lumbrical muscles and the interossei.

physical therapy. When the nerve has been sectioned, the surgical procedure of primary suture is sometimes indicated. When length must be gained to overcome a gap, the nerve may with advantage be transposed to a position anterior to the epicondyle. The results of nerve suture are imperfect, since, as a rule, neither motor nor sensory losses are completely restored. In late traumatic neuritis immobilization may produce satisfactory temporary improvement, but for permanent cure it is often necessary to perform an anterior transposition of the ulnar nerve at the elbow. The results of this operation are excellent in most cases.

Median nerve

Etiology. The commonest causes of median nerve paralysis are injuries from penetrating or lacerating wounds and primary or secondary involvement in association with supracondylar fractures of the humerus. In the forearm the median nerve may be compressed by scar tissue or, rarely, by the pronator teres *(pronator syndrome)*. At the wrist a median paralysis sometimes follows traumatic lesions such as transverse laceration of the soft tissues, severely displaced Colles' fracture, or anterior dislocation of the lunate bone. Also, at the wrist the nerve may be compressed (1) in the volar carpal tunnel, as a result of trauma or arthritis, producing the *carpal tunnel syndrome*, and (2) as a result of the flexion-ulnar deviation position *(Cotton-Loder position)* in the treatment of Colles' fracture.

Clinical picture. Lesions in the arm or at the elbow cause paralysis of most of the flexors of the wrist and fingers, of the pronators of the forearm, the abductor-opponens group of the thumb, and the two lateral lumbrical muscles. Flattening of the thenar eminence is a conspicuous sign. The little finger and ring finger can be flexed through the ulnar supply to the profundus, but the patient cannot make a tight fist or pronate the forearm (Fig. 148). Power in the opponens pollicis muscle, which must be carefully differentiated from the adductor pollicis, is lost. In lesions at the wrist this loss of opponens and abductor brevis power is the most valuable diagnostic feature. The sensory loss is the same at whatever level the nerve is divided; it usually

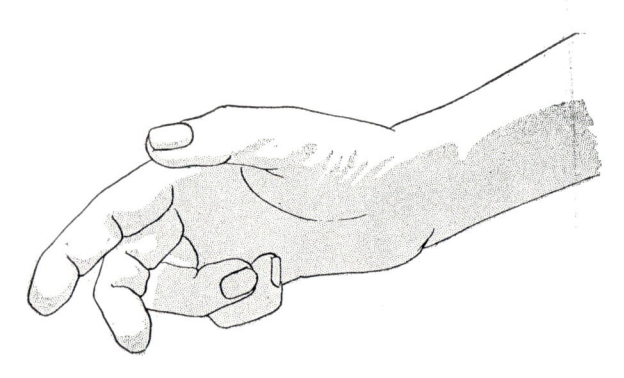

Fig. 148. Paralysis of median nerve, showing inability to flex fully the index finger and middle finger.

involves the thumb, the index finger, the middle finger, and the lateral half of the ring finger. The nails may be atrophic and the skin shiny and dry. Incomplete division of the median nerve frequently results in causalgia. Compression of the nerve in the carpal tunnel is accompanied by tingling pain and numbness in the hand over the median nerve distribution and, if unrelieved, is followed by atrophy of the thenar eminence. Tinel's sign may be positive. With dorsiflexion of the wrist, paresthesia may occur; it may be relieved by volar flexion. Sometimes these evidences of a median nerve disturbance may develop several years after a wrist fracture has resulted in bony deformity; this condition is called *late median nerve palsy*.

Treatment. After lacerating wounds it is often possible to perform a primary nerve suture. The technic must be scrupulous, owing to the likelihood of incomplete recovery and the development of causalgia. For traumatic neuritis, neurolysis is often sufficient. Splinting, to prevent stretching of the weakened muscles, and physical therapy are important parts of the treatment. The results of suture of the median nerve are more favorable than in the case of the ulnar nerve; however, the recovery is usually incomplete. For the carpal tunnel syndrome, the transverse ligament of the carpus usually requires section, but in mild cases simple splinting may relieve the symptoms. In irreparable lesions of the median nerve, tendon transplantations may be of benefit.

Lumbosacral plexus and cauda equina
Lumbosacral plexus

The trunks of the lumbosacral plexus may be injured by penetrating wounds, fractures, inflammatory conditions, and tumors of the pelvic wall or viscera. The management of these conditions consists primarily of treating the causative lesions. Rarely compression by the fetal head is said to cause plexus symptoms. More common is the entity of *maternal obstetric palsy*, in which sciatic pain and sometimes peroneal paralysis and sensory changes are the result presumably of stretching of the lumbosacral trunks during a difficult labor. The prognosis for spontaneous recovery is good. Nonsurgical treatment, consisting of a foot-drop brace and physical therapy, should be employed. Very rarely, after a difficult birth, the infant may show temporary signs of a traction injury of the lumbosacral plexus analogous to the familiar stretching of the brachial plexus that produces obstetric paralysis of the upper extremity.

Cauda equina and conus medullaris

These structures may be injured in penetrating wounds or by severe trauma with or without fracture of the lumbar vertebrae or sacrum. Motor and sensory losses may be slight or very extensive, depending upon the extent of the trauma and the level involved. The complete *cauda equina syndrome* includes a total flaccid paralysis of both lower extremities, paralysis of the sphincters of rectum and bladder, and anesthesia of the buttocks, the perineum, the entire posterior aspect of the legs, and the feet. The complete *conus medullaris syndrome,* resulting from involvement of the five fused sacral segments of the spinal cord, consists of paralysis of the sphincters and anesthesia in a saddle-shaped area of the buttocks and perineum. In most of the cases the only practicable therapy is nonsurgical. Rarely an exploratory laminectomy is indicated.

In rare instances the cauda equina syndrome may result from the midline protrusion of a nucleus pulposus; in such cases early surgical intervention is important.

Sciatic nerve

Etiology. The sciatic nerve is involved commonly in gunshot wounds, and occasionally in displaced fractures of the pelvis or femur and dislocations of the hip. It is sometimes injured during a closed reduction for traumatic or congenital dislocation of the hip or during a manipulation of the hip and low back for sciatic pain. In infants a common cause of sciatic injury is the accidental injection of medication into the nerve; intramuscular injections in young children are given more safely in the anterior thigh muscles than in the buttocks.

Clinical picture. Complete division causes a total paralysis of all muscles below the knee, and of the hamstrings also if the lesion is above the middle third of the thigh. In partial division the common peroneal fibers are most often injured. The outstanding motor sign of sciatic paralysis is *foot drop* or inability to carry out active dorsiflexion of the ankle. Also lost is active dorsiflexion of the toes. The *steppage gait* of foot drop is characteristic. The paralyzed muscles develop severe atrophy. Sensation is lost in the foot, except for its medial surface, and in the lateral aspect of the leg. Trophic ulcers are very likely to develop at points of pressure on the sole and may extend deeply to involve the bones. After incomplete division the sciatic nerve is prone to develop the syndrome of causalgia.

Treatment. Conservative treatment consists of physical therapy and of braces to prevent foot drop and contractures, such as the Cabot splint for use at night and an ankle brace, fitted with a spring or right-angle stop joint, for use when walking. Surgical exploration and repair must sometimes be undertaken when satisfactory return of nerve function does not take place, but recovery is always slow and the results are usually disappointing. During and after operation the optimal position for relief of tension upon the nerve—hyperextension of the hip and flexion of the knee—should be preserved. At times advanced trophic changes and ulceration may make amputation of the extremity necessary.

Common peroneal nerve

Etiology. As the common peroneal nerve winds superficially about the neck of the fibula it may be injured by (1) lacerating wounds; (2) sudden compression from a blow; (3) gradual compression from an ill-fitting cast; (4) laceration, edema, or cicatricial involvement associated with fracture or osteotomy of the upper end of the fibula, and sometimes of the tibia; or

(5) stretching associated with the correction of a knee flexion contracture of long duration.

Clinical picture. The motor signs consist of paralysis of the anterior tibial, peroneal, and long extensor muscle groups with resulting foot drop. As in the case of the radial nerve, the usual result of trivial as well as of major injuries is complete motor paralysis. In high lesions sensation is lost over an area situated on the lateral aspect of the leg and the dorsum of the foot.

Treatment. Especial attention should be paid to the prevention or correction of foot drop. In most cases there is no indication for operation. When the signs of complete interruption are present after severe injuries, however, early exploration and suture are indicated. When the nerve lesion is irreparable, foot stabilization and tendon transplantation may improve the gait.

Tibial nerve

Injuries of the tibial nerve are uncommon; they are caused usually by penetrating wounds. Division causes paralysis of the plantar flexors and of the intrinsic muscles of the foot and a loss of sensation over the sole, the lateral surface of the heel, and the plantar surface of the toes. Vasomotor disturbances and trophic ulcers, particularly in the sole of the foot, may form serious complications. The treatment is based upon the usual principles.

Femoral nerve and obturator nerve

Division of either of these nerves is excessively rare. Section of the *femoral nerve* causes paralysis of the quadriceps muscle, together with slight sensory losses in thigh and leg. The power of extending the knee may be partially restored by transplantation of one or two of the hamstring tendons and the iliotibial band into the patella. Division of the *obturator nerve* causes an adductor paralysis without significant sensory changes.

NEURITIS

In addition to acute traumatic injuries, peripheral nerves are subject to a variety of chronic irritative disturbances. These disorders, while of interest to orthopaedic surgeons, are primarily of neurologic character and can be mentioned here only briefly and in their relationship to disease of the bones and joints.

Chronic irritative disorders of the peripheral nerves may be grouped conveniently into two classes: (1) traumatic neuritis, in which the causative factor is chronic mechanical injury, and (2) toxic neuritis, in which the nerve is affected by the presence of some deleterious chemical agent or toxin. Since such toxic substances are usually of systemic distribution, toxic neuritis is likely to involve more than one nerve, in which case it is known as *multiple neuritis* or *polyneuritis*.

Traumatic neuritis

The symptoms and signs of traumatic neuritis vary with the degree of nerve irritation. There may be motor paralysis, as well as pain, sensory disturbances, tenderness along the nerve trunk, and trophic changes. Well-recognized forms of traumatic neuritis are those from prolonged hanging of the arm over the back of a chair or the edge of a bed or from the continuous pressure of a cervical rib. *Crutch palsy*, a partial paralysis of the radial nerve from pressure of a crutch in the axilla, is a common example. The sciatic symptoms often found in association with mechanical derangement in the low back can be interpreted on a similar basis. Irritation of the lateral femoral cutaneous nerve produces a burning discomfort and hypesthesia over the anterolateral aspect of the thigh; the condition is termed *meralgia paraesthetica*. Paralysis of varying degree, resulting from pressure upon the common peroneal nerve as it winds about the head of the fibula, sometimes follows the application of a poorly padded or tightly fitting leg cast. The treatment of these lesions consists in removing the offending mechanical factor, in protecting the weakened muscles with braces when necessary, and in using daily physical therapy to encourage the return of function and to prevent atrophy and contracture.

Toxic neuritis

Although the subject of toxic neuritis is primarily of medical interest, the orthopaedic surgeon is often called upon to aid in the prevention of deformity and the restoration of function. In most of these cases disturbances of sensation, tenderness along the nerve trunk, and motor losses are observed, and the distribution may be symmetrical in the two corresponding extremities. Pathologically the chief change is a degeneration of the neuraxons, and the prognosis for recovery, usually good with adequate treatment, depends upon the extent to which this degeneration is followed by interstitial fibrosis. A common cause of toxic neuritis is poisoning by metals, such as lead or arsenic, or by organic compounds, such as methyl or ethyl alcohol or carbon monoxide. Other common causative agents are the toxins of infectious diseases, such as that of diphtheria. The treatment of toxic neuritis is primarily medical and preventive, but, when paralysis has developed, rest in supportive apparatus and subsequent physical therapy are indicated.

Serum neuritis

A rare form of toxic neuritis may develop after the injection of prophylactic or therapeutic serum, such as that used for tetanus or diphtheria.

Clinical picture. Usually the patient develops an intense serum reaction several days following the injection. A few days later severe pain is experienced in the arms and other parts of the body, and after several more days weakness may become noticeable. The paralysis is almost invariably located about the shoulder girdle without relationship to the site of serum injection.

Treatment. The treatment is rest and protection for the weakened muscles by means of braces and, in the convalescent stage, daily physical therapy. The prognosis for recovery of muscle power is only fair, especially if muscle atrophy has occurred. Surgical procedures of the types employed for poliomyelitis are to be considered when the recovery of muscle power is inadequate.

GUILLAIN-BARRÉ SYNDROME

This form of polyneuritis is characterized by a slowly progressive, symmetrical, ascending motor weakness often confused with poliomyelitis. The cerebrospinal fluid usually shows changes in albumin content, increased protein, and a low or normal cell count; this triad is not found in poliomyelitis.

Etiology. The etiology is unknown. The syndrome frequently develops a few days or weeks after a mild infection and is associated with or subsequent to many virus, toxic, or bacterial diseases. Some patients, however, have no associated or antecedent illness.

Clinical picture. The onset is gradual with initial paresthesias. Pain may be present in the extremities, with muscle and nerve trunk tenderness; there may be mild signs of meningeal irritation. A symmetrical paralysis follows, requiring days or weeks to develop. The first manifestation may be a paralysis of the muscles of the upper extremities or face. Proximal muscle groups tend to be involved more than the distal ones. The second, third, fourth, and sixth cranial nerves are commonly involved. The muscles become flaccid, and tendon reflexes disappear. There may be sphincter disturbances. Fever is usually absent, but respiratory complications may occur.

Differential diagnosis. Differential diagnosis includes consideration of other types of polyneuritis, as well as poliomyelitis and acute ascending myelitis.

Treatment and prognosis. In the early stages, bed rest, an adequate nutritional intake, medication for pain, and proper bowel and bladder care are indicated. If the respiration is embarrassed, a respirator may be necessary, and possibly a tracheotomy. Moist or dry heat should be used over the tender and painful areas, and early, active exercises should be carried out daily through the range of painless joint motion. Recovery is usually complete but may take many months. If residual paralysis results, the treatment should be the same as that outlined for poliomyelitis.

NEURALGIA

Although the term "neuralgia" may be correctly used to denote the symptom of pain arising from any irritative lesion of a nerve, it is too often applied loosely in a quasidiagnostic sense to any painful lesion whatever. This practice is to be condemned, since it tends to obscure the true diagnosis and to lead to inefficient treatment. Although it cannot be proved that pain never arises idiopathically in a nerve free from demonstrable organic lesion, it is far better in each case to avoid use of the term "neuralgia" and to preserve an open mind for the consideration of better-known and more effectively treated entities.

HEREDITARY MUSCULAR ATROPHY OF PERONEAL TYPE (CHARCOT-MARIE-TOOTH DISEASE)

This type of progressive atrophy and paralysis, caused by degenerative changes in the peripheral nerves, begins clinically with involvement of the peroneal muscles. It usually makes its appearance between the ages of 5 and 10 years, affects boys more commonly than girls, and shows a familial tendency. Often a slight shortening of the heel cord and equinovarus deformity are the first changes. Slight stumbling and unsteadiness of gait develop and become progressively worse. There may be cramps in the legs. The hands and forearms may become involved. A clawfoot (Fig. 244) or clawhand (Fig. 147) often develops. The atrophy slowly progresses upward but never extends above the elbows or the middle of the thighs. The reflexes are hypoactive or absent, Babinski's sign is absent, and numbness is occasionally present.

Treatment. Surgical lengthening of the Achilles tendon may lessen the deformity of the ankle and foot and improve the gait for several years. The operation should be followed by systematic exercises. Occasionally it is advisable to support the feet and ankles with braces in order to prevent the development of severe equinovarus deformity. For patients in whom the disease is advancing only slowly, subtalar arthrodesis is sometimes indicated. With the arthrodesis it is sometimes advisable to transfer the anterior tibial tendon laterally on the dorsum of the foot.

Involvement of muscles

PROGRESSIVE MUSCULAR DYSTROPHY (PRIMARY MYOPATHY)

The term "progressive muscular dystrophy" is commonly used to include a number of neuromuscular disorders, the most common of which is *pseudohypertrophic muscular dystrophy.*

This affection appears most frequently at about the age of 5 years and is seen almost exclusively in boys. Symmetrical progressive muscular atrophy is accompanied by apparent hypertrophy of the muscles; the enlargement is usually most marked in the legs and forearms, whereas atrophy is more noticeable about the shoulder girdle. The increase in size is due to hypertrophy of the muscle fibers, which is quickly followed by increase in the size and number of sarcolemmal nuclei, splitting of the fibers, increase of connective tissue, and deposition of fat. Microscopically the muscle may look like a fatty tumor with little resemblance to muscle. The etiology is unknown; it may be an intrinsic nutritional defect of the muscles. In about 60% of the cases the disease is hereditary.

Clinical picture. Often the first evidence of progressive muscular dystrophy is weakness of the legs and resultant fatigue. As the condition advances, the child stands with an obvious increase of the lumbar lordosis, walks with a peculiar waddling gait, has difficulty in climbing steps, and falls frequently. Weakness of the extensor muscles of the legs and trunk is

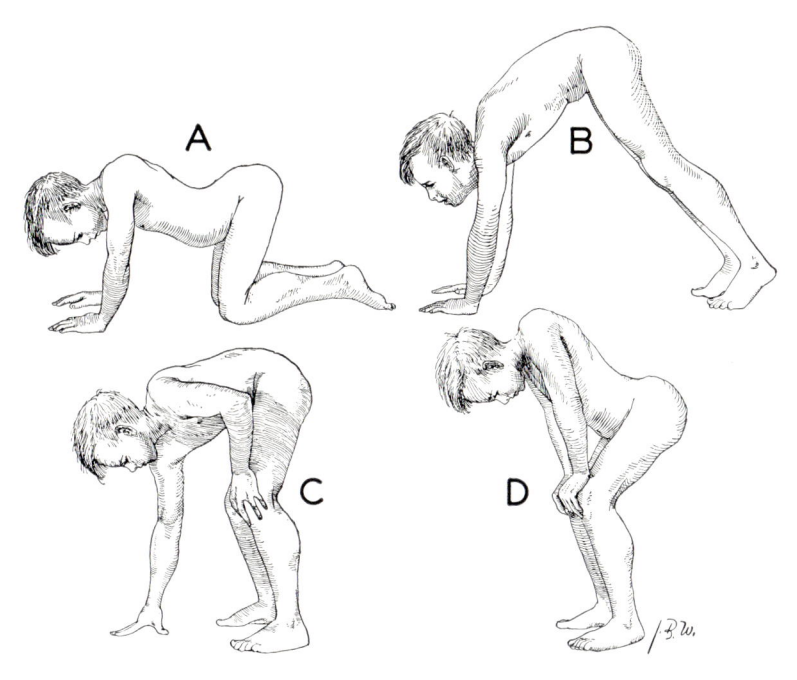

Fig. 149. Progressive muscular dystrophy. Characteristic method of rising to a standing position, the arms being used to push the body erect (Gowers' sign). Note the increased lumbar lordosis, relaxed shoulder girdle, and enlarged calves.

characteristic. On attempting to get up from the floor the patient usually climbs laboriously upon his legs and thighs (Gowers' sign, Fig. 149).

Weakness about the shoulder girdle is characteristic also; when it is marked, the affection is sometimes spoken of as *facioscapulohumeral dystrophy (Landouzy-Déjerine type of progressive muscular dystrophy)*. When the patient is lifted by the examiner, with his hands under the armpits, the patient may slip through because of weakness of chest and shoulder muscles. This type of dystrophy is as frequent in girls as in boys and appears usually about puberty. There may be facial weakness with inability to close the eyes or to whistle, a masklike facial expression, and winging of the scapulae. The reflexes may be hypoactive. Sensation is unimpaired.

Diagnosis. The diagnosis is made from the history, the characteristic clinical appearance, and the findings on physical examination. Because of the waddling gait progressive muscular dystrophy may be confused with bilateral congenital dislocation of the hip, excessive lumbar lordosis, or congenital coxa vara. Occasionally it is to be differentiated from poliomyelitis.

Prognosis. By the age of 12 years extreme disability is usually present, and later the patient dies of intercurrent infection. A common course is gradual progression of the disease in the six to twelve years after its onset, until the patient becomes severely crippled. Occasionally, for no obvious reason, the disease is arrested before the disability becomes severe. Arrest is more likely to occur in the facioscapulohumeral type than in the pseudohypertrophic type of dystrophy.

Treatment. There is great psychologic value in treatment to prevent or minimize deformity. Systematic exercises are usually indicated. If the Achilles tendons are contracted, surgical lengthening will make walking easier. However, care must be taken to avoid prolonged immobilization in a cast following surgery. Active motion and exercises should be started at the earliest possible moment. Braces are indicated when the ankles are weak and unstable. It may be advisable to support the back by means of a brace or corset.

Although active research is being done in this field, no specific medication has yet been found which will arrest or ameliorate the disease.

CHAPTER 13

Tumors

Tumors and tumorlike affections of bone

BONE TUMORS AND LESIONS that simulate bone tumors clinically, pathologically, or in both respects, together make up a large and complex group of orthopaedic affections. Some of the individual entities are uncommon or rare. Some are of trivial import to the patient's welfare, others of the gravest significance. Accordingly the diagnosis, which is often difficult, must be made with the greatest care, and the treatment must be thoughtfully planned and executed.

When a patient's history and physical findings suggest the possibility of a bone tumor, roentgenograms should be made promptly. When despite evaluation of the combined clinical and roentgenographic findings the diagnosis remains uncertain, biopsy should be done promptly. It is often advisable to have the microscopic slides reviewed by a pathologist especially experienced in interpreting bone lesions. Only then is the orthopaedic surgeon ready to formulate and carry out the treatment that will be best for his patient. In the case of malignant bone neoplasms the treatment must be started without unnecessary delay and with aggressiveness sufficient to eradicate all parts of the tumor.

Classification. Although several excellent classifications of the tumors and tumorlike affections of bone are available, none can be entirely satisfactory until the obscurities now surrounding the origin and nature of many of these lesions have been clarified. The following classification, based on that of Lichtenstein, groups the most important bone tumors according to presumptive tissue of origin and benign or malignant nature:

	Tissue of origin	*Benign*	*Malignant*
1.	Osteoblastic	Osteoma Osteoid-osteoma Osteoblastoma	Osteogenic sarcoma
2.	Cartilaginous	Chondroma Chondroblastoma Chondromyxoid fibroma	Chondrosarcoma
3.	Nonosteoblastic connective tissue	Nonosteogenic fibroma Benign giant cell tumor	Fibrosarcoma Malignant giant cell tumor

Continued on next page.

	Tissue of origin—cont'd	Benign—cont'd	Malignant—cont'd
4.	Mesenchymal connective tissue		Ewing's sarcoma
5.	Hematopoietic		Multiple myeloma Malignant lymphoma
6.	Nerve	Neurofibroma Neurilemmoma	
7.	Vascular	Hemangioma Hemangiopericytoma	Hemangioendothelioma
8.	Fat cell	Lipoma	Liposarcoma

Since limitation of space prohibits description of all of these entities, the more common tumors and tumorlike affections of bone will be discussed according to the following outline:

Benign
1. Osteoma, chondroma, and osteochondroma
2. Osteoid-osteoma
3. Nonosteogenic fibroma
4. Giant cell tumor
5. Bone cyst

Malignant
1. Osteogenic sarcoma
2. Chondrosarcoma
3. Ewing's sarcoma
4. Multiple myeloma
5. Tumors metastasizing to bone

In addition to the entities enumerated in this simple classification, there are a number of less common new growths of bone which deserve mention. *Hemangioma* is common as a small, asymptomatic, innocuous lesion, of questionably neoplastic nature, in vertebral bodies; it occurs occasionally as an expansile tumor of a single vertebra that may cause paraplegia by posterior extension and collapse. *Benign chondroblastoma (Codman's tumor)* is an uncommon neoplasm that arises in epiphyseal cartilage, usually near the end of adolescence. *Chondromyxoid fibroma* is an uncommon benign tumor seen most often in the tibia in adolescents or young adults. Although the histologic findings in benign chondroblastoma and chondromyxoid fibroma may suggest malignancy, the clinical course of these tumors is benign; accordingly it is imperative that they be diagnosed accurately and treated by excision rather than amputation.

Chordoma, a rare malignant tumor arising from remnants of the embryonic notochord, occurs about the base of the skull or in the sacrococcygeal region and is characterized by bone destruction, slow growth, and encroachment on the surrounding tissues. Chordoma of the sacrococcygeal area must be distinguished from teratoma and from other tumors, primary or metastatic, which arise not infrequently in this location.

Adamantinoma, a slowly growing tumor of obscure histogenesis, occurs rarely in the limb bones, where it is seen almost exclusively in the tibia. *Aneurysmal bone cyst*, which is probably a disorder of the vasculature of the bone marrow, may require differentiation from bone tumors. It is a painful solitary lesion, commonest in the long bones or vertebrae in the second and third decades of life; the lesion is often a shell-like bony protrusion filled with a spongy mass of channels containing circulating blood; treatment by excision, curettement, or irradiation is usually curative.

Benign tumors and tumorlike affections of bone
OSTEOMA, CHONDROMA, AND OSTEOCHONDROMA

Osteoma

A benign tumor composed chiefly of bone is called an osteoma. The term *exostosis* is often used synonymously with osteoma but is better restricted to localized benign bony overgrowths that can be interpreted as the result of reaction to a local chronic irritation, such as calcaneal spurs or the multiple exostoses associated with osteoarthritis. Osteomas may be cancellous or compact and extremely hard. Microscopically tissue from an osteoma may be indistinguishable from normal bone. Osteomas seldom involve the extremities or spine; they occur most often in the skull, where they may grow slowly to protrude into the orbits, paranasal sinuses, or mouth and cause symptoms from local pressure. The treatment of osteoma is excision, and, if the extirpation is complete, no recurrence need be anticipated.

Chondroma

A benign tumor composed chiefly of cartilage is called a chondroma. These tumors usually arise within the medullary cavity and are termed *enchondromas*. Frequently several bones are involved simultaneously by *multiple enchondromas*. Enchondromas are found most often in phalanges, metacarpals, and metatarsals and occasionally in the humerus, femur, and other bones. They occur most often in patients between the ages of 20 and

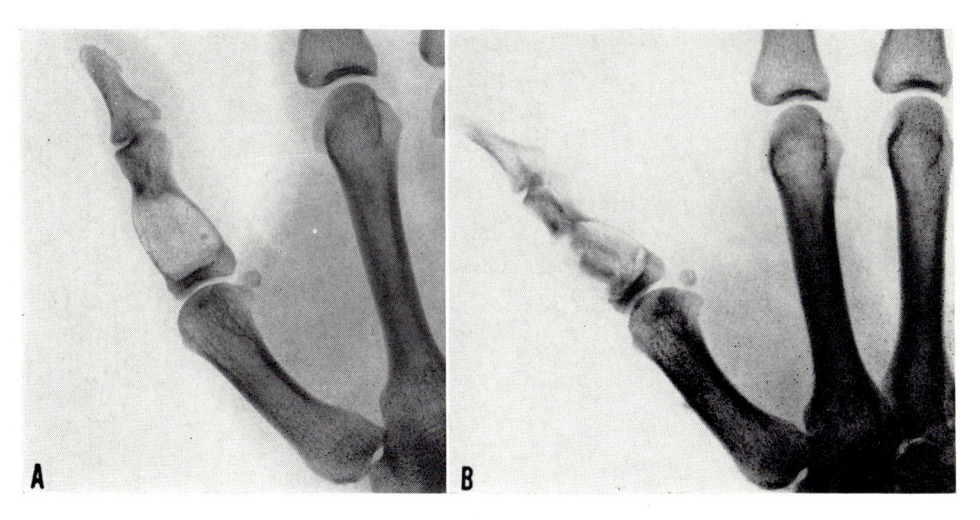

Fig. 150. Roentgenograms of enchondroma of proximal phalanx of thumb in a man 30 years of age. **A**, Note rounded radiolucent area with thinned overlying cortex. **B**, One week after excision of tumor and packing of cavity with small grafts from the ilium.

266 Handbook of orthopaedic surgery

30 years. The clinical picture is that of a slowly growing tumor, producing as a rule only slight discomfort. Pathologic fracture may initiate the symptoms. The characteristic roentgenograms (Fig. 150) show a rounded area of decreased density with a smooth outline, often expanding beneath a narrow shell of cortical bone. Enchondromas of large tubular bones occasionally undergo malignant transformation to chondrosarcomas. The treatment of chondroma is excision, after which it is usually advisable to pack the resulting cavity with small bone grafts.

Osteochondroma

Osteochondromas are the most common benign tumors of bone. Called by Jaffe and Lichtenstein *osteocartilaginous exostoses,* osteochondromas are hamartomas rather than true tumors, their growth usually ceasing simultaneously with that of the bones in which they have arisen. Multiple osteochondromas, often associated with skeletal deformity, form a distinct clinical entity of hereditary nature, which has been discussed (p. 107) under the subject of general affections of the skeleton.

Osteochondromas occur usually in persons between the ages of 10 and 25 years and typically are situated near the ends of the long bones, where they form pedunculated bony overgrowths, the apices of which are covered by a layer of cartilage. The cartilaginous surface may be lobulated or roughened, and the protuberance is often covered, especially when in the vicinity of an overlying tendon, by a well-developed adventitious bursa containing fluid of synovial type. The symptoms produced by these growths are usually slight. Swelling is often the patient's only complaint, although there may be discomfort in the adjacent joint. The duration of symptoms is usually long, and the tumor may eventually reach considerable size. The commonest location for these growths is near the adjacent ends of the femur and tibia or at the upper end of the humerus, although they are

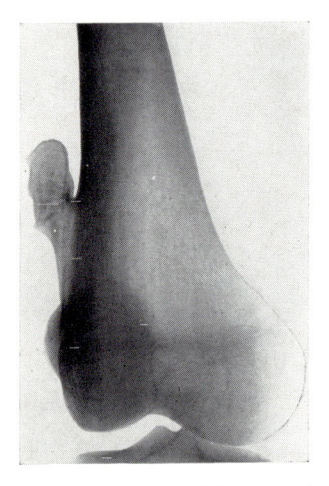

Fig. 151. Roentgenogram of osteochondroma of lower end of the femur in patient 12 years of age.

not uncommon in other sites. Of the flat bones the scapula is most frequently involved. Roentgenograms show the typical picture of an osseous base or pedicle of normal bone density, springing directly from the cortex of the underlying bone and capped by an expanded area showing irregular calcification (Fig. 151). Microscopically the tumors present bone of normal appearance covered by a layer of calcifying cartilage, which in turn may be bordered by a thin layer of fibrous tissue. The treatment is excision. Since osteochondromas rarely become malignant, operation is not always necessary; however, any large osteochondroma in a location prone to traumatization should be removed. If excision is not done, periodic roentgenographic examination should be made, particularly in the older age groups, to determine whether changes suggestive of malignancy are present.

OSTEOID-OSTEOMA

Osteoid-osteoma is a small, benign osteogenic lesion that occurs in either cortical or spongy bone, frequently near the articular portion. It has been found most often in persons between the ages of 10 and 25 years. When arising in the shaft of a long bone it usually provokes a deposition of bone either beneath the periosteum or in the medulla. Although osteoid-osteoma may arise in almost any bone, the femur and tibia are the commonest sites.

Pathology. In the early stage the lesion may consist largely of a vascular mesenchymal substratum, closely packed with osteoblasts and containing occasional osteoclasts. Later, intercellular substance develops between the osteoblasts, forming patches of osteoid tissue or numerous osteoid trabeculae, from which the name of the tumor is taken. This osteoid is gradually calcified, being converted into atypical dense bone that has the microscopic appearance of an osteoma rather than an osteoid tumor. Surrounding this lesion is always found a sclerotic osseous zone which is slow in making its appearance and in which no microscopic evidence of inflammation has been observed.

Clinical picture. The principal complaint is local pain that has been present for several months. The pain is mild at first and then increases in intensity until it is severe enough to wake the patient at night; usually it can be relieved, however, by aspirin. There may be stiffness and weakness in the adjacent muscles, and a limp if the lesion is in a bone of the lower extremity. Localized swelling and tenderness may be present, but there is no elevation of body temperature.

Roentgenographic picture. The involved bone shows a small, rarefied, well-circumscribed area, which is usually oval or round; in the center of this area there may be a minute shadow of increased density. This is surrounded by dense bone which, if the lesion is in the cortex, may extend several inches above or below the point of the original lesion (Fig. 152). Later, the entire lesion may become calcified.

Differential diagnosis. Osteoid-osteoma may be confused with chronic nonsuppurative sclerosing osteomyelitis or with Brodie's abscess. It is also to be differentiated from syphilis and from sclerosing osteogenic sarcoma.

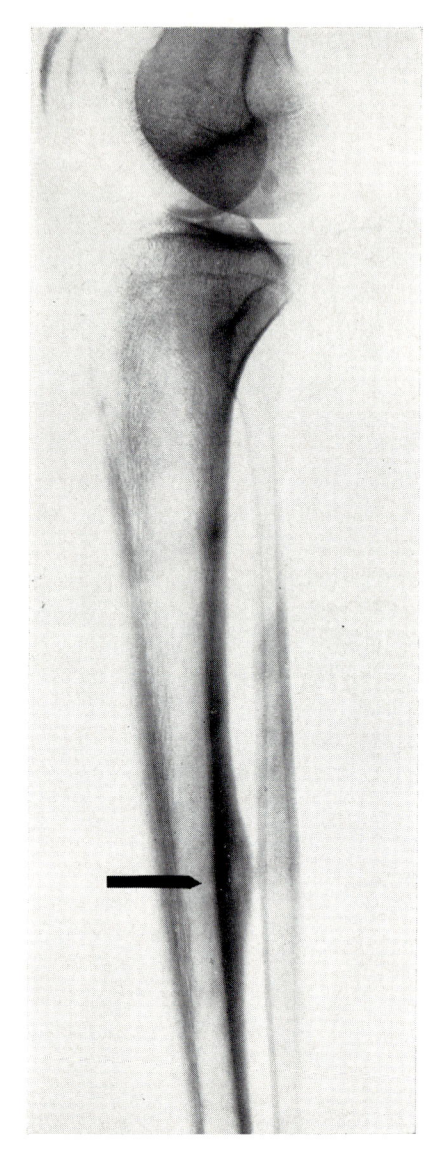

Fig. 152. Lateral roentgenogram showing osteoid-osteoma of tibial shaft. Note the small rarefied area surrounded by osteosclerosis and subperiosteal new bone.

Treatment. The best treatment is complete excision of the lesion and the adjacent sclerotic bone. Replacement with small bone grafts may be indicated.

NONOSTEOGENIC FIBROMA (NONOSSIFYING FIBROMA)

Nonosteogenic fibroma is a common, circumscribed, benign lesion seen near the ends of the diaphyses of long bones, most often in the lower extremities of children and young adults. These lesions are usually innocuous, asymptomatic, and discovered incidentally on roentgenographic examination. Larger nonosteogenic fibromas, however, sometimes lead to pathologic fracture. Grossly these lesions consist of circumscribed yellow-brown fibrous tissue underlying thinned cortex; microscopically they contain bundles of connective tissue cells, a few multinucleated giant cells, and frequently lipoid-containing foam cells. The typical roentgenographic appearance (Fig. 153) is a sharply demarcated, eccentric, loculated area of rarefaction. It is believed that many if not all of these lesions are obliterated in a few years by gradual ingrowth of bone from their periphery.

Differential diagnosis. Nonosteogenic fibroma must be distinguished from giant cell tumor, bone cyst, fibrous dysplasia, enchondroma, and eosinophilic granuloma. This can often be done without biopsy by consideration of the clinical and roentgenographic details.

Treatment. Asymptomatic, typical nonosteogenic fibromas require only extended observation. Unusually large, symptomatic, or questionable lesions should be treated by excision or curettement, after which the defect may be packed with small bone grafts.

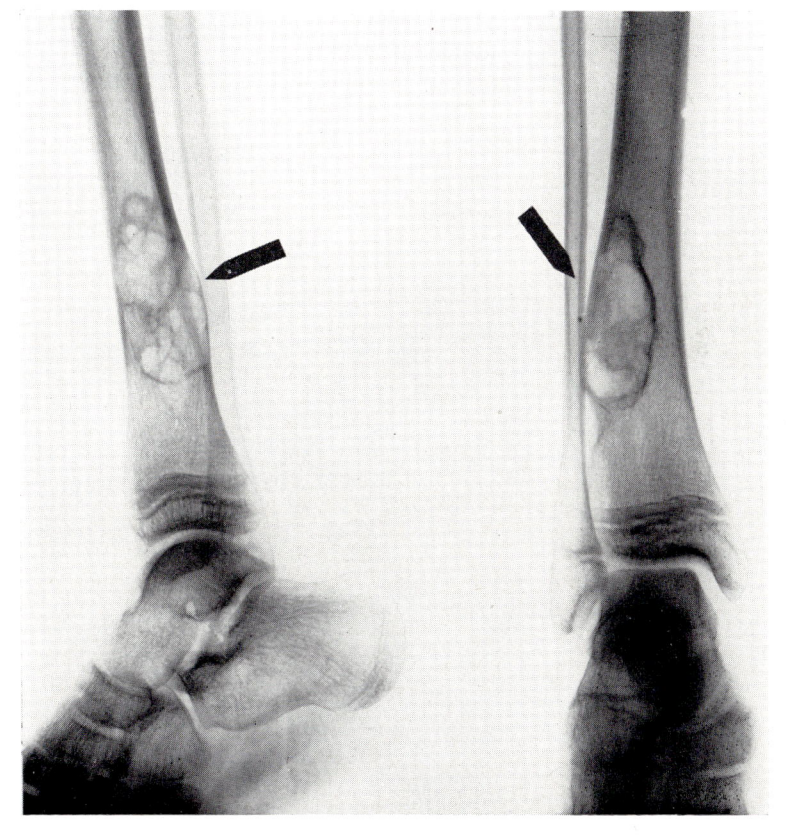

Fig. 153. Lateral and anteroposterior roentgenograms of nonosteogenic fibroma of tibial shaft in 10-year-old child. The treatment consisted of curettement and packing with small bone grafts.

GIANT CELL TUMOR (OSTEOCLASTOMA)

Giant cell tumor of bone is a slowly growing lesion, seen usually in the epiphyseal region of a long bone in young adults, causing swelling with little pain and appearing in roentgenograms as an eccentric area of bone destruction. In recent years giant cell tumor has come to be recognized as a less common and more serious lesion than it was formerly considered. These tumors do not have a uniform clinical course. Most are considered benign, but many recur after curettement and some become frankly malignant.

Pathology. Giant cell tumor begins typically as a circumscribed growth occupying an eccentric position within the end of a long bone. The lower end of the femur, upper end of the tibia, and lower end of the radius are most commonly involved. As growth slowly advances, the overlying cortex is expanded and thinned. Lines of relative thickening of the involved cortical bone, often continuous with fibrous septa extending into the tumor, may produce the roentgenographic appearance of trabeculation.

Grossly the tumor tissue is of brownish red appearance and friable consistency, with areas of fibrosis and of hemorrhagic softening. Microscopically the tumor consists of a vascularized network of fusiform and ovoid stromal cells, among which appear many multinucleated giant cells.

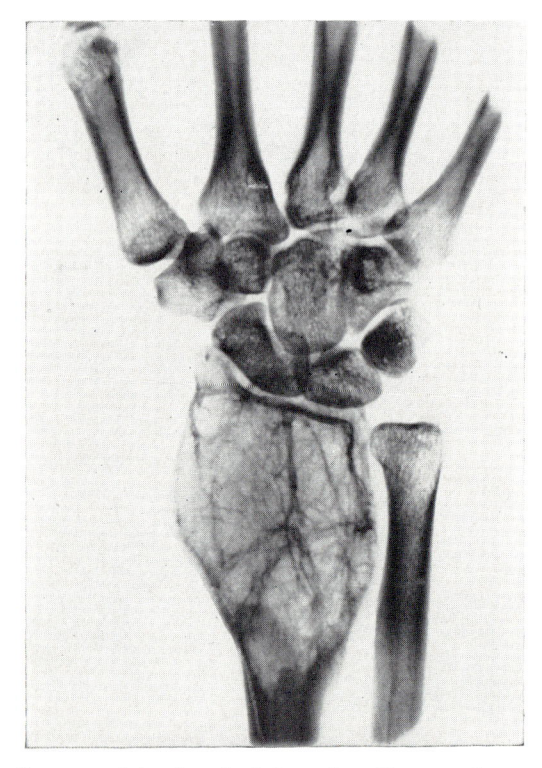

Fig. 154. Giant cell tumor of distal end of the radius. Note rarefaction, trabeculated appearance, and the expansion and thinning of the cortex.

The nuclei of the giant cells are rather uniform, tend to occupy the center of the cell, and may number fifty or more in a single cell.

Clinical picture. Giant cell tumor occurs usually in persons between the ages of 20 and 35 years. In many cases a history of local trauma can be obtained, but trauma has no proved importance in the etiology. Pain of moderate severity is usual and may be associated with slight tenderness. Increase in size is very gradual and may go long unnoticed. Occasionally pathologic fracture occurs.

Roentgenographic picture. Characteristically the giant cell tumor presents an area of radiolucency in the epiphyseal region of a long bone with expansion and thinning of the overlying cortex (Fig. 154). The rarefaction often extends to, but does not invade, the articular cartilage of the adjacent joint. Evidence of subperiosteal new bone formation is minimal.

Treatment and prognosis. Biopsy is indicated to establish the diagnosis and disclose any stromal atypism suggestive of malignant tendency. As a rule the involved bone should be partially or completely excised and replaced, when necessary, by bone grafting or transplantation. In such cases the prognosis for cure is good. Curettement and packing with small bone grafts involves risk of recurrence. When the tumor is in an inaccessible location, roentgentherapy may prove curative but may be followed some years later by the development of sarcoma. Recurrent giant cell tumors should be treated less conservatively than primary ones.

BONE CYST

The simple or solitary bone cyst is not a tumor but is conveniently considered here because of its clinical similarity to certain bone tumors and its consequent importance in differential diagnosis. The typical bone cyst is a slowly growing, fluid-filled lesion occurring in childhood near one end of the diaphysis of a long bone. Its etiology is unknown.

Pathology. Most bone cysts occur in the proximal portion of the humeral shaft. They are seen also in the upper and lower ends of the femoral and tibial shafts and the upper end of the fibular shaft, and occasionally in other bones. Cortical bone overlying the cyst may be extremely thin and fragile. Although the cyst is unilocular, its wall may be traversed by narrow ridges of bone. The cyst commonly has a delicate connective tissue lining; it usually contains an amber fluid. When the cyst wall has been recently fractured, the fluid may be discolored by blood and contain degenerating coagula.

Clinical picture. Bone cyst is a disease of late childhood, the majority of cases occurring in children between the ages of 10 and 15 years although occasional cysts are found even in individuals over 20 years of age. Usually the first symptoms are occasioned by fracture, which takes place on slight traumatization of the thinned cortex.

Roentgenographic picture. The roentgenographic appearance of a single or, less typically, a multilocular central bone defect occurring in the di-

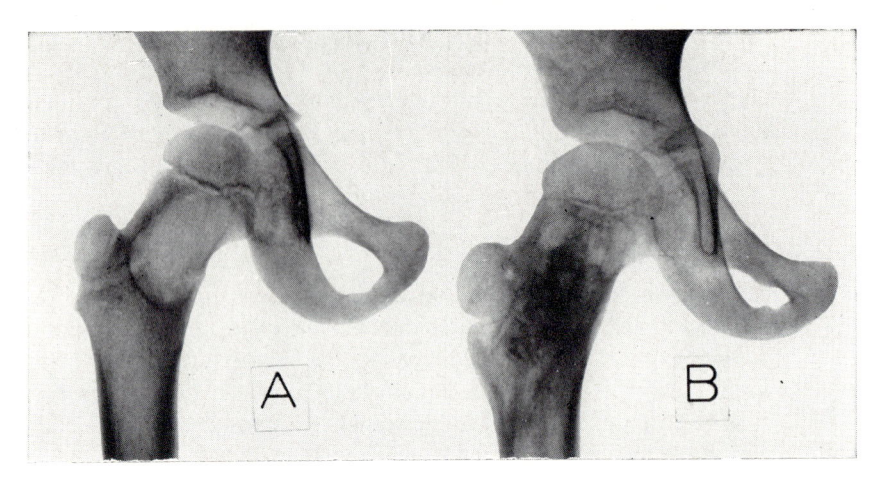

Fig. 155. Roentgenograms of solitary bone cyst in femoral neck of a child 10 years of age. **A**, Before operation. **B**, Six months after curettement and packing with bone chips taken from an iliac wing.

aphysis, with a smooth and intact outline formed by thinned and often slightly expanded cortical bone, is characteristic (Fig. 155).

Treatment and prognosis. When fracture has occurred through a bone cyst, treatment of the fracture is occasionally followed by spontaneous obliteration of the cyst. Ordinarily the treatment of bone cyst is thorough curettement and packing of the cavity with numerous small grafts of healthy bone, preferably from the ilium (Fig. 155). Irradiation is ineffective and may be followed by sarcoma. With careful treatment the prognosis is good; however, the recurrence rate is about 25%. Cysts most likely to recur are those nearest the epiphyseal plate.

Malignant tumors of bone

OSTEOGENIC SARCOMA (OSTEOSARCOMA)

Osteogenic sarcoma is perhaps the most important member of the entire bone tumor group, since it is the commonest primary malignant neoplasm of bone. Typically it occurs near the end of the diaphysis of a long bone in late childhood or early adult life. It is characterized clinically by early and severe pain, together with a rapidly increasing swelling. Radiographically both osteolysis and osteogenesis are usually present, although occasionally either may occur alone; invasion of the soft tissues may be conspicuous. Metastasis occurs early, and the prognosis for life, despite early and efficient treatment, is unfavorable. The five-year survival rate is probably 5 to 10%.

Pathology. The upper tibia, lower femur, and upper humerus are the most common sites of osteogenic sarcoma, although involvement of other bones, including those of the axial skeleton, is not infrequent. Pathologically there is considerable variation among the individual tumors of this large group. Microscopically the diagnostic findings are a frankly sarcomatous stroma and the production of osteoid and bone by the tumor cells. The typical cell of osteogenic sarcoma is spindle-shaped, and in the more malignant tumors hyperchromatism, pleomorphism, mitotic figures, and true tumor giant cells are frequent. Small islands of newly formed bone are common, together with areas of tumor cartilage in various stages of differentiation.

Clinical picture. Osteogenic sarcoma is commonest in children and young adults. It occasionally occurs in later adult years; in such cases an underlying osteitis deformans may be present. Pain is as a rule the first symptom. It is usually persistent even at rest. A history of local trauma is usually obtained, but injury is thought to play no part in causing the tumor. Noticeable swelling (Fig. 156, A) and secondary limitation of motion in the adjacent joint soon follow. The more rapidly growing tumors are likely to show distended superficial veins and an increase in surface tem-

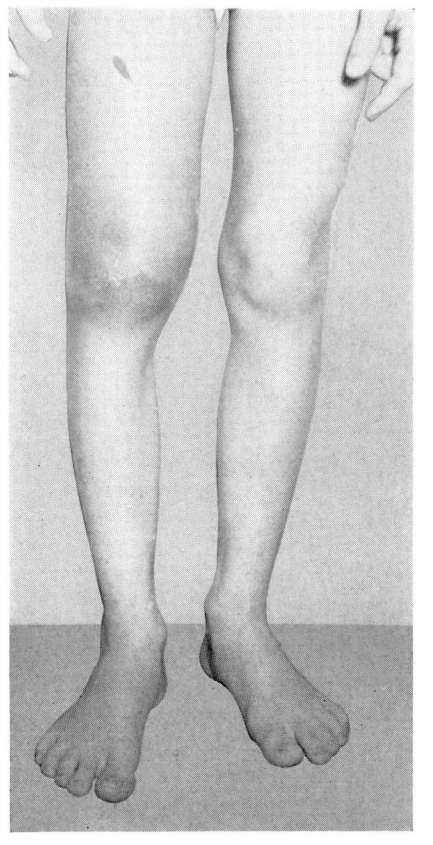

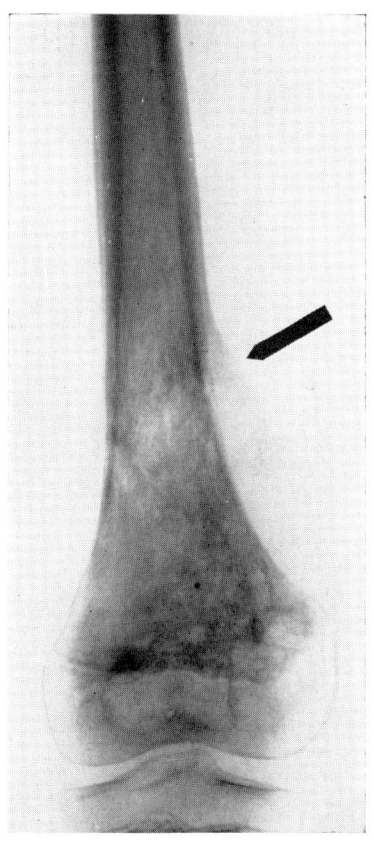

Fig. 156. Osteogenic sarcoma of lower end of right femur in boy 10 years of age. **A,** Note enlargement of right knee and thigh and discoloration of skin about the knee. **B,** Roentgenogram of femur showing moth-eaten appearance of metaphysis, subperiosteal new bone, and Codman's triangle (arrow). A hip disarticulation was done; the patient died of metastases eighteen months later.

274   Handbook of orthopaedic surgery

perature. Other cases are less typical in onset and in their early stages are differentiated only with difficulty from the other bone tumors and from low-grade inflammatory conditions.

Roentgenographic picture. Areas both of bone destruction and of new bone formation are usually visible. Small spicules of bone at right angles to the shaft (Fig. 157) are frequently conspicuous; they are not specific for osteogenic sarcoma. In advanced cases there is evidence of irregular invasion of the surrounding soft tissues (Figs. 156, B, and 158).

Treatment and prognosis. Early definitive diagnosis and treatment are of the utmost importance. The prognosis is always unfavorable because of early metastasis to the lungs, but amputation of the extremity, if performed early, can be expected to result occasionally in cure. Even after the recognition of pulmonary metastases, amputation is often advisable in order to

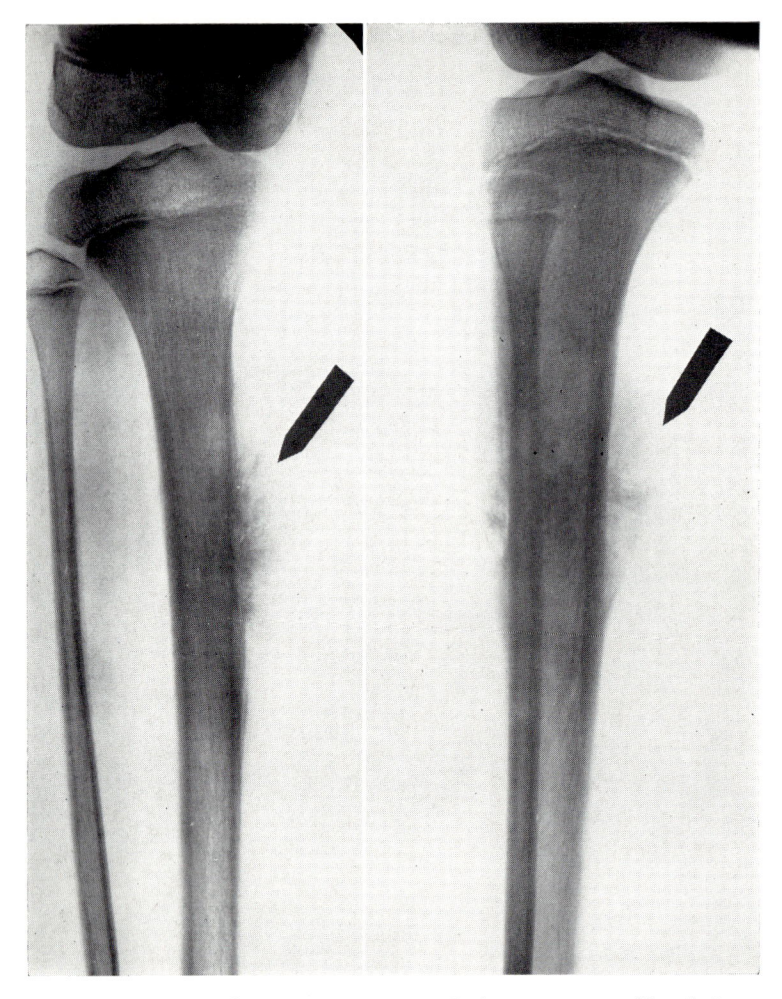

Fig. 157. Roentgenograms of osteogenic sarcoma of tibia in 10-year-old girl. In proximal third of tibia note indistinctly outlined new bone and changes in density of the shaft.

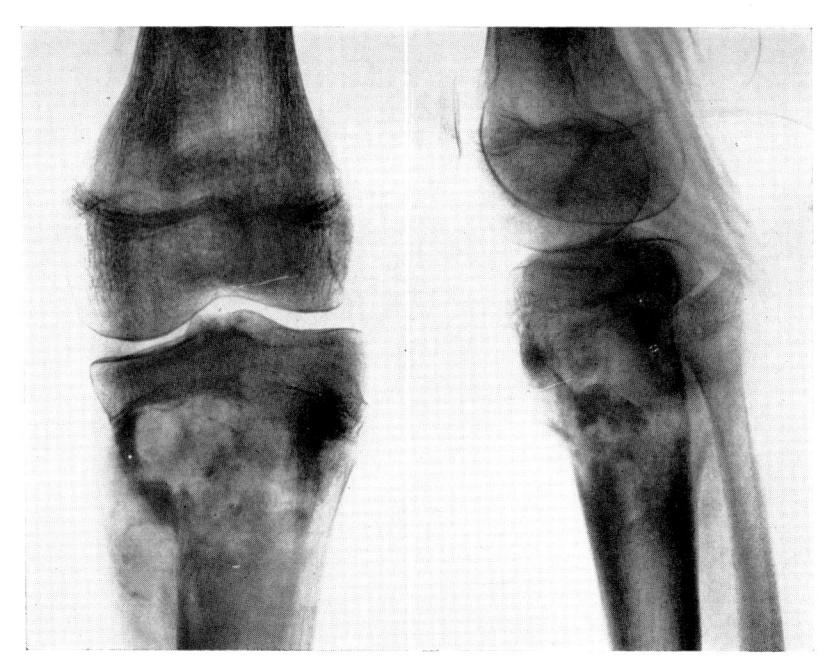

Fig. 158. Anteroposterior and oblique roentgenograms of osteogenic sarcoma of tibia with pathologic fracture, in patient 13 years of age. Note areas of increased and decreased density in upper tibia, new bone extending into the soft tissues, and slight angulation with break in continuity of the medial cortex of the tibia. Note also that the destructive process has not crossed the epiphyseal plate.

remove a painful lesion which may ultimately undergo pathologic fracture, ulceration, and hemorrhage. As a rule radiotherapy is considered to have no advantage over surgical ablation; it may, however, be used as an adjunct. In advanced cases roentgentherapy is usually advised, but it cannot be expected to accomplish more than a temporary retardation of the malignant process.

CHONDROSARCOMA

Chondrosarcoma is a malignant tumor that develops from cartilage cells; it is about half as common as osteogenic sarcoma.

Pathology. *Central chondrosarcomas* arise in the interior of a bone, sometimes from the malignant transformation of an enchondroma of a long, tubular bone. *Peripheral chondrosarcomas,* developing on the surface of a bone, may arise from malignant change in osteochondromas.

Grossly the tissue of a chondrosarcoma is usually recognizable as cartilage. Microscopically the diagnosis of malignancy may be difficult, requiring generous biopsy material and experienced interpretation.

Clinical picture. Chondrosarcoma is a tumor of middle age. It is seen most commonly in the femur, humerus, tibia, pelvic bones, and scapula. Chondrosarcomas usually grow slowly, causing pain and swelling, and may reach considerable size.

Roentgenographic picture. Chondrosarcoma usually appears in roentgenograms as a bulky mass of soft tissue density, containing irregular, blotchy areas of more opaque calcification. Uncalcified intraosseous areas of the tumor are relatively radiolucent.

Treatment and prognosis. Since chondrosarcoma is usually slow to metastasize, its prognosis ordinarily is far better than that of osteogenic sarcoma. The treatment is surgical, amputation or wide excision being indicated as soon as the histologic diagnosis has been made. Chondrosarcomas are not radiosensitive.

EWING'S SARCOMA

Ewing's sarcoma, called also *Ewing's tumor*, is an uncommon malignant tumor of medullary origin that often simulates a low-grade osteomyelitis, with an onset characterized by pain, tenderness, fever, and leukocytosis. It is primarily bone-destructive, causing osteogenesis only by periosteal reaction. The tumor is at first most susceptible to irradiation but usually this response is only temporary and metastasis and death soon supervene.

Pathology. The typical site of origin of Ewing's sarcoma is near the middle of the shaft of a long bone. The tumor occurs in the femur more commonly than in any other bone. It also occurs in the flat bones. Grossly the main mass of the tumor often lies subperiosteally but outside the thickened and eroded cortex. The histogenesis of these tumors is obscure. Microscopically the tumor may show areas of closely packed small polyhedral cells with scant cytoplasm and dense round or oval nuclei. There is no intercellular stroma. Connective tissue septa form a network dividing the tumor tissue into rounded areas, and many large vascular spaces containing blood and lined by tumor cells may be present. Differentiation from neuroblastoma, reticulum cell sarcoma, and anaplastic carcinoma may be extremely difficult.

Clinical picture. Ewing's sarcoma is most frequently encountered in patients between the ages of 10 and 25 years. A history of incidental trauma is often obtained. Pain is an early and distressing symptom although there may be periods of complete freedom from discomfort. There is often a constitutional reaction suggesting a low-grade inflammatory process. Palpation may reveal a smooth fusiform tumor continuous with the bone and of slight or extreme tenderness. Temporary subsidence of the pain and tenderness is believed to be due to relief of tension when the tumor has broken through the periosteum. In advanced cases there may be symptoms from metastases to the lungs or to bones, particularly the skull.

Roentgenographic picture. The roentgenographic appearance often is similar to that of a subacute or chronic osteomyelitis and must be carefully differentiated. In very early cases condensation of reacting bone about small areas of destruction may be visible. Some cases show widening of the shaft from the formation of reactive endosteal and subperiosteal bone in layers parallel to its long axis (Fig. 159). In later stages, areas of bone destruction are evident.

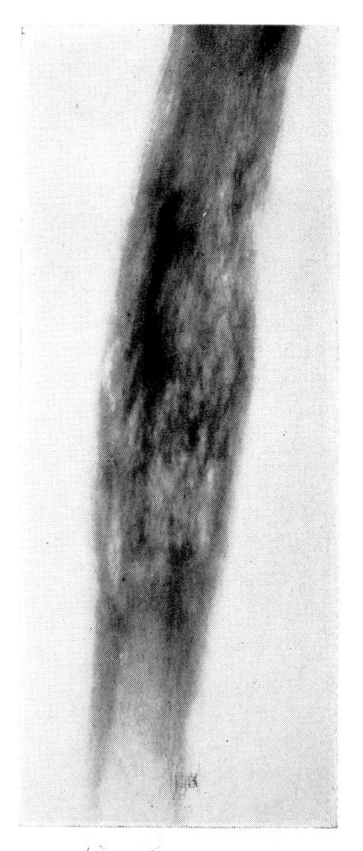

Fig. 159. Lateral roentgenogram showing Ewing's sarcoma of femoral shaft. Note areas of decreased and of increased density, obliteration of the medullary cavity, and thickening of the shaft.

Treatment and prognosis. Since Ewing's sarcoma is markedly sensitive to irradiation, roentgentherapy is often considered the best treatment. Even early radical operation offers little chance of cure. A combination of irradiation and surgery is considered by many authorities to be the treatment of choice at the present time. With any form of therapy, death is likely to occur not later than a very few years after the appearance of metastatic tumors.

MULTIPLE MYELOMA

Multiple myeloma is a highly malignant tumor of bone marrow origin, arising in middle adult life and most commonly affecting the bones of the axial skeleton. The lesions, which are entirely bone-destructive, present roentgenographically a characteristic punched-out appearance. Multiple myeloma is highly sensitive to irradiation, but the ultimate outcome is uniformly fatal.

Pathology. Ribs, sternum, skull, and vertebrae are the most common sites of multiple myeloma. Many bones may be found to be involved simultaneously or in quick succession, and in advanced cases the distribution is

278 *Handbook of orthopaedic surgery*

widespread. The tumor begins in the medullary cavity and extends rapidly, replacing the normal bone marrow. The cortical bone is also invaded and usually shows many discrete areas of destruction. There is no bone formation other than a slight widening of the shaft from periosteal reaction. The process may extend to perforation of the periosteum and invasion of surrounding soft tissues. The typical cells resemble plasma cells in appearance.

Clinical picture. Multiple myelomas are commonest among males in the age group of from 40 to 60 years. In contrast to the other bone sarcomas, this tumor does not produce characteristic early symptoms. The onset is insidious, and vague pain, swelling, signs of local pressure, or pathologic fracture, commonly of a rib or vertebra, may be the first manifestation. In an occasional case the osseous changes may at first be limited for some time to a single bone. In later stages the pain may become more marked. Anemia resulting from invasion of the bone marrow, severe cachexia, and a slight febrile reaction are present in advanced cases. Sternal puncture may demonstrate myeloma cells. *Bence Jones albuminuria* is a valuable confirmatory finding but is frequently absent. The serum protein may be high because of an excess of globulin. Kidney function is often impaired.

Roentgenographic picture. Multiple punched-out areas appearing in the

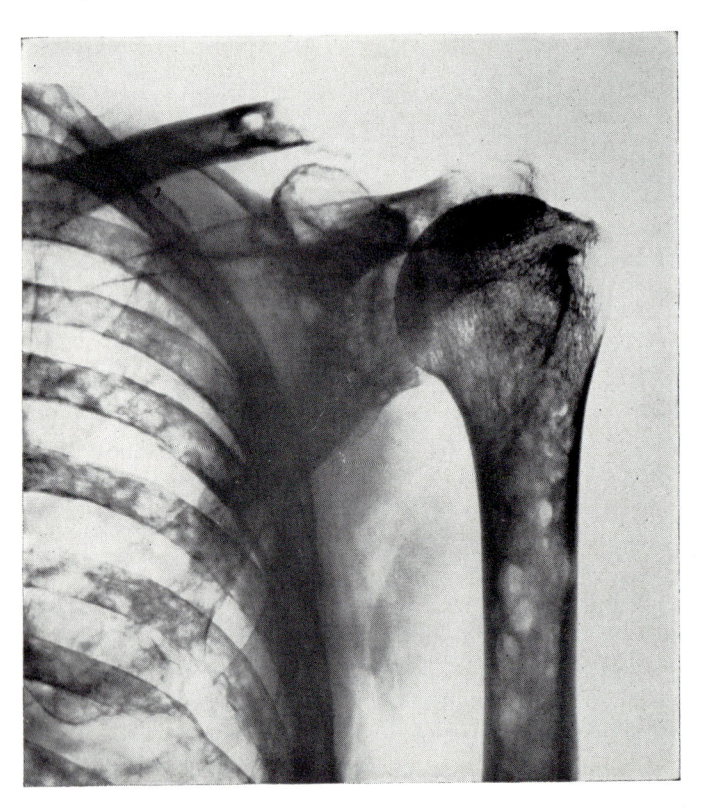

Fig. 160. Roentgenogram showing multiple myeloma. Note small punched-out areas in ribs, scapula, and humerus and complete disappearance of the outer end of the clavicle.

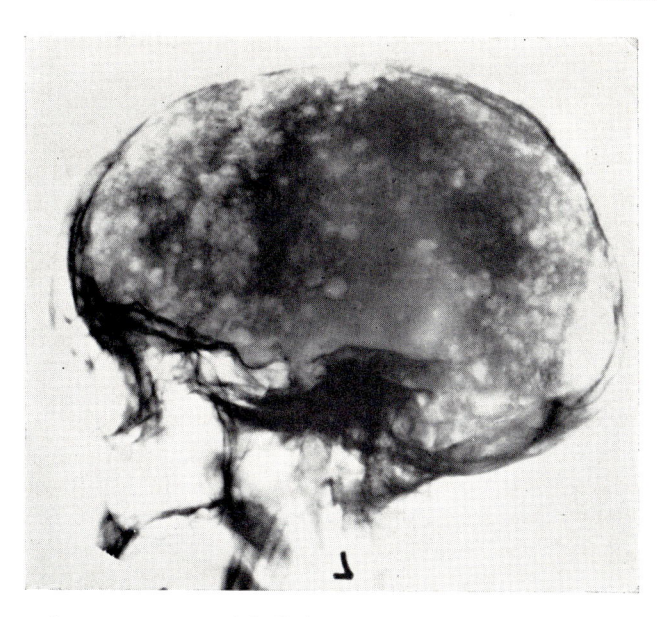

Fig. 161. Lateral roentgenogram of skull showing multiple myeloma (same case as shown in Fig. 160). Note multiple small punched-out areas.

bones of the axial skeleton are characteristic of multiple myeloma (Figs. 160 and 161) but must be differentiated from similar lesions produced by metastasis from osteolytic carcinoma of visceral origin.

Treatment and prognosis. As a rule, the central situation or the multiplicity of the bones involved contraindicates surgical treatment; painful involvement of a long bone may occasionally make amputation the treatment of choice. Multiple myeloma is highly susceptible to irradiation, which should be employed to the limit determined by the resultant leukopenia. Urethane or cortisone may relieve the pain, inhibit the tumor process, and prolong life to some extent. Immobilization may be indicated to prevent or treat pathologic fracture. The prognosis is uniformly unfavorable, the average duration of life being approximately three years, although instances of survival for as long as ten years or more have been recorded.

TUMORS METASTASIZING TO BONE

In the diagnosis of bone tumors the possibility of involvement of bone by metastasis or by direct extension from a tumor that is primary elsewhere must always be kept in mind. Bone metastases are most common in carcinomas of the breast, lungs, prostate gland, and kidneys, and are also frequent in cancer of the thyroid gland, gastrointestinal tract, and female genitalia. Erosive changes in the bones may occur in the leukemias and in Hodgkin's disease.

Pathology. The most common sites to be involved by metastatic tumors are the upper end of the femur, the pelvis (Fig. 162), vertebrae, ribs, skull, and humerus. Metastatic tumors are rare below the elbows and the knees.

280   *Handbook of orthopaedic surgery*

Metastases from renal carcinomas are usually osteolytic; those from the breast are predominantly osteolytic, although they may present areas of bone formation as well. In cancer of the prostate gland, bone metastases of osteoplastic nature occurring in the pelvis and lumbar spine are typical. The histologic appearance of bone metastases depends upon the histogenesis of the primary tumor but is often not sufficiently characteristic to provide a basis for specific diagnosis.

Clinical picture. The clinical appearance of metastatic bone tumor is not uniform. The age of the patient, as a rule, is of aid in rendering primary bone sarcoma other than multiple myeloma unlikely. There is often a history of preceding operation upon breast or prostate gland. Pain may be an early symptom and often occurs before there is roentgenographic evidence of bone involvement. In some cases, on the other hand, pathologic fracture is the first clinical sign (Fig. 163). This is most common in metastases from cancer of the breast. The presence of lung metastases is to be suspected and may be a valuable point in ruling out multiple myeloma. The alkaline phosphatase may be elevated.

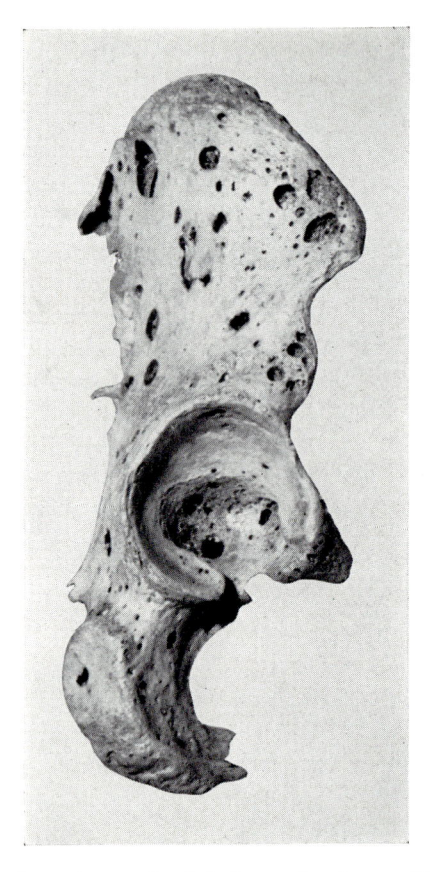

Fig. 162. Photograph of specimen of pelvic bone showing multiple punched-out areas of metastases.

Tumors 281

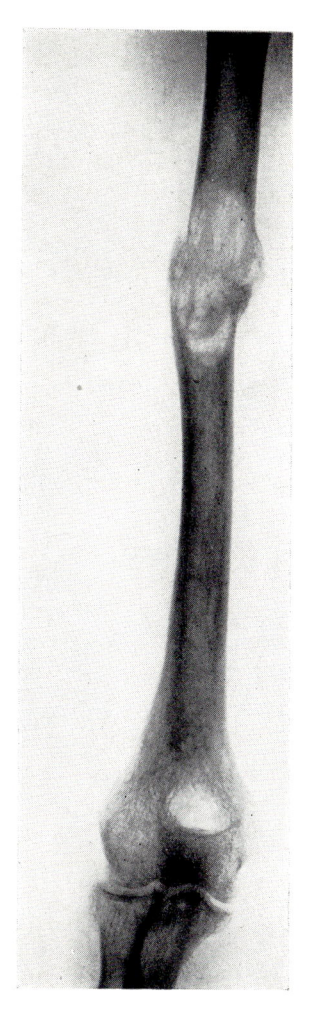

Fig. 163. Roentgenogram showing pathologic fracture of humerus in metastatic lesion from carcinoma of the breast. Note localized, well-demarcated area of bone destruction.

Roentgenographic picture. The areas of involvement are often multiple. The appearance of the bone varies with the type of the original tumor. Punched-out areas of bone destruction without new bone formation are frequent in the osteolytic tumors (Fig. 163), whereas in the case of metastases from the prostate gland a diffuse increase of density is the rule.

Treatment and prognosis. Biopsy should usually be performed if the diagnosis is uncertain. Irradiation can do much to relieve the pain caused by metastatic tumors and in the case of the more radiosensitive growths may prolong life. Cortisone sometimes affords relief of pain. Pain caused by bone metastases from carcinoma of the prostate gland can be relieved by orchidectomy and the administration of estrogen. Bone metastases from breast cancer may be favorably influenced by sterilization, adrenalectomy, or the administration of hormones, and metastases from thyroid cancer may respond temporarily to the use of radioactive iodine. Cytotoxic chemotherapy, when given with care to control its undesirable effects, may be helpful. Traction, intramedullary nailing, cast, or corset may be indicated for a pathologic fracture. Although the prognosis is uniformly unfavorable, palliative treatment can do much to relieve the patient's discomfort.

Tumors of joints, tendons, tendon sheaths, and bursae

True neoplasms of joint structures, of tendons and tendon sheaths, and of bursae are uncommon or rare. They may be simulated by several non-neoplastic entities that deserve mention.

Within the joints occur *lipomas* and *hemangiomas,* arising from fatty connective tissue and its blood vessels. *Osteochondromatosis* (p. 404) is probably to be regarded as a self-limited metaplastic process rather than a neoplasm; it occurs most commonly in the knee but is also seen in other joints and gives rise to multiple loose bodies. *Pigmented villonodular synovitis* (p. 405) is regarded by some observers as a neoplasm. So-called giant cell tumors of the synovium may be manifestations of pigmented villonodular synovitis. Cartilage cysts, such as those of the lateral meniscus of the knee (p. 398) probably arise through mucoid degeneration rather than neoplasia. A joint may be invaded by a malignant tumor of the articular end of one of its component bones. The only primary malignant tumor that arises within joints with any frequency is the *synovial sarcoma,* or synovioma. Synovial sarcomas are seen most often in or about the knee, are composed of a spindle cell stroma containing characteristic clefts, tend to recur locally after excision and to metastasize, and carry an extremely grave prognosis.

Tendons may be involved by tumors of adjacent structures or by tumorlike granulomatous or degenerative processes but do not produce true neoplasms. Tendon sheaths and bursae, with lining membranes so similar to that of joints, are subject to the same tumors and tumorlike lesions that involve joints. So-called giant cell tumors occur frequently about tendon sheaths, especially in the hand and wrist; these are small, dense nodules whose nature is probably granulomatous rather than neoplastic. Ganglia of tendon sheaths and joints (p. 477) probably result from the myxoid degeneration of connective tissue rather than from neoplasia.

Diagnosis and treatment. Accurate diagnosis of tumors of the joints, tendons, tendon sheaths, and bursae is often impossible prior to exploration. The treatment is surgical and varies with the clinical and microscopic characteristics of the individual tumor. Most small, circumscribed growths should be removed with a margin of surrounding tissue. Synovectomy is sometimes indicated for diffuse involvement. Every patient with a joint tumor must be observed carefully for evidence of a recurrent lesion. When the diagnosis of malignancy is established, resort must usually be made to radical surgery, possibly combined with irradiation.

Tumors of muscles and fasciae

Although soft tissue tumors are encountered clinically with great frequency in muscular regions of the extremities and the trunk, these new growths arise almost invariably from mesoblastic derivatives other than muscle. Although cases of *myoblastoma* and *rhabdomyosarcoma*, tumors derived from voluntary striated muscle cells, have been reported, their rarity makes them of little clinical importance. The great majority of the subcutaneous soft tissue tumors are derived from cells of connective tissue, of fatty, or of endothelial type. Of these, the benign varieties are *fibroma, lipoma,* and *angioma,* and the only malignant new growth of common occurrence is *fibrosarcoma.*

FIBROMA, LIPOMA, AND ANGIOMA

These benign tumors may arise at a subcutaneous level or deep within the musculature. They grow very slowly, cause few symptoms, and may be noted early as small nontender nodules or only much later after having attained considerable size. *Fibromas* are encapsulated and are palpable as firm circumscribed masses, often movable to some extent on the underlying tissue; they are particularly common in the hands and feet. *Lipomas* possess little or no capsule; they may be either circumscribed or diffuse and of irregular contour. *Angiomas* are of less frequent occurrence and have been described particularly as arising in the muscles of the extremities. Unlike fibromas and lipomas, they may extend locally and involve the surrounding tissues.

In diagnosis these tumors must be differentiated from masses of similar clinical appearance that may occur at corresponding sites; for instance, lipoma of the popliteal fossa may be distinguished only with difficulty from distention of the gastrocnemio-semimembranosus bursa. Their differentiation from the malignant fibrosarcoma is occasionally difficult, and the diagnosis is sometimes established only by exploration.

The treatment of these benign tumors is excision. Recurrence need not be feared in the case of lipoma but must be kept in mind after the excision of fibromas. Any involvement of surrounding structures by an angioma necessitates wide excision and prolonged observation to rule out recurrence.

FIBROSARCOMA

Pathologically the fibrosarcomas of nonvisceral origin can be divided into several varieties according to the cellular morphology, but clinically they form a single important group with well-marked characteristics.

Fibrosarcoma may occur at any age but is commonest in the fifth decade. It is particularly likely to occur in the lower third of the thigh, in the forearm, or in the abdominal wall. A history of suddenly increased rapidity of growth or of recurrence after surgical removal suggests the diagnosis of malignancy. Fibrosarcomas are typically of firm consistency and because of the involvement of surrounding fascial structures are relatively immobile.

284   *Handbook of orthopaedic surgery*

Metastases usually develop late, especially in the lungs, and in advanced stages are characteristically widespread.

When malignancy is suspected, biopsy is always warranted. The treatment should consist of early, wide, and thorough excision of the tumor. The usual tendency is toward a too conservative removal, which favors recurrence. Irradiation is usually ineffective. When the tumor is situated in an extremity, amputation is often the best treatment.

Tumors of nerves

True *neuroma*, a tumor derived from nerve elements rather than from their investing connective tissue sheaths, occurs so rarely as to be of little clinical importance. *Neurofibroma*, which arises in association with peripheral nerves and is composed of cells derived from some part of the nerve sheaths, is, however, very common. By special staining, many of these tumors may be shown to contain little or no tissue of true nerve origin, and failure to demonstrate the presence of nerve fibers or ganglion cells does not invalidate the diagnosis of neurofibroma. Indeed it is held by many oncologists that most fibromas and fibrosarcomas are of neurogenic origin and are more properly termed *neurofibromas* and *neurofibrosarcomas*.

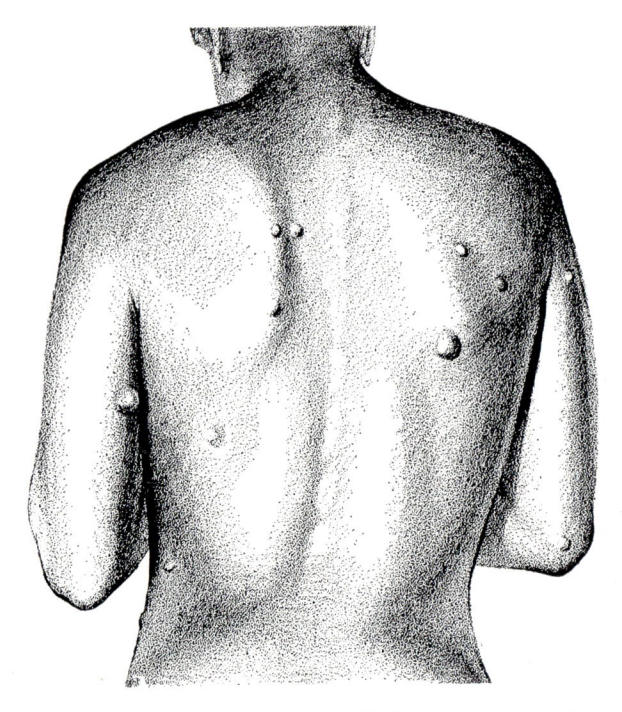

Fig. 164. Neurofibromatosis (von Recklinghausen's disease). Note multiple small tumor masses on back and arms. These pedunculated soft tissue tumors are associated with scattered areas of light brown skin pigmentation (café au lait spots), not shown in this drawing.

Of the tumors that tend to occur in close relationship to nerve trunks, two varieties may be distinguished: (1) *solitary neurofibroma* and (2) *multiple neurofibromas,* called also *neurofibromatosis* and *von Recklinghausen's disease.* Intermediate clinical types are common.

SOLITARY NEUROFIBROMA

A solitary neurofibroma is usually a firm, nontender, slowly growing mass attached to one of the larger nerves but not as a rule interfering with its function. When malignancy is present, growth is more rapid, the tumor mass becomes fixed, and nerve irritation or block may develop. Surgical removal of the tumor is indicated. In the presence of malignant changes wide excision should be carried out. In advanced cases of neurofibrosarcoma excision may be impossible, and amputation, as a palliative measure, may be indicated.

NEUROFIBROMATOSIS (VON RECKLINGHAUSEN'S DISEASE)

Neurofibromatosis, or von Recklinghausen's disease, which is of hereditary nature and slightly more common in males, is characterized by the gradual development of numerous pedunculated soft tissue tumors (Fig. 164) and by the frequent association of small scattered areas of skin pigmentation with smooth edges, which are called café au lait spots. The tumors vary greatly in number and size and lie in the subcutaneous tissue or skin of any or all parts of the body. A large diffuse mass may develop about the head or neck and form an unsightly, drooping fold of skin and soft tissue. Tumors attached to deeper nerve trunks, such as the sciatic nerve, as well as intraspinal tumors, are seen not infrequently. Bone changes secondary to involvement of the local nerves are often observed; scoliosis is a frequent finding.

The tumors tend to progress slowly and to cause few symptoms except from local mechanical pressure. They possess, however, a definite tendency toward malignant change, and the ultimate outcome is often fatal. Excision of deforming or disabling growths must be done with the realization that removal is often followed by the appearance of recurrent tumors of heightened malignancy.

CHAPTER 14

Fracture deformities

IN A SHORT TEXTBOOK of this type there is insufficient space for presentation of the methods of treating recent or fresh fractures. An introductory discussion of the *principles* of fracture management, however, will be found in the Appendix (p. 485).

It is important to understand the unsatisfactory results, or *fracture deformities,* which sometimes follow the treatment of fresh fractures. The physician should know what treatment can be employed to restore involved areas to the best possible structural and functional status and know also what measures can be taken to minimize the frequency of these unsatisfactory results. This chapter includes a discussion of the following subjects: (1) the repair of fractures, (2) delayed union, (3) nonunion, and (4) malunion.

REPAIR OF FRACTURES

Following fracture, blood extravasates into the spaces between the bone fragments, into surrounding soft tissue and the bone marrow, about the periosteum and endosteum, and into the haversian canals. As in the repair of wounds, healing begins with the clotting of this extravasated blood. Organization of the hematoma begins within twenty-four hours. The blood clot is invaded by granulation tissue, which consists of a loose meshwork of capillaries and young fibroblasts. The torn ends of periosteum and of endosteum and the bone marrow adjoining the fracture line supply cells that proliferate and differentiate into fibrous connective tissue, fibrocartilage, and hyaline cartilage, all of which take part in the formation of new bone. Undifferentiated cells of the marrow also contribute to the new bone formation.

New bone formation begins in young individuals on the inner and outer surfaces of the damaged bone within the first forty-eight hours. At the time of injury elevation of the periosteum from the bone surface occurs and extends for a variable distance above and below the fracture. This tearing away of periosteum is a strong stimulus for proliferation of the cells in its

Fracture deformities   287

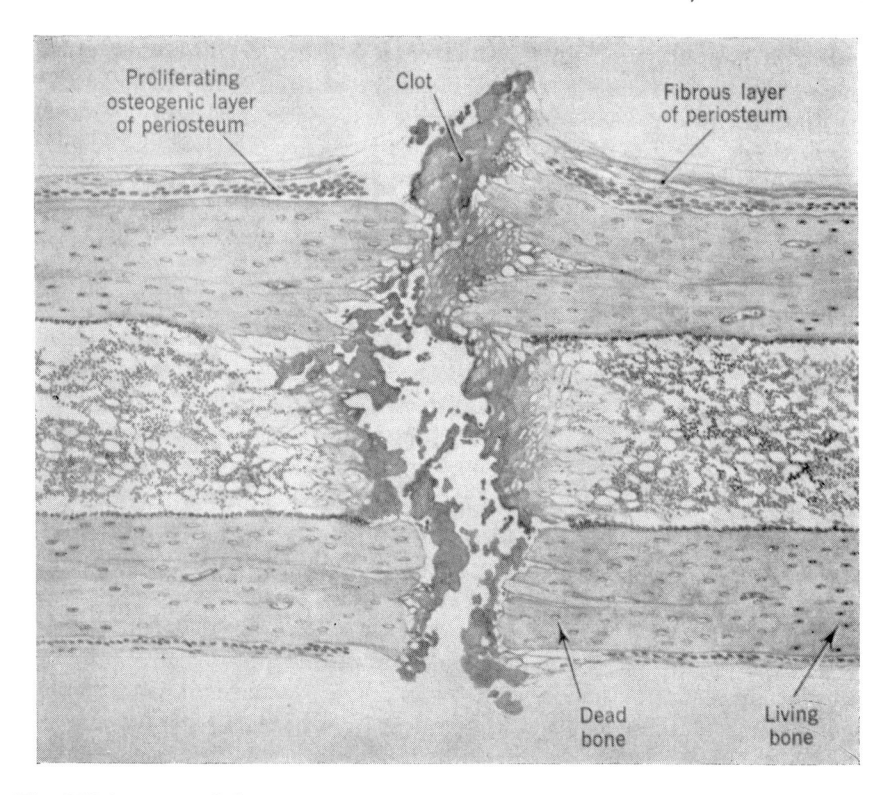

Fig. 165. Drawing of the microscopic appearance of a longitudinal section of a fractured rabbit rib in which healing had taken place for forty-eight hours. The drawing was made sufficiently out of perspective to permit both a considerable area and cell detail to be shown. (From Ham and Harris: In Bourne, editor: The biochemistry and physiology of bone, New York, 1956, Academic Press, Inc.)

deeper layers, and microscopic evidence of new bone formation by these cells may be seen within two days after injury (Fig. 165). While this new bone formation is noted quite early at a distance from the fracture site, cells in the immediate vicinity of the fracture may produce a cartilaginous or fibrocartilaginous tissue. The amount of callus varies with the type, location, duration, age, and treatment of the fracture. In an undisplaced linear fracture, callus may be minimal and is predominantly bone. Fractures in the shafts of young bones tend to produce an abundance of callus, especially if some movement takes place during healing. In early stages such callus may be predominantly cartilage. The presence of cartilage in the callus may result directly from motion at the fracture, or it may be secondary to the rapid and overabundant cellular proliferation resulting from such motion. When cellular proliferation is rapid it may outstrip its blood supply. Cells of the osteogenic series tend to differentiate into bone when oxygen tension (blood supply) is adequate and into cartilage when oxygen tension is low. Mature cartilage callus later undergoes changes (Fig. 166) similar to those seen in enchondral ossification at the epiphyseal

288   Handbook of orthopaedic surgery

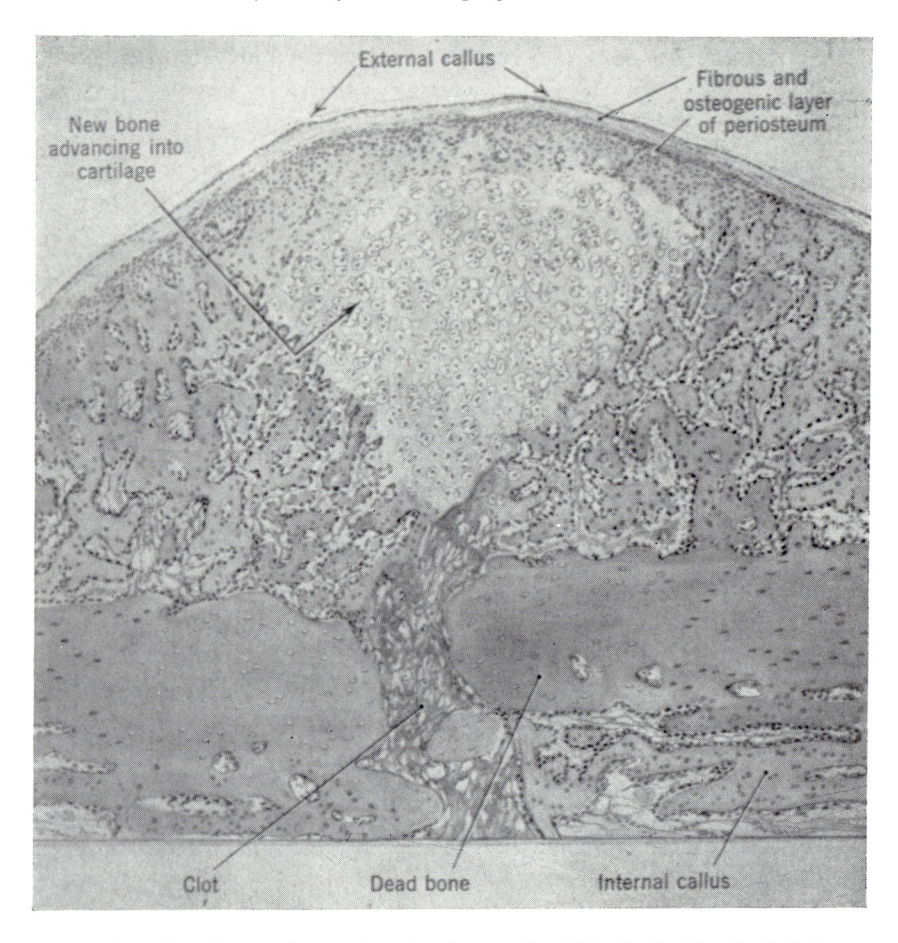

Fig. 166. Drawing of part of a section of a fractured rabbit rib that has healed for two weeks, illustrating the external callus to advantage and showing that the cartilage in it is being replaced by bone along a V-shaped line. Some clot, still unorganized, can be seen. (From Ham and Harris: In Bourne, editor: The biochemistry and physiology of bone, New York, 1956, Academic Press, Inc.)

line and is replaced by bone. Finally the structure of the new bone becomes adapted, according to Wolff's law, to the stresses and strains to which it is subjected.

The shape of the callus and the volume of tissue required to bridge a fracture depend upon the amount of bone damage and displacement. The healing time is directly proportional to the total volume of damaged bone and the breadth of the fracture defect. Some impacted fractures heal in a few weeks, whereas displaced fractures may require months or years for healing. With contact of the fractured bone ends, the humerus and forearm bones may unite in three months. The femur and tibia normally may require six months. Spiral fractures, with fragments of greater surface area, heal more rapidly than transverse fractures. The child generally produces more callus and heals a fracture faster than the adult. Beyond puberty, however, age has much less influence on the rate of fracture healing.

Growing callus is calcified like cartilage and bone elsewhere in the skeleton. New bone ordinarily begins to calcify in the callus as soon as it is formed, provided that sufficient concentrations of calcium and phosphate ions are present in the blood plasma. Whenever a calcifiable tissue is encountered, calcium is deposited at the line of contact with the osteogenic tissue or bone. In the calcification process, when calcium is to be deposited in the bones, it moves first from the plasma to the intercellular fluid and thence is deposited in locations suitable for calcification. As calcium is being deposited in one or more places in the skeleton, it is being withdrawn from other places; the entire "plasma to intercellular fluid to bone" system remains in a state of dynamic equilibrium. The levels of serum calcium, inorganic phosphorus, and alkaline phosphatase are not appreciably altered during fracture healing.

In 1923 Robison announced that he had found the enzyme *phosphatase*, at the site of bone repair; he assumed that the action of the enzyme was critical in the phenomenon of calcification. Recently, attention has been called to the high phosphatase content of osteoclasts and to the possibility that the enzyme plays a part in resorption, perhaps by mediating the synthesis of phosphoric esters. Except for the localization of phosphatase in the cartilage matrix, its distribution in the cellular elements of bone and cartilage, including the cytoplasm and perhaps also the nucleus, does not suggest any direct relationship to the deposition of bone salt. Especially striking is its absence from calcifiable bone matrix, as in rickets, at a time when the surrounding osteoblasts are rich in the enzyme. McLean and Urist have concluded that phosphatase plays no part in calcification; however, they believe there is a possibility that phosphatase is concerned with preparation of the matrix.

The search for a substance that will stimulate the healing of fractures has motivated much research on the effects of minerals, vitamins, and hormones upon callus formation. Thus far, no effective agent either to suppress or to stimulate bone repair has been found.

DELAYED UNION

Delayed union is said to be present when a fracture fails to consolidate in the time usually required for union to take place. In delayed union the processes of bone repair are retarded but are still going on and, with sufficient time, will produce firm union without surgical treatment.

The period required for bone consolidation after fracture varies considerably in different individuals and under different circumstances. Delayed union is said to be present in the tibia if a closed fracture does not become clinically firm in twenty weeks (Fig. 167); in the humerus, in ten weeks; and in the femur, in twenty weeks. These are common sites of delayed union.

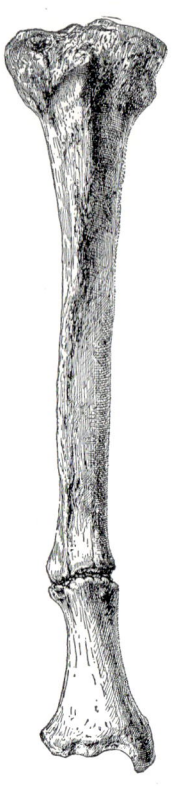

Fig. 167. Delayed union of fracture of tibia. (Drawing from specimen.)

The causes of delayed union are as follows:
1. Inaccurate reduction
2. Inadequate or interrupted immobilization
3. Severe local traumatization
4. Impairment of circulation following open operation
5. Infection, as in compound fractures
6. Loss of bone substance, such as might occur in compound fractures after free excision of devitalized fragments
7. Distraction or separation of fragments caused by excessive traction, a frequent sequel to too strong skeletal traction, or by improperly applied internal fixation

Treatment. Delayed union can best be avoided by (1) an early, accurate, and gentle reduction and immobilization, uncomplicated by circulatory impairment from pressure of the splint or unnecessary surgical interference; (2) avoidance of the repeated traumatization of unnecessary attempts to perfect the alignment; (3) frequent observation of cases in skeletal traction to forestall separation of the fragments; (4) sound judgment and technic in the use of internal fixation; and (5) protection against undue strain upon the fracture line, especially in the lower extremity.

The treatment of delayed union should be directed toward correction of recognizable factors which may be contributing to the delay. The type and quality of immobilization should be checked. An ill-fitting, inadequate cast should be replaced by a snug, well-applied cast including, in most instances, the joints above and below the fracture. Infection should be treated according to methods discussed in Chapter 6. Patients will often ask whether they should drink milk or take calcium pills to speed healing. There is no evidence that supplementary dietary calcium has any effect on the healing rate of fractures. The body reserves of calcium are tremendous. The surfaces of bone crystals throughout the body are in constant equilibrium with the body fluids. This surface area has been estimated as greater than 200 square meters per gram of bone. Actually when a normally active person is immobilized in a cast there is some generalized bone resorption, which creates an excess of mobilized calcium. Delayed union calls for relatively long immobilization and for patience on the part of patient and physician. In delayed union of the tibia or femur, weight bearing in a walking cast often seems to accelerate union.

NONUNION

Nonunion is present when the processes of bone repair, after having failed to produce firm union, have ceased completely. Unless this situation is changed radically by treatment, the nonunion will continue as a permanent and, in most instances, a severely disabling condition.

No fracture should be considered ununited until at least six months after the date of injury. Even after eight months or more have elapsed, firm union will occasionally take place without surgical aid.

Etiology. Nonunion may result from the following:
1. Separation of the fragments, which is the most common cause
2. Loss of bone substance, resulting from extrusion or excision of small fragments in open fractures
3. Inadequate fixation, allowing excessive motion at the site of fracture, such as might result from ineffective plating or nailing
4. Repeated manipulation to improve the position, causing disturbances of the circulation
5. Interposition of soft parts such as muscle and fascia between the fragments
6. Infection, which may develop following an open fracture or open reduction
7. Impairment of circulation by injury of the nutrient vessels or other sources of blood supply at the time of the original injury or at open reduction

Pathology. The fragments may be connected by a fibrous or fibrocartilaginous tissue, or there may be a pseudarthrosis between the fragments with the formation of a thick bursal sac containing synovial fluid, in which rice bodies may be present. The ends of the fragments usually consist of hard, sclerotic, eburnated bone; they may, on the other hand, become

292 *Handbook of orthopaedic surgery*

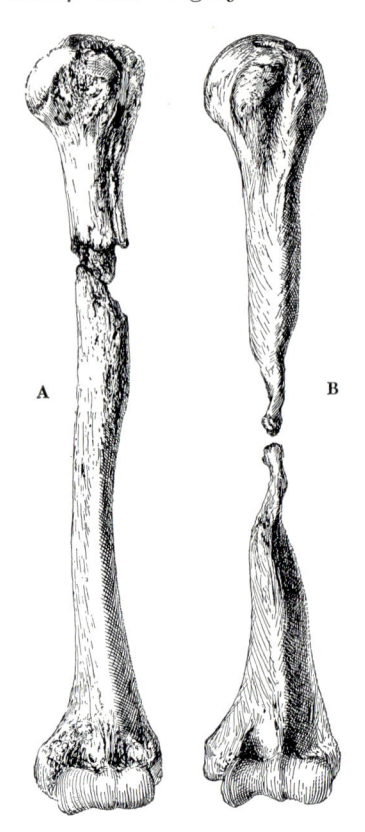

Fig. 168. Nonunion of fracture of humerus. **A,** Common type with moderate bone absorption. **B,** Pencil-point type characterized by extreme absorption. (Drawings from specimens.)

porous, atrophic, and cone-shaped (Fig. 168). There may be excessive callus limited entirely to one fragment, usually the proximal.

Clinical picture. Mobility at the site of fracture varies widely. In some cases it is slight and hardly demonstrable, whereas in others, and particularly in pseudarthroses, there may be excessive movement in all directions. The pathologic mobility may be obvious when the patient attempts to move the extremity. Occasionally motion elicits pain, but usually little discomfort is associated with the motion of a pseudarthrosis. In cases of nonunion in the lower extremity there are often pain on weight bearing and a slight amount of swelling following activity. Pain and swelling are more conspicuous when there is little mobility between the fragments than when, as in pseudarthroses, the mobility is great. Muscle atrophy is extreme and joint function may be limited. Especially great is the loss of mobility of the knee joint which may accompany an ununited fracture of the femur.

Treatment. The treatment consists of the use of braces or of surgery. Braces are entirely palliative and are used primarily to prevent deformity and to relieve strain and accompanying pain. In ununited fracture of the humerus, a closely fitting laced leather cuff extending from the shoulder to the elbow will improve the function of the arm. A Thomas walking caliper splint fitted with a molded leather cuff for the thigh will brace an ununited fracture of the femur sufficiently to permit the patient to walk. A similar brace may be used for ununited fracture of the tibia; it should be fitted with a leather cuff that has been molded closely to the leg from knee to ankle.

When nonunion follows the frank infection of an open fracture, surgical treatment should usually be delayed three to six months following the healing of the wound, since the development of infection in a wound containing transplanted bone often means complete failure of the surgical work. The use of chemotherapy and antibiotics, however, has made it possible to shorten the waiting period in some cases. It is often advisable to perform the operation of bone grafting in two stages. In the first stage the potentially infected scar tissue should be thoroughly excised and the hard, eburnated ends of the bone fragments removed. Infected, scarred, or poorly nourished skin areas should be removed and replaced, preferably by a single skin graft of pedicle, flap, or split-thickness type. If healing takes place without signs of infection, a bone graft operation may be performed several weeks later.

Most ununited fractures require a bone transplant before union can be obtained. When the bed is being prepared for the graft, all surrounding scar tissue and sclerotic bone should be removed until healthy bleeding occurs from the bone ends and from the surrounding soft tissues.

What happens to transplanted bone has been and continues to be extensively studied. In the case of autogenous cortical bone transplants it is known that the vast majority of the osteocytes die. Perhaps a very few of the transplanted cells survive, but new bone is formed by cells already near the fracture site. The graft becomes incorporated by this new bone and is invaded by blood vessels. Over a period of time the necrotic bone of the graft is resorbed. New bone may be formed as rapidly as the graft is removed, the fracture being bridged by this new bone as it replaces the graft. Under unfavorable circumstances graft resorption is not accompanied by new bone formation and the nonunion persists. In transplants of autogenous cancellous bone it is possible that more of the transplanted bone cells survive, for they are more accessible to the blood supply at the fracture site. Osteoblasts on the surfaces of the trabeculae of the cancellous graft may take some part in the new bone formation that bridges the fracture.

Autogenous bone is superior to homologous bone for transplantation when satisfactory grafts can be obtained. However, in some instances insufficient autogenous bone is obtainable and it is necessary to use another source. Bone banks are available as such a source. Bank bone is taken under sterile conditions from the cadaver, from amputated limbs, or from excess bone removed at operation; it is preserved by freezing or freeze-drying in sterile containers, or by storage in antiseptic solutions. At opera-

294   *Handbook of orthopaedic surgery*

tion a piece of bone of approximately the needed size is taken from the container and used in the same manner as an autogenous transplant.

Several types of bone graft are in common use. Choice of the most effective graft for the individual case depends largely upon the site of nonunion, the condition of the ends of the bone fragments, and the training and experience of the orthopaedic surgeon. The more important types of bone graft are the (1) massive onlay, (2) inlay, (3) cancellous, (4) multiple, and (5) osteoperiosteal grafts.

Massive onlay graft. The massive onlay graft (Fig. 169), taken usually from the tibia, may include the periosteum as well as the full thickness of the cortex. The bed is prepared across the fragment ends by removing

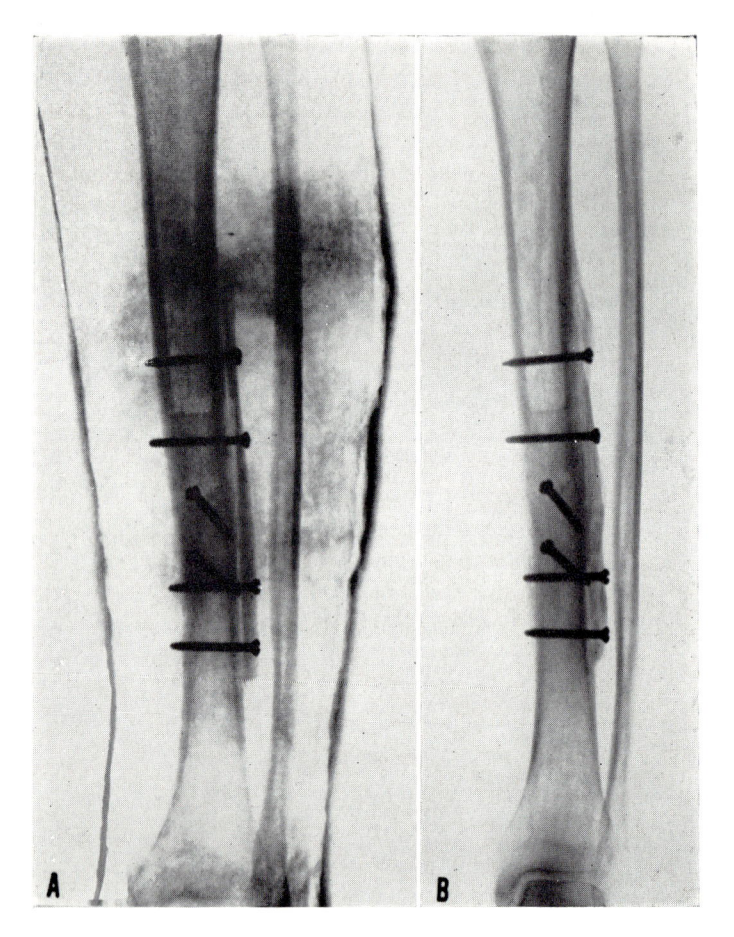

Fig. 169. Roentgenograms of onlay bone graft for ununited fracture of tibial shaft. **A,** Massive cortical graft from proximal half of tibia has been fixed across fracture site with two transverse screws in each fragment. The two middle screws transfix the oblique ends of the fracture fragments. Note cast, which is essential for further immobilization during the healing period. **B,** Six months after operation. Note consolidation of onlay graft with tibial shaft.

the periosteum and outer cortex. No attempt is made to place the graft in contact with the endosteum or medullary cavity. As a rule, fixation is best secured by the use of Vitallium or stainless steel screws long enough to traverse both cortices. Onlay grafts produce very satisfactory results in the hands of surgeons who are experienced in the technic that their application requires.

The *dual graft*, described by Boyd, comprises two massive onlay grafts that span the defect on opposite surfaces of the fractured bone. They are fixed firmly by screws going through both grafts and both cortices. Dual grafts are particularly useful for the more difficult cases of nonunion.

The *subperiosteal onlay graft* of Phemister is excellent for certain cases with little displacement of the fragments. The periosteum is lifted on both sides of an ununited fracture, which has been approached through healthy tissue, and a rigid graft 7 to 12 cm. in length for an ununited shaft is inserted beneath the periosteum. The nonunion site is not disturbed, and no internal fixation is used.

Inlay graft. The inlay graft, popularized by Albee, includes periosteum, cortex, and endosteum and is spoken of as a full-thickness or cortical graft. The bed for the graft is usually prepared in the fragments with the same double-bladed motor saw which is used to cut the graft. In fracture of the lower third of the tibia, a sliding inlay graft, which requires no second operative procedure for obtaining the transplant, may be most suitable. It is cut from the upper fragment, is slid into a bed across the defect, and according to the usual current technic is fixed firmly in place with screws.

Cancellous graft. A cancellous graft consists of spongy bone, usually taken from the crest or wing of the ilium. The circulation is more readily re-established through its cancellous structures than through the dense bone of a cortical graft, and union takes place in less time. It is the most useful type of nonrigid graft.

Multiple grafts. Frequently it is wise to place many long, thin strips of bone across the fracture line as a supplement to metallic internal fixation or a massive graft. Such strips, taken from an iliac wing, are chiefly cancellous but may include a thin layer of cortical bone.

Osteoperiosteal graft. The osteoperiosteal graft is usually taken from the anteromedial surface of the tibia or from a rib in such manner as to include the periosteum and a thin layer of small adherent chips of cortical bone. The particular advantage of this graft is that it is pliable and can be molded to fit the contour of the fragments and the defect.

Other measures. Many ununited fractures require metallic internal fixation at the time of bone grafting. In addition the fragments should usually be immobilized by means of ample and well-molded plaster splints or a cast. Bleeding from the denuded bone surfaces always occurs, and care must be taken postoperatively that this does not cause excessive pressure and ischemia. A properly padded cast which is elevated on pillows postoperatively does not usually require splitting; if it must be cut to relieve pressure, complete temporary bivalving is the safest method. After grafting of a major

296   *Handbook of orthopaedic surgery*

bone of an extremity a cast should be worn until there is roentgenographic evidence of enough bone formation to ensure union. This period varies with the site of the graft and the bone involved; it is usually from twelve to twenty-four weeks. The plaster should then be bivalved and active exercises started.

Congenital fractures and nonunion

A defect in the bony continuity resembling an ununited fracture or pseudarthrosis is occasionally demonstrable in the bone of an infant immediately after birth. Lesions of this type can be differentiated by means of

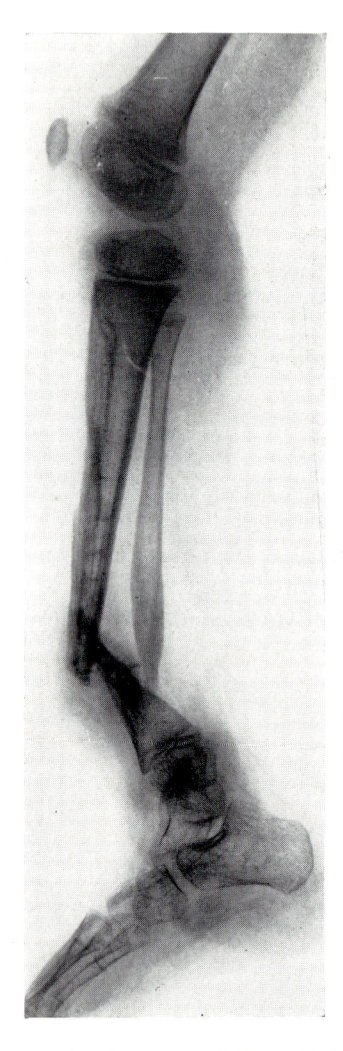

Fig. 170. Lateral roentgenogram showing congenital pseudarthrosis of the tibia in a boy 7 years of age. Two bone graft operations had been performed without union. Note thin, tapered fragment ends and atrophy of all bony structures. (Courtesy Dr. R. H. Hutchinson.)

roentgenograms from fractures occurring during delivery. Their etiology is unknown. They may result from a congenital deficiency of bone production. These fractures are rare, are seen in the tibia much more often than in other bones (Fig. 170), and unfortunately are very resistant to treatment. Three types of poorly united congenital fractures have been recognized: (1) those which are quite unstable at birth; (2) those which present a feeble malunion and which later are very easily fractured; and (3) those with a feeble union in good position; these also are easily refractured.

Attempts to induce union of these fractures, especially those of the first type, have often been unsuccessful. The fresh homologous dual graft of Boyd, however, allows early operation and occasionally has given good results. The grafts are best taken from a person closely related to the patient.

The treatment of massive defects of the long bones

Extensive loss of continuity in the shaft or at one end of a long bone is seen occasionally as the result of a severely comminuted open fracture, radical resection of bone for a malignant tumor, failure of bone regeneration in osteomyelitis, or a congenital anomaly. The replacement of a large defect in the continuity of the bone or the creation of a new bony structure to replace the absent end of the bone constitutes a problem much more difficult than the ordinary bone grafting for nonunion. Such cases must be considered individually, and great care must be exercised in selecting the operation most suitable for improving the function of the disabled extremity.

It is essential that certain conditions be fulfilled before the reconstructive bone operation is performed. Any infection that may be present must first be eliminated. Poorly nourished skin and scars must be replaced with healthy tissues by means of plastic surgical procedures. The nutrition, mobility, and strength of the extremity must be restored as nearly as possible to normal by means of physical therapy, and the general physical condition and motivation of the patient must be good.

The technic of the reconstructive bone operation varies with details of the individual case. In the lower extremity extensive defects may often be successfully bridged by a massive sliding onlay or inlay graft, by a massive graft from the tibia of the opposite leg, or by use of the shaft of the fibula as a graft. A dual graft is often indicated. In most instances the cortical graft should be supplemented by the addition of a considerable amount of cancellous bone; this may be taken conveniently from the ilium. The ribs also form a useful source of autogenous grafts. When the tibial shaft is involved, it is sometimes advisable to transfer the shaft of the fibula into the ends of the tibia, above and below (p. 300), without exposing the tibial defect.

In the upper extremity length is not an essential consideration. It is often advisable to approximate the ends of the fragments rather than attempt the spanning of a large defect in the humerus. The entire upper part of the fibula may be used to replace a lost portion of the humerus or radius. In rare instances of extensive defect of the shaft of the radius, a transference of the distal end of the radius to the shaft of the ulna may be indicated.

Nonunion of individual bones
Neck of the femur

Although nonunion of femoral neck fractures is much less common than before the introduction of technics of internal fixation by Smith-Petersen and others about thirty years ago, it still occurs in approximately 15% of the cases (Figs. 171 and 172). The reasons for nonunion of the neck of the femur are (1) an anatomically meager blood supply, and (2) difficulty in securing accurate approximation and rigid immobilization of the fragments.

The outstanding manifestations of nonunion of fracture of the neck of the femur are (1) pain in the hip on weight bearing; (2) shortening and, as a rule, external rotation of the lower extremity; and (3) grating in the hip on motion. Additional complicating factors that may be present include ischemic necrosis of the femoral head, which appears roentgenographically

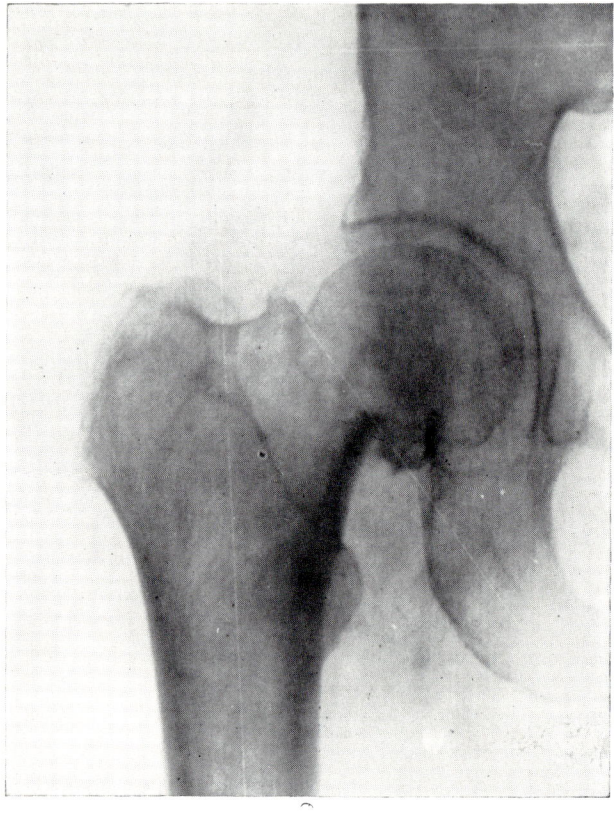

Fig. 171. Roentgenogram showing ununited fracture of the neck of the femur. Note upward displacement of distal fragment. Similar density of the head and neck suggests at least partial viability of the head.

Fracture deformities 299

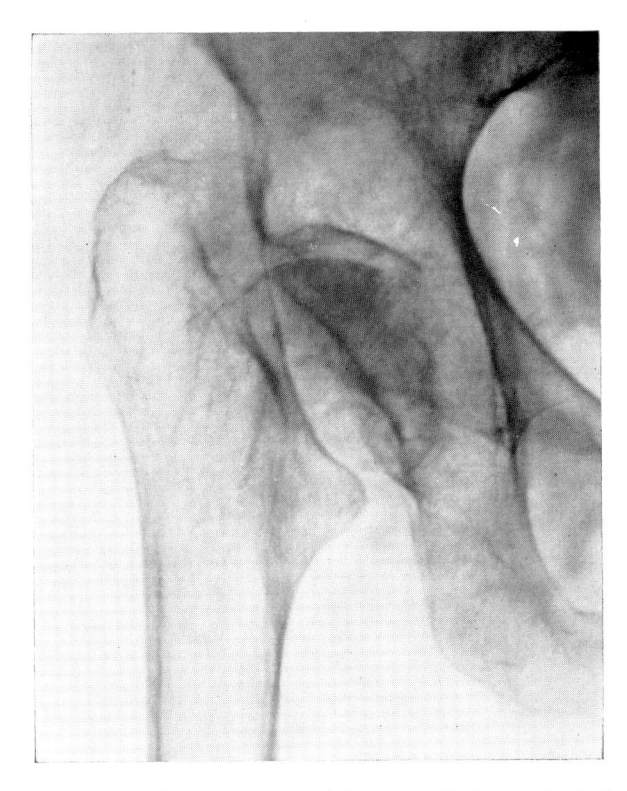

Fig. 172. Roentgenogram showing ununited fracture of the neck of the femur with marked upward displacement of the distal fragment four years after unsuccessful nailing of the fresh fracture in a patient 80 years of age. Femoral neck has disappeared. Relatively dense areas of the head suggest nonviability.

as changes in the density of the head, and osteoarthritis, which may restrict the mobility of the head in the acetabulum.

Treatment. Operation is required, and no one procedure is suitable for use in all cases. The patient's general condition and the details at the fracture site must be given careful consideration. In individuals under 60 years of age who are in good condition and who do not show severe ischemic necrosis of the femoral head or marked absorption of the distal fragment, a *bone peg* operation may be followed by solid union. In the Albee type of bone peg operation the hip joint is opened, the fibrous tissue is removed, and the fragments are freshened on either side and approximated. A peg graft taken from the crest of the tibia is then inserted through the greater trochanter far into the neck and head. For additional strength a three-flange nail may be inserted alongside the graft. The results of this operation in selected cases have been satisfactory in leading to union and return of function.

When the fragments are not widely displaced and the femoral head is viable, an osteotomy just above the lesser trochanter with medial displacement of the distal fragment, according to technics described by Dickson,

McMurray, Blount, and others, may be indicated. Such osteotomies result in good hip function in many of the cases.

When the patient is over 70 years old, it may be advisable to abandon the effort to secure union and to replace the femoral head with a long-stemmed metal prosthesis (Fig. 126). This operation has the advantage of allowing the patient to return quickly to walking. However, normal hip function is usually not regained; the patient should be advised preoperatively that for most walking a cane or a crutch will be required.

Shaft of the femur

Nonunion of the shaft of the femur is fairly common. If the fragments are overriding, it may be best to begin the treatment with a period of skeletal traction. When the fracture is near the middle of the shaft, the usual surgical treatment consists of trimming the fragment ends to bleeding bone, securing their approximation and fixation with an intramedullary nail, and surrounding the fracture site with multiple cancellous grafts taken from the ilium. For additional fixation a double spica cast, extending down to the knee of the well leg, is often necessary.

Patella

Nonunion of patellar fragments rarely occurs after good initial treatment of the fracture. Fibrous union is compatible with satisfactory knee function unless the fragments are considerably displaced. In diagnosis, the developmental anomaly of bipartite patella (p. 52) must be excluded. Knee disability associated with the nonunion of displaced fragments may be relieved by excision of the patellar fragments, any indicated revision of the quadriceps tendon, and a program of active knee exercises started after adequate tendon healing has taken place.

Tibia and fibula

In the experience of many authors the lower third of the tibia is the most common site of nonunion (Fig. 173). A contributing cause may be meager circulation over the flat medial surface of the tibia. In some cases the intact or healed fibula may prevent close approximation of the tibial fragments. The sliding inlay type of graft is often used at this site, or a large onlay graft may be placed on the posterior or lateral aspect of the tibia, which makes it possible to cover the transplant with healthy muscle tissue. Nonunion of the fibular shaft occurs rarely and requires no treatment.

Surgical transference of the shaft of the fibula into the tibia above and below the level of the ununited fracture is sometimes preferable to the use of a free graft. This transference is particularly useful if the tibial defect is large or chronically infected as a sequel of open fracture or osteomyelitis. The operation is usually carried out in two stages. The postoperative cast, which is worn for several months, must often be followed by a brace to protect the fibular transplant until it has undergone sufficient hypertrophy to withstand the stresses normally placed upon the tibia.

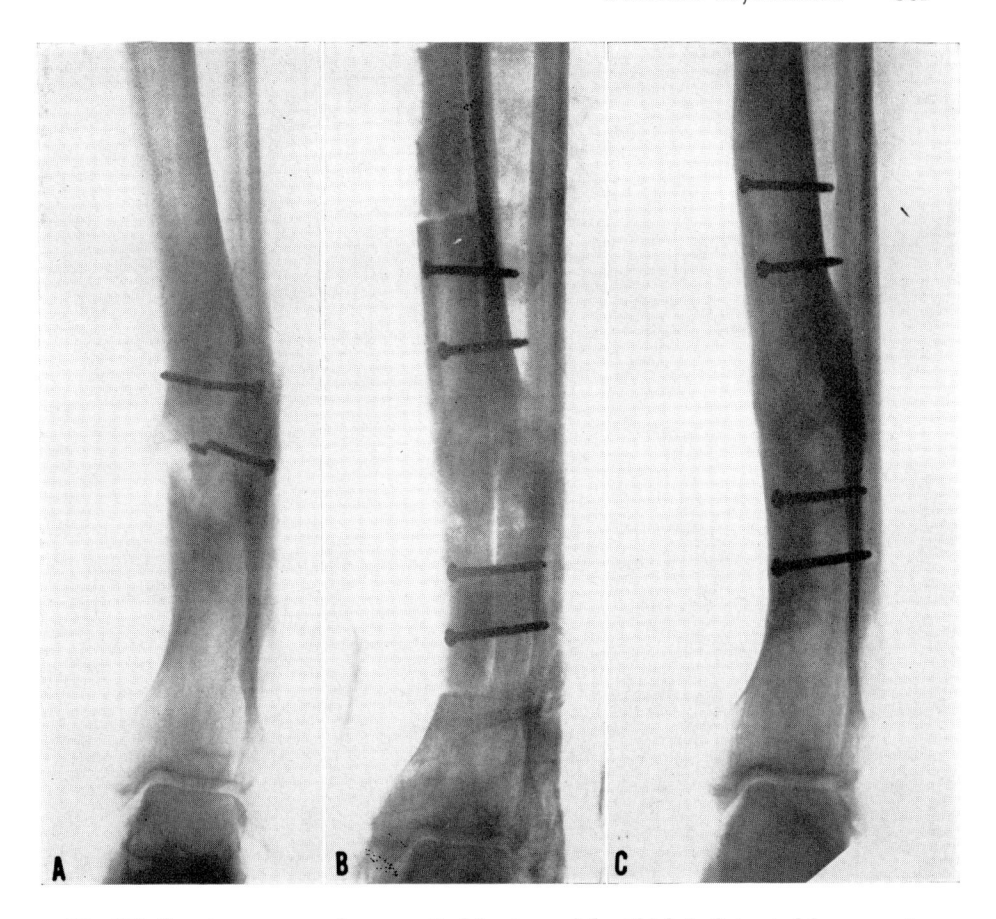

Fig. 173. Roentgenograms of an ununited fracture of the tibial shaft treated by a massive cortical bone graft. **A,** One year after fracture. Failure of previous treatment is indicated by nonunion, angulation, extensive sclerosis of fragment ends, and broken screws. **B,** Several days after graft operation, which consisted of taking a massive segment from the proximal part of the tibial shaft, placing it in a bed prepared across the old fracture site, and fixing it with two screws in each fragment. **C,** Eighteen months after graft operation. Note strong bone healing throughout tibial shaft.

Ununited fracture of the tibial malleolus should be treated surgically if causing symptoms. If the malleolar fragment is quite small it may be excised. If larger, it should be replaced and fixed by a screw; the addition of a small bone graft is often helpful.

Clavicle

Occasionally an ununited fracture of the clavicle is observed. As a rule no treatment is indicated, since the disability is slight and internal fixation and grafting do not always succeed in producing union. When symptoms are associated with an ununited fracture near the lateral end of the clavicle, the lateral fragment may be excised.

Humerus

Ununited fractures of the middle third of the humerus are relatively common and are usually the result of inadequate initial approximation and immobilization of the fragments.

Nonunion of the shaft of the humerus is often treated by the *step-cut operation,* a splicing of the refreshened and fitted ends of the fragments, plus internal fixation by means of screws, sutures, or an intramedullary nail. Some surgeons prefer simple osteotomies and internal fixation. To either operation the addition of autogenous iliac grafts is advisable. In difficult cases massive onlay grafts fixed by screws form an excellent means of inducing union.

Ununited fracture of the lateral condyle of the humerus, with resulting valgus deformity of the elbow, should be treated by replacing the condyle and fixing it with a screw, nail, or threaded Kirschner wire. Small osteoperiosteal grafts placed posteriorly are often advisable to facilitate bony union in this location. Small ununited fragments of the lateral or the medial condyle that cause pain and grating in the elbow should be excised.

Radius and ulna

For nonunion of both bones of the forearm, the fixation of onlay grafts, done through separate incisions to avoid radioulnar synostosis, is usually best effected with screws. Alternatively, alignment of the fragments can often be maintained conveniently by the insertion of an intramedullary nail or pin, after which cancellous strips of iliac bone are packed about the fracture sites. Ununited fracture of the radius or the ulna alone is more common. If the fracture is in the lower third of the radius, an inlay or onlay graft may be used, the distal end of the graft being sharpened and driven into the cancellous bone of the distal fragment. Ununited fracture of the lower third of the radius is often accompanied by an unsightly prominence of the lower end of the ulna, which may be resected. Ununited fracture of the ulna near the elbow is usually best treated by dual onlay grafts.

Carpus and metacarpus

Ununited fracture of the scaphoid bone occurs frequently, resulting presumably from lack of immobilization and from poor blood supply; the scaphoid has three articulating surfaces, and only two small nonarticulating surfaces through which the blood vessels enter. A great many "sprained wrists" with prolonged disability will on roentgenographic study show an ununited fracture of the scaphoid. With several months of immobilization by means of a plaster cast that includes the thumb and holds the wrist in slight dorsiflexion and radial deviation, many old fractures of the scaphoid bone will unite. When union cannot be obtained by immobilization alone, bone grafting may be indicated. In some instances excision of one or both fragments or excision of the radial styloid process leads to improved function and less pain in the wrist. If a nonunion of long duration is attended by pain and arthritic changes in the adjacent bones, arthrodesis of the wrist may be indicated.

Ununited fractures of the metacarpal bones are uncommon. They may be treated by open reduction, temporary internal fixation with intramedullary wires, and grafting with small strips of cancellous bone from the ilium.

MALUNION

Union in poor position is usually caused by (1) failure to secure accurate reduction or (2) failure to maintain effective immobilization for a sufficient length of time. Malunion is thus the outcome of unsuccessful treatment. The principal evidences of malunion are (1) a shortening of the extremity due to overriding of the fragments (Fig. 174), (2) a deformity due to angulation of the fragments, (3) an abnormal rotation of the fragments with relation to each other, and (4) an abnormal limitation of joint motion due to a bone block.

Malunion of individual bones
Femur

Malunion of the neck of the femur is infrequent as compared with nonunion. However, malunion of intertrochanteric fractures is quite common, while nonunion is seldom seen. Malunion may take place with the thigh externally rotated and adducted, with resultant coxa vara, retroversion of the femoral neck, and shortening. The deformity causes a limp and a tendency to tire quickly. Its correction may require an intertrochanteric osteotomy.

At times fractures about the hip unite with irregularities that cause pain upon walking. For symptomatic relief such cases may require arthroplasty, reconstruction operation, or arthrodesis.

After fracture of the shaft of the femur, anterolateral angulation or rotation of the shaft may develop as a result of weight bearing before the callus has become firm. It is sometimes possible to correct this type of deformity by manipulation. If the fracture has become solid an osteotomy is indicated. An intramedullary nail may be used to maintain the corrected alignment, and cancellous grafts from the ilium are usually indicated. It is advisable to mobilize the stiffened joints before operation by the use of physical therapy. When overriding has caused appreciable shortening (Fig. 174), it may be best to perform an osteotomy at the old fracture line, use skeletal traction until the shortening has been overcome, and then carry out open reduction, internal fixation, and grafting.

Following fracture of one of the condyles of the femur, a varus or valgus deformity of the knee may develop. In many instances this can be corrected by supracondylar osteotomy.

Patella

Occasionally a fractured patella unites with a rough articular surface, which causes considerable pain and disability. The surgical treatment con-

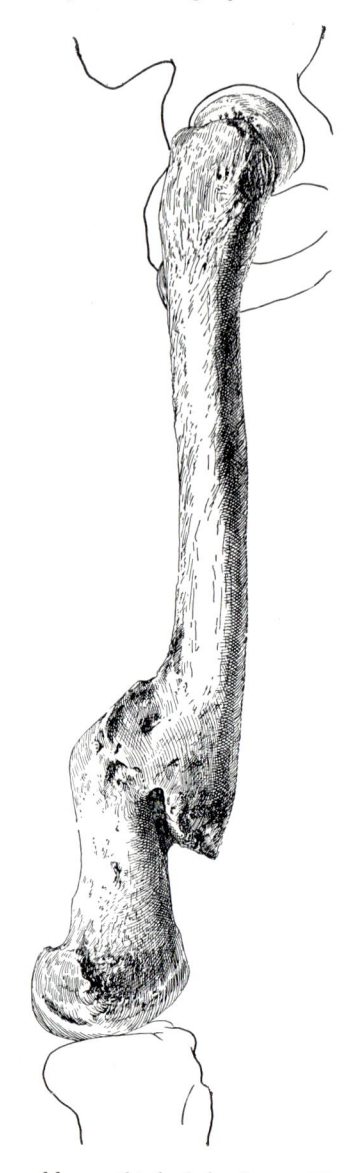

Fig. 174. Malunited fracture of lower third of the femur. The overriding fragments have become firmly united. (Drawing from specimen.)

sists of smoothing the posterior surface of the patella or excising the entire bone. If the quadriceps muscle has become contracted, excising the surrounding scar tissue or lengthening the quadriceps tendon will improve the range of knee motion.

Tibia and fibula

Occasionally a depressed fracture of the lateral or the medial condyle of the tibia leaves irregular or displaced joint surfaces and abnormal weight-bearing lines that give rise to severe pain and disability on weight bearing. It may be possible to elevate and fix the depressed fragment and to remove the irregularities about the tibial plateau. After the depressed fragment has been elevated, the space beneath it should be packed with bone chips. In less favorable cases arthrodesis or arthroplasty of the knee is indicated. The type of operation should depend largely upon the age, physical condition, temperament, and occupation of the patient.

Fractures of the tibial and fibular shafts may unite with unsightly and disabling angulation. In order to correct the deformity, osteotomy may be performed through the site of angulation. After osteotomy of the middle or lower thirds, internal fixation and grafting are advisable. With moderate angulation a supramalleolar osteotomy to correct the angle of the ankle joint surface to the weight-bearing axis of the leg may be preferable. A rotation deformity of the foot and leg below the site of fracture sometimes follows failure to align the fragments accurately at the original reduction. Such rotation deformity can be completely corrected by osteotomy.

Ankle

Malunion of fractures of the lower end of the tibia and fibula results in severe disability. The foot usually becomes fixed in marked valgus with abnormal prominence of the medial malleolus (Fig. 175). The Achilles tendon may become contracted. Pain on weight bearing is severe. At the original reduction of a fracture of the lower end of the tibia and fibula, the

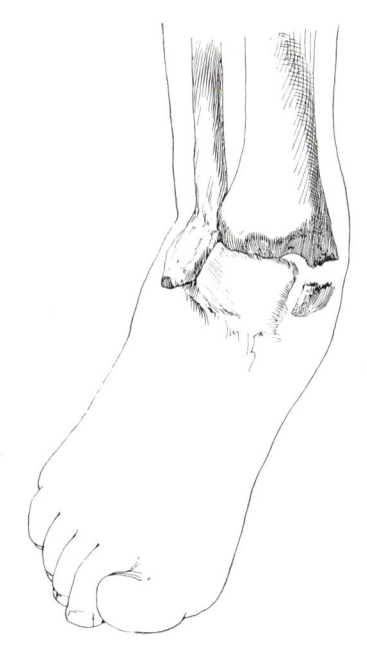

Fig. 175. Old fracture-dislocation of ankle with malunion of fibular fracture, nonunion of fractured tibial malleolus, and abduction and lateral displacement of the foot (malunited Pott's fracture).

talus should be so placed against the medial malleolus that the longitudinal axis of the tibia bisects at a right angle the transverse diameter of the upper articular surface of the talus. If this anatomic relationship can be maintained and there is minimal injury of the articular surfaces, permanent disability seldom results.

In cases of malunion with only slight displacement, the pain and disability may be relieved by a longitudinal arch support and ankle bandages. This treatment, however, is only palliative. In adults most malunited fractures involving the lower articular surfaces of the tibia and fibula require open operation.

In cases of only a few weeks' standing, it may be possible to break the beginning union by means of a Thomas wrench and to correct the deformity by manipulation. In cases of longer duration the fractured surfaces should be separated at open operation. Care must be taken to examine the posterior margin of the tibia ("posterior malleolus"), and if this is significantly displaced its position should be corrected. It is usually necessary to retain the corrected position of the fragments by means of an autogenous bone peg, screw, or nail.

In old cases a reconstruction operation is sometimes indicated. It may be necessary to perform an osteotomy at the old fracture line in the fibula before the talus and foot can be mobilized and brought into alignment. In an eversion fracture of the lower end of the tibia and fibula it is sometimes advisable to place a bone graft across the defect between the fragments of the fibula. For associated nonunion of a fracture of the tibial malleolus, it may be necessary to excise the pseudarthrosis and fix the fragment to the tibia with a bone peg, screw, or nail. The Achilles tendon occasionally requires lengthening.

The persistence of severe pain in a patient over 45 years of age, due in large measure to traumatic arthritis, is an indication for arthrodesis of the ankle joint. After reconstruction operations there is always the danger of traumatic arthritis, particularly if the posterior margin of the tibia has been displaced, and an arthrodesis, producing a stiff but painless ankle, is in most instances the preferable procedure. Arthrodesis involves removal of all joint surfaces, bone grafting, and immobilization of the ankle with the foot in functional position.

Following a displacement and reposition of the distal epiphysis of the tibia, the epiphysis may unite prematurely, resulting in the gradual development of a varus deformity of the foot and a marked prominence of the lower end of the fibula. The treatment is similar to that of malunited fracture and should be done early.

Talus

Malunion of a fracture of the talus is likely to produce an equinus or equinovarus deformity. Persistent pain and disability following fracture of the talus are indications for a triple arthrodesis (Fig. 134). If the ankle and the subtalar joints are involved, a pantalar arthrodesis may be advisable.

Calcaneus

Before the introduction of the methods of Cotton and, later, of Böhler for the treatment of fresh fractures of the calcaneus, attempt was seldom made to correct the bone compression that often accompanies the fracture. Malunion of these fractures results in (1) broadening of the heel; (2) piling up of bone beneath both malleoli, particularly the lateral; (3) abduction deformity of the foot; and (4) in many instances, pes planus. The patient seldom regains the normal range of inversion and eversion of the foot.

In the milder cases it is occasionally possible to correct some of the eversion deformity by means of forcible manipulation. This may result, however, in a chronically painful subtalar joint. Longitudinal arch supports, Thomas heels elevated on the medial side, and ankle supports may afford partial symptomatic relief. Surgical treatment is more effective. Arthrodesis of the subtalar joint, removal of the excess bone beneath the malleoli, and smoothing of the bony projections on the inferior surface of the calcaneus are to be advised. The results of this type of operation are quite satisfactory. Subtalar motion is lost, but there is only slight deformity, and the patient walks with little or no pain. In recent years severely comminuted fractures of the calcaneus have been treated in some clinics by triple arthrodesis immediately after the injury.

Metatarsus

Occasionally following fracture of a metatarsal an irregular mass of bone may become prominent on the sole of the foot because of plantar angulation. For this type of lesion it is advisable to osteotomize the metatarsal, remove the excess bone with its projecting spurs, fix the fragments in accurate approximation with an intramedullary wire, add small cancellous grafts, and immobilize the foot in a plaster boot. When the patient starts walking, a pad should be fitted under the injured metatarsal bone to prevent recurrence of its plantar angulation.

Clavicle and scapula

In most instances deformity from malunion of the clavicle is well tolerated and no treatment is necessary. Any sharp, disfiguring spurs should be resected. Malunited fractures of the clavicle or scapula sometimes result in limitation of motion of the shoulder. Such stiffness can be improved by physical therapy, traction, and gentle manipulation. Resection of the outer end of the clavicle (Mumford operation), for pain in the acromioclavicular joint following an old fracture or dislocation, may be followed by complete relief of the symptoms.

Humerus

Operation for malunited fracture of the upper end of the humerus is seldom indicated. Occasionally, however, the removal of sharp bony spurs and edges is necessary. Stiffness of the shoulder may be improved by exercises or gentle manipulation under anesthesia. Resection of the head of the

308   *Handbook of orthopaedic surgery*

humerus seldom results in a satisfactorily functioning shoulder. It is only occasionally necessary to perform an operation for malunion of the shaft of the humerus. An osteotomy may be indicated to correct an extreme angulation or rotation deformity.

The lower end of the humerus and the elbow are often involved in malunited fractures. Unreduced or incompletely reduced supracondylar fractures may restrict joint motion. Bony spurs that project anteriorly into the joint and limit its range of motion may be resected. The operation should be followed by a program of supervised active exercise. The increase in range of motion is often slow.

In children, unreduced fracture of the lateral condyle is usually followed by the development of a marked valgus deformity of the elbow (Fig. 176, A). Delayed ulnar palsy, or late traumatic ulnar neuritis, from friction or stretching of the nerve (p. 253) frequently accompanies a severe cubitus valgus. For correction of the deformity a supracondylar wedge osteotomy of the humerus with replacement or removal of the detached lateral condyle is often necessary (Fig. 177). Varus deformity of the elbow (Fig. 176, B), which often follows an incompletely reduced supracondylar fracture, is sometimes an indication for a similar type of osteotomy.

Occasionally following fracture about the elbow joint, a mass of new bone may form in the olecranon fossa and prevent normal extension of the elbow. Removal of the excess bone may be followed by improvement of mobility. Occasionally, following a severely comminuted fracture involving the joint surfaces, complete or partial ankylosis develops.

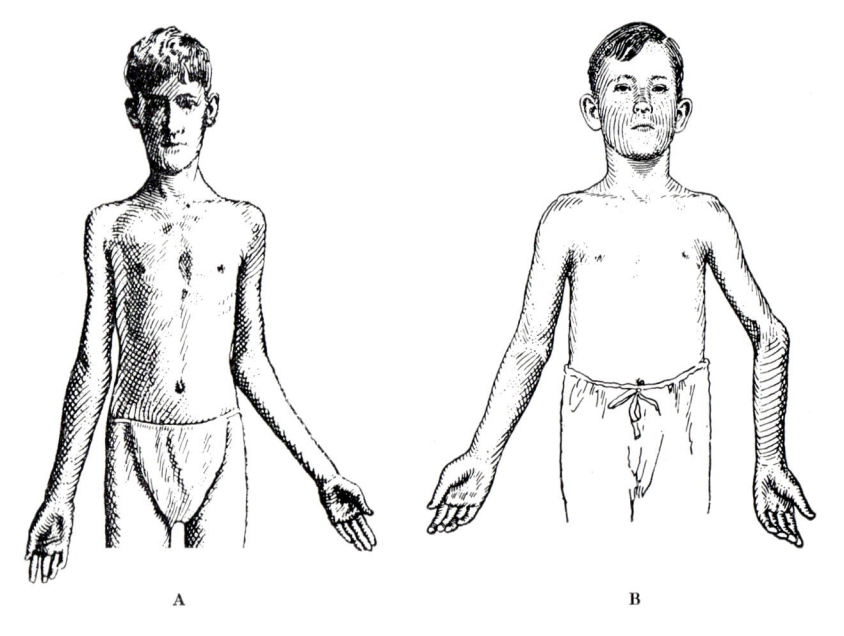

Fig. 176. **A,** Malunited fracture of lower end of left humerus, showing cubitus valgus. **B,** Malunited fracture of lower end of left humerus, showing cubitus varus.

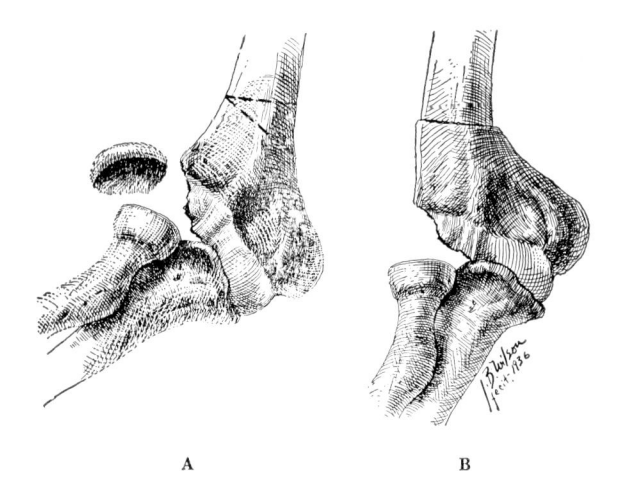

Fig. 177. A, Valgus deformity of elbow resulting from malunited fracture of lower end of humerus and ununited fracture of its lateral condyle. B, After operation, which included removal of the detached lateral condyle and a supracondylar wedge osteotomy.

For this type of lesion an arthroplasty or reconstruction operation may be indicated.

In association with fracture or dislocation about the elbow joint a mass of bone may form in the brachialis muscle *(traumatic myositis ossificans,* p. 468). This bony mass may be directly connected with the periosteum of the lower end of the humerus. If spontaneous absorption fails to take place after prolonged rest and conservative therapy, the mass of new bone should be excised with as little traumatization of the surrounding tissues as possible. If the excess bone is removed too soon, it may recur; excision should not be attempted until at least six months after the injury.

After operations upon the elbow the recovery of joint motion is notably slow.

Radius and ulna

Malunited fracture of the head of the radius often causes severe disability. Rotation of the forearm is restricted, and extension of the elbow may be impaired. In such cases the head and neck of the radius should be completely excised. Small comminuted fragments of the head of the radius may have become lodged in the joint and at operation must be carefully removed. Because of the disturbance of forearm growth, the head of the radius should not be excised in children.

The combination of fracture of the upper third of the ulna and dislocation of the head of the radius, first described by Monteggia in 1814, is frequently seen. This type of injury may be followed by an unsightly deformity due to outward angulation of the upper third of the ulna. In these cases it is advisable to osteotomize the ulna, correct the alignment, and fix the fragments with a massive or dual onlay graft, an intramedullary pin, or a metal plate. The dislocation of the head of the radius should be reduced, especially if the patient is a child, and a new annular ligament should be constructed to maintain the reduction. When local conditions in the adult are unfavorable for the fashioning of such a ligament, the head of the radius may be excised.

Malunion or even nonunion of fractures of the olecranon often results in little or no limitation of elbow function.

Fracture of both bones of the forearm may be followed by a radioulnar synostosis, which prevents rotation. In such cases the excess bone may be resected and fascia or fat placed between the radius and the ulna. If the operation is indicated, it should be done promptly to minimize the accompanying muscle atrophy.

When fracture of both bones has been followed by severe angulation and overriding but firm union, osteotomies at the sites of angulation are indicated for correction of the deformity. It is usually necessary to hold the fragments in apposition by means of massive onlay bone grafts, intramedullary pins, or metal plates.

Wrist

In the reduction of a Colles' fracture, whether recent or old, particular attention should be paid to the alignment of the joint surface of the radius. Normally a line drawn anteroposteriorly across the articular surface of the lower end of the radius forms anteriorly an angle of from 70 to 80 degrees with the longitudinal axis of the radius, and a line drawn laterally across the articular surface of the lower end of the radius forms radially an angle of from 105 to 110 degrees with the longitudinal axis of the radius. These relationships must be restored before a Colles' fracture can be considered adequately reduced. The most common cause of a poor functional result is failure to correct adequately the deformity of radial deviation.

Fibrosis and stiffness of the metacarpophalangeal and interphalangeal joints are often observed after immobilization of the wrist for a fresh Colles' fracture and may cause greater disability than the fracture itself. This is especially true in older people. It is essential to start motion of the fingers and thumb soon after the injury. In fractures about the wrist joint, and especially in Colles' fracture, it is important that the splints should not be carried posteriorly beyond the knuckles or anteriorly beyond the middle of the palm. If the fracture has been properly reduced and immobilized, the danger of slipping is not significantly increased by movement of the fingers and thumb. Following Colles' fracture in old people, stiffness of the elbow and shoulder is also a common finding. During the course of treatment these joints should be put through their full range of motion actively once or twice a day.

Unreduced Colles' fracture or displacement of the distal radial epiphysis causes an unsightly deformity. There is usually a "silver-fork deformity," marked prominence of the lower end of the ulna, and radial deviation of

Fracture deformities 311

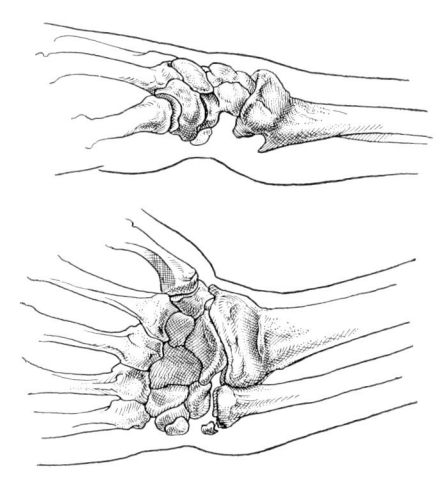

Fig. 178. Malunited fracture of lower end of the radius (malunited Colles' fracture). Note dorsal displacement of distal fragment, posterior tilting of articular surface of radius, radial deviation of hand, prominence of distal end of ulna, and ununited fracture of ulnar styloid process.

the wrist (Fig. 178). The deformity is accompanied by pain, restriction of wrist and finger motion and forearm rotation, and considerable disability of the hand.

In early cases it may be possible to reduce the deformity by the use of a Thomas wrench. This procedure should be carried out without the use of excessive force. When the deformity cannot be reduced easily by manipulation, a wedge of bone should be removed from the volar surface of the lower end of the radius and the alignment corrected. Internal fixation with wire or pin is useful to prevent postoperative slipping of the small distal fragment. When there is undue prominence of the lower end of the ulna and especially when it is associated with pain, restriction of pronation and supination, and shortening of the radius, the projecting bone, which may be more than an inch in length, should be removed at the same operation. Occasionally when the prominent lower end of the ulna is extremely mobile, its removal, together with a portion of the lower end of the shaft, will result in improved function of the wrist.

Unreduced dislocation of the lunate bone is sometimes observed among old injuries of the wrist (p. 482). The lunate bone should be excised.

Hand

Malunion of a fracture of the base of the first metacarpal involving the carpometacarpal joint (Bennett's fracture) may cause serious disability. Secondary arthritic changes in this joint result in pain on grasping or pinching movements. In recent injuries, an open reduction, removal of excess callus, and internal fixation may restore normal alignment. In older cases arthrodesis of the carpometacarpal joint may be indicated.

Angulation of a metacarpal shaft due to malunion is a common finding in pugilists. The deformity can be corrected by osteotomy. After osteotomy an intramedullary wire is useful for temporary immobilization of the fragments. As a rule little need be done for the "prize-fighter's knuckle," which is a malunited fracture of a metacarpal neck, since the disability is slight. Fractures about the phalangeal joints, such as are found in "baseball fingers" (p. 473), are seldom improved by operation. The fragments are often too small to be replaced accurately and fixed securely.

Pelvis

Occasionally stiffness and pain in the hip may persist following fracture of the pelvis, particularly if the acetabulum has been involved. Restriction of activity and the use of cane or crutches may relieve the symptoms in mild cases and in sedentary individuals. If the pain persists, and if secondary arthritic changes are obvious, it is wise to consider an arthroplasty or arthrodesis. The choice of procedure depends chiefly upon the age and occupation of the individual.

Spine

Following a severe injury of the back it is not uncommon for compression of one or more vertebral bodies to be discovered as a late manifestation. The lesion may evidence itself by kyphosis associated with considerable pain and disability in the back. The fracture is particularly likely to be overlooked unless good lateral roentgenograms are made following the injury. In rare cases, however, fracture may not be evident in films taken immediately after the injury but may appear several days later when postural stresses have increased the deformity of the weakened vertebral body. After any type of severe trauma, particularly that associated with an automobile or industrial accident, which is followed by any back pain whatever, it is wise to make anteroposterior and lateral roentgenograms.

In most instances compression fractures of the lumbar or dorsal spine that unite with slight or moderate malalignment cause little or no disability. Persistent or recurrent symptoms may be attributable to malunion involving the vertebral arch and affecting the facet joints. When pain and disability are associated with an old vertebral fracture, treatment consisting of bed rest for several weeks, followed by the use of a plaster jacket or brace for several months, may lead to symptomatic relief. In some cases with persistent pain, however, an arthrodesis of the injured segment of the spine should be done.

In the case of an old injury of the cervical spine it may be necessary for the patient to remain recumbent with head traction, obtained with a halter or skull tongs, for several weeks and then to wear a plaster collar and later a Thomas leather collar. Rarely is arthrodesis of the cervical spine indicated unless a persistent or recurrent dislocation is associated with the fracture.

COMMENT

In this chapter an attempt has been made to point out the deformities and disabilities that sometimes follow fractures despite the best efforts of the physician who is treating the patient. In the patient's mind a fear of permanent crippling may be paramount, and anything short of perfect cosmetic and functional recovery tragic. Unfortunately, some degree of permanent disability is an inevitable result of certain fractures, and the healing of fractures is fraught with serious complications. There should be close cooperation between the orthopaedic surgeon, who is primarily interested in bone injury and the restoration of function, and the physician who is treating a broken bone along with innumerable conditions foreign to the management of fractures. State industrial accident commissions and insurance companies, which reckon these injuries in dollars and cents, have come to realize the savings in compensation benefits when fractures are treated by the orthopaedic and trauma specialist. The public is gradually recognizing this and in many sections is demanding the services and consultations of doctors who have been especially trained in fracture work. It is the duty of every medical student who is anticipating practice and of every practitioner of medicine to equip himself with a knowledge of the principles of treating fractures, of preventing fracture complications when possible, and of minimizing the disabling effects of unavoidable fracture deformities.

CHAPTER 15

Amputations, prostheses, and braces

FAMILIARITY with the closely related subjects of amputations, prostheses, and braces comes from detailed study of the problems of individual patients. Underlying the treatment of every patient, however, are certain principles that lend themselves to brief presentation.

AMPUTATIONS AND PROSTHESES

Amputations may be congenital (Fig. 179), traumatic, ischemic, or surgical in origin. Surgical amputation is an ancient procedure. At first glance it may appear a purely destructive measure, incompatible with recognized orthopaedic principles of physical conservation and restoration. Usually, however, amputation is only the essential first step in a series of measures designed to achieve finally the maximum rehabilitation of the patient. The surgeon who plans an amputation should be prepared not only to execute the surgical operation but also to deal—early and late—with the patient's psychologic problems, to provide efficient postoperative care including physical therapy and preparation of the stump for use of the prosthesis, to direct the proper selection and fitting of the prosthesis and adequate training in its use, to guide the patient's return to employment, and to carry out a medical follow-up which may last for many years. Such considerations emphasize the close relationship that exists between amputations and reconstructive orthopaedic surgery.

Indications. Surgical amputation should be done when in the considered judgment of physician and patient the patient's welfare will be significantly improved by the removal of an irreparably damaged, deformed, dangerous, painful, or useless part of the body. When the blood supply of a limb has been lost and cannot be restored, amputation is always necessary. In permanent, irreparable loss of nerve supply, amputation is occasionally indicated to remove an extremity or part of an extremity that may be useless, unsightly, and subject to chronic ulceration and other trophic changes. The commonest reasons for amputation are: (1) trauma, (2) vascular accident or disease, (3) infection, (4) tumor, (5) congenital anomaly, and (6) thermal, chemical, or electrical injury.

Trauma. Amputation is indicated when severe trauma has so destroyed the blood supply or so damaged the tissues of an extremity that gangrene

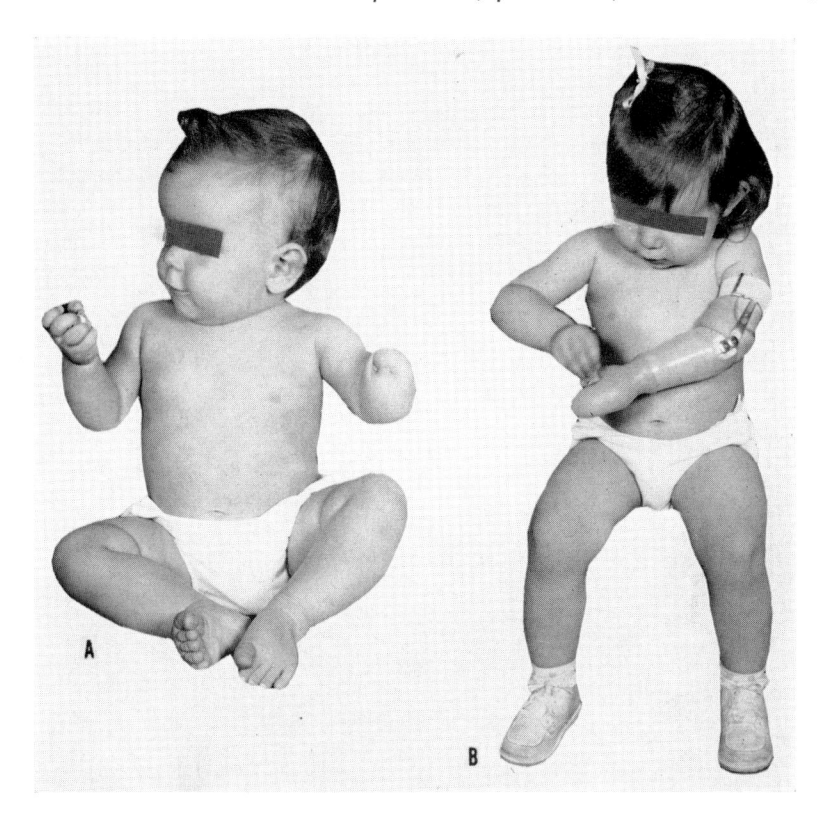

Fig. 179. A, Congenital left below-elbow amputation in a girl 11 months of age. B, Eight months later, patient has become accustomed to the use of a simple mitten prosthesis.

is inevitable or useful reconstruction impossible. For the evaluation of such wounds, careful examination and mature judgment are essential.

Vascular accident or disease. Local blood supply, especially in the lower extremities, may be destroyed suddenly by thrombosis or embolism, or gradually by peripheral vascular disease such as arteriosclerosis or thromboangiitis obliterans. When an adequate blood supply cannot be maintained or restored by treatment, amputation is indicated. The decision may be modified by the patient's general condition, his age, and the circulatory status of his opposite extremity.

Infection. In acute fulminating infections that endanger life by central spread and that cannot be controlled by less radical means, amputation is indicated. The most common of these infections is gas gangrene of high virulence.

In chronic infection, such as a draining osteomyelitis of long standing which has not responded to medical and ordinary surgical treatment, amputation may be indicated because of either local or systemic sequelae. Systemic complications, which include amyloidosis, glomerular nephritis, and bacterial endocarditis, may prove fatal unless amputation is done. Local sequelae of chronic infection that may make amputation and the fitting of a prosthesis advisable include mutilating loss of muscle or bone, deforming contractures and ankylosis, chronic ulceration, painful scars, ischemic changes, persistent sinuses, and the development of carcinoma about sinuses. In adults, extensive tuberculosis of the foot or ankle with multiple sinuses is a form of chronic infection often best treated by amputation.

Amputations for infection and its sequelae are becoming less frequent as improved methods for the control of sepsis are devised and adopted.

Tumor. Amputation is frequently indicated when an extremity is involved by a primary malignant tumor, of which osteogenic sarcoma is a classical example. Amputation should not be done, however, until it has been ascertained, usually by biopsy, that the tumor is definitely malignant and that it cannot be treated satisfactorily by measures such as resection or irradiation. If metastasis has not occurred, amputation may be curative. When the tumor has already metastasized, amputation may still be the treatment of choice as a palliative measure to relieve pain, improve systemic status, and obviate ulceration, infection, hemorrhage, and pathologic fracture.

For certain late, extensive benign tumors of the extremities, amputation may be indicated when excision of the tumor would cause loss of function of the limb.

Congenital anomaly. Several types of congenital anomaly are best treated by amputation. Supernumerary fingers or toes form a clear example: amputation is indicated when they impair appearance or function. Congenital absence of distal parts of an extremity may require amputation for the modeling of a stump satisfactory for a prosthesis. Congenital absence of a long bone should be treated by amputation when the affected extremity cannot be salvaged by reconstructive surgery.

Thermal, chemical, or electrical injury. Extensive, severe tissue damage from excessive heat or cold or from chemical or electrical burns may necessitate amputation.

Types of surgical amputation. Amputation performed through a joint is called *disarticulation.* Amputation in which the surface of the wound is not covered with skin but left unclosed is termed *open amputation.* This is a temporary amputation, used for the control of actual or potential infection, and must usually be followed by a surgical closure. *Closed amputation* is usually a final or definitive amputation performed to create a stump that can be used effectively with a prosthesis.

Amputations through or distal to the metacarpus or the metatarsus are called *minor amputations.* At these levels, an artificial limb will not be worn and the stump should be so planned that as much as possible of its function is retained or recreated. All amputations proximal to the metacarpals or metatarsals are termed *major amputations.* They are designed primarily to produce a stump suitable for an artificial limb.

Amputations of the upper extremity. Recent improvements in artificial limbs have made it possible to fit properly any level of the upper extremity, provided that the condition of the stump is satisfactory. The site of election has become the most distal point at which sound surgical principles permit the formation of a satisfactory amputation stump. The ideal levels of amputation are those which have proved most functional, without a prosthesis in the case of minor amputations and with a prosthesis in the case of major ones.

In amputations of the upper extremity, the basic objective is to maintain function or to substitute for lost function. At the level of the fingers and metacarpals, amputations are designed to retain the most useful elements for grasp, pinch, and hook. At higher levels the surgeon attempts to create a stump suitable for supporting and activating a prosthesis comfortably and capable of withstanding the trauma occasioned by its use.

In amputations through the fingers as much as possible of their length and useful mobility should be retained. When a finger tip is lost, the bone end should be covered with a well-cushioned tactile pad by means of a full-thickness skin flap or graft. In amputations through the distal half of the terminal phalanx the fingernail should be preserved, if possible. It is extremely important that no part of the thumb be sacrificed unless absolutely necessary. Total loss of the thumb, the loss of multiple digits, and amputations in the metacarpus and carpus are individual problems as regards the choice of procedure best suited for restoring the complex function of the hand.

Above the metacarpals, the entire carpus should be retained when possible, since it will be extremely useful to the patient with or without a prosthesis. Disarticulation at the wrist has the advantages that the prosthesis need not include the elbow joint and that pronation and supination are retained. In amputations through the forearm, as much length as possible should as a rule be preserved. The usual prosthesis is hinged at the elbow and includes a forearm socket with a wrist unit to which a prosthetic hand or a hook may be attached interchangeably. The hook is more useful than the hand. It can be opened by the pull of a cable attached to a harness about the patient's opposite shoulder and closed by rubber bands about its base.

Disarticulation at the elbow is uncommon. Above-elbow amputations (Fig. 180) are most satisfactory at the supracondylar level; above this, functional efficiency becomes less as the shoulder is approached, and at least two inches of bone stump should remain below the anterior axillary fold. In amputations at the shoulder, the head and neck of the humerus should whenever possible be preserved to minimize disfigurement. Interscapulothoracic or forequarter amputation, a severely deforming procedure including removal of the entire shoulder girdle, is sometimes required in the treatment of malignant disease.

In *cineplastic amputations*, used occasionally in the upper extremity, the power of one or more of the patient's muscles, transmitted by means of a small peg traversing a muscle tunnel lined by skin, is used to activate the hand mechanism of the prosthesis. The commonest example is use of the biceps as a motor after short below-elbow amputation. Successful cine-

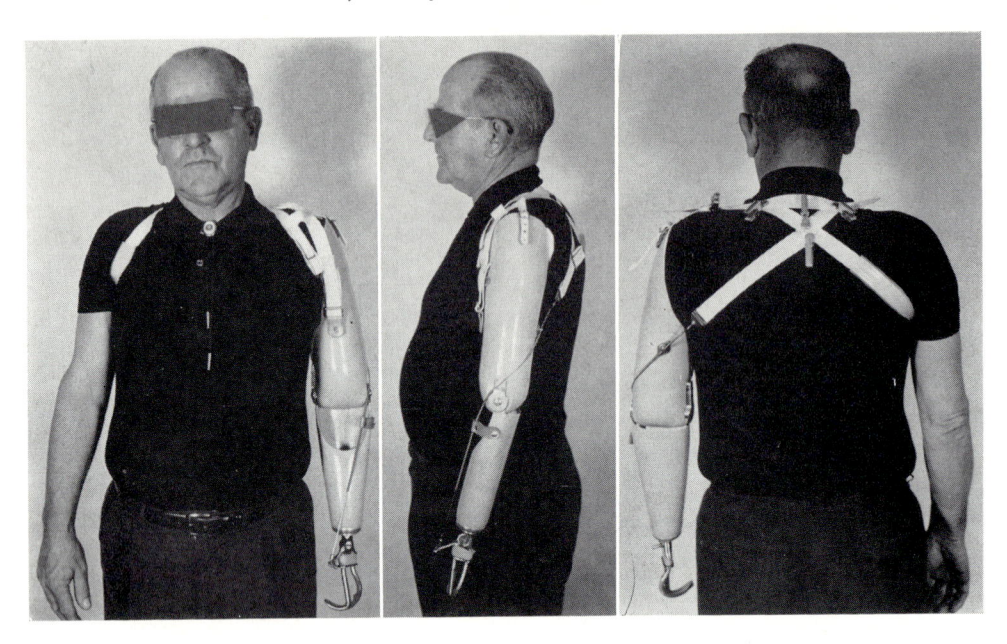

Fig. 180. Amputee with prosthesis for above-elbow stump. Dorrance hook is opened by cable and closed by elastic band. (Prosthesis is just being fitted; clamps on the harness are temporary.)

plasties require a careful selection of patients and the combined, skillful efforts of surgeon, prosthetist, and physical or occupational therapist.

In the *Krukenberg operation* the forearm stump, after a below-elbow amputation, is converted into a crude pinching mechanism by separating the lower ends of radius and ulna and covering them with soft tissues. No prosthesis is used. Because of its unsightliness the Krukenberg stump has not become popular. However, the fact that it possesses both tactile sensation and pinching function makes it the best expedient in certain situations, such as that of the blind, bilateral forearm amputee.

Amputations of the lower extremity. Amputations of the lower extremity are about three times as common as those of the upper extremity. The most important requirement of the lower extremity stump is that it be able to bear weight in standing and in walking. Depending upon the level of amputation, weight may be borne on the end of the stump (end-bearing), the metaphyseal flare of the tibia (side-bearing), or the ischial tuberosity. It is desirable that the weight-bearing area be as large as possible and covered with skin that is free from scar and capable of withstanding pressure.

The most common levels for amputation in the lower extremity are shown in Fig. 181.

Amputation of the great toe does not significantly impair standing or unhurried walking. Disarticulation of the second toe leads to hallux valgus. Loss of the three smaller toes does not cause appreciable disability. In

Amputations, prostheses, and braces 319

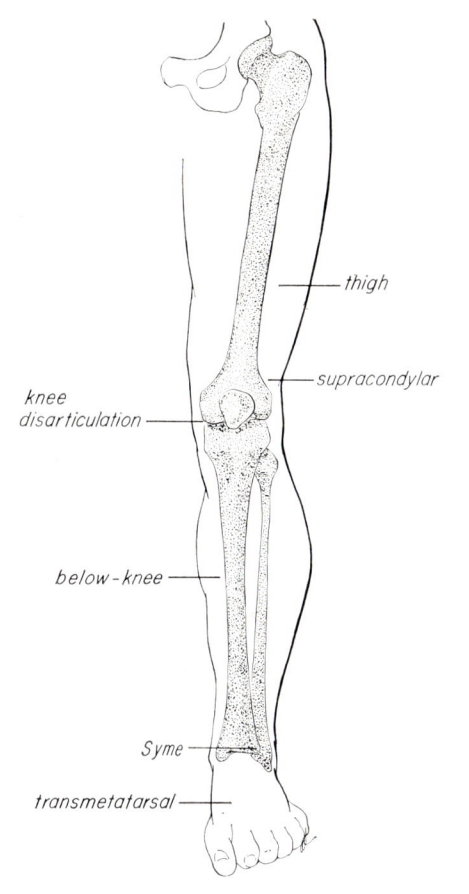

Fig. 181. Common levels for amputation of the lower limb. These levels have proved relatively favorable for subsequent function.

transmetatarsal amputations as much length as possible should be preserved. These amputations require no prosthesis; the end of the shoe may be filled with sponge rubber on a removable insole, and for better weight distribution a metatarsal bar may be used.

Experience has shown that there is no ideal level of amputation between the metatarsal bones and the middle third of the leg. Lisfranc's disarticulation at the tarsometatarsal level and Chopart's amputation through the talonavicular and calcaneocuboid joints have become obsolete because by distorting the muscular balance of the foot they produce intractable deformity. The amputations of Boyd and of Pirogoff include tibiocalcaneal fusion. The Syme amputation, which is often followed by a very satisfactory result, covers the cut end of the tibia ¼ inch above the ankle joint with thick, tough plantar skin. Its prosthesis includes only a below-knee molded plastic socket, an ankle mechanism, and a foot. Since both the bulbous stump and the prosthesis are unsightly, the Syme amputation is a better procedure for men than for women.

320   *Handbook of orthopaedic surgery*

Above the Syme level, the below-knee stump is side-bearing and should be about 6 inches in length. Longer stumps fit prostheses poorly and are liable to circulatory difficulties. The fibula should be 1¼ inches shorter than the tibia. In stumps of 3 inches or less the fibula should be completely excised for better fit. Very short below-knee stumps may be improved by sectioning the hamstring tendons or may be made end-bearing by the use of a bent-knee prosthesis. The usual below-knee prosthesis has consisted of a leather thigh corset laced in front, lateral hinges at the knee, and a shin piece simulating the normal leg, enclosing the stump-fitting socket and connected to the ankle mechanism and foot. The recently developed patellar ligament-bearing, cuff-suspension prosthesis (Fig. 182) eliminates in most cases the need of thigh corset and knee hinges.

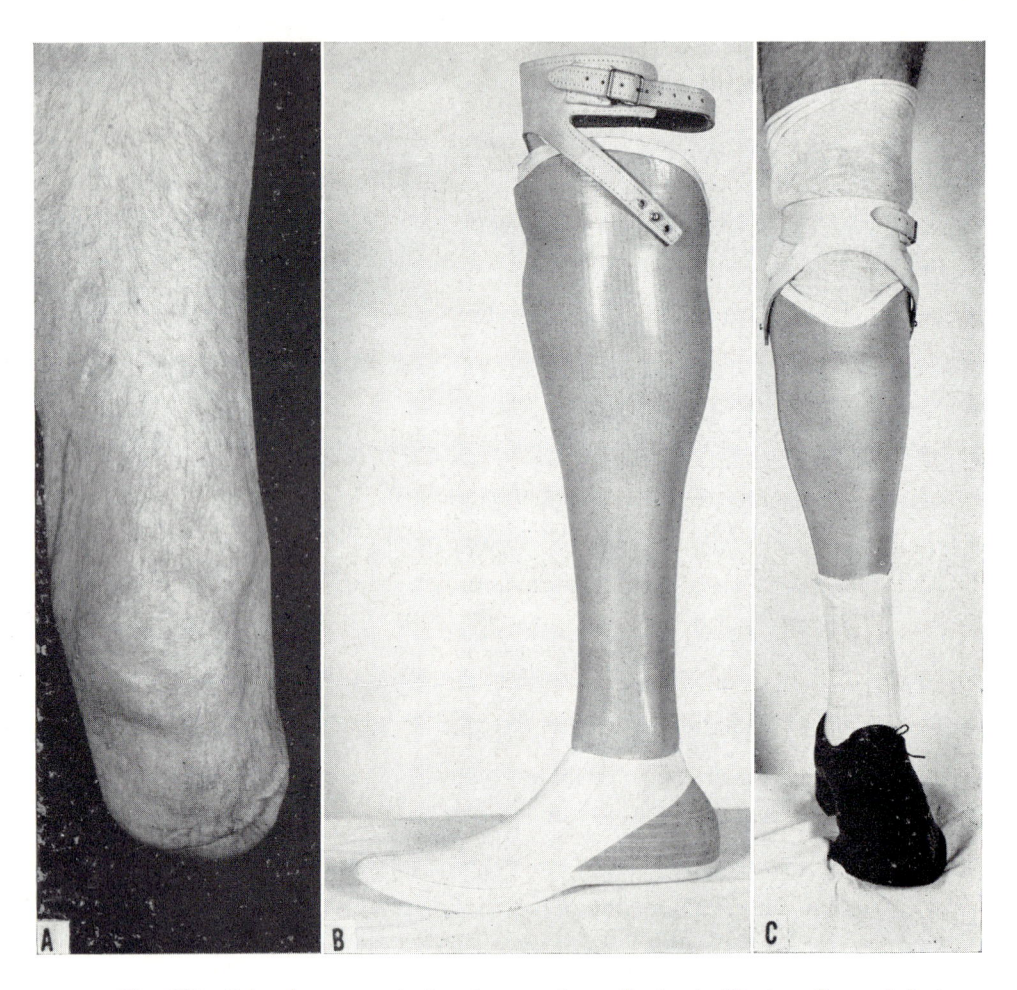

Fig. 182. Below-knee amputation stump and prosthesis. **A**, Short, well-rounded stump is covered by healthy skin. **B**, Plastic prosthesis with leather cuff and solid-ankle, cushion-heel (SACH) foot. **C**, Prosthesis is suspended by cuff over stump sock at the supracondylar level of the thigh.

Disarticulation of the knee and supracondylar amputation produce good end-bearing stumps. Because the disarticulation stump is sometimes difficult to fit satisfactorily with a prosthesis, the supracondylar amputation is more frequently used. The cut distal end of the femur may be covered by tendon (the Kirk, Callander, and Slocum amputations) or by the denuded articular aspect of the patella (Gritti-Stokes amputation).

In amputations above the supracondylar level, the ideal stump extends about 11 inches below the tip of the greater trochanter, providing a long lever arm for the prosthesis but allowing room for its knee mechanism. Above this level, the difficulty of fitting the prosthesis increases as the stump length decreases. Since up-and-down motion takes place within the prosthesis with each step, it is important that the skin over the end of the stump be neither tight nor redundant. The conventional above-knee prosthesis includes an ischial weight-bearing thigh socket and is held to the body by pelvic or shoulder harness. The newer suction socket prosthesis, also ischial-bearing, is often preferable for satisfactory stumps. An air-escape valve is placed in the lower part of its thigh socket, and no attachment above the thigh is required.

Disarticulation of the hip is sometimes indicated, chiefly in the presence of malignancy, but leaves a smooth stump that is difficult to fit satisfactorily with a prosthesis. When the upper end of the femur can be preserved, it aids in retaining the tilting-table socket of an ischial-bearing, flexed-hip prosthesis.

Hindquarter amputation, carried out through the symphysis pubis anteriorly and adjacent to the sacroiliac joint posteriorly, is a major surgical procedure, after which the provision of a satisfactory prosthesis is difficult and sometimes impossible. It is occasionally indicated for the eradication of malignant or massive benign tumors of the hip or iliac regions.

Amputations in children. Of the entire group of orthopaedically crippled children, amputees make up an important and increasing segment with great rehabilitation potential. Most of these amputations are either traumatic or congenital in origin. In addition certain other congenital anomalies of the extremities, such as severe unilateral shortening, are frequently best treated by the fitting of a prosthesis, with or without prior surgical amputation.

In children, the object of amputation and the fitting of a prosthesis is to facilitate early function, to enhance appearance, and at the same time to produce an optimal stump for maturity.

A major postoperative complication of amputations in children is overgrowth of bone as compared with the soft tissues of the stump. This may lead to perforation of the skin and secondary infection of low grade. Such overgrowth occurs most commonly in the humerus, fibula, or tibia and is of unknown cause. It appears to be of endosteal origin; attempts to prevent or correct it by the surgical arrest of epiphyseal growth are not indicated. The usual treatment is reamputation of the bony stump. The stump complications of shortness, scarring of the skin, bony spurs, and neuromas, which so often lead to disabling symptoms in adults, cause little difficulty in children, and phantom limb sensations are temporary and painless.

Prostheses for children are of standard types with minor technical variations. It is important that they be comfortable and simple. Early fitting tends to minimize psychologic difficulties. The upper extremity amputee may be fitted with a simple mitten prosthesis (Fig. 179) as early as 6 months of age; the lower extremity amputee should begin to use a prosthesis at normal standing age. The prosthetic training of children is often less time-consuming than that of adults. The child amputee and his prosthesis should be re-examined at frequent intervals.

Preparation for the prosthesis. The period between sound healing of the surgical wound and the fitting of the prosthesis is occupied by several measures; some of these are begun immediately after the operation, and all are of the greatest importance in the final rehabilitation of the amputee. They include explanation and encouragement; proper positioning of the limb to prevent contractures; massage of the stump to mobilize the scar, decrease tenderness, and improve vascularity; active exercise to strengthen muscles and mobilize joints; and firm, smooth elastic bandaging to prevent edema and shrink the stump to contours that will remain relatively constant.

Selection of the prosthesis. The prosthesis should be carefully chosen with due regard not only to the stump but also to the personal and occupational needs of the individual patient. This always calls for the closest co-operation between orthopaedic surgeon, patient, and prosthetist. The assistance of a physiatrist or a physical therapist is often desirable, and in amputee centers the consulting team may include also an occupational therapist, vocational counselor, psychologist, and social worker.

Training in use of the prosthesis. Without sound prosthetic training, few persons who have had major amputations will acquire satisfactory use of the prosthesis and none is likely to achieve an optimal functional result. Longer periods of training are required for upper extremity than for lower extremity amputees, for bilateral than for unilateral amputees, and for adults than for children. The amputee must learn efficient control of stump and prosthesis as a unit in the activities of his daily living and in the demands of his occupation. He is best taught, under the surgeon's supervision, by physical therapists and occupational therapists experienced in work with amputees and prostheses.

Disabilities of the amputation stump. Amputation stumps are subject to many early complications and late disabilities. Some of these difficulties are attributable to ill-advised surgical or prosthetic factors; others arise from recognized but unpreventable causes; and still others are of unknown pathogenesis. Frequent among late disabilities of the stump are ulcerations, infections, and noninfectious conditions characterized by pain or tenderness.

Ulceration of the stump is usually associated with ischemia and secondary infection; it often develops along the surgical scar. Ulceration may arise from several causes, including excessive postoperative scarring and the friction, tension, and pressure exerted by the prosthesis. The ulcer should usually be treated by local rest, elevation, and hot compresses until it is clean and the skin about it appears healthy. The ulcer, a narrow rim of skin surrounding it, and its entire scarred base should then be excised; if necessary the underlying bony stump is shortened to allow closure of healthy soft tissues without tension.

The unfavorable circulatory and mechanical influences present in amputation stumps predispose them to the development of *infection*. Early infection of low grade frequently produces pain in the stump before clinical signs of sepsis appear. Common forms of infection include cellulitis, abscesses, sinus tracts, and osteomyelitis. These lesions are treated according to established surgical principles, the final step usually consisting of plastic closure of the stump after all diseased or redundant tissue has been removed.

The normally proliferating end of a sectioned nerve, especially when it becomes involved in scar tissue and subjected to tensions and pressures from the prosthesis, may become a *painful amputation neuroma*. Surgical excision of neuroma and scar is indicated. The nerve should be resected at a higher level and its end allowed to retract into normal tissue. In some cases it may be advisable simply to interrupt the nerve well above the level of amputation, with care to produce no anesthesia of the stump.

Phantom limb sensations follow almost all amputations. Usually the phantom limb is painless and temporary or intermittent. The *painful phantom limb* is a serious sequel of amputation. Its pathogenesis has not been established, and its treatment is unsatisfactory. Resection of a neuroma, procaine blocks, sympathectomy, and chordotomy are among the therapeutic measures frequently but often unsuccessfully used.

Hyperesthesia of the stump, unassociated with the phantom limb phenomenon, is another recognized complication of unknown etiology. It is not relieved by local treatment of the stump; after reamputation it recurs at the higher level. Sympathetic blocks are sometimes helpful.

BRACES

Orthopaedic braces are mechanical supports used for the relief of pain, the improvement of motor function, and the prevention and correction of deformity. Since every brace must meet needs peculiar to an individual patient, braces are necessarily of many different types and degrees of complexity. To all varieties, however, certain principles apply.

Principles of bracing. The chief function of most braces is to relieve weakened structures of undesirable stresses by passively restricting motion, tension, or pressure. Thus a back brace (Figs. 99 and 202), by restricting spinal mobility, may relieve pain arising from a damaged intervertebral disk; a shoulder brace (Figs. 145 and 183), by restricting adduction, may provide relaxation for a temporarily paralyzed deltoid muscle; and an ischial-bearing brace (Fig. 215), by taking body weight off the lower extremity, may prevent the crushing of a femoral head weakened by coxa plana.

Varying degrees of protection from stress are afforded by braces of

324   Handbook of orthopaedic surgery

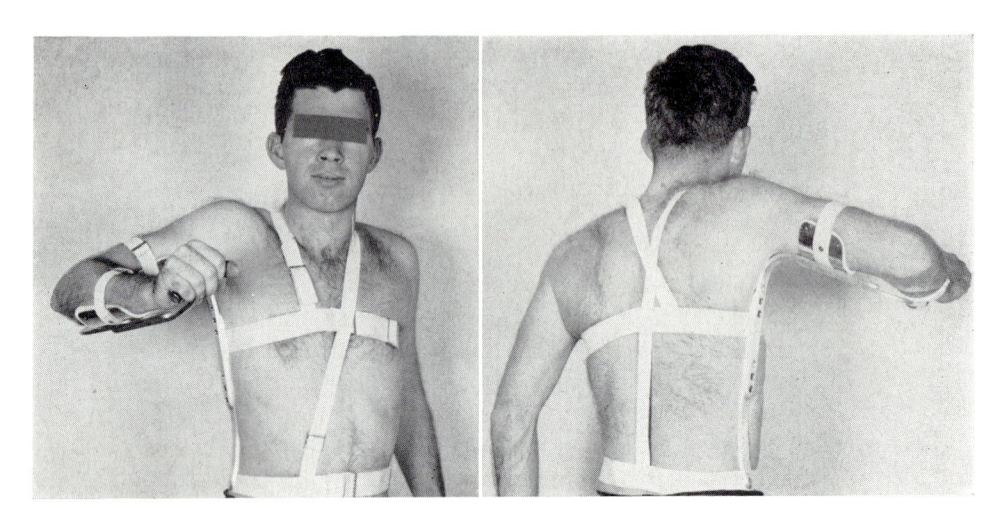

Fig. 183. Brace for supporting the right shoulder in abduction.

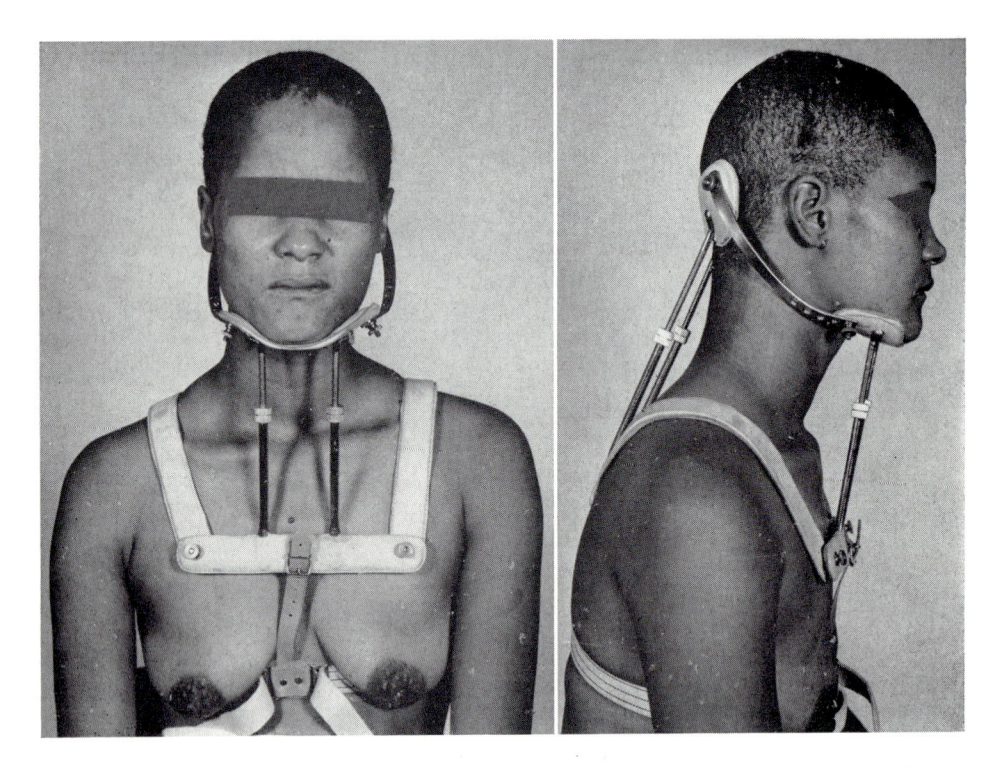

Fig. 184. Turnbuckle brace for the neck. Adjustment of the four turnbuckles facilitates effective support and slight distraction. A brace of this type should be available in hospital emergency rooms for early protection of the patient with injury of the cervical spine.

Amputations, prostheses, and braces 325

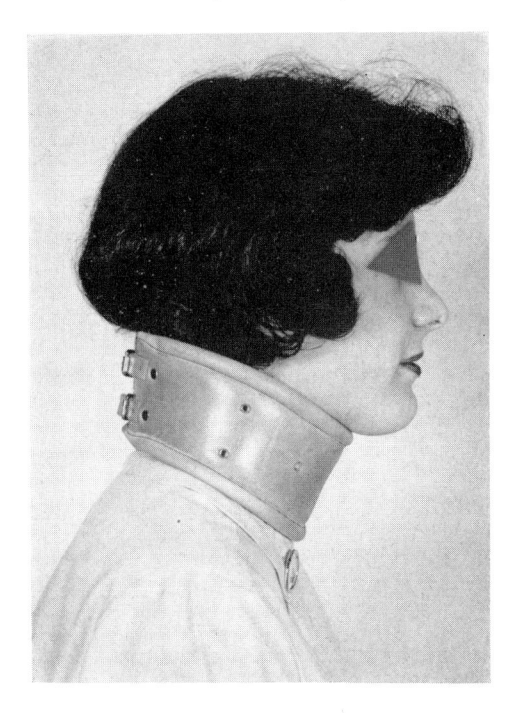

Fig. 185. Thomas collar (modified). This light, inexpensive collar provides adequate support in minor disabilities of the neck.

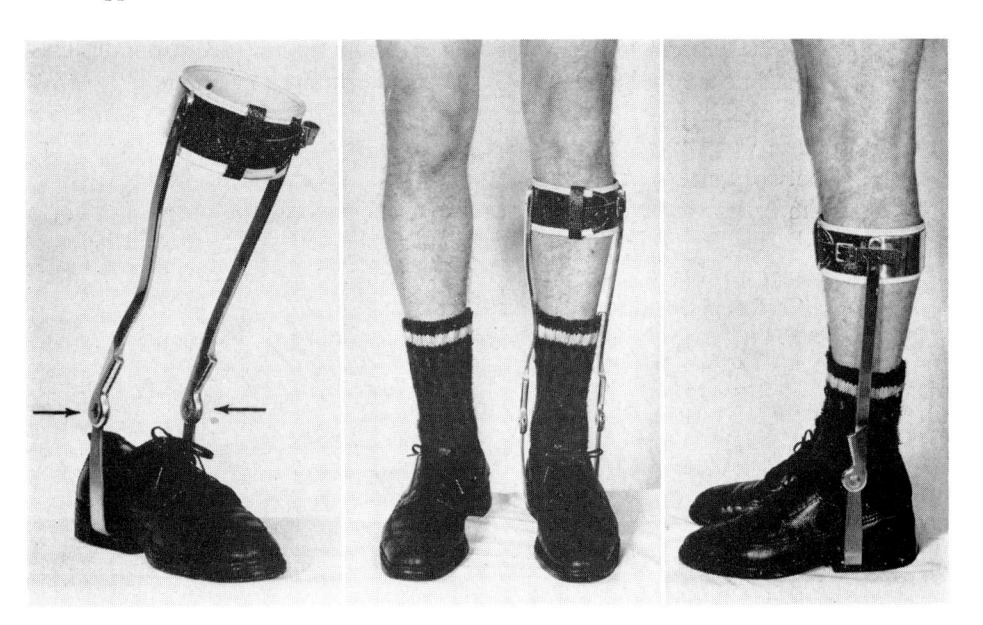

Fig. 186. Spring foot-drop brace. When weak dorsiflexor muscles are overbalanced by stronger plantar flexors, the adjustable spring at the ankle hinge of each upright (Klenzak joint, Pope Foundation, Inc.) is used to supply passive dorsiflexion and so prevent foot drop and an equinus limp.

differing design. Thus a neck brace with four turnbuckles (Fig. 184) is required for adequate immobilization and support of the severely injured or potentially dangerous cervical spine, whereas a cylindrical Thomas collar (Fig. 185) will provide sufficient restriction of motion for a less serious or less acute disability.

In more complex braces the principle of an active corrective force is often utilized. This is usually done by incorporating a metal spring or elastic band to produce the desired self-adjusting tension or pressure. A wrist brace fitted with wires and rubber bands is useful for stretching early flexion or extension contractures of the fingers. An ankle brace fitted with a spring mechanism favoring dorsiflexion (Fig. 186) is often indicated for paralytic foot drop. Braces which incorporate an active corrective force are helpful not only in overcoming contractures but also in providing power to balance that of unopposed muscles, facilitating therapeutic exercise of the involved structures. Bunnell pioneered the development of extremely useful devices of this type, suited to the needs of various disabilities of the hand and its digits. Such dynamic or physiologic splinting is especially useful in the preoperative and postoperative treatment of the disabled hand.

In recent years the application of these principles has been further developed in the field of *functional bracing* of the permanently paralyzed upper extremity. When sufficient experience and facilities are available, it is possible by means of individually designed bracing to restore useful function even in the presence of severe weakness and disability.

The prescription of braces. Having determined the details of his patient's need of a brace, the physician selects from available types that which best combines utility, comfort, strength, durability, lightness, cleanliness, and economy. Many bracing problems call for the closest cooperation between orthopaedist, patient, and the brace-maker or orthotist. On delivery the brace frequently requires minor adjustment for the individual patient, who also must be instructed in its application and use. If the brace is to be worn for a long period, arrangement for subsequent examinations, adjustments, and repairs must be made.

CHAPTER 16

Affections of the spine and thorax

IN THIS CHAPTER abnormal curvatures of the spine and deformities of the chest are discussed. Affections of the lumbosacral region are so common and so important that they have been placed in a separate chapter under the heading "Affections of the low back."

Affections of the spine
SCOLIOSIS

Definition. In scoliosis or lateral curvature of the spine a series of vertebrae is persistently deviated from the normal spinal axis; the lateral deviation is invariably accompanied by some degree of rotation of the vertebrae. Scoliosis is a deformity rather than a disease and is often secondary to pathologic changes outside the spine.

Incidence. Lateral curvature is one of the most common deformities of the spine. Its onset occurs usually during the years of growth. The factors which result in scoliosis are often established long before the child reaches school age, and definite deformity is usually recognizable before the age of 14 years. In early school ages scoliosis is slightly more common in boys, but during adolescence it occurs three to five times as often in girls. In a recent survey in Delaware, scoliosis of mild to severe degree was found in 19 per 1000 (1.9%) of 50,000 chest roentgenograms in a population over 14 years of age.

Classification and etiology. For purposes of description, cases of scoliosis can be conveniently classified in two ways: (1) according to the causative agent and (2) according to the shape and level of the curvature.

The etiologic classification is necessarily imperfect, since our knowledge of the causes of scoliosis is incomplete. One large group is made up of patients whose spinal curvature is a result of temporary postural influences. Such *postural or functional scoliosis* (Fig. 187) is not accompanied by asymmetrical changes in the individual structures of the spine and is relatively easy to correct. *Structural scoliosis* (Fig. 188), on the other hand, is characterized by definite morphologic abnormalities, and it is with this

328 Handbook of orthopaedic surgery

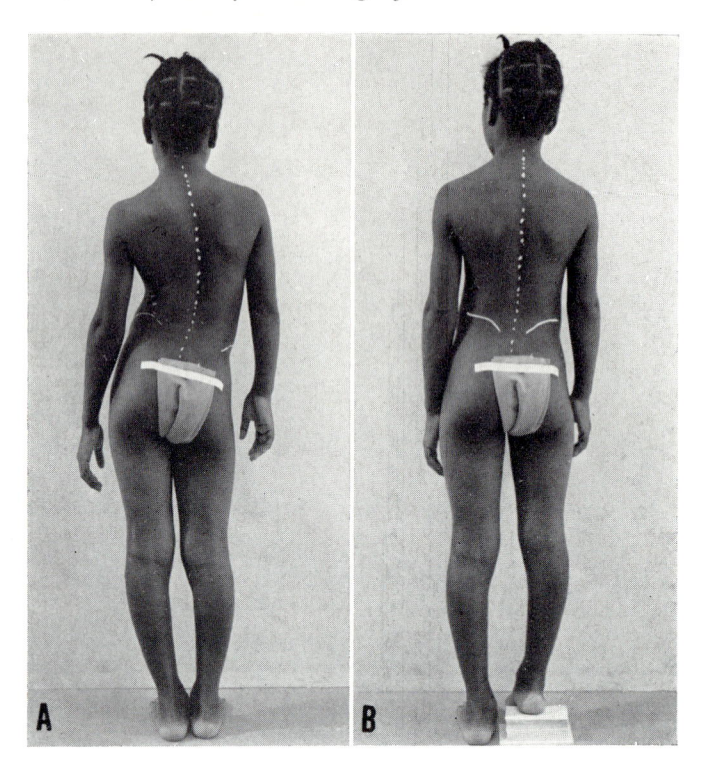

Fig. 187. Postural scoliosis in 11-year-old girl with congenital hemihypertrophy, the left limbs being longer than the right. **A,** Note right C-shaped scoliosis secondary to inequality of leg length. **B,** Note correction of postural scoliosis when shortness of right leg is compensated by elevation of right foot.

group of cases that therapeutic effort is most concerned. It is possible that some cases of functional scoliosis in children may progress, develop morphologic changes, and so undergo transition into the structural type.

The causes of structural scoliosis are numerous. In crippled children's clinics, *congenital scoliosis* is common (Fig. 189). A clear example of this type is scoliosis associated with the presence of a hemivertebra. Another common cause of structural scoliosis is asymmetrical paralysis of the trunk muscles, which destroys the normal balance of the supporting musculature. Such *paralytic scoliosis* is seen frequently after poliomyelitis and less often in other neurologic affections, such as infantile spinal muscular atrophy and progressive muscular dystrophy. Structural scoliosis occurs also in neurofibromatosis, in bone-softening affections such as rickets and osteomalacia, and, especially in children, after unilateral thoracic conditions such as thoracoplasty and chronic empyema. In many instances of scoliosis, however, the pathogenesis is unknown. In such cases, called *idiopathic scoliosis*, the underlying factor may be a functional weakness or insufficiency of the spine or the musculature, or asymmetrical growth at the epiphyseal plates of the vertebrae. Uncommonly a scoliosis of unknown origin, called *con-*

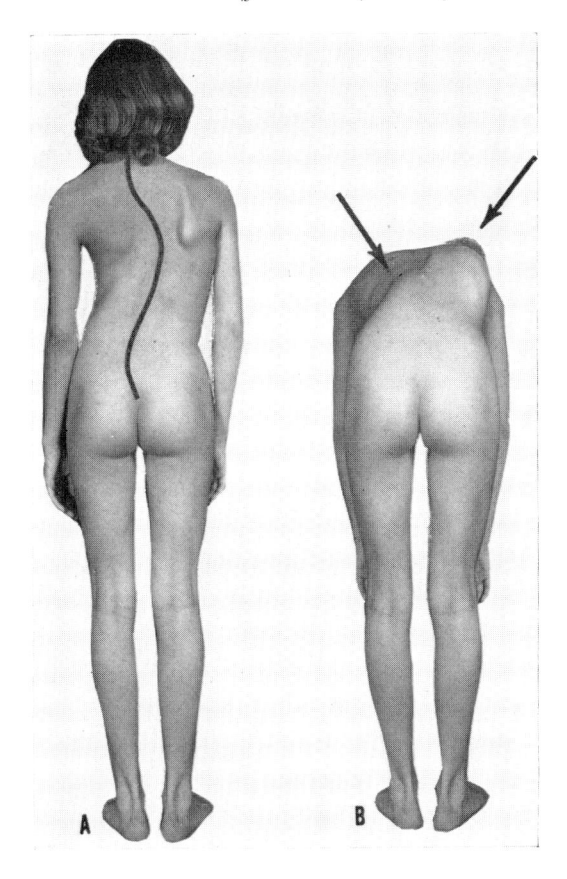

Fig. 188. Structural scoliosis in 13-year-old girl. **A,** Note the right thoracic, left lumbar curvature and the prominence of the lower part of the right scapula. **B,** Posterior prominences of the back, associated with vertebral rotation, are accentuated when the spine is flexed.

genital idiopathic scoliosis, develops at 2 or 3 years of age and may progress to cause severe deformity.

In the regional classification of scoliosis, three types of curvature are outstanding. These are (1) the **C**-shaped, left total curve, with its apex usually at the lower dorsal level, which is usually postural, paralytic, or congenital in origin; (2) the **S**-shaped compound curve, consisting usually of a primary right dorsal curve and secondary left cervical and left lumbar curves, which is often idiopathic in type; and (3) primary left or right lumbar curvature, which may be caused by forward slipping of a vertebral body on one side as a result of a defective lower lumbar intervertebral facet. Other varieties of lateral curvature are less common.

Pathology. The extent of the pathologic changes varies with the degree of lateral curvature. All the structures of the concave side are compressed or shortened, while those of the convex side may remain normal or become lengthened (Fig. 190). The apical vertebra, situated at the middle of the

330   *Handbook of orthopaedic surgery*

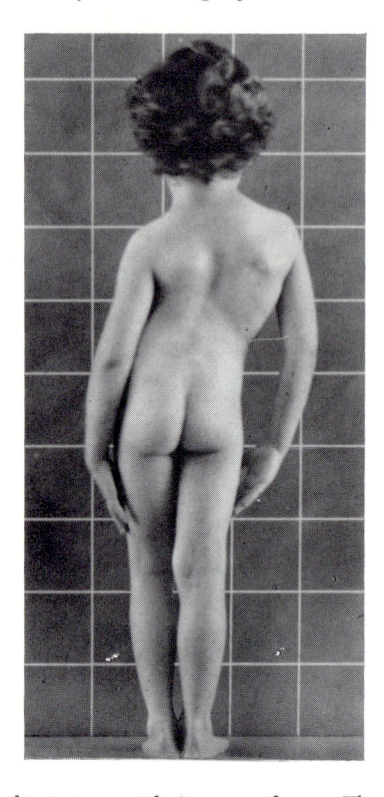

Fig. 189. Congenital scoliosis in a girl 4 years of age. The roentgenograms showed multiple congenital anomalies of vertebrae and ribs.

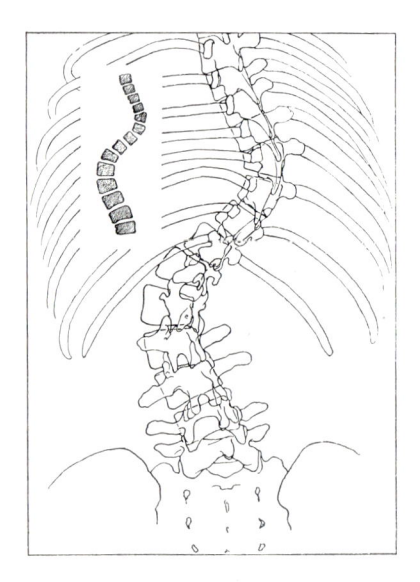

Fig. 190. Structural scoliosis. Note rotation of vertebrae and wedging of vertebral bodies. The wedging is diagrammed in the inset. (Tracing from roentgenogram.)

curve, shows the greatest change, being wedge-shaped and most rotated. Those above and below it undergo similar but less marked changes. The intervertebral disks are compressed on the side of the concavity and may bulge on the opposite side as a result of the pressure. The anterior longitudinal ligament is thickened on the concave side and thinned on the convex side. As the deformity increases, proliferation of bone takes place; later, ossification of the ligaments may occur. Rarely such changes may progress until the spine becomes ankylosed at the level of greatest distortion by the fusion of two or three vertebrae. In severe, late cases the muscles may become atrophic and on section exhibit fatty and fibrous degeneration. Because of rotation of the vertebrae, which is invariably present, the ribs on the side of the convexity are thrust backward with an increase in their angularity; this produces a so-called "razor back" deformity. When the curve affects the lower part of the spine, the pelvis may be distorted. Changes in the anterior chest wall include a flattening and diminution of thoracic capacity on the convex side of the curve and a prominence and increased capacity on the concave side. All of the organs of the chest and abdomen may be distorted by the abnormal pressure and stress put upon them by changes in the shape of the thorax (Fig. 191).

Clinical picture. As a rule there is no complaint until deformity of the back is noticed, and, since the deformity is of very gradual development, it may reach considerable proportions before its presence is observed. The patient may be brought to the doctor because of a high shoulder, a prominent hip, or a projecting shoulder blade. When the patient is a young girl, the fitting of a dress may first call attention to the deformity. Occasionally the child may complain of fatigue and backache before a deformity is noted. As the scoliosis increases, the discomfort may become more marked. Pain developing in the lumbar region may be due to pressure of the ribs upon the crest of the ilium. There may be shortness of breath, from diminished respiratory capacity, and gastrointestinal disturbances from crowding of the abdominal organs. In patients with only slight deformity, however, symptoms usually do not occur until middle age or later.

The physical examination should include careful note of the following points: (1) inspection of the natural, relaxed standing position; (2) estimation of the shape and degree of spinal curvature, the number of vertebrae involved, and the level and extent of the maximum deviation; (3) estimation of the degree of rotation or twisting of the vertebrae; and (4) estima-

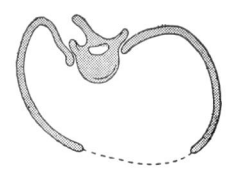

Fig. 191. Cross section of thorax in scoliosis, showing distortion of ribs associated with rotation of the vertebra. (After Hoffa.)

tion of the amount of spinal flexibility. Each of these findings is important in determining the treatment.

In the majority of cases of structural scoliosis the backward rotation is on the side of the convexity, the slight prominence of the ribs posteriorly causing a corresponding asymmetry of the thorax (Fig. 188, *B*). The shoulder on the side of the convexity is elevated and anterior with respect to the other shoulder. In left total scoliosis the deformity is a long curvature with its convexity to the left. In cases of purely postural character the curvature can be straightened voluntarily and undergoes complete spontaneous correction during recumbency. Right total scoliosis is much less common than left.

The compound or **S**-shaped type of curve is found in most cases of so-called idiopathic scoliosis and in approximately 30% of the entire group of scoliosis patients. The deformity consists most often of a primary dorsal curve convex to the right and of secondary cervical and lumbar curves convex to the left. The curvature cannot be corrected voluntarily and in recumbency may be less pronounced but does not disappear. The asymmetry and rotation may be severe. The rotation deformity is best observed when the patient leans sharply forward.

Simple lumbar scoliosis is most commonly convex to the left with its apex at the level of the second lumbar vertebra. The iliac crest is more prominent on the side of the concavity, whereas there is fullness of the back on the side of the convexity. This type of scoliosis usually does not progress to a severe deformity. Single dorsal curves tend to develop accentuation of the normal dorsal kyphosis, a rotation deformity, and secondary curves in the cervical and lumbar regions.

Diagnosis. Since scoliosis is not a primary disease of the spine but the resultant of certain mechanical forces exerted upon it, the examiner must attempt to determine the basic etiologic factor. Careful history and physical examination, together with good roentgenograms, are essential. The roentgenograms may show the character of the curve, the degree of distortion of individual vertebrae, and the presence of bony defects. The degree of curvature should be measured on the roentgenograms by a standard method and recorded (Fig. 192). Similar roentgenograms and measurements, made several months later, should be compared with those of the initial examination to demonstrate whether the curvature is increasing or is static.

Prognosis. Structural scoliosis is essentially a self-limited condition; in most cases progression of the curvature ceases spontaneously by the age of 15 years in girls and 16 years in boys. A useful roentgenographic guide, described by Risser, is the fact that idiopathic scoliosis does not increase after the iliac crests have been fully capped by their apophyses.

In many cases of structural scoliosis, however, the deformity tends to progress rapidly during the growing period of childhood and therefore constitutes a serious therapeutic problem until arrest of any advancing curvature can be assured. Every case demands careful attention and supervision over a long period of time. Pain is a common finding in adult scoliosis,

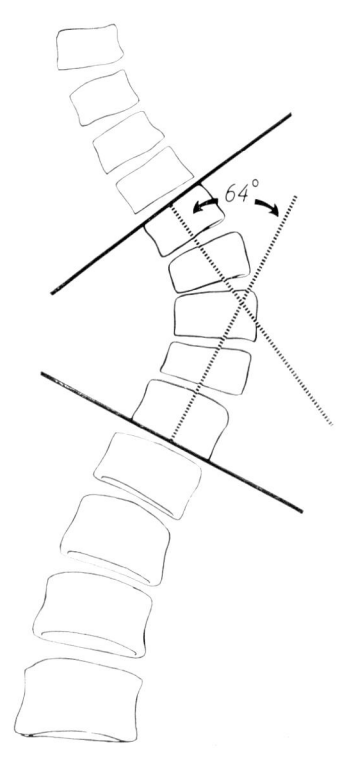

Fig. 192. Measurement of scoliotic curve by method of J. R. Cobb. Highest vertebra is that with the disk below it wider on the convex side and the disk above wider on the concave side; the lowest vertebra has the disk above it wider on the convex side and the disk below it wider on the concave side. Intersecting perpendiculars determine the angle of curvature. The Ferguson method of measuring scoliotic curvature utilizes lines drawn from the centers of the bodies of the highest and lowest vertebrae of the curve to the center of the body of the middle vertebra of the curve.

appearing in about two thirds of the cases, very often in the fourth decade of life.

Without treatment the postural curvatures may remain stationary, as may the deformities of structural scoliosis in adults, but the structural curvatures in growing children often increase to cause severe deformity and disability.

With treatment, scoliosis of the postural type may be completely cured. The structural type in young children may be prevented from becoming worse and often may be greatly improved; rarely, however, is complete correction of the curvature obtained.

The earlier the treatment is started, the better the prognosis. The C-shaped curvatures are more amenable to treatment than are the compound or S-shaped curves. Thoracic curves become more deforming than lumbar curves; in children thoracogenic scoliosis tends to progress to severe deformity despite any form of treatment.

Treatment. With these prognostic considerations in mind, the treatment of scoliosis must be suited to the age, type of curvature, and other characteristics of the individual patient.

The basic principles are (1) to prevent the increase of scoliosis, when the tendency toward curvature is recognized at an early stage; (2) to overcome rigidity of the spine and improve balance of the trunk, when the deformity has become established, by means of mobilizing exercises; (3) to secure as much correction of the deformity as possible; (4) to develop sufficient muscle strength, if possible, to maintain the correction; (5) to supply artificial support of the spine when the muscle strength is inadequate to maintain the correction; and (6) to prevent overfatigue and other deleterious influences that might lead to an increase of the curvature.

Prophylactic treatment. Recognition of the earliest stage of scoliosis is essential. Prophylactic treatment is usually concerned with the preschool child rather than the older girl or boy. Any recognizable underlying cause of scoliosis should be treated. Improper postural influences in school, such as a poorly designed school desk, do not cause scoliosis but may aggravate an existing disorder. Unilateral defects of sight or hearing may play an etiologic role and should be corrected. The child who has had infantile paralysis must be observed at intervals for a number of years to rule out the development of paralytic scoliosis. Exercises may be prescribed to maintain the mobility of the spine and to improve the balance of the trunk muscles. When an increase of the curvature is considered likely, the patient should be examined at frequent intervals.

Treatment of established scoliosis. The treatment of most cases of scoliotic deformity falls into three mutually complementary stages: (1) *mobilization* of contracted structures by means of exercises, (2) *correction* of the curvature by application of straightening forces, and (3) *maintenance* of the correction by brace or spinal fusion. The technical procedures by which these objects are best attained vary with the characteristics of the individual case. The following methods are in common use:

1. *Corrective exercises alone:* How effective are exercises in the treatment of structural scoliosis is debatable. Properly chosen and supervised exercises may mobilize the curved portions of the spine in selected cases and strengthen certain muscle groups to aid in maintaining improved position. As muscular weakness often accompanies the deformity and as maintenance of the improved position of the spine may require greater muscle strength than was present before correction, it seems important that an attempt be made to increase the power of the supporting musculature. Corrective exercises should be performed for from one to two hours daily; they are best carried out under careful direction in a gymnasium and should be continued for many months. After an adequate period of supervision the exercises may be carried on at home. No improvement is to be expected unless the patient is willing to work faithfully with the exercises. Any increase of the deformity necessitates change to a different method of treatment.

2. *Corrective exercises, traction, and back supports:* Periods of recum-

bency with or without head and pelvic traction and repeated short periods of vertical head halter traction with the patient sitting are sometimes combined with exercises and back supports in initial treatment. Most braces and body jackets are quite ineffective in controlling structural scoliosis. However, a closely fitting plastic jacket, made over a plaster mold of the trunk taken while the patient is suspended vertically by a head halter, may often be used to advantage. Such a support should be worn almost constantly except while the patient is engaged in scoliosis exercises. Such a combination of exercises and special back supports may be especially suitable for patients whose curvatures are slight and increasing only slowly, and whose ages are close to that of spinal maturity.

3. *Corrective plaster jackets and braces:* The deformities of structural scoliosis can be greatly improved by forceful mechanical means. For permanent improvement such forceful correction must usually be followed by an extensive arthrodesis of the spine. Such a therapeutic program is long and arduous for the patient and requires much experience on the part of the orthopaedist, as well as specialized mechanical aids; it is indicated in only a small percentage of scoliosis patients.

Gradual straightening of the curvature can be accomplished by utilizing the principle of a hinged jacket. For this the turnbuckle plaster jacket of Risser is widely used. It consists of a body cast which incorporates one or both thighs and the head and neck and which is provided with anterior and posterior hinges and a turnbuckle on the side of the concavity; after correction has gradually been effected, stabilization usually is secured by means of surgical fusion performed through a window in the back of the cast.

More rapid improvement of the curvature can sometimes be secured by combining longitudinal traction with pressure over the apex of the convexity. The localizer body cast of Risser is applied with the patient on a special frame provided with attachments for exerting head traction, pelvic traction, and localized pressure posterolaterally over the rib angulation.

Of the many and diverse types of braces that have been devised for the treatment of scoliosis, the most effective is the Milwaukee or Blount brace. It incorporates both distraction, by adjustable uprights extending from head to pelvis, and adjustable posterolateral pressure over the thoracic prominence. In it the patient can lie down, sit, stand, and walk. This brace may be used as a corrective and holding support in milder, nonsurgical cases, as well as before and after spinal arthrodesis.

4. *Surgical treatment:* The operation of spinal fusion is the most effective means of maintaining permanently the correction of structural scoliosis (Figs. 193 and 194). Stabilizing operations are indicated when rapid increase or recurrence of the curvature cannot be prevented by the use of other methods. In many clinics operation is advocated for all forms of paralytic scoliosis, for increasing idiopathic scoliosis, and for any other type that is accompanied by marked deformity in adolescence. As a rule only about 5% of the cases are severe enough to require fusion.

The spinal fusion may be done in one or more stages after maximum cor-

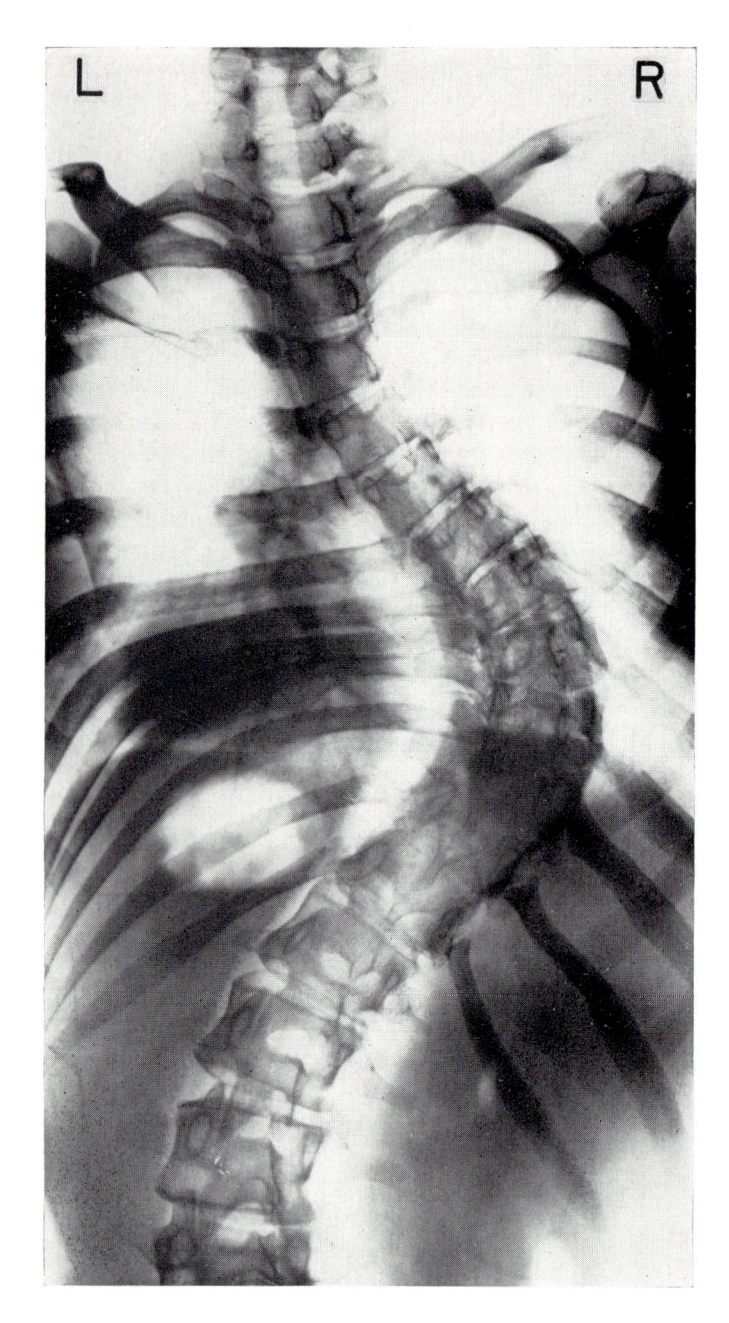

Fig. 193. Roentgenogram of idiopathic scoliosis, in a 15-year-old girl, before treatment; angulation of right dorsal curve, as measured by the method of Cobb, is approximately 85 degrees.

Affections of the spine and thorax 337

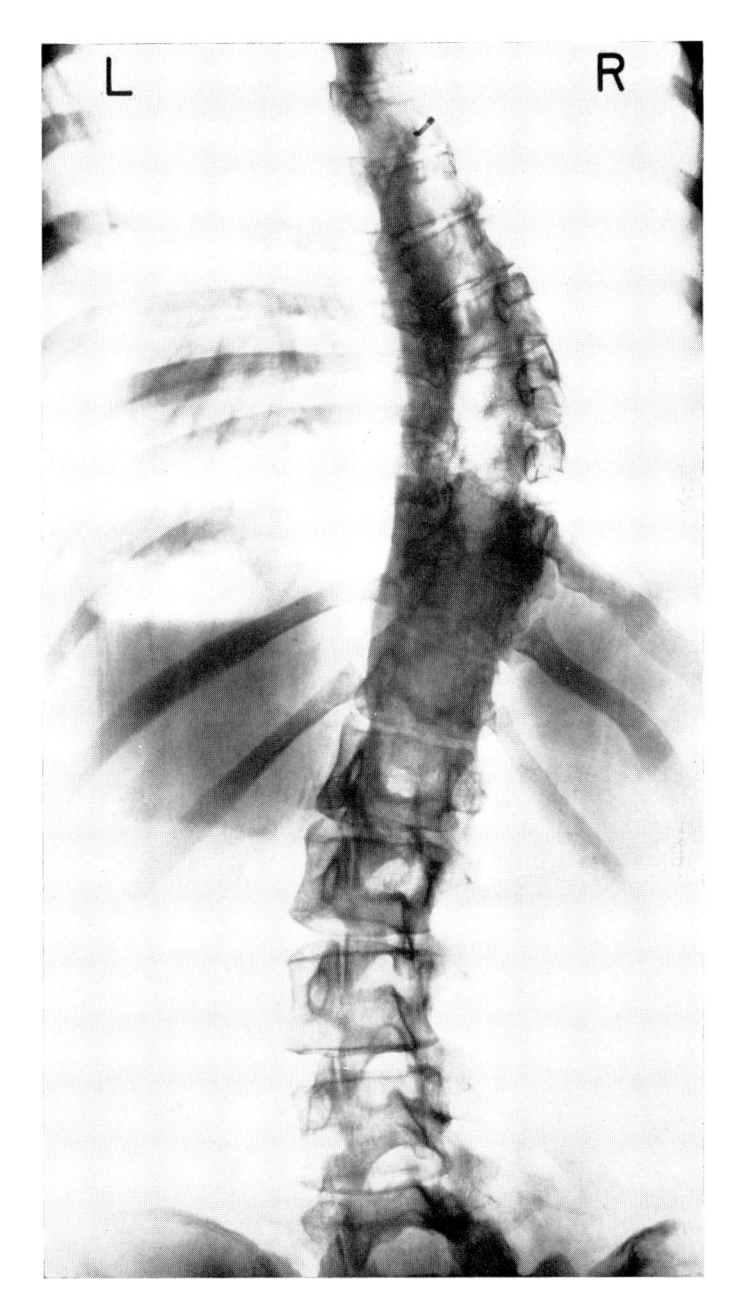

Fig. 194. Roentgenogram of patient shown in Fig. 193, two and one half years later, after correction in turnbuckle jacket and posterior arthrodesis extending from fourth thoracic to second lumbar vertebra. Angulation, by Cobb measurement, is now 40 degrees.

rection of the curvature has been obtained. Alternatively the arthrodesis may precede correction, since straightening of the curvature is facilitated by the temporary increase of spinal mobility after operation. Surgical fusion of a long segment of the spine, the level depending upon the details of the individual curvature, may be carried out according to the Hibbs technic (Fig. 96) or according to a modification of this method with reinforcement by autogenous iliac bone.

Most spinal fusions for scoliosis should be followed by rest in bed, preferably in a plaster cast or Milwaukee brace, for a period of from three to six months, after which an ambulatory plaster jacket or strong spinal brace should be worn for an additional period of six months or more, until roentgenograms show a solid column of bone sufficiently strong to maintain permanent correction of the curvature. The patient must then be followed at intervals for a number of years, during which any recurrent increase of curvature suggests that there is a pseudarthrosis, or failure of fusion, which should be explored surgically and repaired.

Recently developed technics for treating scoliosis by the surgical insertion of metal appliances to exert distracting and contracting forces directly on the vertebrae show considerable promise but as yet have not been thoroughly evaluated. In paralytic scoliosis associated with asymmetrical weakness of the muscles of the abdomen, much improvement may result from surgical reinforcement of the weakened abdominal muscles by the use of long strips of fascia lata *(Lowman operation)*.

KYPHOSIS (ROUND BACK)

Anteroposterior curvature of the spine in which the convexity is directed posteriorly is called *kyphosis*. The thoracic and sacral levels of the normal spine exhibit this type of curvature. Posterior convexity of abnormal degree results from pathologic changes located primarily in the vertebral bodies, the intervertebral disks, or the supporting musculature.

Kyphotic deformity occurs not uncommonly in children and young adults. The most frequent cause is faulty posture. Kyphosis resulting from diseases such as tuberculosis or chronic arthritis has been described in preceding chapters. Other entities that may cause kyphosis in youth include *vertebral epiphysitis* and *vertebral osteochondritis*.

Kyphotic deformity seen in middle or late age groups is often termed *adult round back*. Its causes include postural influences and common bone and joint diseases, as well as degenerative spinal lesions peculiar to adult years.

Vertebral epiphysitis (Scheuermann's disease, adolescent kyphosis)

The term *vertebral epiphysitis* has been applied to a chronic affection of the epiphyses of the vertebral bodies that is evidenced clinically by fatigue, backache, and kyphosis of gradual development (Fig. 195). The process always involves a number of contiguous vertebrae and usually is most marked in the lower or middle portion of the dorsal spine. Vertebral

Affections of the spine and thorax 339

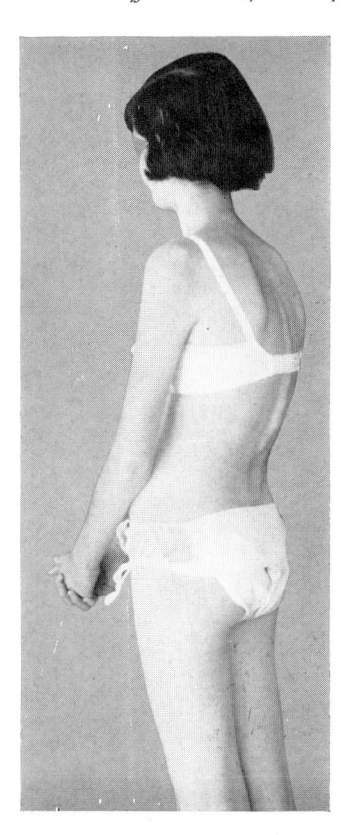

Fig. 195. Vertebral epiphysitis in 11-year-old girl, showing pronounced dorsal kyphosis and poor posture. This patient was treated for two years with postural exercises and bracing.

epiphysitis makes its appearance at puberty and is self-limited, its active course lasting usually for two or three years.

Etiology. Roentgenographic evidence suggests that the process is a disturbance of the ossification of the epiphyses. The etiologic agent has not been established. Hypotheses of the causation include (1) inadequate circulation associated with rapid growth, similar to that sometimes believed to occur in coxa plana, and (2) disturbance of epiphyseal growth by protrusion of the intervertebral disks through deficient cartilage plates. Relatively greater weight on the anterior part of the vertebral bodies, resulting from the kyphosis and present during the growth period, may increase the deformity.

Roentgenographic picture. In early cases the bone edges above and below the intervertebral spaces are ill-defined and of uneven density. The epiphyses are irregular in outline, particularly at their anterior edges, and may appear fragmented. As healing takes place, the fragmentation disappears, and the bone outlines become relatively more distinct but remain irregular. The vetebral bodies are wedged anteriorly and the interbody spaces distorted (Fig. 196). Localized indentations of the spongiosa, resulting from protrusions of nuclear material through defects in the cartilage plates and called *Schmorl's nodes,* may be seen. There is often a visible horizontal cleft in the middle portion of the vertebral body, extending from the anterior margin posteriorly for about two thirds of the depth of the body. In most normal children such clefts disappear before the tenth year of age.

Clinical picture. The symptoms usually begin between the ages of 12 and 16 years. The first subjective evidence may be fatigue and pain in the back. Undue prominence of the spinous processes of the vertebrae may be noticed, especially at the lower dorsal and upper lumbar levels, and gradual development of kyphosis takes place. Compensatory increase of lumbar lordosis may be noticeable. The deformity persists in recumbency. Stiffness and tenderness may be present throughout the spine. Expansion of the chest is abnormally restricted. The affection sometimes progresses to the point of severe disability, whereas in other cases it causes few or no symptoms. In later years osteoarthritic changes and backache may develop.

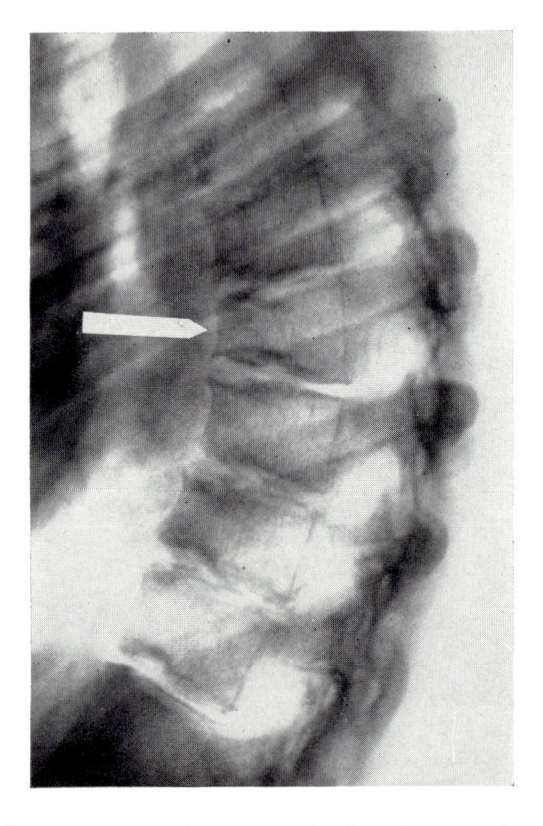

Fig. 196. Lateral roentgenogram showing vertebral epiphysitis in boy 14 years of age. Note the narrowing or wedging of the anterior portion of some of the vertebral bodies and the irregularity of their superior and inferior surfaces.

Diagnosis. Vertebral epiphysitis is to be distinguished from tuberculosis of the spine. In tuberculosis there is marked spinal rigidity, which is never striking in epiphysitis, and the roentgenograms show localized bone destruction and an angular rather than a rounded kyphosis. Vertebral epiphysitis is also to be differentiated from osteochondritis, which develops at an earlier age and is localized to a single vertebral body.

Treatment. The therapy depends upon the severity of the symptoms. In milder cases it may be advisable to have the patient limit activities that put stresses on his spine, use a fracture board without pillow, and carry out kyphosis exercises. It is sometimes necessary to support the spine by means of a brace or plaster jacket. Occasionally, recumbency upon a Bradford or a Whitman frame, followed by the use of a brace or plaster jacket, may be advisable. In an occasional case, persistent pain in later years is an indication for spinal arthrodesis.

Vertebral osteochondritis (vertebra plana, Calvé's disease)

Vertebral osteochondritis is an uncommon affection, occurring usually in the dorsal spine of children between 2 and 12 years of age and characterized by pathologic changes that are almost always localized in a single vertebral body. It has been considered an ischemic necrosis somewhat analogous to that of the femoral head in coxa plana (p. 374); however, in recent years histologic examinations have shown that in many if not all of these cases the vertebral lesion may be a pathologic fracture secondary to a benign destructive process such as eosinophilic granuloma.

Roentgenographic picture. The affected vertebral body may appear fragmented or eroded; it becomes uniformly flattened or wedge-shaped. Adjacent disk spaces are normal or thickened. With healing the affected body increases in density; in a young child it may regain considerable height as growth progresses.

Clinical picture. Pain, fatigue, and an angular kyphosis are characteristic. Muscle spasm and tenderness may also be present.

Diagnosis. The differential diagnosis should include eosinophilic granuloma, tuberculosis, tumor, solitary cyst, compression fracture, congenital anomaly, and vertebral epiphysitis. Lesions in bones other than the affected vertebra should be excluded by roentgenograms. Biopsy may be advisable.

Treatment. Rest in recumbency is indicated. The patient may be placed upon a frame in hyperextension with head and pelvic traction (Fig. 95) for a period of several weeks. A brace or plaster jacket should then be used until roentgenograms show the lesion healed. Rarely it may be advisable to stabilize the spine by arthrodesis.

Adult round back

Etiology. Adult round back may be due to faulty posture alone or to an occupation that requires constant flexion of the spine; to old age with its constant atrophy of the intervertebral disks *(senile kyphosis);* to atrophy of the vertebral bodies *(postmenopausal* and *senile osteoporosis);* or to a pathologic entity such as chronic arthritis, osteitis deformans, poliomyelitis, fracture, metastatic tumor, tuberculosis, or other diseases that affect the spine. Atrophy of the intervertebral disks sometimes takes place in middle life; it may progress to cause a single, long kyphosis with flattening of the lumbar and cervical portions of the spine and forward projection of the head.

Pathology. In adult round back due to lesions of the intervertebral fibrocartilages, the pathologic changes that occur in the disks are characteristic. The normal disk, as demonstrated by Schmorl, comprises a central portion, the *nucleus pulposus,* consisting of a semifluid medium under pressure, and a peripheral portion, the *annulus fibrosus,* which forms a fibrocartilaginous capsule. Two thin plates of hyaline cartilage separate the disk from the bones above and below; these cartilage plates are in contact with the superior and inferior surfaces of the vertebral bodies. In 30% of all adult spines, localized protrusions of nuclear material through the cartilage plates and into the spongy bone of the vertebral bodies *(Schmorl's nodes)* have been found. These lesions may occur in any case of abnormal anteroposterior spinal curvature, whether in a child or in an adult. They are also seen in the absence of clinical deformity.

Gradual thinning or collapse of the intervertebral disks allows adjacent vertebral bodies to become approximated. Altered local stresses lead to new bone formation about the edges of the vertebral bodies. If in addition the anterior portion of the cartilage plates is destroyed, bridges of new bone may develop across the intervertebral spaces, resulting in ankylosis.

In adult round back from senile osteoporosis the disks remain relatively normal, but the spongy bone within the vertebral body becomes atrophic and the cortex becomes thinned. Disuse atrophy may play a part. In the thoracic spine the vertebral bodies may become wedge-shaped, while in the lumbar region they may assume a biconcave or hourglass contour as seen in lateral roentgenograms. The osteoporosis may lead to pathologic compression fractures of the vertebral bodies (Fig. 81), which may further increase the kyphosis.

Clinical picture. The deformity of kyphosis is of characteristic appearance and may be associated with considerable pain, weakness of the back, and general fatigue. The aching and tiring of the back usually occur below the apex of the kyphosis. Seldom is there any localized tenderness; it is usually present, however, in senile osteoporosis with recent compression fracture.

Treatment. Attempt should be made to maintain correct posture; exercises to strengthen the muscles of the back and abdomen and to expand the chest will sometimes aid in accomplishing this. In more advanced cases it may be necessary to apply a light spinal brace or corset. If the symptoms are located in the cervical spine, a Thomas collar (Fig. 185) may be used to support the head and so relieve the constant dragging sensation. In some cases a period of immobilization on a Bradford or Whitman frame is advisable, and, rarely, arthrodesis of the spine may be indicated for the relief of intractable backache. In postmenopausal and senile osteoporosis, the administration of sex hormones will usually relieve the back symptoms but may induce undesirable side effects.

LORDOSIS (HOLLOW BACK)

Anteroposterior curvature of the spine in which the concavity is directed posteriorly is termed *lordosis*. Cervical and lumbar levels of the spine normally exhibit lordosis. Abnormal degrees of lordosis are usually secondary to other deformity of the spine or to deformities of the lower limbs. Lordosis is often found in association with flexion contracture of the hip, congenital dislocation of the hip, coxa vara, progressive muscular dystrophy, paralysis from poliomyelitis, obesity of the abdomen, dorsal kyphosis, and shortening of the Achilles tendons. Some cases are idiopathic, no cause being recognizable.

Clinical picture. Constant aching throughout the lower part of the back, protrusion of the abdomen, and generalized fatigue are often present. Asymptomatic lordosis is fairly common in young children.

Treatment and prognosis. Therapy should include general postural exercises with particular effort to strengthen the abdominal and the gluteal muscles. In adults, a strong support for the back with a lower abdominal pad may be helpful. The result of treatment is often complete relief of the backache, but usually the improvement will not be permanent unless the pathologic factor underlying the deformity can be remedied.

FAULTY POSTURE

Faulty posture is always undesirable from the cosmetic standpoint, frequently causes symptoms such as chronic backache, and may lead over a period of many years to permanent degenerative changes in joints. Faulty spinal posture is often associated with postural defects about the shoulders, hips, knees, and feet; its correction tends to improve postural relationships in the extremities.

Criteria of good posture. In good standing posture (Fig. 197, A) the thoracic spine is slightly convex posteriorly while the cervical and lumbar levels are slightly concave posteriorly. There is moderate forward inclination of the pelvis. The spine shows no lateral deviation. There is no lateral asymmetry of shoulders or hips. The shoulder joints lie in the mid-axillary plane of the body. The hips and knees are extended at the neutral zero position. The patellae face directly forward; the feet diverge anteriorly and show little or no pronation. The line of weight bearing which passes through the mastoid process falls across the greater trochanter, the tibial tuberosity, and the fifth metatarsal base.

When applied to individual patients, these criteria of good posture may require modification because of variations in age, body build, and nutrition.

Physiology of posture. The standing position, which is a composite depending on the position of each joint, is maintained by tonic contraction of

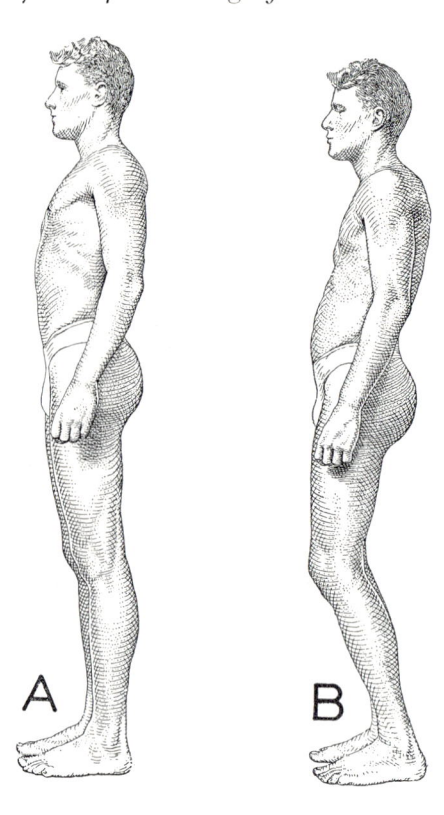

Fig. 197. Posture in a young adult. **A**, Excellent; **B**, faulty. In **B** note increased inclination of the pelvis, increased anteroposterior curvatures of the spine, round shoulders, flat chest, protruding abdomen, and flexed knees.

the muscles. Tonic contraction, or postural tone, is produced by the successive activity of small groups of muscle fibers that are stimulated reflexly by the central nervous system on receiving afferent impulses from muscles, tendons, eyes, ears, and skin.

Erect posture is dependent largely upon maintenance of the balance of pelvis on femoral heads by the hip extensors (glutei, hamstrings, and posterior adductors) and the hip flexors (iliopsoas, rectus femoris, and anterior adductors). Anteroposterior curvatures of the spine vary with the pelvic inclination, determined chiefly by these hip muscles, and with the balance between the spinal extensor (erector spinae) and the spinal flexors (psoas and abdominal muscles).

Etiology of faulty posture. Ascribed causes of faulty posture include (1) muscular weakness and (2) psychosomatic influences. It seems probable that in the individual case either or both may be responsible. Faulty posture is seen with malnutrition, after prolonged illness, and during periods of rapid growth of the long bones; it is common also in individuals who are depressed or careless of personal appearance. As Wiles puts it, posture is a reflection of personality as well as physique.

Clinical picture. The common picture of faulty posture includes increased inclination of the pelvis, accompanied by excessive lumbar lordosis and rounding of the thoracic spine (Fig. 197, *B*). The head protrudes forward, the shoulders are rounded and drooped, and the vertebral borders of the scapulae are prominent. The chest is flat and the abdomen sags forward, particularly in its lower half. Commonly associated are slight internal rotation of the hips, valgus and slight flexion deformities of the knees, and valgus deformities of the feet.

Faulty posture is seen chiefly in two types of patients: (1) children and adolescents who are often asymptomatic, and (2) adults who complain of chronic aching and pain. The symptoms probably arise from tension in ligaments inadequately protected by muscular action, or from degenerative changes in joints produced by long periods of malpositioning.

Treatment. Before ascribing a patient's complaint to faulty posture, one must rule out, by a careful clinical and laboratory study, any other possible cause for the symptoms. When the diagnostic studies have been completed, however, many cases will remain in which the symptoms and signs can be ascribed to defective posture alone.

The first step in treatment is to secure the patient's cooperation and motivation in a program of posture training. He should then be given a clear idea of the defects which are present and of the proper mechanical relationships which are to be gained. The objective is his acquisition of improved postural habits. The patient must be taught that the influence of any system of corrective exercises will depend upon their being executed while all parts of the body are in proper mechanical relationship. A system of muscle training exercises for daily use is then to be adopted, suited to the characteristics of the individual case and so graduated as to lead by easy stages to the desired endurance level. When pain is a factor, light corrective braces may be worn between exercises, but it must be emphasized that such apparatus is only a temporary expedient, is to be discarded as soon as possible, and in most instances serves chiefly as a reminder to the wearer that only by his own effort will his posture be permanently corrected. As muscular vigor begins to return, the relief and gratitude exhibited by many of these patients, whose chronic distress has been the result simply of careless and defective posture, is striking. With the physical improvement there develop often an increased mental independence and vigor that make the weeks or months of muscle training a distinctly worthwhile investment. Proper postural habits once acquired will usually be retained with a minimum of effort.

Biophysics of the locomotor system. No discussion of the postural relationships of the body at rest can be complete without calling attention to the vastly more complex subject of the physiology, normal and pathologic, of the body in motion.

The biomechanics of the locomotor system has become a subject of increasing interest. The older studies of posture (Goldthwait) and the theoretical mechanics of normal and pathologic locomotion (Steindler) have been followed by experimental technics (Schwartz, Saunders, and Inman) which involve time and force analysis of the stance and swing phases of gait by methods that include photography, force plate analysis, strain gauge technics, and electromyography. Each muscle used in gait has been studied to reveal the exact time and force of its contraction with relation to the stance or the swing phase. Such data have been applied in the analysis of normal variations as well as in conditions involving paralysis, tendon transferences, and the use of prostheses. Investigation of subjects such as the expenditure of energy in locomotion, the use of isometric muscle contraction at optimal muscle length, effective changes in lever arms, and the engineering characteristics of bone, tendon, and muscle will undoubtedly lead to great advances in understanding the physiology of the locomotor system and in treating orthopaedic patients.

Deformities of the thorax

Slight deformities and asymmetries of the thorax are common, cause no disability, and often require no treatment. Such deformities, including flat chest associated with round back, can be made less apparent if exercises are prescribed to improve the posture and to build up the pectoral muscles and shoulder girdle.

The more serious deformities of the chest are almost certainly congenital in origin and are probably interrelated. They are always associated with overgrowth of the ribs. Often several members of a family, more commonly the males, are affected; they may have chest deformities of differing types.

PIGEON BREAST (PECTUS CARINATUM)

In the chest deformity known as pigeon breast, the sternum projects forward and downward like the keel of a boat (Fig. 198). This increases the anteroposterior diameter of the thorax, impairs the effectiveness of coughing, and restricts the volume of ventilation. Premature development of emphysema or cor pulmonale sometimes results from severe degrees of pigeon breast.

Treatment. Mild deformities can be made less noticeable by exercise, which increases the strength and size of the pectoral muscles. The more severe deformities require thoracic surgery, the affected costal cartilages and the xiphoid process being resected and the sternum replaced in normal position. The cosmetic and functional results are gratifying.

FUNNEL CHEST (PECTUS EXCAVATUM)

Funnel chest (Fig. 199) is the mirror image of pigeon breast, the sternum being pushed posteriorly by overgrowth of the ribs. The anteroposterior diameter of the thorax is decreased. The heart is often displaced into the left side of the chest. Shortening of the central tendon of the diaphragm has been considered the cause of the deformity, but there is little evidence to support this concept. Severe forms of funnel chest can result in kyphosis,

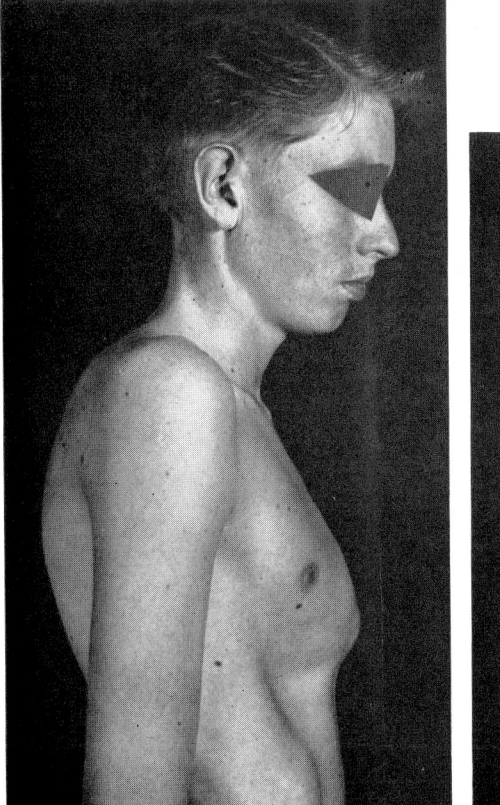

Affections of the spine and thorax 347

Fig. 198
Fig. 199 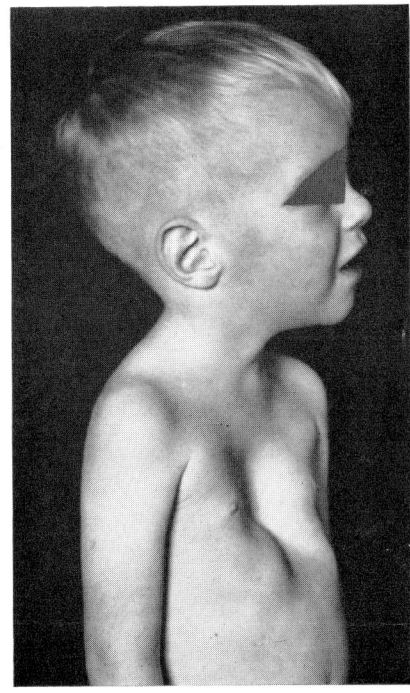

Fig. 198. Pigeon breast (pectus carinatum) in 19-year-old boy. Note projection of lower portion of sternum and deformity of ribs.

Fig. 199. Funnel chest (pectus excavatum) in 3-year-old boy. Note depression of sternum and deformity of ribs.

repeated respiratory infections, wheezing respirations, cardiac arrhythmias, and premature emphysema. Funnel chest may produce considerable disfigurement in both boys and girls; it may cause the youth to avoid circumstances where he must remove his shirt, and the girl to shun normal social contacts.

Treatment. In mild cases exercises to improve posture and build up the shoulder girdle and pectoral muscles will greatly improve the patient's appearance. More severe cases require a thoracic surgical procedure similar to that for pectus carinatum. The deformed costal cartilages and xiphoid process are resected, and the sternum is restored to proper position. In the seriously disabled patient the improvement following this operation is often dramatic.

CHAPTER 17

Affections of the low back

THE TERM "affections of the low back" is used in this chapter to include ligamentous and muscular strains, spondylolisthesis, intervertebral disk lesions, and several less serious disorders involving the lower part of the back.

The frequency with which affections of the low back are encountered brings them constantly to the attention of every practitioner of medicine. Patients whose low back pain is caused by visceral rather than musculoskeletal lesions or is an hysterical conversion symptom associated with tension, nervousness, and chronic fatigue are problems for the internist and psychiatrist, respectively, rather than the orthopaedist. However, low back pain, with or without sciatic pain, is the commonest complaint with which orthopaedic surgeons are confronted in adults. The variety of bone, joint, muscle, ligament, and nerve lesions which may cause low back pain and the difficulties encountered in their treatment make these affections formidable orthopaedic problems. In each case the diagnosis and treatment must be based upon a careful evaluation of the clinical and roentgenographic findings in the light of available information on the various recognized types of low back lesions.

Classification. For convenience of description, cases characterized by low back pain may be discussed according to the following outline:

1. Lesions peculiar to the low back
    (a) Ligamentous and muscular strains of the normal low back. Of these, the syndrome of lumbosacral strain resulting from acute or chronic traumatic influences is the most important.
    (b) Abnormalities of the bony structure of the low back. Among these are congenital anomalies, spondylolisthesis, and prespondylolisthesis.
    (c) Lesions of the lumbar intervertebral disks.
    (d) Other lesions of muscle and fascia.
2. Common osteoarticular lesions of infectious, neoplastic, or traumatic nature affecting the low back.
3. Visceral lesions that may cause low back pain.

LIGAMENTOUS AND MUSCULAR STRAINS OF THE NORMAL LOW BACK

The majority of cases of low back pain of orthopaedic nature fall into this group. The mechanism of injury is either an episode of trauma or a continued mechanical strain of postural or occupational type. It has been reported that 80% of low back pain is caused by mechanical strain. In many cases the lesion is presumably a tear or stretching of ligaments that support and limit the mobility of a joint. There is considerable evidence that in some cases the lesion is a tear of the posterior longitudinal ligament, a tear of the annulus fibrosus, or traumatic changes within the disk substance. Muscle injury may be associated. The hemorrhage and organization which follow an injury may cause the ligaments to lose their normal tension and strength and so lead to a state of chronic relaxation which predisposes the joints to further injury. During pregnancy temporary relaxation of the ligaments of the sacroiliac joints occurs normally.

The lumbosacral joint, situated at the critical level between movable and immovable portions of the spine, is particularly liable to injury from forces applied in an obliquely anteroposterior direction, as in violent flexion or hyperextension of the spine, falls upon the buttocks, and gravitational stresses associated with excessive lordosis. Lumbosacral sprains are therefore very frequently encountered. The sacroiliac joints, on the other hand, are large in area and protected by strong ligamentous structures; little motion can be demonstrated in them (5 degrees in young women). They may nevertheless be injured occasionally by violence applied to the low back in a rotary or obliquely lateral manner.

Clinical picture. The symptoms and physical signs are very similar to those of other affections of the low back and warrant detailed analysis. Many of these symptoms and signs are identical with those of rupture of an intervertebral disk, which are described on pp. 364-366.

Localized pain. Pain in the low back is the outstanding symptom. The discomfort is often localized to a single area. At times it is generalized across the whole back, however, and the area of maximum intensity may shift from one side to the other. If pain in the low back is precipitated or aggravated by motion, it will in most instances be relieved by recumbency.

Radiating pain. Radiation of pain into the lower extremities is a frequent symptom in low back affections. Such pain may be (1) radicular or (2) somatic. (1) *Radicular pain* results from nerve root irritation. The most common cause of root irritation is rupture of an intervertebral disk, which will be discussed later in this chapter. The root may also be irritated mechanically in a narrow, irregular intervertebral foramen, or by local inflammatory or neoplastic processes. Radicular pain tends to be sharp, shooting, and fairly well localized to a dermatomal pattern. (2) *Somatic pain* arises within ligamentous and muscular tissue. It is of diffuse, deep, aching character. Such pain may be produced by injecting small amounts of hypertonic salt solution into the lumbar paravertebral muscles, fairly constant areas of radiation to the lower extremities being demonstrable. Deep segmental pain commonly extends into the gluteal region and into the posterior or lateral aspect of the thigh. Radiation below the knee is less common. It is probable that the occasional good results from injecting tender areas in the back with a local anesthetic are produced by blockage of this pain mechanism.

Tenderness. There is usually localized pain on firm pressure over the affected area. When the lumbosacral joint is involved the tenderness may be most acute over the lumbosacral supraspinous ligament, but it may be present over the iliolumbar ligament of either side or generalized across the whole low back. When the sacroiliac structures are affected tenderness may be present about the inferior sacroiliac ligaments and the greater sciatic notch.

Muscle spasm. In patients who are having low back pain there is often marked spasm of the lumbar muscles. The spasm may be equal on the two sides; it is often asymmetrical, however, causing curvature of the spinal column, the so-called "sciatic scoliosis" (Fig. 200). Spasm may be present also in the hamstring muscles, making it impossible to flex the hip while the knee is extended. There also may be spasm of the tensor fasciae latae muscle and contracture of the fascia lata.

Abnormal limitation of mobility. There is usually marked limitation of

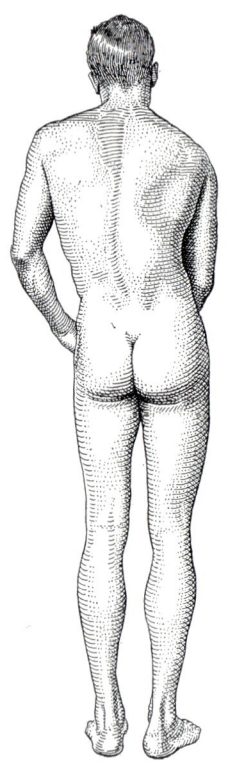

Fig. 200. Lateral curvature of the lumbar spine in acute affection of the low back (sciatic scoliosis).

motion, from muscle spasm, especially in acute cases. Tests of mobility dependent upon the localization of the muscle spasm are of value in differential diagnosis and should be carried out with the patient in the standing, sitting, and lying positions. In the standing position, flexion and hyperextension may be sharply limited. Rotation of the lower portion of the spine is often restricted, the patient being able to turn slightly more toward the normal side than toward the affected side. Flexion in the sitting position may be definitely restricted. In acute low back affections the lumbar spine is often flattened.

Special tests of passive mobility. A number of passive mobility tests have been devised or popularized by various observers and are of value in the clinical analysis of low back affections. Among tests in common use are the following:

1. Extreme flexion of both thighs upon the abdomen, with the knees flexed, places the lumbosacral joint under flexion stress while causing no unilateral rotary stress of the sacroiliac joints or stretching of the sciatic nerves. Lumbosacral pain produced by this maneuver is therefore suggestive of a disorder of the lumbosacral joint.

2. Straight leg-raising, i.e., flexion of the hip while the knee is held in extension (Fig. 201), stretches the sciatic nerve and places a rotary and flexion stress upon the low back structures. It causes pain when sciatic irritation is present.

3. When the hip of the affected side is flexed, extension of the knee will cause pain in the affected side of the low back; this pain is accentuated by dorsiflexion of the foot (Lasègue's sign). The mechanism is similar to that of the preceding test.

4. Contracture of the iliotibial band may be demonstrated by the following test: the patient lies on his sound side with the thighs flexed enough to obliterate the normal lumbar lordosis; grasping the ankle lightly with one

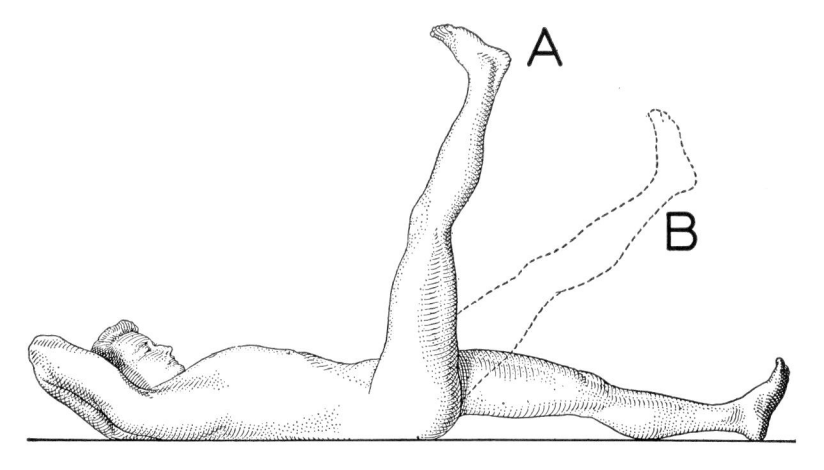

Fig. 201. Straight leg-raisign test. **A,** Normal limit of hip flexion with knee extended. **B,** Limitation of hip flexion due to pain in the presence of sciatic irritation.

hand and steadying the hip with the other, the examiner flexes the knee to a right angle, abducts the hip widely, and extends the hip. If the iliotibial band is shortened, the hip tends to remain passively abducted (Ober sign).

5. Forceful and prolonged lateral compression of the iliac crests, while placing no stress upon the lumbosacral joint, sometimes produces pain in an affected sacroiliac joint.

Roentgenographic examination. Roentgenograms are often of little help toward making a positive diagnosis. They are of great assistance, however, in ruling out conditions such as neoplasms, pyogenic infections, or tuberculosis. The presence of bony anomalies, such as sacralization of the last lumbar vertebra (Figs. 203 and 204), should be looked for. Occasionally calcification is seen within the iliolumbar ligaments. In lumbosacral affections the plane and smoothness of the articular facets, the width of the intervertebral disk spaces, and the degree of the lumbosacral angle are to be noted. Arthritic spurring and bridging may be seen. The roentgenograms should include anteroposterior, lateral, and oblique views. A search for defects of the isthmus or pars interarticularis should be made, and any forward displacement of a vertebral body should be noted. The examiner should also look for destructive changes and increased bone density about the sacroiliac joints.

Differential diagnosis. Ligamentous and muscular disorders of the low back must frequently be differentiated from (1) arthritis of the lumbar spine or sacroiliac joints, (2) fracture of the body or processes of a lumbar vertebra, (3) spondylolisthesis and prespondylolisthesis, (4) injury of an intervertebral disk, (5) tuberculosis and other infections, (6) malignancy, (7) tender fatty and fibrous nodules overlying ligaments and muscles, (8) hysteria, and (9) malingering. When the diagnosis is being made, the visceral diseases that may cause low back pain must be considered. A history of aggravation of the pain by exercise and of relief during recumbency suggests that the symptoms are of osteoarticular rather than visceral origin.

Treatment. Brief presentation of the more important therapeutic principles and their clinical application will be made. In the majority of cases nonsurgical treatment of ambulatory or recumbent type is indicated. In certain selected cases, however, surgical treatment is to be preferred.

Nonsurgical treatment. The principles of the treatment of ligament and of muscle injuries of the low back are essentially the same. The primary requisite is rest and support. In the acute phase uninterrupted recumbency is most helpful; the patient should lie supine in bed upon a firm mattress or on a thin mattress that is separated from the bedsprings by a fracture board. Frequently it is advisable to apply traction to one or both legs in order to relieve muscle spasm and pain. Traction may be obtained by applying straps to either side of a pelvic belt; 16 to 20 pounds can be applied in this manner with the foot of the bed elevated 4 to 6 inches. Recumbency may sometimes be made more effective by placing a pillow under the knees or under the painful portion of the back. Recumbency should continue until pain and muscle spasm subside. It is often advisable to accompany the rest in bed with local heat and massage, maintaining constant warmth over the painful area by means of an electric pad or a hot-water bottle. Aspirin may be helpful. Acute cases attended by muscle spasm may be relieved by muscle relaxant drugs. If there is a point of acute tenderness, its injection with a local anesthetic or hydrocortisone may be very helpful. In moderately acute cases in which the symptoms improve rapidly with recumbency, it is usually possible to allow gradual return to walking in one or two weeks, at which time the back may be firmly strapped with adhesive plaster or supported with a snugly fitting low back brace or corset (Fig. 202). In sacroiliac affections the support should exert lateral compression upon the ilia but need not extend above their crests, whereas in the much more common lumbosacral affections it should extend from the lower buttock crease to the spine of the tenth dorsal vertebra. Occasionally it is necessary to obtain still stronger support by the application of a light plaster cast. Such a cast should be well molded to the patient's torso and should extend well down over the iliac crests.

When walking is allowed, it is sometimes desirable to have the patient begin with crutches. Often an acute case will become chronic if weight bearing without proper support of the back is allowed too soon. A program of posture exercises to increase the strength of the back and abdominal muscles, often started before the patient begins to walk, is increased as he becomes more active. Too much emphasis cannot be placed upon the necessity of warning the patient to be careful about lifting and bending. He should not be allowed to return to strenuous work until the prescribed exer-

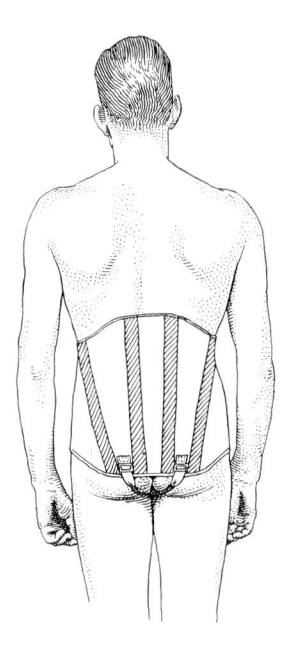

Fig. 202. Lumbosacral support made of heavy canvas with stays of spring steel. This wide belt may be used for low back affections which do not require rigid bracing.

cises can be performed without causing pain. If a contributing factor such as faulty posture or obesity is present, especial attention should be given to its correction. Manipulation of the lumbar spine is advocated by some physicians; it is discussed further in the section on lesions of the lumbar intervertebral disks.

Cases of only moderate severity may be treated without the initial period of recumbency.

Surgical treatment. When a thorough trial of conservative treatment fails to produce adequate and lasting relief of low back pain, lumbosacral arthrodesis should be considered. Seldom is it indicated, however, in the absence of demonstrable abnormality in the low back structures, and the patient for whom arthrodesis is contemplated must be very carefully evaluated. Surgical treatment is ordinarily contraindicated unless the patient is psychologically sound, uninfluenced by compensation or insurance expectations, and strongly motivated toward recovery and return to activity. Applying a plaster body jacket and observing the patient's response while he wears it, ambulatory, for perhaps six weeks will sometimes facilitate the evaluation of pertinent physical and psychologic factors. The orthopaedist must also keep in mind the facts that arthrodesis does not always produce solid fusion and that solid fusion does not produce a normal back. These considerations should be weighed and discussed preoperatively with the patient.

Arthrodesis is ordinarily done by a modification of the Hibbs technic (Fig. 96), and the addition of an iliac prop-graft at the lumbosacral level, as advocated by Bosworth, may be most helpful. Postoperatively it is essential to provide a period of recumbency, external support, and prohibition of strenuous activity sufficiently long for strong bony union to take place. Six to twelve months of such protection of the back may be required.

ABNORMALITIES OF THE BONY STRUCTURE OF THE LOW BACK

A great many of the patients with low back pain present roentgenographic evidence of anomalous bony development. In interpreting the relationship of these abnormalities to the clinical symptoms, the examiner must remember that similar anomalies are often present in individuals who are symptom-free. Nevertheless, some statistical studies support the natural inference that certain anomalies of the bony structure of the low back render it somewhat less stable than the normal back and more inclined through faulty mechanics to development of the ligamentous and muscular affections that have been described.

The most common bony anomalies of the low back are shown in Fig. 203. They include sacralization of the last lumbar vertebra; elongation of the transverse process of the last lumbar vertebra; defects of the laminae (spina bifida occulta); variations of the spinous processes, the lumbosacral angle, and the articular facets; constitutional variations; and isthmus defects. Isthmus defects are an essential factor in spondylolisthesis, which is an important cause of low back pain.

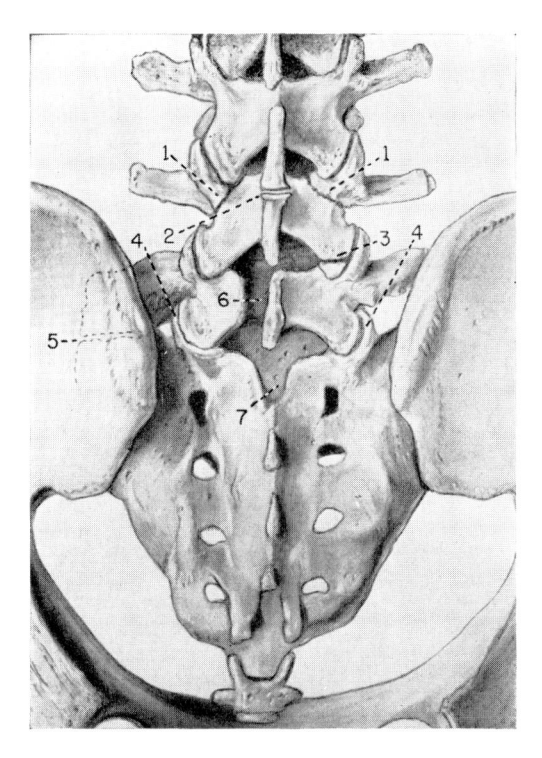

Fig. 203. Common congenital anomalies of the lumbosacral region: 1, bilateral isthmus defect; 2, impingement of third and fourth lumbar spinous processes; 3, laminar fissure at articular facet; 4, abnormal plane of articular facets; 5, sacralization of fifth lumbar transverse process with pseudarthrosis; 6, spina bifida occulta of fifth lumbar vertebra; 7, spina bifida occulta of first sacral segment. (From Freiberg, J. A.: In Bancroft, F. W., and Marble, H. C., editors: Surgical treatment of the motor-skeletal system, Philadelphia, 1951, J. B. Lippincott Co.)

Sacralization of the last lumbar vertebra

A bony conformation in which one or both of the transverse processes of the last lumbar vertebra are long and wing-shaped and articulate with the sacrum, the ilium, or both (Fig. 204) is termed sacralization of the last lumbar vertebra. The condition is more often bilateral than unilateral; it is found in 3.5% of all individuals. If radiating leg pain accompanies unilateral sacralization, the pain is usually down the side opposite the sacralization. A lumbosacral fusion may be indicated if conservative measures have failed to relieve the pain and intervertebral disk rupture has been ruled out.

Elongation of the transverse process of the last lumbar vertebra

Abnormally long fifth lumbar transverse processes are found in many cases of low back pain. Such processes may occasionally impinge upon the ilium, and the resulting friction may give rise to the formation of a painful bursa.

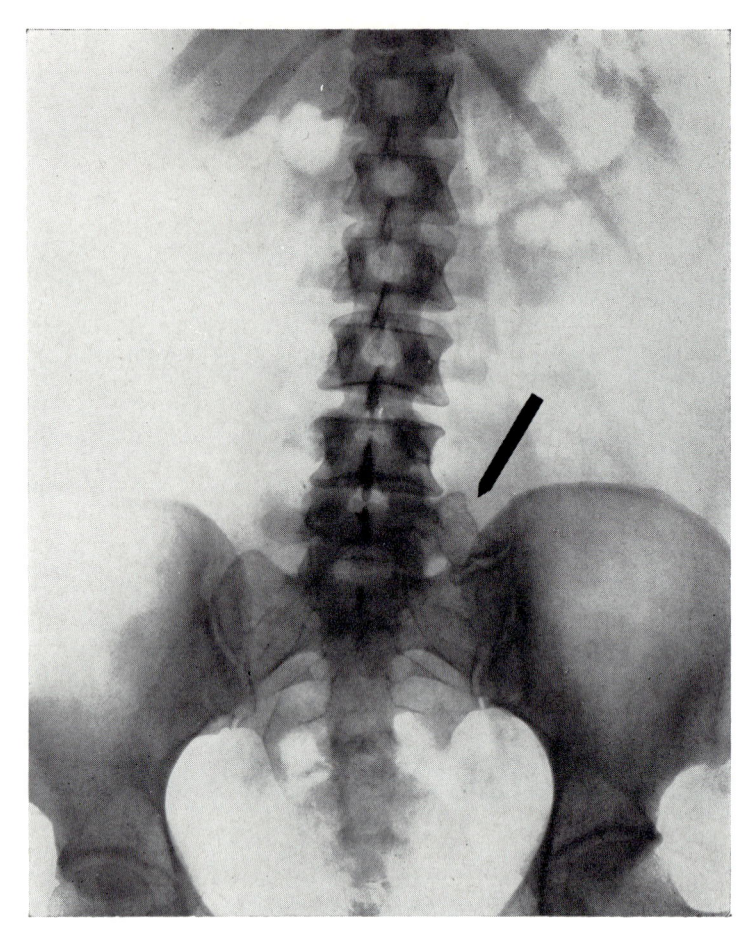

Fig. 204. Roentgenogram showing congenital anomalies of the lumbar spine. The left transverse process of the lowest of six lumbar vertebrae is sacralized.

Defects of the laminae (spina bifida occulta)

Clefts are frequently found in the vertebral laminae (Fig. 205) and may be associated with underdevelopment of the supporting ligaments. Partial or complete lack of fusion between the laminae of the last lumbar vertebra or of the first sacral segment is common; this imperfection has been found in 5% or more of all spines examined by roentgenograms. There is little evidence of any precise relationship between mild degrees of spina bifida and mechanical low back pain. A patient with low back pain whose roentgenograms show such an anomaly should be treated along the principles discussed under back pain of ligamentous or muscular origin.

Variations of the spinous processes

When the neural arch has failed to fuse, the spinous process may be attached to only one lamina. In other instances a spinous process associated

Affections of the low back 357

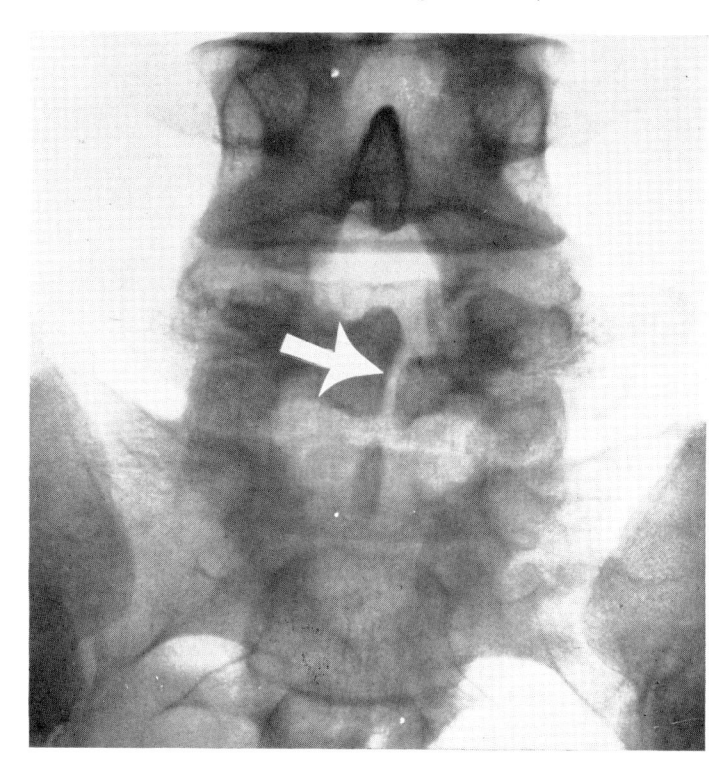

Fig. 205. Roentgenogram showing spina bifida occulta of the fifth lumbar vertebra. Note cleft in the laminal arch.

with normal laminae may be large and elongated so that it touches the spinous process of the vertebra above or below. There may be an associated increase in the normal lumbar lordosis. Constant irritation caused by this friction may give rise to the formation of a painful bursa. The symptoms can usually be relieved without resort to surgical treatment.

Variations of the lumbosacral angle

Wide variations of the angle between the upper surface of the sacrum and the horizontal plane when the patient is standing are not uncommon. Increase of the lumbosacral angle is often associated with the so-called horizontal sacrum and excessive lordosis. In such backs the lumbosacral joint is prone to injury from strain, with the subsequent formation of small bony spurs about the margins of the vertebral bodies. The treatment is the same as that of lumbosacral sprain.

Variations of the articular facets

Variations in the size and plane of these small but important joint surfaces are common (Fig. 203). The facets between the last lumbar vertebra and the sacrum are particularly prone to such asymmetries. Their significance as a cause of low back pain has not been proved.

Constitutional variations

The entire structure of the spine varies with the development of the body as a whole. In the tall, thin type the presence of a sixth lumbar vertebra is not uncommon, whereas short, stocky individuals sometimes have only four lumbar vertebrae. Low back pain is common in individuals with long, narrow backs or with flat backs. The treatment is the same as that of lumbosacral sprain.

Isthmus defects

Absence of bony continuity at the pars interarticularis, or isthmus, of the fifth lumbar vertebra is found in about 5% of adult skeletons. It is called *spondylolysis;* when bilateral it is also termed *prespondylolisthesis.* The defect is more often bilateral than unilateral. It may lead to low back pain and spondylolisthesis. Its treatment is the same as that of spondylolisthesis.

SPONDYLOLISTHESIS

Spondylolisthesis is a forward displacement of the fifth lumbar vertebra and spinal column upon the sacrum (Fig. 206) or, less commonly, of the fourth lumbar vertebra and spinal column upon the fifth lumbar vertebra. In approximately 85% of the cases the fifth lumbar vertebra is displaced on the sacrum. Apparent posterior projection of the last lumbar vertebra on the sacrum is sometimes demonstrable in lateral roentgenograms but of no

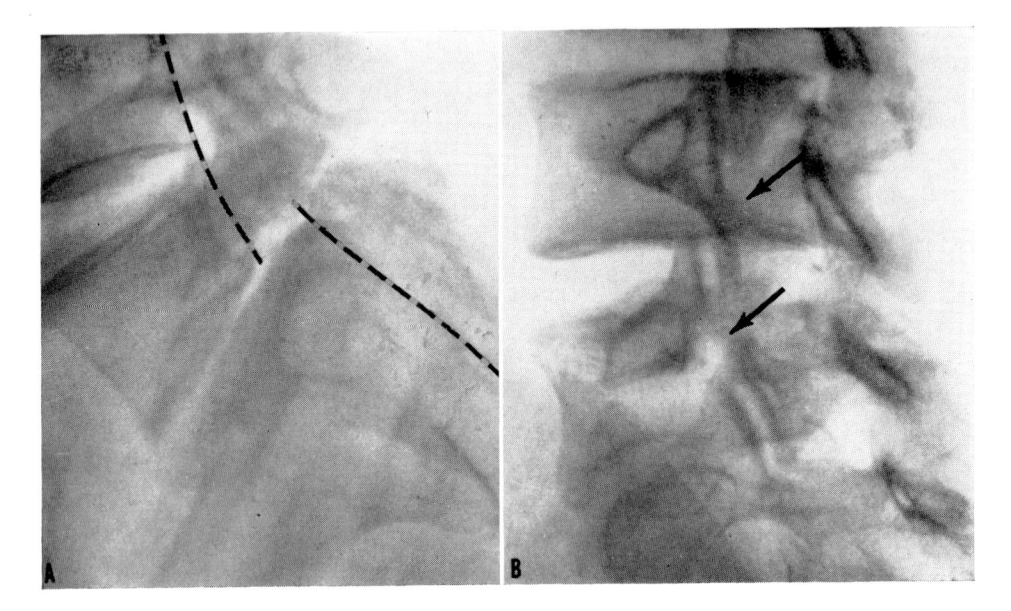

Fig. 206. Spondylolisthesis. **A,** Lateral roentgenogram. Note forward slipping of fifth lumbar vertebra upon the sacrum (shown by interrupted line). **B,** Oblique roentgenogram. Note intact isthmus of fourth lumbar vertebra and defect in isthmus of the fifth lumbar vertebra.

clinical significance. Slight actual posterior displacement, constituting the reverse of the usual spondylolisthesis, is probably related to settling of the vertebra in the presence of degenerative disk disease.

Etiology. The underlying cause of spondylolisthesis is an absence of bony continuity at each isthmus, the narrowest part of the neural arch. The pathogenesis of isthmus defects has not been established; they are believed to result from fracture, possibly at birth, or from anomalous development of the vertebra. The defect may represent an ununited fatigue fracture. Bilateral isthmus defects divide the vertebra into two separate pieces of bone. The anterior portion is made up of the body, pedicles, transverse processes, and superior articular processes. The posterior portion, often referred to as a separate neural arch, consists of the laminae, the inferior articular processes, and the spinous process. When a bilateral fifth lumbar isthmus defect is present, the bony anchorage of the vertebral column to its base on the sacrum is lost and its stability is altogether dependent upon the ligaments. The presence of a bilateral isthmus defect without forward displacement of the vertebral body, called *prespondylolisthesis* or *spondylolysis,* is thought to be a cause of low back pain.

Although the slipping or listhesis may be caused by a single severe injury, chronic postural strains are probably far more often responsible. Contributing mechanical factors are the mobility of the lumbosacral joint and the inclination of the upper sacral surface. Progressive increase of slipping in adults is uncommon; it may, however, occur in children. The symptoms are associated with narrowing of the intervertebral disk, degenerative changes in the disk, and proliferative bone changes about the intervertebral foramina.

Rarely the body of a vertebra together with its intact neural arch may become displaced forward when articular facet lesions are present; this condition has been termed *pseudospondylolisthesis* or *articular spondylolisthesis.* The displacement may produce symptoms of pressure upon the roots of the cauda equina.

Clinical picture. Pain may be severe, slight, or entirely absent. It is often well localized in the lumbosacral joint region but may radiate down one or both legs along the course of the sciatic nerve and especially into the distribution of the peroneal nerves. There is often complaint of stiffness of the back, and all of the symptoms become worse with exercise and strain. Prior to the onset of frank symptoms there may have been recurrent episodes of low back fatigue and weakness. Upon examination the low back appears lordotic. The spinous process of the detached neural arch is prominent on palpation and often is evident on inspection. There is a tender depression just above it. The sacrum is much nearer vertical than normally. In cases of extensive slipping, the torso is shortened, the ribs may rest upon the iliac crests, and the abdomen may protrude. In severe cases the pelvic inclination is decreased and the body is swayed backward. There may be marked limitation of anteroposterior motion in the affected area and considerable spasm of the erector spinae muscles. There may also be spasm of the hamstring muscles. When the condition is severe, the gait is sometimes awkward and waddling.

Spondylolisthesis is frequently found in women and is an important complication of pregnancy.

Diagnosis. Because of similarities in the clinical appearances of the back, spondylolisthesis of severe degree is occasionally confused with congenital dislocation of the hip, tuberculosis of the lumbar spine, and rickets. It may be impossible to differentiate clinically between spondylolisthesis with slight displacement and lumbosacral sprain or ruptured intervertebral disk. In spondylolisthesis the roentgenograms show the pathognomonic findings, however, of isthmus defects, seen best in oblique views, and the unmistakable forward slipping of the body of one vertebra on another.

Treatment. For cases in which the symptoms are trivial, no treatment is indicated other than posture exercises and precaution against overexertion or injury. When moderate symptoms are present, immobilization of the spine in a flexed position, by means of a plaster cast extending from the lower part of the thighs to above the costal margins, will relieve most of the acute pain. The cast should be followed by a back brace. In the milder cases an ambulatory plaster jacket or brace, together with posture exercises to strengthen the muscles of the back, may be adequate treatment. The majority of cases of spondylolisthesis can be treated by conservative means of this type.

When there is progressive increase of pain or recurrence of acute episodes of trauma that the patient cannot well avoid, surgical fusion of the last two or three lumbar vertebrae to the sacrum may be indicated. This should be followed by from six to twelve weeks of recumbency and then by a brace for a period of from six months to a year following the date of operation. The functional results are usually satisfactory. In the rare cases in which there is evidence of pressure upon the cauda equina, laminectomy should be carried out.

LESIONS OF THE LUMBAR INTERVERTEBRAL DISKS

In the lower lumbar region, degenerative changes in the intervertebral disks are a frequent cause of back pain, and rupture of disk material posteriorly is the most common cause of sciatic pain, or sciatica. Although these lesions do not necessarily affect the general health of the patient, they often result in prolonged disability. As an economic problem disk disease is enormous, for it frequently affects the wage earner and results in the loss of many man-hours of work. In addition, in some instances a person with a ruptured disk finds himself unable to return to his previous occupation and must seek training in another field.

Etiology and pathology. Before considering the clinical picture referred to as "ruptured disk," one should review the anatomy and the pathologic changes associated with aging and with trauma. The intervertebral disk consists of the nucleus pulposus, surrounded by the annulus fibrosus and enclosed above and below by the cartilaginous end-plates of the vertebral

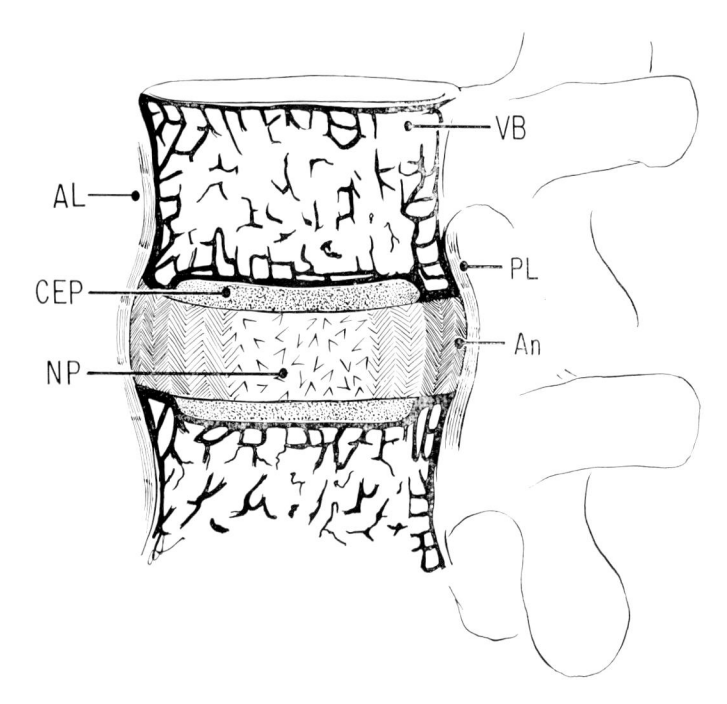

Fig. 207. Diagram of normal disk and adjacent vertebrae. **AL**, Anterior longitudinal ligament; **CEP**, cartilage end-plate; **NP**, nucleus pulposus; **VB**, vertebral body; **PL**, posterior longitudinal ligament; **An**, annulus fibrosus.

bodies (Fig. 207). The disk is reinforced by the strong anterior longitudinal ligament in front and by the posterior longitudinal ligament in back. These structures, along with the adjacent margins of the vertebral bodies, undergo characteristic, progressive changes from the beginning to the end of life. It is often impossible to distinguish sharply between what should be considered the normal aging process and what should be called pathologic.

In early life the nucleus pulposus is a gelatinous material with strong water-binding properties. Cells of notochordal origin are present in very young disks but gradually disappear. At its periphery the nucleus is more fibrous, blending with the annulus. Centrally its ultrastructure has been shown to consist of a network of fine collagen fibrils surrounded by mucopolysaccharide (principally chondroitin sulfates). The latter material accounts for the water-binding property; at birth the nucleus pulposus is 88% water. As age increases, the water content decreases; this change is associated with and is probably the result of a decrease in mucopolysaccharide. The collagen content increases at the expense of the mucopolysaccharide. Thus as age progresses the nucleus becomes more fibrous and loses some of its hydrodynamic properties. The young, healthy nucleus acts as a hydraulic shock absorber between two vertebral bodies. Since it is essentially a fluid, stresses placed upon it are equally distributed in all directions to the fibers of the annulus and to the cartilaginous end-plates, regardless of the position of adjacent vertebrae in relation to each other. Thus the danger of excess stress in any one area is minimized. As the disk loses some of these fluid properties with age, excessive localized stresses may occur and result in pathologic changes.

The annulus fibrosus surrounds the nucleus pulposus as a series of concentric fibrocartilaginous lamellae. The fibers of the lamellae run obliquely from one vertebra to the other, alternating in direction in adjacent lamellae. The peripheral fibers insert directly into the bony rim of the vertebral body as *Sharpey's fibers*. The more central fibers insert into the cartilaginous end-plates. The fibers of the annulus blend in front with the strong anterior longitudinal ligament and behind with the weaker and narrower posterior longitudinal ligament. Age changes become apparent in the annulus during the third decade of life, at which time the fibers become coarse and fissures appear in the lamellae. Thinning of the disks occurs as age advances. The thinning may be a very gradual process or may be abrupt. The causes of the decrease in disk material are several. Progressive dehydration and fibrosis of the nucleus pulposus is one; rupture of the annulus fibrosus with extrusion of disk material is another. In osteoporosis, nuclear material may compress the cartilaginous end-plates, causing the centra to become biconcave. Actual ruptures of the cartilaginous end-plates may occur. A discrete amount of nuclear material may protrude into the vertebral body as a *Schmorl's node*.

Associated with thinning of the disks and the aging changes in the nucleus and annulus, reactive changes occur about the margins of the vertebral bodies (Fig. 208). Bony spurring or lipping develops. This is similar to the

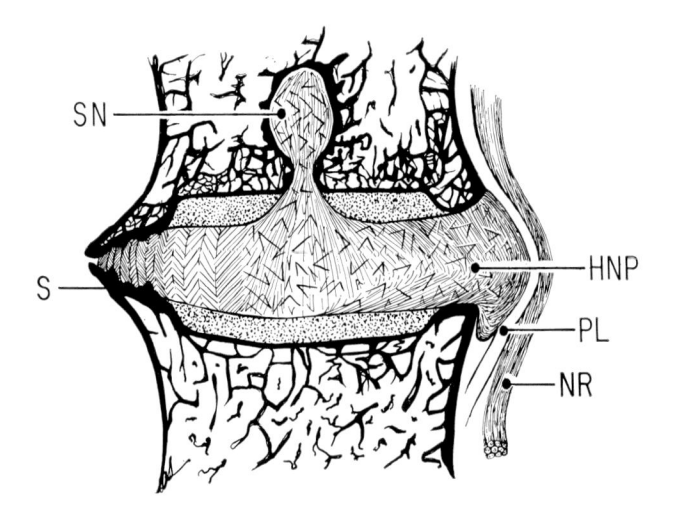

Fig. 208. Diagram of several lesions that may be associated with degenerative disk disease: marginal lipping, demonstrated by anterior bony spur, **S**; herniation of nuclear material through the cartilage end-plate into the vertebral body, forming a Schmorl's node, **SN**; posterior herniation of nucleus pulposus, **HNP**, beneath the posterior longitudinal ligament, **PL**, displacing the nerve root, **NR**.

lipping seen in osteoarthritis, but since synovial joints are not involved some authors prefer to refer to this process as *spondylosis* or *spondylophytosis*. The entire complex of changes noted here is sometimes referred to as *degenerative disk disease*. While these changes are related to aging and to wear and tear, other factors are probably involved. Why some individuals show extensive degenerative disk disease at an early age whereas others fail to do so has not been answered satisfactorily. The role of trauma in disk rupture is sometimes difficult to ascertain. Rupture of a normal disk is probably uncommon. Acute disk rupture is usually the result of a combination of acute trauma and pre-existing degenerative changes. When the degenerative changes are minimal, one may assume that relatively severe trauma is required to cause rupture. When degenerative changes in the annulus are advanced, minimal trauma such as simple forward bending may cause rupture.

As degenerative changes in the disk occur, and provided that an acute rupture does not cause nerve root pressure, the patient may experience only mild or moderate back pain and stiffness. It is probable that many cases classified under lumbosacral sprain are actually manifestations of early degenerative disk disease. In most instances the degenerative changes cause few symptoms unless the back is put under abnormal strain. It is rare, however, for an individual to pass through adult life without having experienced some back discomfort. As the degenerative changes become more advanced, the disks thinner, and the marginal lipping more marked, a certain amount of stability results from fibrosis and the approximation of adjacent vertebrae. At this stage, back symptoms may be minimal or absent; one often sees individuals in late adult life with extensive spondylosis and disk narrowing but no back complaints. These people have rather stiff backs but experience little discomfort on ordinary activity.

The herniation of nuclear material often occurs after the onset of degenerative changes but before they reach an advanced stage. Most disk ruptures occur in the third and fourth decades, which represent the most active period of adult life. The rupture may take place through the cartilaginous end-plate or through the annulus. Ruptures through the annulus usually occur in its thin, posterior portion. Disk herniation that does not involve a nerve root may result in back pain without sciatica. From the clinical standpoint, however, diagnosis of ruptured disk is made only when nerve root symptoms are present.

The herniation of nuclear material usually occurs through a small rent or tear in the annulus just lateral to the posterior midline (Fig. 209). Posterior midline ruptures are less common because the posterior longitudinal ligament is thickest in its mid-portion. The nuclear material, in the form of a bulge 5 to 15 millimeters in diameter beneath the fibers of the posterior longitudinal ligament, pushes and stretches the overlying nerve root to produce sciatic pain. Most disk herniations in the lumbar spine occur at the two lowest interspaces. Disk ruptures at the L_4-L_5 level usually involve the fifth lumbar root, which emerges between L_5 and the sacrum; ruptures at

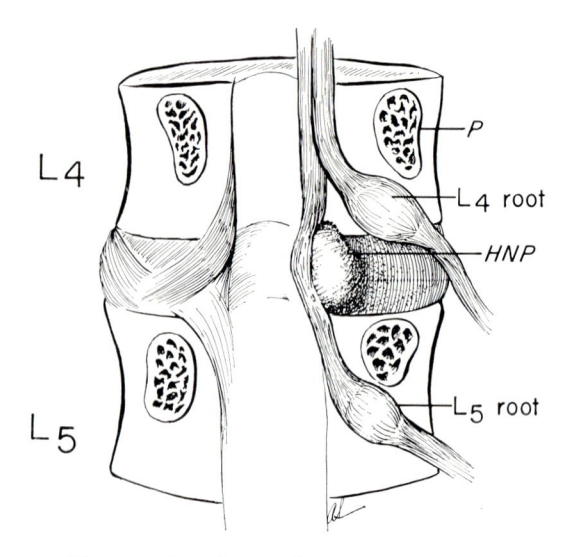

Fig. 209. Diagram of herniated nucleus pulposus, **HNP**, as seen from the back with spinous processes and laminae removed from the pedicles, **P**. Note that the disk protrusion between the fourth and fifth lumbar vertebrae impinges upon the fifth lumbar nerve root.

the lumbosacral level frequently involve the first sacral root, which leaves the spine between the first and second sacral segments.

Clinical picture. The patient's primary complaint is pain in the low back and leg. The pain is usually first noted in the back, and the onset may be either abrupt or gradual. Frequently the patient gives a history of previous attacks of nonradiating back pain diagnosed as lumbosacral strains. In some cases, but by no means the majority, the onset is associated with significant trauma. Such trauma may occur when the patient is helping to lift a heavy object and the entire load is suddenly forced upon him. He may experience an immediate snapping sensation in the low back, presumably from the acute rupture of an annulus. Other patients may date the onset to a catching sensation in the back as they were stooping; still others cannot date the onset but have become aware of gradually increasing low back discomfort. The leg pain usually appears from a few days to several weeks after the onset of back pain, but in some instances the two are associated from the beginning, and occasionally the patient complains of leg pain alone. The extremity pain is often of two types: (1) a deep, aching pain extending to the thigh and leg, and (2) a sharp, lancinating pain shooting down the extremity to the lateral side of the leg and ankle and even into certain toes. Both back pain and leg pain are aggravated by spinal motion and by factors, such as coughing or sneezing, which increase the intracranial pressure. The patient may complain also of numbness in his foot or toes, and occasionally of weakness and instability of the foot and ankle.

On examination the back is found to be held stiffly. The lumbar lordosis is flattened and often reversed. The lumbar spine may be shifted to the left or right (*sciatic scoliosis*, Fig. 200). The scoliosis may be toward or away from the painful side, the direction apparently being determined by the relationship of the protruded disk to the nerve root. If the protrusion is lateral to the root, the curvature will be to the side opposite the lesion. If the protrusion lies medial to the root, the curvature is to the same side as the lesion. Thus the back assumes the curvature most favorable to the relief of root pressure. Palpation of the back discloses tightness of the lumbar muscles from spasm, and tenderness usually localized to the interspinous ligaments of the lowest one or two lumbar segments.

Abnormalities in the lower extremities result from irritation and injury of the nerve root. Since as a rule the root is not completely destroyed by the disk protrusion, the findings are variable. Damage to the nerve root is manifested by muscle weakness and atrophy, reflex changes, and hypesthesia and other sensory disturbances. Since the first sacral root usually supplies sensation to the lateral aspect of the leg and foot, hypesthesia in this area suggests a disk protrusion at the lumbosacral level. The Achilles reflex is also supplied at this level; accordingly an absent or diminished ankle jerk is frequently found with lumbosacral disk lesions. Involvement of the fifth lumbar root by a protrusion at the L_4-L_5 level may produce hypesthesia of the dorsum of the foot and first two toes, as well as weakness of the extensor of the great toe. Motor impairment is quite variable, however, and may be so slight that it can be detected only by special tests such as electromyography. Disk herniations above the fourth lumbar vertebra, which are uncommon, may involve roots making up the femoral nerve; accordingly they may be associated with anterior thigh pain and alterations in the knee jerk. Although disk herniations may be noted at several levels simultaneously and although a large single herniation may affect more than one root, neurologic changes involving multiple roots are suggestive of other lesions, such as spinal cord tumors.

Signs of nerve root irritation may be demonstrated by any method of increasing tension upon the root. Of these the straight leg-raising test is the most obvious. The sacral plexus roots making up the sciatic nerve join within the pelvis to emerge through the sciatic foramen posteriorly. The sciatic nerve passes down the posterior aspect of the thigh to continue as the tibial nerve and terminate as its medial and lateral plantar branches. As the extremity, with the knee fully extended, is flexed at the hip, tension on the nerve is increased; actual movement of the roots within the foramina may be demonstrated in anatomic preparations, and a small manometer placed beneath the root will register a positive pressure. Thus straight leg-raising stretches the already taut root over the ruptured disk and causes an increase of pain. There are numerous variations of this confirmatory test. When the extremity has been raised to the point where pain is first noted, the patient may be asked to strain, cough, or flex his neck, or his foot may be passively dorsiflexed by the examiner, and increased sciatic pain will result. If the hip and knee are flexed and the knee then extended to the point of discomfort, the posterior tibial nerve can often be felt as a tight band in the middle of the popliteal space. A gentle flick of the nerve by the examiner's thumb may then send pain shooting up to the buttock or down to the foot.

Diagnosis. Presumptive diagnosis of intervertebral disk rupture is made on the history and physical findings. It must be remembered, however, that most of the findings are based only upon the presence of nerve root irritation. Although disk herniation is the causative lesion in the great majority of cases with root irritation at the lowest two lumbar segments, the list of conditions that have been found to mimic disk rupture is quite long. Metastatic tumors, tumors of the cauda equina or of individual nerve roots, and bone tumors primary in the spine have all been found to produce symptoms and signs very similar to those of a ruptured disk. Inflammatory conditions such as spinal tuberculosis, vertebral osteomyelitis, and Strümpell-Marie arthritis can cause irritation of a single nerve root. Many of these affections can be brought to light by means of a careful history and physical examination. The history of a mastectomy several years before, or of a little blood in the sputum, should stand out as a red flag, for it may be the physician's only warning that this "ruptured disk" is actually metastatic carcinoma from breast or lung. Some of these conditions may be ruled in or out on the basis of routine spinal roentgenograms. In other instances, particularly when the history and physical findings are atypical or suggest involvement of more than one nerve root, myelography may be necessary.

Treatment and prognosis. Since disk herniation is an acute lesion superimposed upon a degenerative process common in greater or lesser degree to all adults, one cannot expect treatment to produce the strong, painless, flexible back of a teen-ager. Accordingly the aim of treatment is to provide relief of pain and a back strong enough to allow the patient to resume his normal occupation. Occasional recurrent symptoms should be expected, and it is possible that disk rupture may occur later at another level. Nevertheless, in the majority of cases, satisfactory relief of the symptoms can be obtained by conservative means. Some of these have been described on p. 352. In the acute stage, rest in bed is the treatment of choice. The majority of patients will be most comfortable in a semi-Fowler's position with spine, hips, and knees slightly flexed. Skin traction applied to the legs or pelvis may help. Many patients can be treated conservatively at home. Those who fail to respond to home treatment can often be relieved successfully by the stricter rest program accomplished in hospital. As the patient's condition improves, exercises to strengthen the abdominal muscles and decrease the lumbar lordosis are quite helpful.

Manipulation has been used in the treatment of the ruptured disk by both qualified and unqualified practitioners. Various forms of manipulation have been advocated, including bilateral forced flexion of the hips and knees on the pelvis with an accompanying rotary movement, bilateral or unilateral straight leg-raising, and hyperextension of the spine or hips. The movements are gross, the lesion small. Nevertheless, in some instances sudden and dramatic relief of pain has been noted. Such relief may have resulted from a slight shift in the position of the nuclear material, or the stretch may have severed the nerve root. Forceful manipulation in patients with osteoporosis, arthritis, or destructive lesions of the vertebrae may cause serious damage.

Certain patients, probably less than one fourth of those with ruptured lumbar disks, require surgical treatment. The indications for disk surgery are (1) severe symptoms that fail to improve on an adequate conservative program, (2) progressive neurologic involvement, and (3) moderately severe symptoms with failure of conservative therapy when economic or other factors make it difficult for the patient to continue nonsurgical treatment. It is unfortunate that many patients believe that surgical removal of the disk, like an appendectomy, eliminates the offending condition. This, of course, is not true. Degenerative disk disease remains, and symptoms arising at other levels are always possible. Surgical treatment usually consists of a partial laminectomy, exposure of the protruding mass, and excision of the mass as well as all nuclear material remaining in the disk. When back symptoms have been a prominent feature, spinal arthrodesis may be carried out at the time of disk surgery. In most instances, however, arthrodesis is unnecessary.

OTHER LESIONS OF MUSCLE AND FASCIA
Myofascitis

Localized areas of tenderness and sometimes induration are occasionally found in the lumbodorsal fascia and its underlying muscle, as well as along the attachments of these structures to the iliac crests. The pathologic nature of these areas is unknown; it seems likely that a number of different factors are involved. The terms "myositis" or "fibrositis" are sometimes used to describe such conditions, but the presence of a microscopically demonstrable inflammatory reaction in the designated tissue is questionable, and perhaps the term "myofascial pain," used by Wiles, is sufficient. Most of these affections respond to the use of local heat and massage. When the lesion is well localized, its infiltration with a local anesthetic may bring relief.

Herniation of fascial fat

Lobules of fat may herniate through small defects in the lumbodorsal fascia. In many instances these fatty nodules are painless; they are frequently palpated as an incidental finding in patients with low back pain of other cause. At times, however, such a nodule is quite tender and is associated with diffuse low back pain. Injection with a local anesthetic relieves both the pain and the tenderness. If the symptoms recur after several such injections, excision of the nodule is recommended.

COMMON OSTEOARTICULAR LESIONS OF INFECTIOUS, NEOPLASTIC, OR TRAUMATIC NATURE

Specific pathologic conditions of the bones and joints, not limited necessarily to the lumbosacral or sacroiliac joints, often cause low back pain directly or lead to an impaired mechanical resistance that may augment the incidence of sprain. Low-grade infections, neoplastic processes, and old fractures are examples. In young adults, Strümpell-Marie arthritis is a frequent cause of low back pain. In stout individuals over 40 years of age, with proliferative bone changes about the joint margins, susceptibility to low back pain following acute or chronic strain is greatly increased, and the symptoms are likely to persist for long periods. Arthritic changes in the lower lumbar and lumbosacral articular facets constitute a common and important cause of low back pain and may be associated with pain that radiates to the legs.

Low back pain is sometimes associated with a localized increase of density in the ilia adjacent to the sacroiliac joints; this condition is usually found in women and has been called *osteitis condensans ilii*. In adolescents sacroiliac symptoms are sometimes associated with roentgenographic changes in the sacroiliac joint surfaces, resembling bone destruction and suggestive of osteochondritis. The postural stresses associated with conditions such as flat feet or inequality of leg length may predispose an individual to low back pain.

VISCERAL LESIONS THAT MAY CAUSE LOW BACK PAIN

Low back pain unassociated with local osteoarticular changes may be caused by any of a wide variety of visceral diseases. This pain, although located definitely over a bone or joint by the patient, is entirely of referred type. A carefully performed history and physical examination will usually reveal the source of the pain. Pain in the low back is particularly common in the course of the following disorders: gastrointestinal, urologic, and gynecologic diseases; lesions of the central nervous system; sciatic neuritis; lesions of the retroperitoneal structures; generalized infectious diseases; and vascular lesions.

Gastrointestinal diseases

Various disorders of the gastrointestinal tract may produce back symptoms. The diagnosis is not easily confused, however, since the symptoms are not usually aggravated by mechanical factors such as bending or lifting. Chronic pancreatitis or posterior perforation of an ulcer may give rise to lumbar pain.

Urologic diseases

Most of the diseases of the genitourinary tract may at times cause moderate or severe low back pain. This is particularly true of the infections and tumors of the prostate gland.

Gynecologic diseases

Tumors of the female pelvic organs, retroversion and retroflexion of the uterus, and endometriosis may lead to referred pain in the low back. Over-emphasis has sometimes been placed on these conditions, however, with the result that gynecologic operations have sometimes been done in the hope of relieving low back pain that was actually of musculoskeletal origin. In very rare instances the sacral plexus has been involved by endometriosis, causing typical sciatica during menstruation.

Lesions of the central nervous system

Tabes, meningitis, syringomyelia, lateral sclerosis, and similar conditions occasionally give rise to pain in the low back. Tumors of the spinal cord are often accompanied by low back pain. Tumors of the cauda equina are likely to be evidenced by pain radiating into one or both legs and by spasm of the hamstring muscles.

Sciatic neuritis

Primary sciatic neuritis, a rare affection, is usually accompanied by pain referred to the low back.

Lesions of the retroperitoneal structures

Infections and tumors in the retroperitoneal area may cause pain in the low back.

Generalized infectious diseases

Diseases such as influenza, undulant fever, and septicemia are often accompanied by pain in the low back.

Vascular lesions

Occlusion of the aorta or the common iliac arteries may cause back, buttock, or thigh pain. Such pain may simulate that of disk disorders. It differs, however, in that it is not aggravated by single motions such as forward bending but, rather, is brought on by more prolonged activity such as walking. Changes in the peripheral pulses and the presence of calcification in roentgenograms of the aorta or iliac arteries are helpful in establishing the diagnosis.

COCCYGODYNIA

Pain about the coccyx and lower part of the sacrum, or coccygodynia, is in many cases a result of sprain of the sacrococcygeal ligaments and often follows a direct blow or fall, such as may be occasioned by sitting down suddenly or sliding down a flight of stairs. It is sometimes caused by sitting for a long period on a hard surface. The pain is not always experienced immediately after the injury but may develop gradually later. Coccygodynia sometimes begins insidiously without evident trauma and may be a result of faulty posture. It is occasionally seen after severe weight loss, when thinning of the buttocks leaves the coccyx relatively unprotected and vulnerable to trauma.

Clinical picture. There is usually an aching, nagging pain located near the sacrococcygeal junction. At times there may be shooting pains in the buttocks or even down into the legs. These pains are especially severe when the patient is sitting on a hard surface or when arising after sitting for any length of time. There may be considerable pain on defecation. When the condition occurs in an individual with a psychoneurotic personality, the symptoms may be markedly exaggerated. Examination shows a tender coccyx, which on rectal examination is sometimes rough and angulated. It may be abnormally mobile or fixed.

Diagnosis. The diagnosis should be made with caution, since pain in the coccygeal region is often associated with arthritis of the low back or with psychoneurosis. Roentgenograms occasionally show deviation of the coccyx forward or to one side as a result of either injury or developmental variation, but identical changes occur in many individuals who have no symptoms.

Treatment. In acute traumatic cases showing displacement of the coccyx, the deformity may be reduced by gentle manipulation, especially if the coccyx has been angulated forward and its motion appears to be restricted. Hot baths, strapping across the buttocks and the low back, and massage may afford considerable relief. The patient should be instructed to sit on cushions or soft chairs. Occasionally, however, sitting upon cushions that are very soft may cause the buttocks to spread and may thus increase the pain. The use of a large rubber ring is sometimes indicated to relieve the pressure occasioned by sitting. An alternative method is to have the patient sit on a firm cushion, which is placed forward in the chair. The application of a thick piece of felt, with an opening cut out over the coccyx to prevent pressure, is another method of treatment. All exercise that increases the pain should be avoided. Injection of a local anesthetic and hydrocortisone in the region of the sacrococcygeal joint has sometimes been helpful.

If the pain cannot be relieved by nonsurgical measures, excision of the coccyx, which can be carried out very simply, will often relieve the patient of all symptoms. Before resort is made to operation, however, great care should be taken to remove all contributing causes of the discomfort, since in occasional cases the diagnosis is somewhat uncertain and the relief of pain following operation is incomplete. If a psychoneurosis is present, it should be treated before surgery is contemplated.

COMMENT

Current treatment of patients with low back pain is not uniformly satisfactory. In some cases the symptoms may be prolonged because of insufficient rest of the back in the acute stage, inadequate support of the back, or too early resumption of activity. With conservative treatment that is efficient and thorough the great majority of mechanical disorders of the back can be relieved without resort to surgery. On the other hand, when a patient is unable to afford a prolonged period of such care, surgical treatment may be desirable for economic reasons to enable him to resume his occupation. One cannot be too cautious, however, in operating upon the back of a patient who has a pending compensation or insurance claim or who shows any evidence of an abnormal psychosomatic state.

Many unorthodox practitioners and cultists thrive on the frequent failure of physicians to appreciate or employ optimal treatment of the common affections that cause low back pain. Most of the cultists' activity involves manipulation to break up adhesions and so relieve pain. The patient may be told that a dislocated joint or bone has been put back into place, a statement which makes a profound impression on the lay mind. Much misunderstanding on the part of the patient will be avoided if the physician can recognize and explain carefully to the patient the true nature of the problems involved in the treatment of low back pain.

CHAPTER 18

Affections of the hip

THE BALL-AND-SOCKET STRUCTURE of the hip joint allows a wide range of motion that is exceeded in no other joint of the body except the shoulder. At the same time a remarkable degree of stability is provided by the close fit of the femoral head into the acetabulum and its deepening lip, the glenoid labrum, and by the support of the strongest capsular ligaments and the thickest musculature of the body. Of all the joints, the hip is most deeply situated. This relative inaccessibility increases the difficulty of diagnosing hip lesions, renders thorough operative exposure of the joint arduous, and so plays a large part in making affections of the hip one of the most challenging parts of orthopaedic surgery.

The blood supply to the femoral head is of crucial importance in disorders of the hip, and especially in relation to hip affections of childhood and adolescence, hip fractures, and hip surgery. Injection studies by Trueta and others have shown that the sources of blood for the femoral head vary with age (Fig. 210). They include (1) retinacular arteries, which arise from the medial circumflex artery, extend up the femoral neck between the bone and its synovial covering, and form the main vascular source throughout life and usually the only source in young children; (2) the artery of the ligamentum teres, arising from the obturator or medial femoral circumflex artery, which is inconstant and supplies at most only a limited segment of the head; and (3) the nutrient artery or arteries of the femoral shaft, which arise from perforating branches of the deep femoral artery, contribute little or no circulation to the epiphysis in children, and may be a supplementary source in some adults. The posterior retinacular arteries, sometimes inaccurately termed capsular arteries, are the chief source of circulation to the femoral head.

The especial affections of the hip that are discussed in this chapter can be grouped conveniently according to the location of the lesion. *Coxa plana* and *slipping of the upper femoral epiphysis* are common and important entities characterized by pathologic changes in the epiphysis or at the epiphyseal plate. *Congenital coxa vara* and *coxa valga,* marked by alterations in the angle of femoral neck to femoral shaft, are less common. *Pathologic dislocation of the hip* and *intrapelvic protrusion of the acetabulum*

Affections of the hip 373

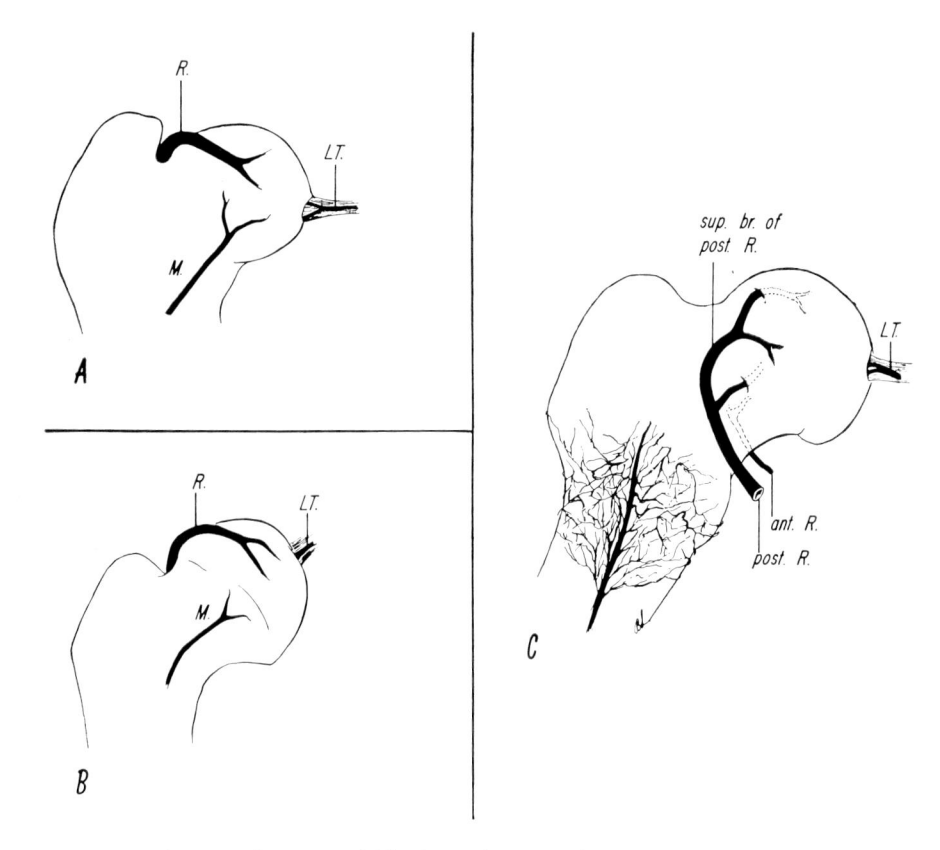

Fig. 210. Schematic drawings of blood supply to the femoral head, of which there are three sources:

(1) Retinacular arteries, **R**, ascend the neck between synovium and bone. Their posterior group, arising from the medial femoral circumflex, includes a superior branch (the lateral epiphyseal artery of Trueta) which is the main vascular supply to the head in adults and usually the only supply in children prior to penetration of the epiphyseal cartilage by the artery of the ligamentum teres. The anterior retinacular artery, from the lateral femoral circumflex, appears to be inconstant and relatively unimportant.

(2) Artery of ligamentum teres, **LT**, arising from obturator, medial femoral circumflex, or both, is present in only 33% of children but over 70% of adults. Never the chief vascular supply to the head, it may be supplementary to the vital supply from the retinacular arteries.

(3) Superior branch of nutrient artery of femoral shaft, **M**, ascends in medullary cavity, traverses metaphysis, and anastomoses with cervical branches of the retinacular arteries. Not crossing epiphyseal plate before age 13 years, it is unimportant as concerns the capital epiphysis in children but a supplementary source for the head in some adults.

A, At birth (anterior view), the retinacular and metaphyseal supplies are constant and that via the ligamentum teres inconstant. **B**, At ages 4 to 7 years (anterior view), the retinacular arteries are usually the only significant supply to the bony epiphysis, since the ligamentum teres and metaphyseal vessels meet cartilaginous barriers. In preadolescence the artery of the ligamentum teres begins to enter the bony epiphysis from above, and in adolescence the metaphyseal arteries begin to enter it from below. **C**, In the adult (posterior view), the head is supplied chiefly by the retinacular arteries, the ligamentum teres and metaphyseal vessels being inconstant or meager contributors.

are characterized by a changed relationship between femur and pelvis. To be remembered also in the diagnosis of hip affections are lesions of the soft tissues, which include *synovitis, bursitis,* and *snapping hip.*

COXA PLANA (LEGG-CALVÉ-PERTHES DISEASE, AVASCULAR NECROSIS OF THE CAPITAL FEMORAL EPIPHYSIS)

Coxa plana is a flattening of the epiphysis of the head of the femur due to osseous changes without primary involvement of the articular cartilage. It was described in 1909 by Legg in Boston and by Waldenström in Sweden, and in 1910 by Calvé in France and Perthes in Germany. Before the affection was recognized as an independent entity these cases were believed to represent a mild form of tuberculosis of the hip.

Coxa plana occurs in children between the ages of 3 and 12 years and is found much more commonly in boys than in girls. Unilateral involvement is more common than bilateral.

Etiology. The cause of the pathologic changes occurring in coxa plana has not been established. Most observers believe that a circulatory disturbance due to trauma or strain is a primary factor. Slight injury of the femoral head, resulting in a disturbance of the circulation between epiphysis and femoral neck, may be responsible. Sometimes children exhibit a partial subluxation of the hip as a result of an unusual shallowness of the acetabulum and an increase in the normal anteversion of the neck of the femur; it has been supposed that weight bearing on abnormal joint structures of this kind may cause the pathologic changes in the femoral head.

Pathology. Massive subchondral necrosis of the bone and marrow of the epiphysis of the femoral head takes place. It is followed by disintegration and absorption of the dead bone and its replacement by new, living bone. Collapse of the head may occur, producing a characteristic flattening. As new bone is formed, healing takes place and the fragmented areas become reorganized into a smooth, regular mass of bone, which rarely, however, regains the shape and appearance of a completely normal epiphysis. The regeneration and return to the normal shape usually become more nearly complete in the younger than in the older child. The articular cartilage usually remains smooth; it continues to grow. The synovial membrane and capsule become thickened.

Clinical picture. The most constant early sign is a limp, which is associated with muscular spasm and may or may not be accompanied by pain. The pain is often referred to the inner side of the thigh or knee. As the disease progresses, the limp persists and may become more severe. The hip suffers slight limitation of all motions, and particularly of internal rotation and abduction. In rare instances all of the symptoms may be exaggerated and the disability may be severe. A moderate flexion and adduction deformity with prominence of the greater trochanter may develop. There is atrophy of the muscles of the hip, thigh, and leg. Thickening of the joint capsule is sometimes palpable, giving a boggy feel, and usually slight shortening of the leg is demonstrable. During the stage of repair the signs and symptoms become less severe and the hip may appear almost normal. Later in life, however, the hip may show evidence of a degenerative process that has the appearance of an osteoarthritis *(malum coxae senilis,* p. 189).

Roentgenographic picture. The stages of degeneration and repair can be visualized by roentgenographic examinations (Figs. 211 to 213). Small areas of resorption appear in the femoral neck adjacent to the epiphyseal plate. In early cases the epiphysis shows thinning or flattening and in many instances "fragmentation." Within the head appear dense areas which become less conspicuous as healing takes place. The neck becomes very broad and short and may present a coxa vara. The acetabulum changes in shape to correspond with the deformity of the femoral head. Two types of deformity of the head are observed: (1) the *cap type,* in which the head of the femur has the appearance of a jockey cap, and (2) the *mushroom type,* in which the entire head is flattened. During the stage of "fragmentation" the epiphysis may contain several bony areas that later, during the stage of "repair," can be seen to coalesce into a single mass of healing bone. Flattening and broadening of the head may cause it to protrude laterally from the acetabulum. The senior author has observed in a high percentage of the cases an increase in the normal anterior torsion of the femur (anteversion), as determined by roentgenograms made with a special positioning technic.

Diagnosis. Coxa plana is to be differentiated from early tuberculosis, rheumatoid arthritis, transient synovitis, slipping of the upper femoral epiphysis, congenital dysplasia of the hip, and congenital coxa vara.

Bilateral coxa plana must also be distinguished from *multiple epiphyseal dysplasia,* an uncommon developmental affection, often familial, which is usually manifested by hip pain and stiffness, as well as roentgenographic changes in the femoral head epiphyses. Commonly the child with multiple epiphyseal dysplasia also shows changes in the knees, stubby digits, and shortness of stature.

Prognosis. Coxa plana is a self-limited disease with a constant tendency toward spontaneous recovery as the cycle of avascular necrosis, revascularization, resorption of necrotic bone, and its replacement by living bone proceeds. The prognosis in the mushroom type of head is better than that in the cap type. It is more favorable in younger children than in older. It has been repeatedly demonstrated that relieving the strain of weight bearing by means of traction, recumbency in plaster or splints, or crutches during the stages of degeneration and repair minimizes the progressive distortion of the head. The symptoms may disappear, but further flattening of the head is likely to develop and persist. The functional end result when weight bearing is prevented is usually very good, but, on the other hand, there may be a permanent limp and restriction of hip motion. Without early treatment, the femoral head and neck may develop marked deformity (Fig. 214), which is likely to lead to severe disability of the hip.

Treatment. The primary consideration is rest, particularly from the

376   *Handbook of orthopaedic surgery*

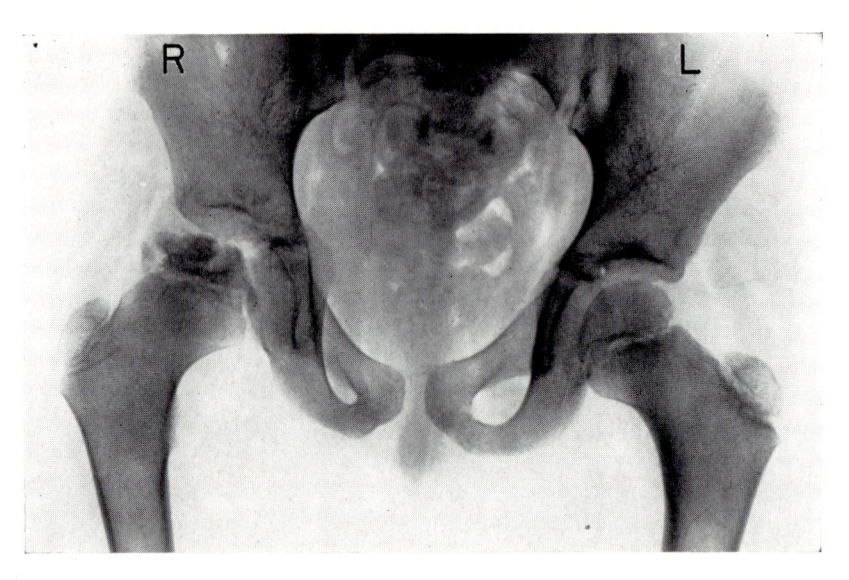

Fig. 211. Roentgenogram of pelvis showing coxa plana of right hip in a boy 8½ years of age. Note fragmentation of right capital epiphysis with areas of increased density and flattening.

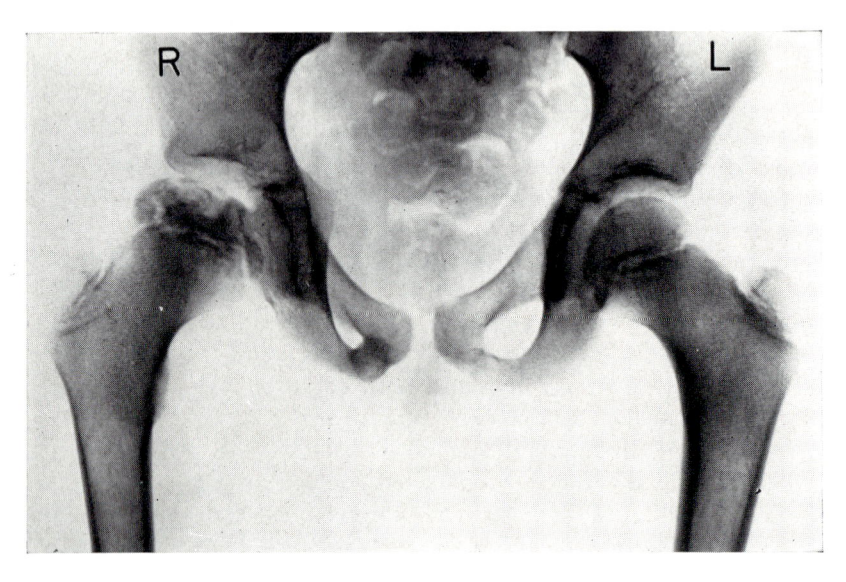

Fig. 212. Roentgenogram of same patient as shown in Fig. 211, nine months later. Note reshaping of right capital epiphysis with new bone formation. Fragmentation is still evident.

Affections of the hip 377

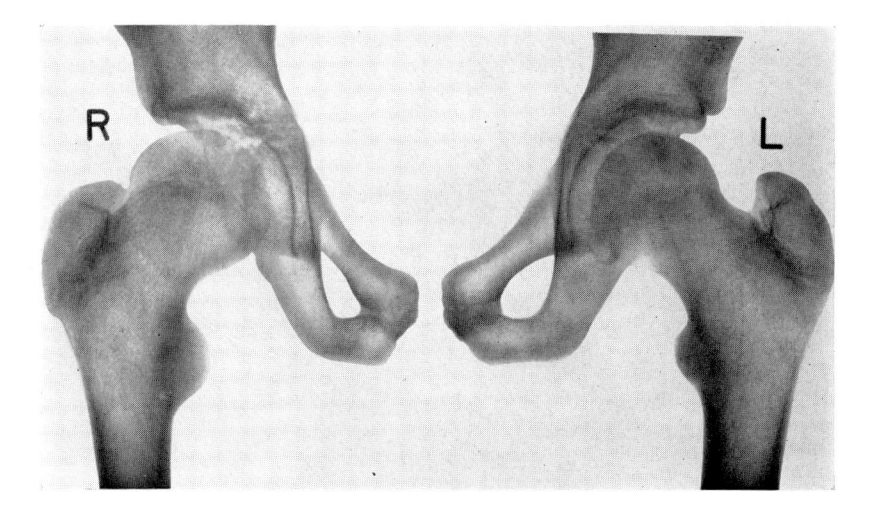

Fig. 213. Roentgenogram of same patient as shown in Figs. 211 and 212, five years after Fig. 211; patient is now 13½ years old. Note well-rounded right femoral head, which is slightly larger than the left. The treatment, which lasted for three years, consisted of traction in recumbency followed by crutches and a hip sling.

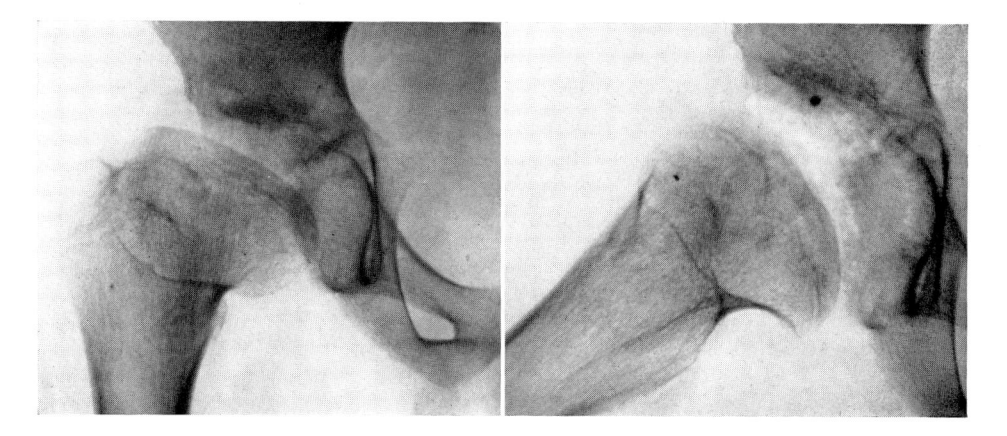

Fig. 214. Anteroposterior and lateral roentgenograms of coxa plana in a 12-year-old boy who had had a limp for three years before being brought to a physician for treatment. Note flat, wide femoral head; short, thick femoral neck; and secondary changes in the acetabulum.

378   Handbook of orthopaedic surgery

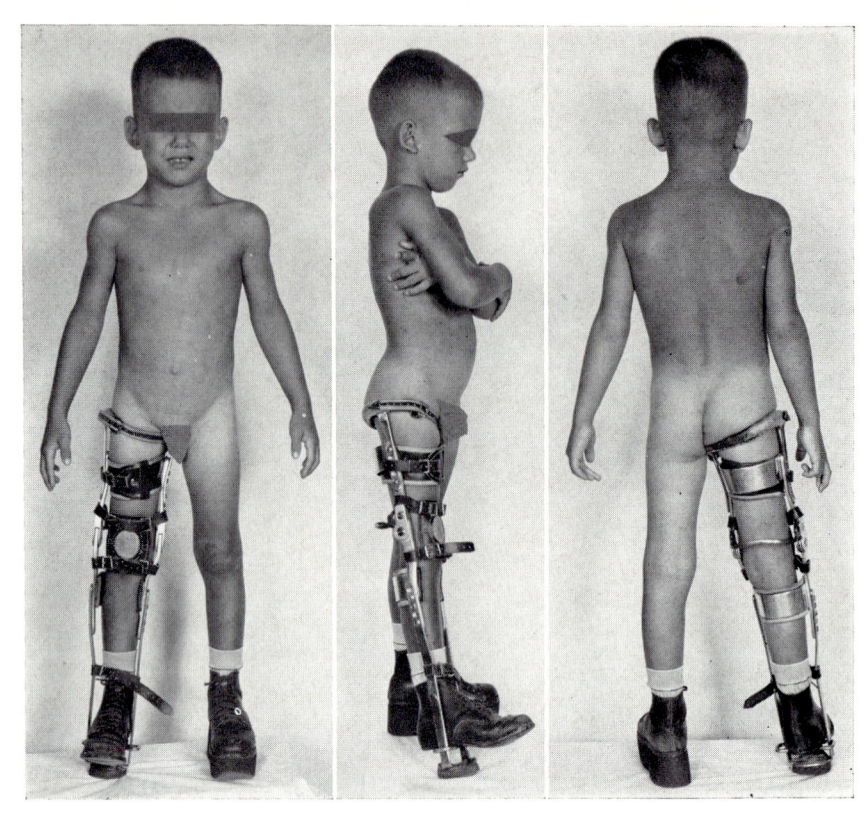

Fig. 215. Ischial weight-bearing brace with knee lock and patten bottom to allow standing and walking without bearing weight on the right hip. To keep the pelvis level, left shoe is elevated.

strain of weight bearing. When pain, muscle spasm, or deformity is present, skin traction is indicated. Rest in bed should be continued until there is no pain or muscle spasm on motion and until there is definite roentgenographic evidence of repair. The hip should then be protected either by the use of a Thomas walking caliper splint that allows no weight bearing through the hip joint (Fig. 215), by the use of crutches accompanied by a high-sole shoe on the sound leg, or by the use of crutches and a sling from the lower leg of the affected side to the shoulder of the opposite side, allowing weight bearing on the sound leg only (Fig. 216). In some children's hospitals skin traction in bed is continued until roentgenographic evidence of nearly complete repair is present, which may be as long as twelve to twenty-four months. Following this treatment, strenuous activity that involves weight bearing should be avoided until the roentgenograms indicate that an end stage of repair has been reached.

COXA VARA

Coxa vara is an abnormality of the upper end of the femur, consisting of a decrease in the neck-shaft angle (angle of inclination) and hence resulting

Affections of the hip 379

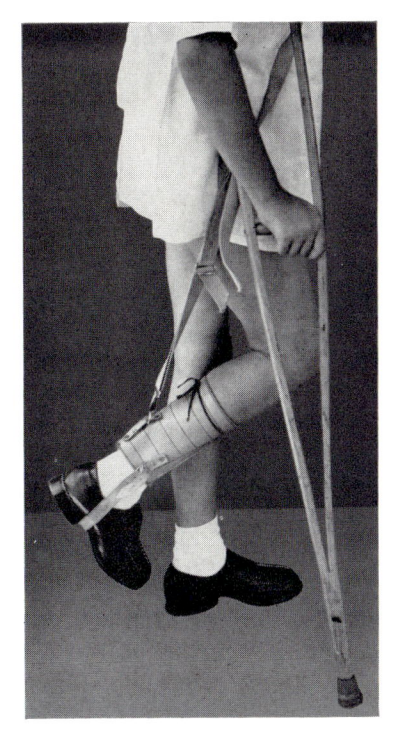

Fig. 216. Snyder-Fort hip sling and crutches. Leg cuff with shoe strap is attached to a strap that circles the opposite shoulder to suspend the hip and knee in flexion and prevent weight bearing on the affected hip.

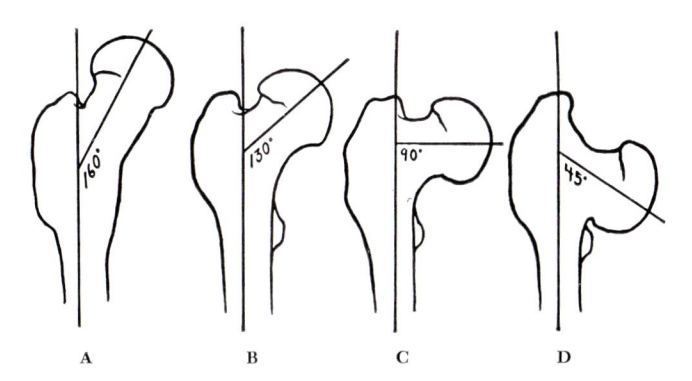

Fig. 217. Angles of femoral neck to shaft. **A**, Coxa valga. **B**, Normal. **C**, Moderate coxa vara. **D**, Severe coxa vara.

380 *Handbook of orthopaedic surgery*

in a shortening of the extremity (Fig. 217). Cases of coxa vara can be classified according to whether the primary anatomic change is in the neck *(cervical)*, in the head *(epiphyseal)*, or in both neck and head *(cervico-epiphyseal)*.

Etiology. Coxa vara may be congenital or acquired. The acquired form is by far the more common. It may develop as a result of rickets, osteomalacia, osteitis deformans, or other bone diseases. It may occur also in the end stages of coxa plana or of congenital dislocation of the hip with or without reduction; it is also seen after slipping of the capital femoral epiphysis, intertrochanteric fracture of the femur that has not been properly reduced and immobilized, and greenstick fracture of the neck of the femur in childhood.

Congenital coxa vara and slipping of the upper femoral epiphysis are of especial interest and importance and will be discussed as separate entities.

CONGENITAL COXA VARA

Congenital coxa vara is usually first observed in early childhood but may not be recognized until later in life. It is usually bilateral and of the cervical type. It is sometimes associated with other congenital defects, especially in the femur.

Etiology. The cause of congenital coxa vara is thought to be a congenital or growth defect of the femoral neck.

Clinical picture. Often the first evidences of the affection appear after an episode of slight trauma. The complaint may be weakness and stiffness in the leg, together with an awkward gait or limp. The range of abduction and internal rotation is usually restricted, while that of adduction and external rotation may be increased. A deformity characterized by prominence of the greater trochanter and external rotation of the extremity may develop. The amount of actual shortening depends upon the extent of the depression of head and neck of the femur on the shaft; it is usually from 2 to 4 cm. Atrophy of the muscles is always marked. There is usually little or no associated pain. At times all of the discomfort is referred to the thigh or knee.

In bilateral coxa vara there may be a characteristic gait, the so-called "duck waddle," in which the body sways from side to side; this is quite similar to the gait seen in bilateral congenital dislocation of the hip.

Roentgenographic picture. In the young child, in addition to the decreased neck-shaft angle, a frequent roentgenographic change is the demarcation of a triangular area of bone in the lower side of the femoral neck close to the head; the epiphyseal line lies on one side of this area, and across the neck on the other side is an abnormal band of decreased density. The head of the femur is situated low in an acetabulum that is often shallow and sloping and that may appear abnormally wide (Fig. 218).

In older cases the depression of the head and neck on the shaft becomes more marked, and the triangular area of bone fuses to the neck to assume

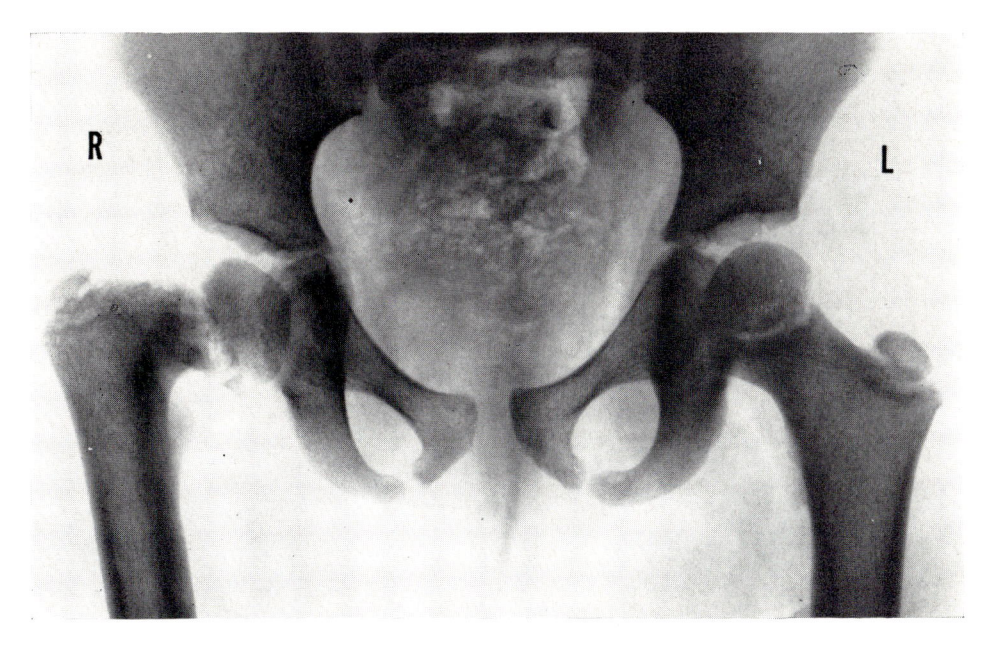

Fig. 218. Roentgenogram of pelvis of 4-year-old girl showing right congenital coxa vara. Note decreased neck-shaft angle and irregular ossification at epiphyseal line.

the appearance of a dependent lip. There is usually a marked upward prominence of the greater trochanter and upper part of the shaft.

Diagnosis. The diagnosis is made from the clinical picture together with the roentgenographic evidence of decrease in the angle of the neck of the femur to its shaft.

Differential diagnosis. Tuberculosis, slipping of the capital femoral epiphysis, congenital dislocation or subluxation of the hip, and coxa plana must be carefully differentiated from congenital coxa vara.

Treatment. When there is little deformity, protection of the hip against unusual weight-bearing stresses constitutes adequate treatment. Fixed adduction deformity should be corrected by an abduction osteotomy through the trochanteric or subtrochanteric area (Figs. 219 and 220). In severe cases in adults, a reconstruction operation or arthrodesis may be indicated for the relief of pain and disability.

SLIPPING OF THE CAPITAL FEMORAL EPIPHYSIS (EPIPHYSEAL OR ADOLESCENT COXA VARA)

Slipping of the upper femoral epiphysis is most often observed in children between 10 and 16 years of age and is more common in boys than in girls. In about 40% of the cases, both hips are affected. In most cases a history of trauma or strain can be elicited, but the traumatic episode is often trivial. Slipping of the upper femoral epiphysis occurs in two types of children: (1) obese children with undeveloped sexual characteristics (Fig. 221) and (2) very tall, thin children. Many of these patients give a his-

382   *Handbook of orthopaedic surgery*

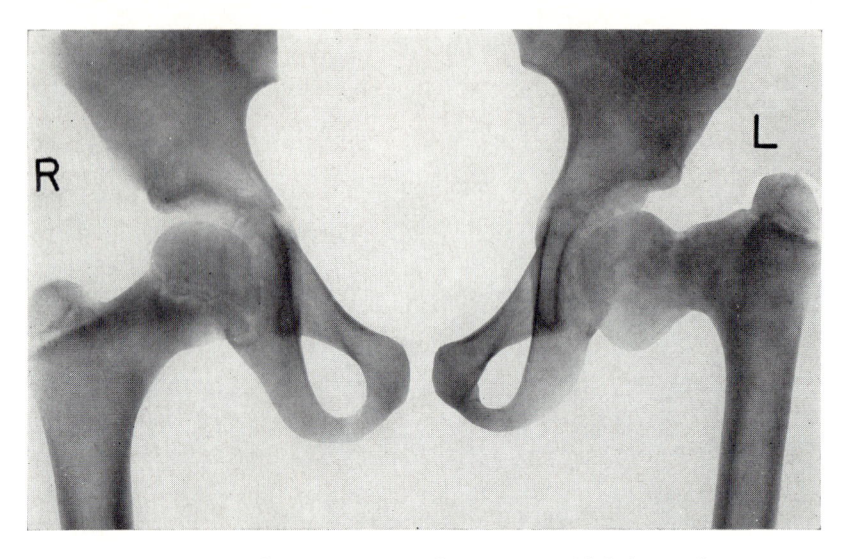

Fig. 219. Roentgenogram showing congenital coxa vara of left hip in boy 11 years of age. The neck-shaft angle of the left femur is 75 degrees as compared with 120 degrees on the right. Note distortion of the epiphysis and neck with prominence of greater trochanter. Left leg is 1 inch shorter than right leg.

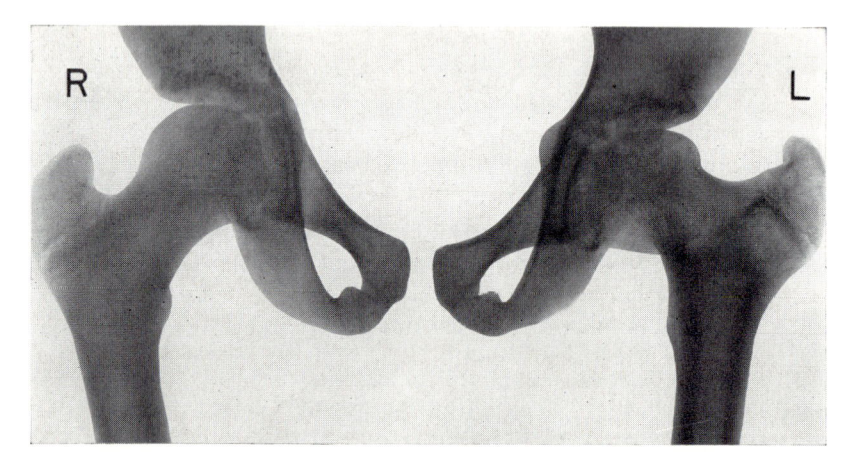

Fig. 220. Roentgenogram showing congenital coxa vara of left hip (same case as shown in Fig. 219) three years following subtrochanteric osteotomy. Neck-shaft angles are now 120 degrees on the left and 125 degrees on the right. Note continued prominence of the left greater trochanter. The leg lengths are equal.

Affections of the hip 383

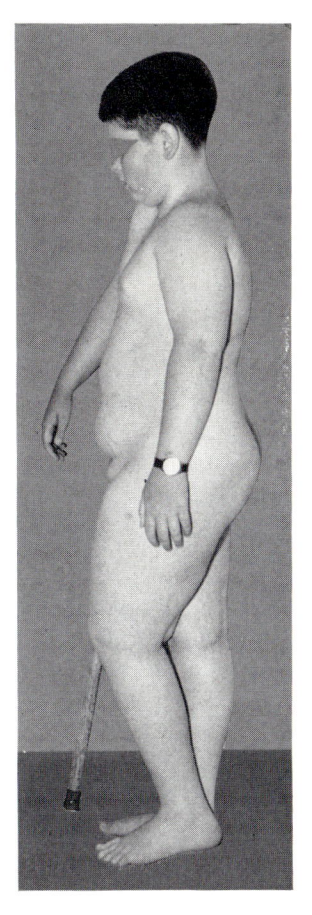

Fig. 221. Tall, obese body type seen frequently in slipping of the upper femoral epiphysis. This 12-year-old boy had slipping of the head of his left femur.

tory of rapid skeletal growth immediately preceding displacement of the epiphysis.

The underlying cause of the epiphyseal slipping is unknown. Endocrine factors may play a part, but no specific endocrine abnormality has yet been proved. The head of the femur becomes displaced downward and backward on the neck (Fig. 222), which retains its normal angle but which later may show roentgenographic evidence of posterior torsion.

Clinical picture. When there is no history of trauma, the onset is usually very gradual, the early symptoms being fatigue after walking or standing and later a slight amount of pain and stiffness, and a limp. The diagnosis should be suspected in any adolescent who has these symptoms and shows a slight restriction of internal rotation of the hip. After trauma the symptoms may either develop immediately or come on gradually. The degree of trauma apparently has little effect on the extent of the disability. The affected extremity gradually becomes shorter and smaller, and the range of

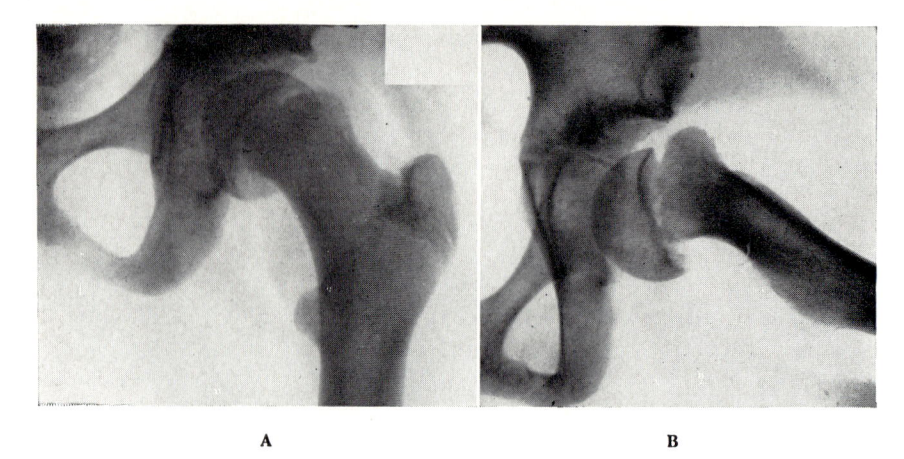

Fig. 222. Anteroposterior, **A**, and lateral, **B**, roentgenograms showing slipping of upper femoral epiphysis in girl 11 years of age. Note upward slipping of the neck of the femur. The head has become displaced downward and backward.

motion, especially of internal rotation and abduction, becomes restricted. Hyperextension may be more easily carried out on the affected side than on the normal. When the affected hip is flexed, it tends to abduct and rotate externally. When the displacement of the epiphysis is marked, the extremity may assume a position of flexion, abduction, and external rotation. At first the discomfort may consist of referred pain in the knee, but later the pain is located in the hip. There is usually pain about the anterior aspect of the hip when the limits of its range of motion are reached. Tenderness may be present about the anterior and lateral aspects of the hip.

Roentgenographic picture. Early slipping can often be recognized in the lateral roentgenogram before it becomes apparent in the anteroposterior view. When further slipping has taken place, the anteroposterior view may show a displacement of the neck upward and forward on the head of the

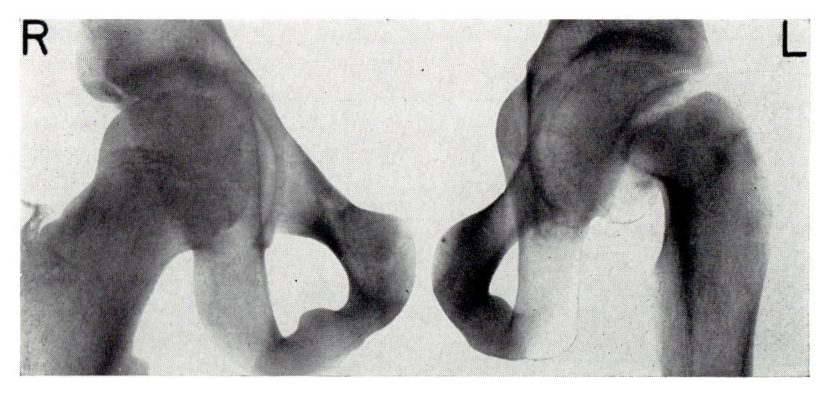

Fig. 223. Anteroposterior roentgenogram showing slipped capital femoral epiphysis of the left hip in a boy 14 years of age. Note upward displacement of neck of femur.

Affections of the hip 385

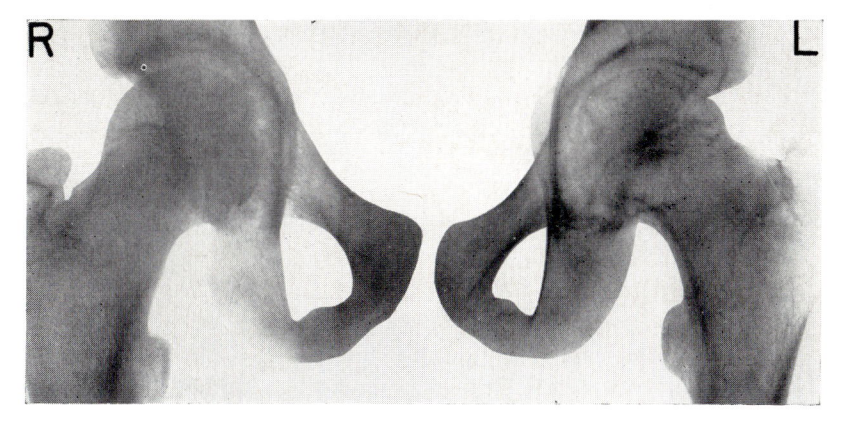

Fig. 224. Roentgenogram of same case as shown in Fig. 223, two months after reduction by skeletal traction and closed manipulation. Note almost normal relationship between capital epiphysis and neck of the femur.

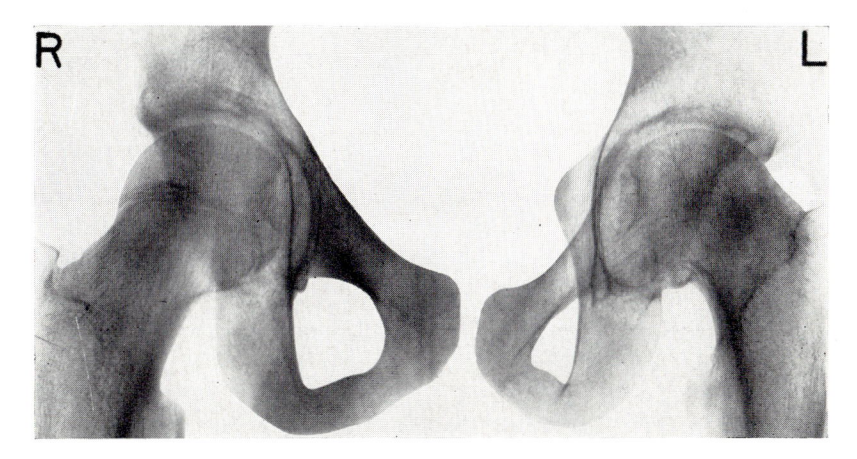

Fig. 225. Roentgenogram of same case as shown in Figs. 223 and 224, eighteen months after closed reduction. In left hip the epiphyseal line has become obliterated, the femoral head is of uneven density, the head and neck are slightly deformed, and slight secondary changes are apparent in the acetabulum. At this time the mobility of the left hip was about half that of the normal right hip.

femur so that the lowest point of the proximal end of the neck projects as a beaklike process (Fig. 223). The upper part of the neck is lengthened, the lower part is shortened, and the whole neck becomes bowed and exhibits coxa vara. New bone may form between the lower border of the neck and the overhanging head. In advanced stages the femoral head appears quite atrophic, especially in its lower half, and the neck is very thick and short. After severe trauma, the roentgenogram may demonstrate complete separation of the head from the neck of the femur.

Diagnosis. Slipping of the upper femoral epiphysis is to be differentiated from early tuberculosis of the hip, coxa plana, congenital coxa vara, subacute infectious processes, and fracture. Roentgenograms are necessary to establish the diagnosis; a lateral view is essential, in addition to the anteroposterior film.

Treatment. The object of treatment is to correct the displacement, when possible with a minimum of trauma, and to maintain the correction until bony union between neck and epiphysis has taken place. For the individual case, the most suitable type of treatment depends upon the degree and duration of the slipping. In some early cases traction, preferably skeletal, in a position of slight abduction and internal rotation for approximately two weeks will reduce the displacement.

The corrected alignment is best maintained by inserting across the epiphyseal plate the multiple pins of Moore or Knowles (Fig. 226) or a Smith-Petersen nail; the pins, being less traumatic, are preferable. Thereafter, to provide freedom from weight bearing, crutches should be used for several months.

Cases with only slight displacement (less than 1 cm. in both anteroposterior and lateral roentgenograms) that is not corrected by a trial period of traction should also be treated by internal fixation with no attempt at forceful correction, since slight malalignment is compatible with satisfactory hip function.

In early cases with moderate or severe displacement of the epiphysis (Figs. 223 to 225), reduction may sometimes be accomplished by the maneuver used for reducing a fractured femoral neck (Leadbetter maneuver), which consists of exerting traction, with the hip and knee flexed, followed by gradual extension, internal rotation, and abduction of the hip. Forceful

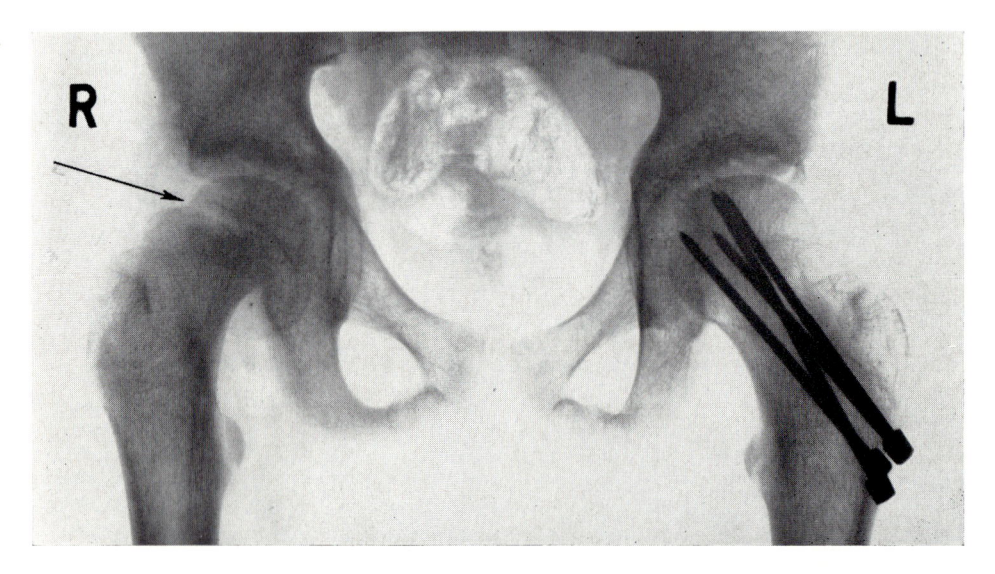

Fig. 226. Roentgenogram of slipped capital femoral epiphyses in 13-year-old boy. Seven months earlier, slipping of the left epiphysis had been reduced by traction and fixed by four Knowles pins. Note slipping of right epiphysis, which was associated with hip pain of two weeks' duration.

manipulation is strongly contraindicated by the danger of causing avascular necrosis of the femoral head by interruption of its blood supply.

In late cases also, manipulation or open reduction is inadvisable because of interference with the blood supply of the epiphysis. The results of open operations on the hip, however well done, are sometimes disappointing. If the deformity is severe, the function of the hip can often be improved by the resection of protruding bone, as suggested by Heyman, or by a transcervical or a subtrochanteric osteotomy. In adult years, an arthrodesis or an arthroplasty may be indicated.

If the patient is obese, his weight should be reduced. In all degrees of slipping, rest of the hip and protection from weight bearing are important. The opposite hip should be watched for any clinical or roentgenographic sign of early slipping, since bilateral involvement is common (Fig. 226).

Prognosis. Cases with slight slipping, treated early, have a favorable prognosis. Late cases with severe displacement often leave a permanent disability despite any form of treatment.

COXA VALGA

Coxa valga is an increase in the angle of the neck of the femur to its shaft, in contrast to coxa vara, which is a decrease of this angle (Fig. 217). Coxa valga tends to produce an increase in the length of the extremity.

Etiology. Coxa valga is most often of congenital origin. The condition is always present in infants before weight bearing is begun. It is sometimes found in association with poliomyelitis, cerebral palsy, pseudohypertrophic muscular dystrophy, congenital dislocation of the hip (Fig. 47), and any other affection of infancy and childhood which has prevented normal weight bearing.

Clinical picture. In extreme cases there is an awkward gait and the thigh is outwardly rotated and abducted. When roentgenograms are being made, the extremity should be held in a neutral position as regards rotation.

Treatment. In most cases no treatment is required. If the patient has not borne weight on the leg and there is no reason for his not bearing weight, he should be encouraged to stand and to walk.

PATHOLOGIC DISLOCATION OF THE HIP

Pathologic dislocation of the hip is not a specific disease entity but a late complication of many affections of the hip. It develops as a result of (1) erosion of bone about the acetabulum, the femoral head, or both, or (2) paralysis of the muscles and relaxation of the other soft tissues around the hip joint. In most cases the head of the femur becomes displaced upward and posteriorly.

Etiology. Tuberculosis of the hip, in which gradual erosion of the acetabulum and destruction of the head of the femur may take place, may result in pathologic dislocation of the hip (Fig. 101). Dislocation often follows pyogenic arthritis or osteomyelitis of the upper end of the femur. In these conditions the dislocation is in large part due to relaxation of the ligamentous supports following distention of the joint capsule by fluid; the relaxed ligaments allow displacement of the head of the femur to the dorsum of the ilium. Pathologic dislocation is occasionally seen in poliomyelitis and cerebral palsy. It may follow the general muscular atrophy of prolonged febrile illness. Occasionally it may accompany rheumatoid arthritis or neuropathic arthropathy. Flexion and adduction of the hip, accompanied by pain and frequently by spasm, are important factors leading to dislocation.

Treatment. Preventive therapy is imperative. The possibility of dislocation should be anticipated and should be guarded against by preventing flexion and adduction. If there is likelihood of displacement, the leg should be kept in traction. As soon as a dislocation is recognized, it should be corrected. Occasionally before reduction can be accomplished, it may be necessary to remove by open operation the fibrous material which has filled the acetabulum. When the dislocation cannot be reduced, it is sometimes advisable to displace the femoral head anteriorly, since this increases the stability of the joint. In selected cases a subtrochanteric osteotomy or a reconstruction operation may be desirable. A shelf operation (Fig. 46) may provide satisfactory stability and is sometimes indicated in dislocation following paralysis. In many cases arthrodesis is the procedure of choice.

INTRAPELVIC PROTRUSION OF THE ACETABULUM (ARTHROKATADYSIS, OTTO PELVIS, PROTRUSIO ACETABULI)

Intrapelvic protrusion of the acetabulum is an uncommon affection of undetermined etiology. In some cases it is of congenital or familial origin. In other instances it is probably secondary to common affections such as rheumatoid or low-grade pyogenic arthritis. It is characterized by a deepen-

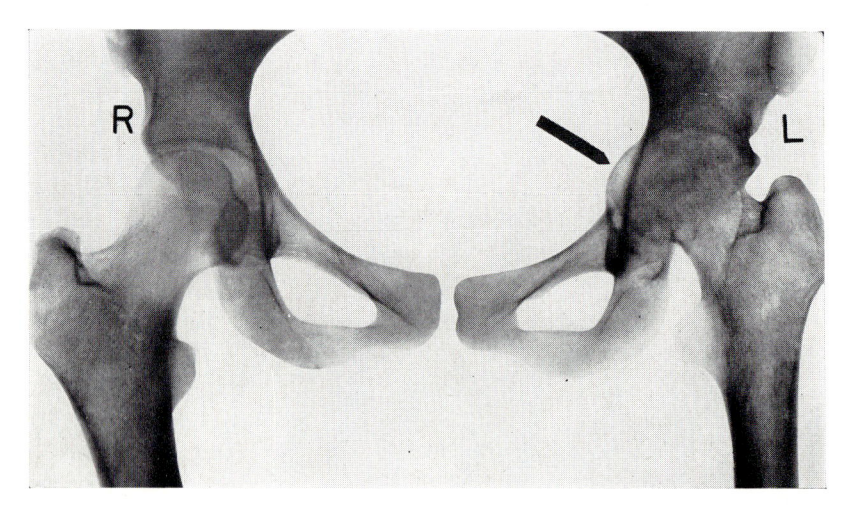

Fig. 227. Roentgenogram showing intrapelvic protrusion of the acetabulum (protrusio acetabuli) in the left hip of a girl 14 years of age. (Courtesy Children's Seashore House, Atlantic City, N. J.)

ing or inward protrusion of the acetabulum, which allows the head of the femur to project farther into the pelvis than normally (Fig. 227). The roentgenograms usually show thinning and eburnation of the walls of the acetabulum, but occasionally there is evidence of increased bone formation; there may be narrowing of the cartilage space. Usually little change occurs in the head of the femur, but occasionally it is irregular or enlarged. The affection is found more often in females than in males and may be either bilateral or unilateral.

Clinical picture. Discomfort and limitation of motion develop gradually over a period of years. Abduction and rotation are especially restricted. There may be little pain until osteoarthritic changes are superimposed. In the end stage, ankylosis of the hip usually results.

Treatment. Little treatment is indicated unless the deformity is accompanied by pain, in which event rest and traction for several weeks, followed by the use of crutches or an ischial weight-bearing brace, may result in symptomatic improvement. Night traction may be used for a long period. If disabling pain persists, arthrodesis or arthroplasty may be indicated.

TRANSIENT SYNOVITIS OF THE HIP

Hip pain and spasm, developing without obvious cause and subsiding after a week or two, may be attributed to a transient synovitis from mild trauma or low-grade, short-lived infection. This obscure affection is usually if not always unilateral and is seen mostly in children.

Clinical picture. There is usually pain upon pressure over the hip joint. Restriction of passive hip mobility by muscle spasm is a constant finding. A limp is usually associated. The hip is often held in a flexed and abducted position.

Diagnosis. Synovitis of the hip joint is to be distinguished from coxa plana, osteomyelitis, pyogenic arthritis, tuberculosis, slipping of the upper femoral epiphysis, and iliopsoas bursitis. Negative roentgenograms support the diagnosis of transient synovitis. If the symptoms persist, additional roentgenograms should be made after an interval of several weeks.

Treatment. Rest and hot applications are indicated. When the pain is severe, fixation in traction, followed briefly by a plaster cast, may be advisable.

BURSITIS IN THE REGION OF THE HIP

Eighteen or more bursae about the hip have been described, but of these only four are of clinical importance. These are the iliopectineal or iliopsoas, the deep trochanteric, the superficial trochanteric, and the ischiogluteal bursae (Fig. 228).

Iliopectineal or iliopsoas bursa

The iliopectineal or iliopsoas bursa is located between the iliopsoas muscle and the iliopectineal eminence, on the anterior surface of the hip joint capsule, and frequently communicates with the joint cavity.

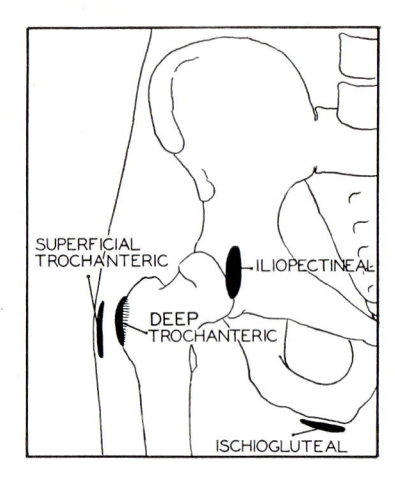

Fig. 228. Most commonly affected bursae about the hip.

Clinical picture. When the iliopectineal bursa is inflamed, tenderness is usually present over the anterior aspect of the hip at about the middle of the inguinal ligament. Pain caused by pressure upon the femoral nerve in this area may radiate down the front of the leg. The hip is usually held in flexion, abduction, and external rotation. Pain is elicited upon attempting to extend, adduct, or internally rotate the hip.

Diagnosis. Femoral hernia, psoas abscess pointing in the groin, synovitis, and infections of the hip joint are to be considered in the differential diagnosis.

Treatment. The patient should be placed at rest in bed with traction applied to the lower extremity. Hot applications should be placed over the area of tenderness on the anterior aspect of the hip. If cellulitis or frank infection is present, antibiotic therapy should be used. The bursitis usually subsides completely within several weeks.

Deep trochanteric bursa

The deep trochanteric bursa is located behind the greater trochanter and in front of the insertion of the gluteus maximus muscle.

When the deep trochanteric bursa is enlarged, the normal depression behind the greater trochanter is obliterated. At this point there may be marked tenderness. The leg is usually held in an abducted and externally rotated position, which relaxes the tension upon the gluteus maximus muscle and the bursa. Pain may radiate down the back of the thigh, and any motion of the hip joint may cause discomfort.

Deep trochanteric bursitis is to be differentiated from infection of the hip joint and from osteomyelitis of the upper end of the femur.

Rest and heat usually constitute adequate treatment. When a pyogenic infection is present, treatment with an appropriate antibiotic is indicated and drainage must be considered. For tuberculous infection complete excision of the bursa is advisable.

Superficial trochanteric bursa

The superficial trochanteric bursa is located between the greater trochanter and the skin.

Tenderness and swelling may be present over the inflamed bursa, but there is no pain on motion of the leg.

The therapy is similar to that outlined for deep trochanteric bursitis.

Ischiogluteal bursa

The ischiogluteal bursa is located superficial to the tuberosity of the ischium. Chronic ischiogluteal bursitis has been called *"weaver's bottom."* It develops in tailors, boatmen, and other individuals whose occupation necessitates prolonged sitting upon hard surfaces.

Tenderness over the tuberosity of the ischium is characteristic, and there may be pain radiating down the back of the thigh along the course of the hamstring muscles.

If the inflammation is not severe, heat and rest will usually cause the symptoms to subside. The use of a pillow or cushioned seat may aid in preventing recurrence. Procaine and hydrocortisone injections may be helpful. Persistence of pain may indicate need for excision of the bursa.

SNAPPING HIP

Snapping hip is an uncommon affection, seen as a rule in young women. With the knee flexed, active internal rotation of the hip will sometimes give rise to a snapping noise. It may be present with every step. It is sometimes caused by the slipping to and fro over the greater trochanter of the iliotibial band or of a fibrous thickening on the deep surface of the gluteus maximus muscle. The snapping can seldom be heard with passive motion. It is annoying rather than painful.

Treatment. As a rule no treatment is indicated, other than explaining to the patient that the snapping is harmless.

CHAPTER 19

Affections of the knee

THE KNEE is the largest joint in the body. In general it is hingelike in character, and its stability is dependent upon (1) an intricate group of strong ligaments and (2) the supporting muscles and tendons. The motions of the knee joint are an extensive anteroposterior, rotatory gliding movement and a very limited axial rotation of the flexed tibia upon the femur. Flexion and extension of the knee take place actually between the semilunar cartilages and the femur. Rotation has been shown to take place between the semilunar cartilages and the tibia.

The knee joint is formed by the articulation of the two rounded condyles of the femur with two shallow depressions in the tibia, which are also called condyles. Between the condyles of the tibia is the tibial spine, which divides to form medial and lateral tubercles. Immediately anterior to the tibial spine is a flattened triangular area on the anterosuperior aspect of the tibia, at the base of which lies the tibial tuberosity. On either side of the joint are strong collateral ligaments that prevent lateral angulation and displacement, and behind the knee is the posterior ligament that forms the floor of the popliteal space. Between the corresponding condyles of femur and tibia are semilunar cartilages or menisci, each of which acts as a wedge-shaped cushion between the tibia and femur and helps to maintain tension in the two cruciate ligaments. The cruciate ligaments extend from the intercondylar notch of the femur to the upper surface of the tibia. The anterior cruciate ligament prevents forward displacement of the tibia, and the posterior cruciate ligament prevents backward displacement. The synovial membrane constitutes the lining of the joint and is continued above into a large anterior pocket called the suprapatellar bursa or quadriceps pouch. Behind the patellar ligament and projecting into the anterior portion of the joint is the infrapatellar fat pad, which is extrasynovial and changes shape with every movement of the joint. This pad is connected with the intercondylar notch of the femur by the ligamentum mucosum. About the joint, in addition to the tendons and muscles, are bursae, blood vessels, and nerves.

INTERNAL DERANGEMENTS OF THE KNEE JOINT

"Internal derangements" is a term commonly applied to those intra- and extra-articular affections of the knee, most often of traumatic origin, which are the result of lesions of the semilunar cartilages, the joint surfaces, the ligaments, the fat pads, or the synovial membrane. The more common derangements include (1) lesions of the semilunar cartilages, (2) rupture of the tibial and fibular collateral ligaments, (3) rupture of the cruciate ligaments, (4) injury of the tibial spine, (5) loose bodies, as in osteochondritis dissecans and synovial chondromatosis, (6) hypertrophy and pinching of the infrapatellar fat pad and synovial membrane, and (7) exostoses.

LESIONS OF THE SEMILUNAR CARTILAGES

Displacements and tears of the semilunar cartilages, or menisci, constitute by far the most frequent type of internal derangement of the knee joint. The medial cartilage is injured from five to fifteen times as frequently as the lateral; the reasons for this are (1) a difference in structure, the medial cartilage being longer, less securely attached, and bifurcated at its anterior pole, and (2) a difference in etiology, the mechanism of injury which causes damage of the medial cartilage being more common than that which affects the lateral. It is convenient to consider the etiology and symptomatology of injuries of each meniscus separately.

Injuries of the medial semilunar cartilage

Etiology. Derangement of the medial semilunar cartilage is usually caused by a sudden internal rotation of the femur upon the fixed tibia while the knee is abducted and flexed. The damage occurs most frequently about the anterior portion of the cartilage. A greater degree of knee flexion at the instant of injury causes the tear to be situated nearer the posterior end of the cartilage. If the anterior portion of the cartilage is torn and slips into the joint, it may lodge between the joint surfaces, prevent complete extension, and give rise to so-called "locking." If the rotary strain is severe, the connection between the cartilage and the tibial collateral ligament may be torn, allowing the cartilage to slip into the joint. With extension of the knee the free border of the cartilage may be caught between the condyles and be split longitudinally. This produces the so-called "bucket-handle" type of cartilage, in which the inner portion may be easily displaced centrally between the joint surfaces and cause "locking." When the joint is "unlocked," the cartilage becomes dislodged from between the articular surfaces.

Pathology. The lesion (Fig. 229) may consist of (1) a tearing of the anterior or posterior part of the cartilage with or without displacement; (2) a transverse tear through the central portion or through any other portion of the cartilage; (3) a longitudinal splitting with or without the displacement characteristic of the "bucket-handle" cartilage; or (4) a simple loosening of the cartilage at its peripheral attachment, allowing it to slip into and out of the joint. Any one of these lesions may give rise to the symptoms of a joint derangement. When the cartilage is partially torn from its peripheral

394   Handbook of orthopaedic surgery

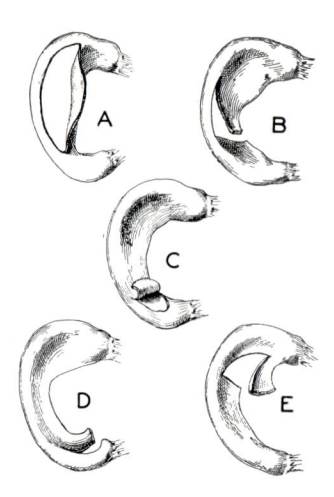

Fig. 229. Types of semilunar cartilage injury. **A,** Longitudinal splitting (bucket-handle type). **B,** Tear of middle third. **C,** Tear of anterior tip. **D,** Longitudinal splitting of anterior third. **E,** Tear of posterior third. (After Henderson.)

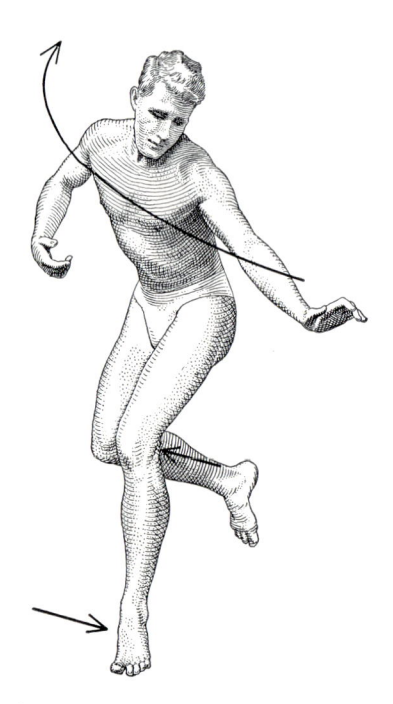

Fig. 230. A mechanism of injury commonly resulting in tear of the medial semilunar cartilage. Note flexion of left knee and violent internal rotation of the femur as the trunk twists to the right while the left tibia and foot are fixed by weight bearing. The anterior portion of the left medial meniscus tends to be displaced posteriorly by the attachment of the tibial collateral ligament and the rotary sweep of the medial femoral condyle.

attachment, it may heal without difficulty if further displacement is prevented. Tears limited to the central rim of the cartilage probably never heal. At operation, the "bucket-handle" lesions are as common as all the other lesions combined.

Clinical picture. An accurate history is most important, since often the diagnosis is based more upon the history than upon the physical findings. A typical history is that of an athlete whose knee is suddenly twisted inward (Fig. 230). Acute pain on the inner side of the knee accompanies the injury, and the athlete is likely to fall to the ground. His knee cannot be straightened, and the joint may swell rapidly. If the leg should be pulled when it is found that he cannot straighten the knee, the athlete may feel something in the knee snap back into place. Instantly he is relieved of the sharp pain and is then usually able to get up and walk. In other instances the history may be that of a coal miner who is working on his knees and who feels something give way in his knee when he turns to shovel coal. Symptoms and signs identical with those of the former case then follow.

If the condition remains untreated, the disability persists for a variable length of time. Following the initial accident the feeling of a slipping within the knee, with pain referred to the medial side of the joint, may recur frequently. Such episodes may be precipitated by external rotation of the foot or abduction of the ankle.

Examination of the affected knee brings to light a number of signs. In acute cases there may be lateral instability and extensive effusion of blood in the joint. In the presence of this effusion it is difficult to diagnose the exact type of injury. As the swelling subsides and the torn capsule heals, the originally unstable knee may gradually regain its stability. Localized tenderness is present at this stage, either about the anterior tip of the medial semilunar cartilage or about the medial or posterior margins of the joint surfaces. Forced adduction often elicits pain on the medial aspect of the knee. If the cartilage remains displaced, full extension will be impossible. A history of partial "locking" is present in approximately 70% of the cases in which the diagnosis can be made definitely. Hamstring muscle spasm often prevents complete extension of the knee and must be differentiated from true "locking." When a posterior tear is accompanied by displacement, it may be impossible to flex the joint fully; this partial "locking" will persist until the dislocation of the cartilage is reduced. Tears of the posterior half of the cartilage may be demonstrated by the McMurray or "click" test: holding the tibia in extreme external rotation and abduction, the examiner slowly extends the knee from the fully flexed position; an appreciable clicking and transient pain indicate the presence of a posterior tear.

When the displacement recurs frequently, the patient always feels insecure. Often a little twist or misstep will again throw the cartilage out of its normal position. The patient may learn to reduce the displacement without assistance. Recurrent displacement is usually accompanied by a moderate increase of joint fluid. The swelling will persist as long as any part of the torn cartilage is irritating the synovial membrane. Occasionally in recurrent cases the meniscus is displaced toward the medial side and a mass can be felt along the medial border of the joint. In such cases the cartilage can usually be pushed in with the fingers. Atrophy of the muscles of the thigh and leg is always present in chronic cases; it is most noticeable in the quadriceps muscle.

Injuries of the lateral semilunar cartilage

The mechanism of injury is the converse of that causing damage of the medial semilunar cartilage. The foot is usually fixed firmly upon the ground, and the femur rotates outward upon the tibia while the knee is adducted and flexed. The pathologic changes are similar to those in injuries of the medial cartilage.

Clinical picture. The symptoms and signs are essentially the same as those of injury of the medial cartilage with the exception that they are referred to the lateral side of the knee and are often less severe. After injury of the lateral cartilage, straightening or fully flexing the knee will at times produce a loud crack or snap that can be felt on the lateral side of the joint as the knee jerks into place. This has occasioned the term "trigger knee." For a posterior tear of the lateral cartilage the McMurray test is the same as that described for the medial cartilage except that the tibia is placed in extreme internal rotation and adduction instead of external rotation and abduction.

Diagnosis. The diagnosis of a derangement of either cartilage is based upon the characteristic history and physical signs. "Locking" is typical but may occur also in other types of internal derangement. Roentgenograms yield little relevant information but should be taken in order to exclude fracture, loose bodies, exostoses, arthritis, and aberrant calcification. In addition to the usual anteroposterior and lateral roentgenograms, a posteroanterior picture should be taken with the knee flexed 90 degrees; this shows the intercondylar space and is sometimes called the "tunnel view." Pneumarthrography, or roentgenographic examination after the injection of air or oxygen into the joint, may provide additional information, but diagnosis based on pneumarthrograms is often unreliable.

Treatment. For derangement of either cartilage the treatment is essentially the same.

If the joint capsule is greatly distended after a recent injury, the fluid should be aspirated, as it is usually bloody and may lead to the formation of adhesions. Application of ice is always helpful in acute knee injuries. If, following an initial injury, the knee is locked, an attempt should be made to reduce the displacement of the cartilage; this may be done by the application of traction or by resort to manipulation. In the case of the medial cartilage the knee should be flexed, abducted, externally rotated, and then quickly internally rotated and extended. For displacement of the lateral cartilage, the knee should be flexed, adducted, internally rotated, and then quickly externally rotated and extended. If the cartilage dislocation can be reduced, the joint should be immobilized for three weeks or more. A dressing of soft glazed cotton rolls, broad splints, and elastic cloth bandages, or a light plaster cast, may be used. Exercise of the quadriceps muscle should always be employed to aid in maintaining muscle tone and strength. Patella-setting exercises with the knee extended should be started early.

If the knee remains weak and stiff after the original displacement, a program of weight-lifting extension exercises is indicated in order to strengthen the muscles and to restore normal mobility. A brace, such as the Jones knee cage or one of its modifications (Fig. 231), may be helpful. If pain and limitation of extension persist, the injured cartilage should be removed.

If the displaced cartilage is unquestionably palpable, if displacement has occurred more than once, or if the symptoms recur after immobilization, an exploratory operation is indicated. It is often impossible to make a specific diagnosis before operation. If it is clinically definite that displacement or laceration of the cartilage has occurred, the operation should not be delayed, for arthritic changes may develop in the joint when a torn meniscus is allowed to remain as an irritant to the synovial membrane and hyaline cartilage. When, on exploration of the joint, the meniscus is found to be loosened or torn in any part it should be removed as completely as possible. In cases of long duration with repeated episodes of knee locking, arthritic changes in the femoral condyle are often found at operation. Such changes are most marked where the articular cartilage of the condyle comes into contact with the torn portion of the meniscus.

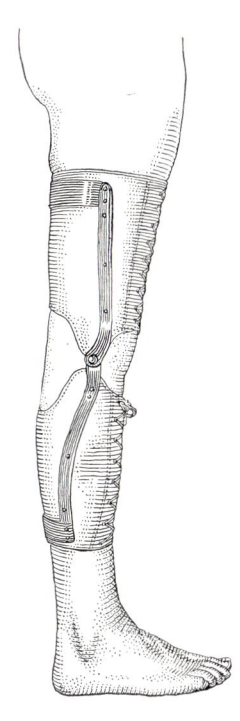

Fig. 231. Modified Jones knee cage for protection and support of injured knee. (After Bennett.)

Instruction and practice in forceful voluntary contraction of the quadriceps muscle should be begun before operation and resumed on the first postoperative day. Weight bearing on the extended knee may be started as early as a day or two after operation. At the end of a week, more strenuous quadriceps exercises are begun; they are continued until normal mobility and strength have been regained. If the meniscus derangement has been accompanied by injury of the knee ligaments, temporary use of a brace may be advisable. Unrestricted exercise should not be allowed until the quadriceps has acquired good strength, which is usually about twelve weeks after operation. Removal of a meniscus does not in itself impair the strength or function of the joint to any appreciable extent.

Cysts of the semilunar cartilages

Semilunar cartilage cysts are six to twelve times as common in the lateral meniscus as in the medial and are found most frequently in the young adult male.

Etiology. The cyst of the semilunar cartilage is thought to represent (1) the end result of a mucoid degenerative process within the cartilage, (2) a congenital defect in the development of the cartilage, or (3) a ganglion-like structure resulting from trauma between the peripheral surface of the cartilage and the synovial membrane.

Pathology. The cysts are more often multiple than single. They contain a soft, gelatinous material and are sometimes lined by cells resembling endothelium.

Clinical picture. The symptoms and signs are similar to those of semilunar cartilage injuries; there is, however, no locking or sudden effusion. Cysts may appear following injury of the knee. Sometimes many years elapse, however, between the injury and the appearance of the cysts. There is sometimes a continuous, dull ache in the affected joint most noticeable at night. The discomfort is always worse after activity and relieved by rest. The typical cyst is found on the lateral side of the joint as a tense, slightly tender swelling, which may become as large as a walnut. It is always more prominent with the knee in extension than in flexion.

Treatment. Complete excision of the cyst and the affected cartilage is indicated. Recurrence of the cyst is common after incomplete excision.

Discoid cartilages

As a result of an uncommon developmental anomaly, the lateral meniscus is sometimes discoid rather than semilunar in form. A discoid cartilage may be present in each knee. It is often associated with a high fibular head.

Clinical picture. The most characteristic clinical feature is a loud click which is felt and heard when the knee joint is flexed or extended; this occurs usually near the limits of knee motion. The joint does not lock. The typical patient is in his teens, has noticed a painless clicking for a variable length of time, and with or without minor trauma of his knee begins to have an aching pain on its lateral aspect and a feeling of weakness in it. Examination confirms the clicking on motion and may disclose tenderness over the lateral cartilage. As the discoid cartilage is thicker than normal, roentgenograms may show a widening of the cartilage space between the lateral condyles of femur and tibia.

Treatment. In the presence of symptoms the treatment is excision of the entire discoid cartilage.

RUPTURE OF THE TIBIAL AND FIBULAR COLLATERAL LIGAMENTS

Etiology. The tibial or medial collateral ligament is ruptured by stresses resulting from forceful eversion of the foot and abduction of the knee, usually when the knee is slightly flexed and the extensor mechanism relaxed. The fibular collateral ligament, less frequently injured, may be ruptured by forceful adduction of the internally rotated knee.

Clinical picture. There is an increase in the lateral mobility of the knee with tenderness over the injured ligament. When the tibial collateral ligament is ruptured, the tenderness is usually greatest over its inferior attachment. There may be an associated increase of joint fluid, swelling, and ecchymosis. Rarely is an unmistakable defect in the region of the affected ligament palpable. Tenderness may be very persistent. On motion of the knee there are definite weakness, instability, and occasionally a sensation of slight catching within the joint.

Treatment. After recent injury of the tibial or fibular collateral ligament the knee should be maintained in complete extension for a period of from three to four weeks. During this time the splints may be removed for daily physical therapy. If the injury is severe, active and passive movements of the joint should not be permitted, but if it is slight they may be allowed. Often the attachment of the medial semilunar cartilage is torn when rupture of the tibial collateral ligament occurs, and in cases of this type it is most important that the knee be put completely at rest. Exercise of the quadriceps muscle should be started immediately after the injury in order to forestall muscle atrophy. These exercises must be carried out frequently and forcefully if knee strength is to be retained. Full weight bearing should not be permitted until there is no tenderness over the torn ligament and no pain on abduction or adduction of the knee. When the patient begins to walk, it is best that a knee brace be applied to prevent excessive lateral motion and hyperextension. The heel of the shoe should be raised ¼ inch on the affected side in order to relieve strain on the ligament. When isolated injuries of the collateral ligaments are carefully treated from the beginning, a complete restoration of function may be expected.

If the acute rupture is complete, as indicated by extreme lateral instability of the knee, or if, despite a vigorous and prolonged course of quadriceps exercises, the knee remains relaxed, surgical repair or reconstruction of the ligament is to be considered. For reinforcement or reconstruction of the fibular ligament a flap of fascia lata and a portion of the biceps tendon may be used. When the tibial collateral ligament is relaxed but not completely ruptured, Mauck's operation of transplanting the distal end of the ligament with its bony attachment downward on the tibia is often successful in improving the stability of the joint. The tibial collateral ligament may be reinforced or reconstructed with the tendons of the gracilis and semitendinosus muscles. The intact semitendinosus tendon may be transplanted into the medial condyle of the femur, as described by Bosworth. The results of these reconstructive operations are generally satisfactory but not so good as the results of prompt surgical repair of the acute complete ruptures.

RUPTURE OF THE CRUCIATE LIGAMENTS

Etiology. The cruciate ligaments are ruptured only by severe trauma. The anterior cruciate ligament may be damaged by the same type of trauma that causes injury of the medial semilunar cartilage, and the posterior cruciate ligament by the same trauma that injures the lateral semilunar cartilage. Forced hyperextension of the knee and internal rotation of the tibia on the femur, with rupture of the tibial collateral ligament, may at the same time produce a rupture of the anterior cruciate ligament. If the ligament itself does not break with this type of violence, avulsion of the medial tubercle of the tibial spine may occur. Any force that displaces the tibia backward on the femur while the knee is flexed may cause rupture of the posterior cruciate ligament. Falling on the flexed knee in such a manner that the force of the impact is received on the upper end of the tibia instead of on the patella may cause rupture of the posterior cruciate ligament. Rupture of either cruciate ligament is always attended by injury of the joint capsule.

Clinical picture. Rupture of a cruciate ligament is followed by great swelling and marked instability of the knee joint. When the anterior cruciate ligament is torn or stretched, the tibia can be displaced forward on the femur. When the posterior cruciate ligament is torn or stretched, the tibia can be displaced backward on the femur when the knee is flexed. Lateral as well as anteroposterior instability may be present. Occasionally both cruciate ligaments are torn; this results in extreme instability and is likely to be associated with complete dislocation of the knee.

In acute cruciate ligament injuries, when early and accurate diagnosis is so important, pain and spasm may obscure the degree of instability and make an examination under anesthesia advisable.

Treatment. In athletic young adults, acute rupture of a cruciate ligament is probably best treated by early surgical repair. Especially is operation indicated when there is injury of the anterior cruciate ligament, tibial collateral ligament, and medial meniscus—the "unhappy triad" of O'Donóghue, in whose hands the results of early operation have been very good.

In older or less vigorous individuals, acute cruciate ligament rupture may be treated by immobilizing the knee in slight flexion, preferably by means of a plaster cast, for a period of at least two months. Immobilization should be followed by a snugly fitting knee cage (Fig. 231), which allows only limited motion.

Operative reconstructions are occasionally done for old injuries of the cruciate ligaments, the anterior ligament sometimes being reconstructed by the use of fascia lata, or the posterior by utilizing the semitendinosus tendon. Unfortunately these procedures cannot be relied upon to restore knee stability of satisfactory degree.

At some stage of treatment all cruciate ligament injuries require a program of vigorous resistive exercises to build up the strength of the quadriceps muscle.

FRACTURE OF THE TIBIAL SPINE

Etiology. Fracture of the tibial spine is usually caused by a mechanism of injury similar to that which results in rupture of the cruciate ligaments. In children this injury is frequently the result of a bicycle accident. Avulsion of the whole tibial spine or of either intercondylar tubercle may occur. With the severe trauma of violent abduction or adduction the whole spine may be broken and one of the intercondylar tubercles depressed. Fracture of the medial tubercle of the spine results from the same type of violence as that which causes injury of the anterior cruciate ligament. The medial tubercle, when detached, usually becomes displaced anteriorly. Fracture of the lateral tubercle of the spine is caused by forcible abduction of the tibia and direct contact with the lateral condyle of the femur.

Clinical picture. Fracture of the tibial spine occurs usually in older children and adolescents. The injury is followed quickly by pain, tenderness, distention of the joint capsule by blood, and inability to extend the knee completely. There is usually a bony block causing "locking," which is an outstanding symptom. There may also be considerable anteroposterior instability of the joint.

Treatment. If little or no displacement of the fragment has occurred, immobilization for four weeks, followed by the use of a knee cage or elastic bandage, may be sufficient. Aspiration should be done before immobilization is effected. Resistive quadriceps exercises should be started early and continued. If the fragment is displaced, it may be possible by means of manipulation to force it back into position; immobilization should then be used for about eight weeks. In many cases, however, open operation is indicated. Small fragments that do not weaken the attachment of the cruciate ligaments may be excised. The aftercare is the same as that of arthrotomy for the removal of a semilunar cartilage. If the fragment is large and includes the attachment of one or both cruciate ligaments, it should be replaced in the upper surface of the tibia and fixed by a single screw or by a suture passed through two drill holes from the anterior tibial cortex to the intercondylar area. This procedure should be followed by immobilization for a period of from eight to twelve weeks.

LOOSE BODIES

Loose bodies are often found in the knee, elbow, and shoulder joints and are frequently referred to as "joint mice." In one reported series the knee was involved in 90% of the cases. The presence of intra-articular loose bodies is more frequently observed in men than in women.

Etiology. Loose bodies may form in the joint as the result of disease or of trauma. They often consist of a structureless fibrinous material; the so-called "rice" or "melon seed" bodies found in association with the chronic synovial reaction of tuberculosis, syphilis, and osteoarthritis are of this type. Occasionally loose bodies arise by the formation and proliferation of cartilage within the synovial villi, forming the so-called synovial chondromas.

Timbrell Fisher has classified loose bodies as (1) those associated with an underlying pathologic process of recognized nature, such as chronic arthritis, tabes dorsalis, tuberculosis, or pyogenic arthritis; (2) those arising from the cartilage or bone of normal joints, such as the loose bodies of osteochondritis dissecans, detached articular ecchondroses, or detached intra-articular epiphyses; and (3) those bodies, such as the synovial chondromas, which follow an obscure pathologic change within the synovial membrane.

Clinical picture. Loose bodies usually cause a chronic intra-articular inflammation that is attended by an increase of joint fluid. There may be an associated weakness and instability of the joint. Following motion there is sometimes a sudden, intense pain, occurring when the loose body becomes wedged between the articular surfaces and causes a "locking" of the joint. In successive episodes of this kind the site of pain may vary widely. Loose bodies that are completely unattached may be found in any part of the joint, and their position may change between successive examinations. This variability of location, commonly determined by roentgenograms, is characteristic. Occasionally the body remains attached by a pedicle, occupies a more constant position in the joint, and can be palpated. Loose bodies can cause all degrees of joint symptoms and disability, from vague pain to extreme swelling and "locking."

Osteochondritis dissecans. Osteochondritis dissecans is a joint affection characterized by ischemic necrosis and partial detachment of a fragment of cartilage and underlying bone from the articular surface (Fig. 232). In advanced cases the fragment is completely detached and its area of origin is recognizable as a shallow crater in one of the articular surfaces. The most common site of osteochondritis dissecans is the lateral portion of the articular surface of the medial condyle of the femur, in the neighborhood of the insertion of the posterior cruciate ligament. Osteochondritis dissecans has been demonstrated also, however, in the ankle, hip, elbow, and shoulder joints. It is seen most commonly in adolescence or early adult life but occurs also in children. Males are affected more frequently than females. The fragmentation is thought by some observers to be the result of trauma, the circulation being impaired and a subsequent disturbance of bone nutrition taking place. It is believed by others to be caused by embolism of minute blood vessels supplying the affected area of bone and cartilage. The symptoms and signs are in general the same as those occurring with other types of loose bodies and include discomfort, weakness, fatigue, and catching or "locking" of the joint. However, when the diagnosis is made in children be-

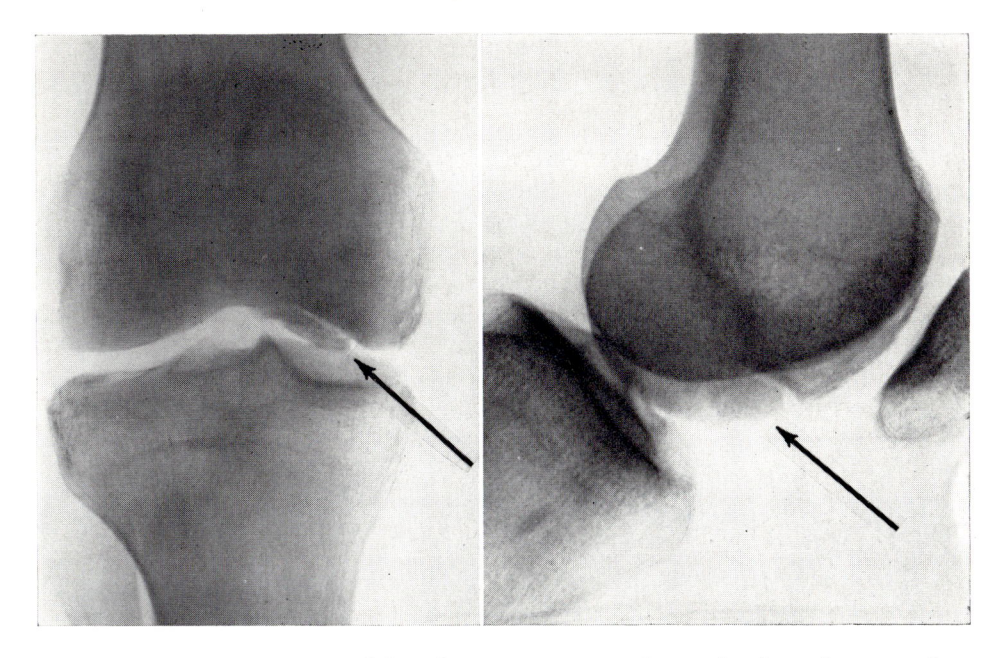

Fig. 232. Anteroposterior and lateral roentgenograms of osteochondritis dissecans of medial condyle of the femur. The small fragment of bone and articular cartilage is only partially detached from the condyle. The patient was a 20-year-old boy.

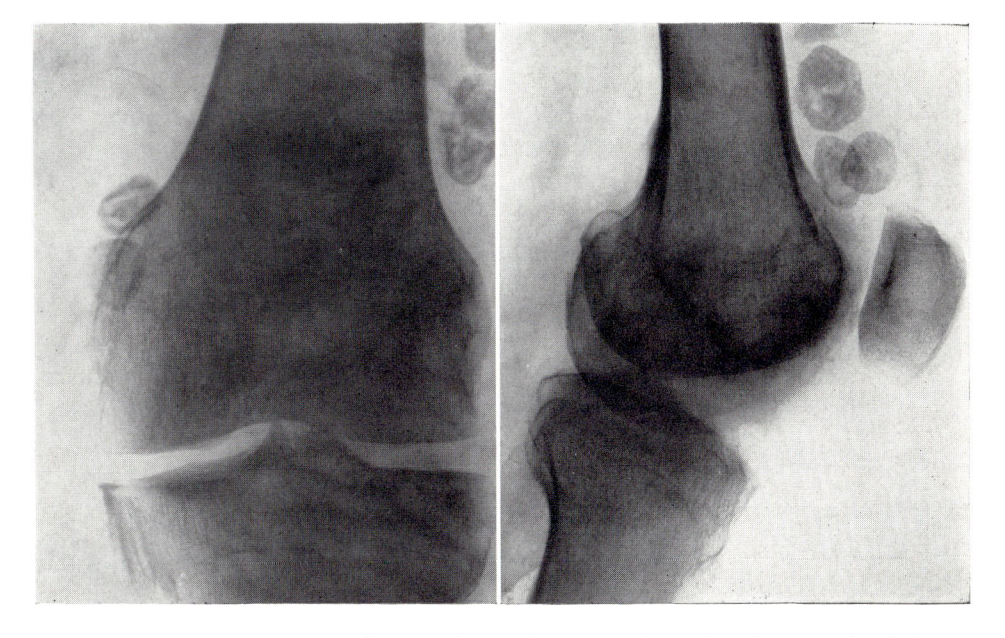

Fig. 233. Roentgenograms of synovial chondromatosis (osteochondromatosis) of the knee, showing characteristic large, rounded loose bodies. The patient was a 39-year-old man.

fore the fragment has separated, complete rest of the joint from weight bearing for several months may bring about a reversal of the pathologic process, followed by complete disappearance of the roentgenographic changes and by clinical cure.

Synovial chondromatosis (osteochondromatosis). In synovial chondromatosis, a rare affection, pedunculated and loose osteocartilaginous bodies arise within the synovial membrane. The knee joint is involved most commonly (Fig. 233). Cartilage cells develop in the synovial villi, presumably as a result of metaplasia of the connective tissue cells. The cartilaginous bodies may occur singly but are usually numerous. Many of them remain attached to the synovial membrane, which often becomes thickly studded with them. The loose bodies frequently show lamination from the deposition of calcium salts; they may possess either a loculated central cavity or a center of bony consistency.

Diagnosis. The diagnosis of intra-articular loose bodies, or *joint mice,* can be made from the history. Roentgenograms demonstrate the presence of loose bodies if they contain calcium or bone.

Treatment. If the loose bodies are producing symptoms of mechanical interference with joint motion, they should be removed. It is often advisable to make a long incision, because of the difficulty of finding the loose bodies and the danger of leaving any within the joint. If the bodies contain calcium, roentgenograms made in the operating room may be helpful. The removal of attached bodies is not technically difficult. Joints in which the synovial changes are generalized are best treated by synovectomy. Loose bodies often occur in the posterior part of the knee joint and require a posteromedial incision into the popliteal space; care must be taken not to injure the popliteal nerves, which should be retracted laterally. The aftercare consists of a short period of immobilization, followed by physical therapy including vigorous active exercise of the weakened muscles.

HYPERTROPHY AND PINCHING OF THE INFRAPATELLAR FAT PAD AND THE SYNOVIAL MEMBRANE

Infrapatellar fat pad

The large pad of fat behind the patellar ligament may rarely be pinched and caught when the knee is extended. With repeated trauma, hemorrhage occurs into the fatty tissue, and a hard organized swelling appears, which may later become calcified. A similar process may take place on either side of the patellar ligament.

Clinical picture. Pinching of the hypertrophic infrapatellar fat pad is associated with pain beneath the patellar ligament. The knee becomes stiff and weak and may show an effusion. Extension may cause a stabbing pain in the anterior aspect of the knee.

Treatment. A trial of nonsurgical therapy is indicated. Raising the heel of the shoe from ½ to 1 inch may afford relief. It may be necessary to apply a hinged knee cage to prevent the last 20 to 30 degrees of extension. Massage and exercises should also be used. If the symptoms persist, surgical exploration and excision of any grossly abnormal part of the fat pad may be helpful.

Synovial membrane

Hypertrophy of the synovial villi is a frequent result of chronic intra-articular inflammation. The villous processes become enlarged and elongated and occasionally form lobulated masses. This may occur in osteoarthritis. Benign proliferation of the synovial membrane is seen also in *pigmented villonodular synovitis*. Although this entity may occur in other joints, as well as in tendon sheaths and bursae, it is seen much more commonly in the knee than in other locations. Pigmented villonodular synovitis may be solitary or diffuse. In the solitary form a single nodule is attached to the synovial lining by a pedicle; such nodules vary in diameter from a few millimeters to several centimeters. In the diffuse form most of the synovial membrane is involved by numerous enlarged villi and nodules. Microscopic sections show hyperplastic synovial tissue containing giant cells, foam cells, and deposits of hemosiderin.

Clinical picture. A solitary lesion often produces symptoms suggesting a loose body, with painful intermittent catching or "locking" followed by effusion. Diffuse lesions cause chronic swelling and mild discomfort in the knee. Palpation may demonstrate thickening of the synovial membrane, increased joint fluid, and in some instances nodules. Aspiration of bloody fluid from a knee that has not been subjected to trauma should suggest the diagnosis of pigmented villonodular synovitis.

Treatment and prognosis. Solitary lesions should be treated by surgical excision. Diffuse lesions, if causing symptoms, require synovectomy. As a rule the lesions do not recur.

EXOSTOSES

Occasionally a joint may become "locked" or obstructed by the slipping of a tendon or muscle over a bony projection. This sometimes occurs, for example, at the posterior part of the knee. A common exostosis about the knee arises from the posteromedial surface of the lower end of the femur and is extra-articular. A sense of discomfort and slipping may accompany every movement. More often, however, the symptoms are trivial. The treatment consists of complete surgical removal of the exostosis.

OSGOOD-SCHLATTER DISEASE (PARTIAL SEPARATION OF THE TIBIAL TUBEROSITY, APOPHYSITIS OF THE TIBIAL TUBEROSITY)

Osgood-Schlatter disease is a partial separation of the tonguelike epiphysis of the tibial tuberosity, apparently caused by the sudden or continued strain placed upon it by the patellar ligament during exercise (Fig. 234). There may be a disturbance of the circulation of the epiphysis, since it often shows fragmentation; however, particles of necrotic bone that have been noted on microscopic examination are probably the result of the separation

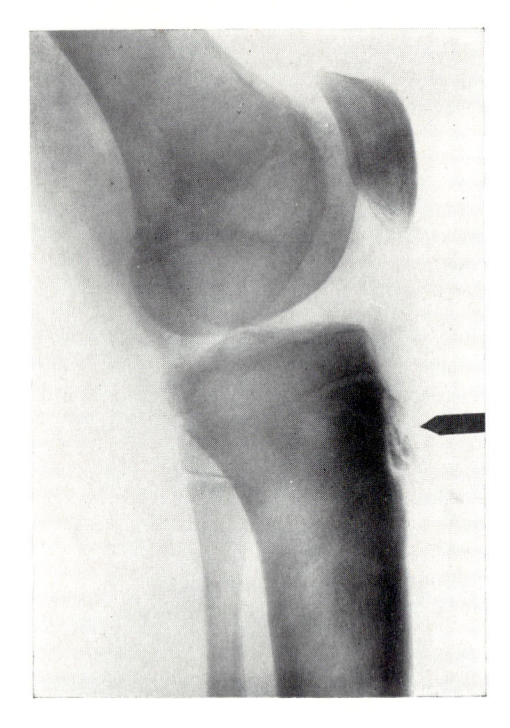

Fig. 234. Lateral roentgenogram of knee showing Osgood-Schlatter disease in a boy 14 years of age. Note prominence and fragmented appearance of the epiphysis of the tibial tuberosity.

rather than of primary avascular necrosis. Osgood-Schlatter disease occurs usually in active boys between 10 and 15 years of age and is especially common among those who ride bicycles. It is frequently bilateral.

Clinical picture. The disorder is associated with pain over the tibial tuberosity when the patellar ligament is tightened on strong extension or actively resisted flexion of the knee. The region of the tuberosity becomes enlarged and often is tender. The symptoms are sometimes acute and the tenderness extreme. Ecchymosis is occasionally observed. There is always aching in the area of the tuberosity on exercise, and particularly on climbing stairs and running.

Roentgenographic picture. The roentgenogram usually shows irregularity and slight separation of the epiphysis of the tibial tuberosity in the early stage and fragmentation of the epiphysis in the later stage. At times, however, little or no change may be visible. A film of the opposite knee may be taken for contrast, but often both knees are affected to the same extent and present an identical roentgenographic appearance.

Prognosis. The outlook for cure is excellent, as progression of the affection is self-limited and the symptoms nearly always respond favorably to treatment.

Treatment. Immobilization in extension by means of splints or a plaster cast for a period of at least five weeks will usually cause the acute symptoms to subside completely, and no additional treatment may be needed. Weight bearing is not prohibited. Following immobilization, it is often advisable not to allow full flexion for an additional period of several months. In the uncommon, persistent case it may be advisable to drill through the tuberosity to the upper end of the tibia in an effort to improve the local circulation. This should not be done unless growth is almost complete, since epiphyseal damage may produce an asymmetrical growth disturbance. In untreated cases a fragment of the epiphysis may remain ununited and later require excision.

RECURRENT OR HABITUAL DISLOCATION OF THE PATELLA (SLIPPING PATELLA)

Recurrent dislocation of the patella occurs more often in females than in males and is usually unilateral. Inherited tendencies resulting in a low lateral condylar ridge are responsible for some of the cases. Recurrent dislocation of the patella is often associated with genu valgum and a general muscular hypotonia of the lower extremities. Direct trauma or strain is usually the precipitating factor.

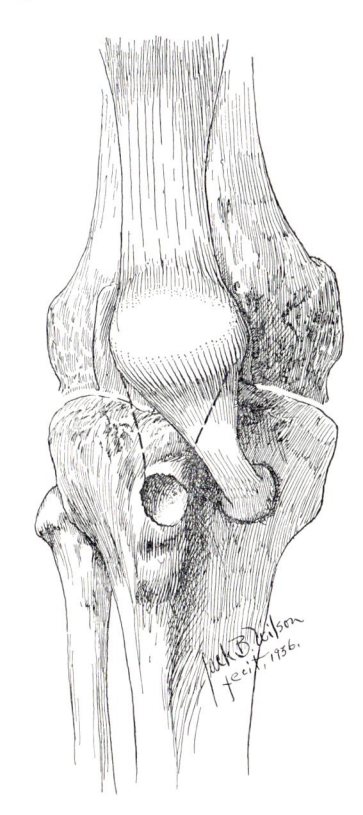

Fig. 235. Operation for recurrent dislocation of patella. The patellar ligament with its bony tibial attachment has been transplanted medially.

Clinical picture. The dislocation is almost always a lateral displacement that occurs on sudden contraction of the quadriceps muscle. It may result from a glancing blow on the medial side of the patella. Immediately following the dislocation, there is a sharp pain which may cause the patient to fall. The pain is particularly severe when the dislocation is infrequent; in some cases the displacement occurs very often and causes little discomfort. Dislocation of the patella may be followed by a slight or moderate amount of effusion into the joint, especially in the early stages of the disorder. The patient invariably complains of a constant feeling of weakness and insecurity and is very timid about taking strenuous exercise.

Treatment. The patella may easily be replaced upon extension of the knee and flexion of the hip. In early cases the leg should be immobilized for a period of from five to six weeks. This may be followed by raising the inner side of the heel ¼ inch, walking with the toes turned in, and strengthening the quadriceps muscle with resistive exercises. In some cases the wearing of a knee cage (Fig. 231) is advisable.

In repeatedly recurrent cases operation is indicated. Numerous surgical procedures involving the use of bone or soft tissue to hold the patella in place have been devised. One of the most successful operations is transplantation of the tibial tuberosity, together with the patellar ligament, from its normal position to the medial side of the anterior surface of the tibia (Fig. 235). The tuberosity may be fixed in its newly prepared bed with a metal screw. After the tibial tuberosity and patellar ligament have been transplanted, it is usually advisable to reef the capsule on the inner aspect of the joint. Occasionally osteotomy is done to correct an associated genu valgum, and in some instances patellectomy may be indicated.

CHONDROMALACIA OF THE PATELLA

Chondromalacia of the patella is a degenerative process of unknown etiology, which involves the cartilage of the articular surface of the patella. The degenerative changes may follow repeated minor or acute severe traumas and often are associated with anomalies of the patella, osteochondritis, and arthritis. The highest incidence of cases is in young adults. When the undersurface of the patella has been examined in arthrotomy of the knee, chondromalacia has been found in approximately 20% of the cases. Seldom is it recognizable in routine roentgenograms of the knee. Articular cartilage changes in the patella have been found in up to 50% of cadavers with supposedly normal knees.

Clinical picture. These patients frequently give a history of having had trauma to the knee, followed by immediate disability and subsequent relief of symptoms. From several months to many years after such an episode there may develop variable pain, catching, instability, "locking," weakness, and swelling in the knee, as well as atrophy of the thigh and tenderness of the patella.

Upon examination there are usually patellar tenderness, subpatellar crepitation, synovial thickening, and effusion.

Treatment. Mild cases should be protected from further injury by strapping or a brace, and isometric quadriceps-strengthening exercises should be instituted. For the advanced case, a partial or total chondrectomy or patellectomy is indicated.

OSSIFICATION OF THE TIBIAL COLLATERAL LIGAMENT (PELLEGRINI-STIEDA DISEASE)

Ossification in the tibial collateral ligament is a fairly common affection, occurring usually in men between the ages of 25 and 40 years. The deposits of new bone usually overlie the medial femoral condyle but have been observed also in the middle portion of the tibial collateral ligament just proximal to the level of the joint space. The ossification may be the result of involvement of the ligament by extension from inflammatory disease in adjacent structures such as bursae, tendons, ligaments, synovia, and bones. Trauma is most often the exciting cause, however, and may be of a single violent type or may consist of repeated minor injuries of the knee joint.

Clinical picture. Following traumatization, the medial aspect of the knee becomes sensitive to pressure, especially about the adductor tubercle. Complete extension of the knee is painful, and the joint is usually held in slight flexion. Slight swelling of the knee may be observed. Occasionally an indurated area can be palpated.

Diagnosis. Dislocation of a semilunar cartilage and other internal derangements of the knee must be excluded before the clinical diagnosis can be made. The roentgenographic picture is pathognomonic.

Prognosis and treatment. In many cases the symptoms subside spontaneously without causing prolonged disability. Nonsurgical treatment consists of rest and support during the acute stage. Physical therapy is helpful but should not be started until all of the acute signs have subsided. The surgical treatment consists of excision of the bony plaque and plastic repair of the ligament. Occasionally the ossified mass recurs following resection, especially if it has been removed before reaching a mature stage.

RUPTURE OF THE QUADRICEPS TENDON AND OF THE PATELLAR LIGAMENT

The quadriceps tendon or the patellar ligament may be ruptured by the same type of violence as that which sometimes causes fracture of the patella, i.e., sudden and violent contraction of the quadriceps muscle when the knee is flexed. Rupture of the tendon or the ligament is a much less common injury, however, than fracture of the patella.

Clinical picture. Rupture of the quadriceps tendon occurs more frequently than rupture of the patellar ligament and is seen most commonly in elderly persons. A definite tender depression can be seen and felt above the superior margin of the patella. The rupture may be associated with bloody effusion into the knee joint and resultant swelling.

Rupture of the patellar ligament results in upward displacement of the patella. A tender depression below the patella may be palpated but usually cannot be seen because of swelling of the infrapatellar fat pad.

Following rupture of either of these structures, active extension of the knee is severely limited. In both conditions active flexion is of normal range but painful, while active extension is impossible in complete rupture and very painful in partial rupture.

Diagnosis. The diagnosis is made from the history and the physical findings. Tendon rupture is to be differentiated from fracture of the patella by roentgenographic examination.

Treatment. The treatment is surgical repair of the rupture. Suture should be followed by immobilization in extension for from six to eight weeks, after which a program of physical therapy including carefully graded exercise in flexion should be instituted.

SNAPPING KNEE

In adults a snapping noise in the knee may be caused by a displacement of the lateral semilunar cartilage, especially if it is of discoid type, or by a sudden slipping of the biceps tendon or the iliotibial band. In early infancy sudden extension of the knee may cause the tibia to spring forward or rotate outward, producing an audible click; the mechanism is presumably a sudden and violent voluntary contraction of the muscular and tendinous structures about the joint. As a rule the symptoms of snapping knee are of trivial nature and there is no disability.

Treatment. Supporting the knee with a brace or plaster splint may result in complete relief.

INTERMITTENT HYDRARTHROSIS (INTERMITTENT SYNOVITIS)

Intermittent hydrarthrosis is an insidious, painless synovitis which appears most often in young women and is characterized by the accumulation of synovial fluid at regular intervals of from five days to a month, each effusion persisting for several days and then regressing spontaneously. It appears most often in the knee but occurs also in the elbow and rarely in other joints. It is not accompanied by increase of local temperature or by pain unless the swelling becomes extremely tense. There is, however, a feeling of stiffness and of slight discomfort about the joint. When the affection has become established, the swelling occurs in regular cycles, so that the patient can foretell exactly when the joint will become swollen. Between periods of swelling, the joint appears in early cases to be normal, but in older cases it may be somewhat boggy and thickened.

Etiology. Intermittent hydrarthrosis is thought by some authorities to be due to an endocrine disturbance. In young women it may be associated with the menstrual cycle. It has been known to disappear completely during pregnancy and to return following the termination of lactation. Other observers have offered the theory that intermittent hydrarthrosis may represent a trophic phase of a vasomotor disorder, since in many respects it resembles a transient angioneurotic edema. The affection has been found to occur in association with the early stages of rheumatoid arthritis. In such cases many of the joints may be involved simultaneously.

Prognosis. The periodic symptoms may continue for years. The outlook for cure is unfavorable except when a controllable causative factor can be found.

Treatment. In many cases the treatment is unsatisfactory. The administration of cortisone or iodides has seemed helpful in some cases. Synovectomy offers an excellent chance for relief of the symptoms in a single joint. In some cases the symptoms have subsided following immobilization in plaster.

BURSITIS

Eighteen or more bursal sacs about the knee have been described, but few of these are of clinical importance (Fig. 236).

The bursae most often affected are the prepatellar, deep infrapatellar, superficial pretibial, and popliteal, as well as variable bursae located beneath the tibial collateral ligament.

Prepatellar bursa

The prepatellar bursa lies anterior to the lower half of the patella and the upper half of the patellar ligament; it occurs more constantly than any other bursa about the knee. It often becomes inflamed from the irritation of repeated or prolonged kneeling. Chronic prepatellar bursitis is spoken of as "housemaid's knee," or "nun's knee."

Deep infrapatellar bursa

The deep infrapatellar bursa is situated between the lower portion of the patellar ligament and the tibia. When the bursa becomes swollen the

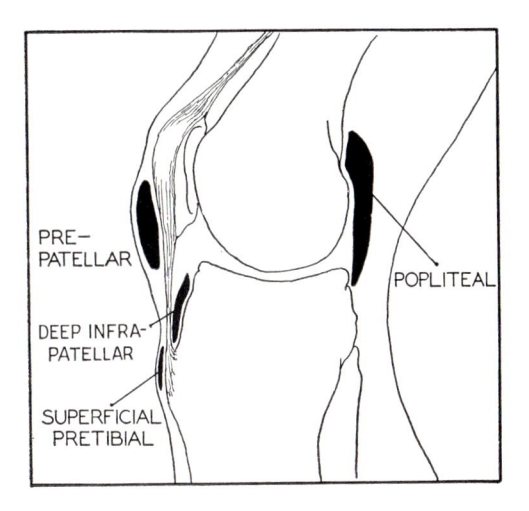

Fig. 236. Most commonly affected bursae about the knee.

normal depressions on either side of the patellar ligament disappear. Active flexion and extension of the knee are painful and limited.

Superficial pretibial bursa

The superficial pretibial bursa overlies the insertion of the patellar ligament into the tibial tuberosity.

Popliteal bursae

The popliteal bursae are found in the popliteal space and are numerous and inconstant. Of these, the *gastrocnemio-semimembranosus bursa* is of most clinical importance, as its distention by fluid is the usual cause of a *popliteal* or *Baker's cyst*. Bursae may develop also about the biceps tendon, and between the semitendinosus and gracilis tendons and the tibia (the *anserina bursa*). Occasionally a tubelike extension of the synovial sac of the knee is present beneath the popliteus muscle. The popliteal bursae are often connected with the synovial cavity of the knee. When enlarged, they stand out as firm, hard swellings when the knee is extended but may disappear when it is flexed. Sudden trauma and strain are important factors in causing symptoms.

Variable bursae beneath the tibial collateral ligament

Variable bursae located beneath the tibial collateral ligament, described by Voshell and Brantigan, may cause localized pain and tenderness, accompanied at times by a visible and palpable swelling.

• • •

Clinical picture. Any of these bursae may develop or enlarge without pain or discomfort. Fatigue and weakness of the knee may gradually appear, especially in affections of the popliteal bursae and of those about the attachment of the patellar ligament. When the bursa becomes distended and tense, the swelling may be accompanied by pain and tenderness of varying degree. The prepatellar bursa is often the seat of an acute pyogenic infection.

Treatment. In most cases the inflammatory symptoms subside with rest of the knee joint and hot applications. If a pyogenic infection is present, aspiration and antibiotic therapy are indicated. The greatly thickened prepatellar bursa resulting from long-standing chronic inflammation or distention is treated by excision. Chronically distended popliteal bursae should also be excised. After the entire sac has been removed the bursa seldom recurs.

INVOLVEMENT OF JOINTS IN HEMOPHILIA

Prolonged and repeated hemorrhage into the knee joint is a common manifestation of hemophilia, a hereditary disease of the blood which occurs in males and is transmitted by females. Involvement of any joint may occur. The knee is most commonly affected, but the ankle, elbow, shoulder, hip, and joints of the fingers are also subject to frequent intra-articular hemorrhages.

Pathology. Repeated hemorrhage into a joint, precipitated by the trauma of motion, weight bearing, or minor external violence, may be followed by incomplete absorption of the blood and later by organization. Degeneration of the articular cartilage, overgrowth of the synovium, and proliferation of bone at the articular edges may take place (Fig. 237). In cases of recent hemorrhage a brown discoloration of the joint surfaces is said to be characteristic. In late cases the pathologic changes may resemble those of rheumatoid arthritis, and the roentgenograms may show areas of spur formation and of cavitation in the atrophic bone. Widening of the intercondylar fossa of the femur is a common finding.

Clinical picture. The patient is a male whose first episode of hemarthrosis has occurred, as a rule, during middle or early childhood. The involvement may be monarticular. In cases of recent hemorrhage the joint capsule is distended, tender, and fluctuant, and motion of the joint causes discomfort. Discoloration of the skin is sometimes observed. Extensive hemorrhage is often accompanied by fever. Use of the joint intensifies the symptoms. Repeated hemorrhage may be followed by chronic swelling, discomfort on motion, muscle atrophy, and contracture. Hemorrhages may occur in any part of the body. The urine often is discolored and contains red blood cells from hemorrhage in the urogenital system.

Diagnosis. Diagnosis of the acute case is made upon the history of

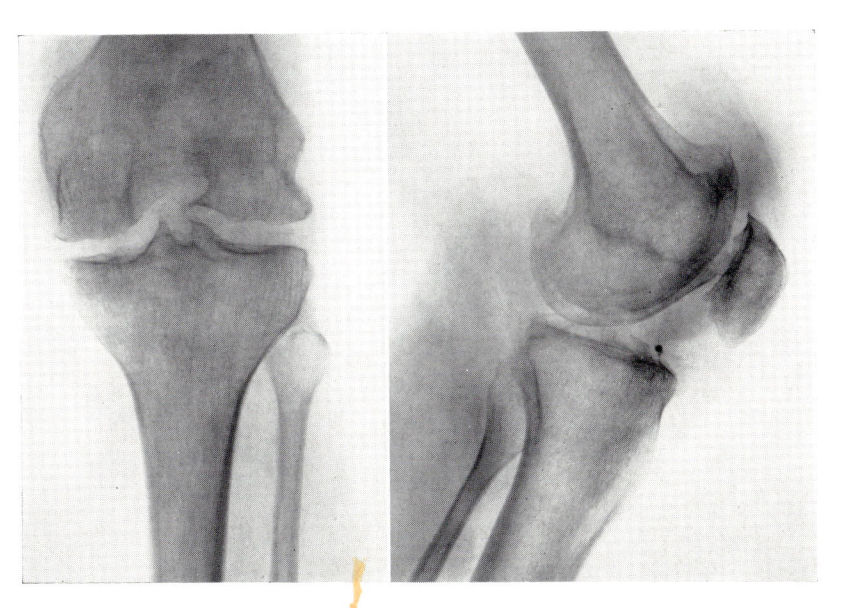

Fig. 237. Roentgenograms of knee of a 29-year-old man, showing characteristic changes in hemophilia. In anteroposterior view note the wide intercondylar fossa and spurs about the tibial spine; the lateral view shows spurs on the articular surface of the patella and about the anterior and posterior margins of the articular surface of the femur.

trivial injury combined with the physical signs of hemarthrosis and is confirmed by the finding of a prolonged coagulation time. Late cases are less characteristic and must be differentiated with care from tuberculosis and chronic arthritis. In the differential diagnosis roentgenograms are of less value than an accurate history and physical examination.

Prognosis. The initial hemorrhage is usually absorbed, and the prognosis for future joint function depends largely upon the patient's cooperation and good fortune in avoiding further episodes of trauma. Successive hemorrhages are likely to be followed by increasing disability, and the affected joint often presents finally a clinical and pathologic picture similar to that of rheumatoid arthritis.

Treatment. In cases of acute hemarthrosis the extremity should be immobilized at once by means of a large cotton pressure dressing and splint. An ice pack should be applied about the affected area. In cases of extensive hemorrhage, transfusion with fresh whole blood or freshly frozen plasma is the most valuable restorative measure. After subsidence of the hemarthrosis, physical therapy, consisting of heat, massage, and gentle motion, should be begun with extreme caution. Protection from further traumatization is essential; when the knee joint is involved, this is often best accomplished by the use of a caliper brace to restrict knee motion and to relieve the stress of weight bearing. In late cases with a deforming contracture, gentle physical therapy should be supplemented by the careful use of traction designed to effect gradual correction with a minimum of traumatization. Injections of hyaluronidase into the joint or hematoma may be made cautiously to promote absorption of the extravasated blood.

CHAPTER 20

Affections of the ankle and foot

THE FUNCTIONS OF THE FOOT are (1) to serve as a support for the weight of the body and (2) to act as a lever in raising and propelling the body forward in walking and running. The muscles of the leg supply the power, and the heads of the metatarsal bones serve as a fulcrum on which the weight is lifted. The foot contains two main arches formed by bones and supported directly by ligaments and indirectly by tendons and muscles. A normal degree of motion and elasticity in these arches is necessary for proper functioning of the foot.

The longitudinal or long arch is made up of two components, the medial and the lateral. The medial component is the more important and comprises the calcaneus, talus, navicular, three cuneiform bones, and the first three metatarsal bones (Fig. 238, A). This arch rests on the head of the first metatarsal and on the calcaneus. The lateral component of the longitudinal arch consists of the calcaneus, the cuboid, and the fourth and fifth metatarsal bones; it is supported behind by the calcaneus and in front by the heads of the fourth and fifth metatarsals. The anterior, transverse, or metatarsal arch is formed by the heads of the five metatarsal bones. Upon weight bearing the anterior arch becomes flattened, but as soon as the weight is removed the metatarsal heads return to their former positions and again form a low arch.

The movements of the foot and ankle are most important in the diagnosis and treatment of disabilities of the foot. The ankle joint permits plantar flexion and dorsiflexion of the foot. The foot is inverted or in the varus position when it is so rotated that its plantar surface faces medially; the foot is everted or in the valgus position when its plantar surface is rotated outward (Fig. 239). These motions occur in the subtalar joint between talus and calcaneus and in the mediotarsal joints, between talus and navicular and between calcaneus and cuboid. The primary motion of the mediotarsal joints, however, is adduction or inward swinging and abduction or outward swinging of the anterior portion of the foot. Pronation of the foot is a combination of eversion and abduction of the anterior portion of the foot; supination is a combination of inversion and adduction.

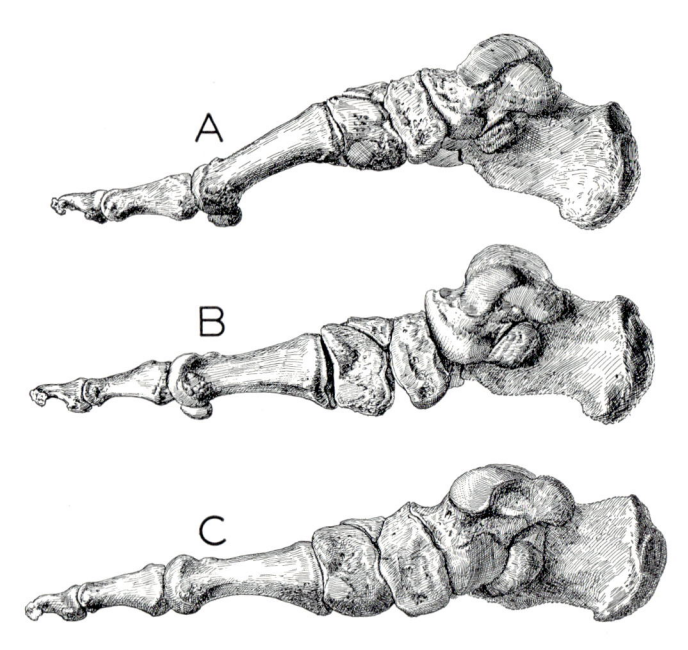

Fig. 238. Medial aspect of bones of foot. **A**, Normal longitudinal arch. **B**, Loss of arch in flexible flatfoot. **C**, Absence of arch in rigid flatfoot, showing adaptive bone changes.

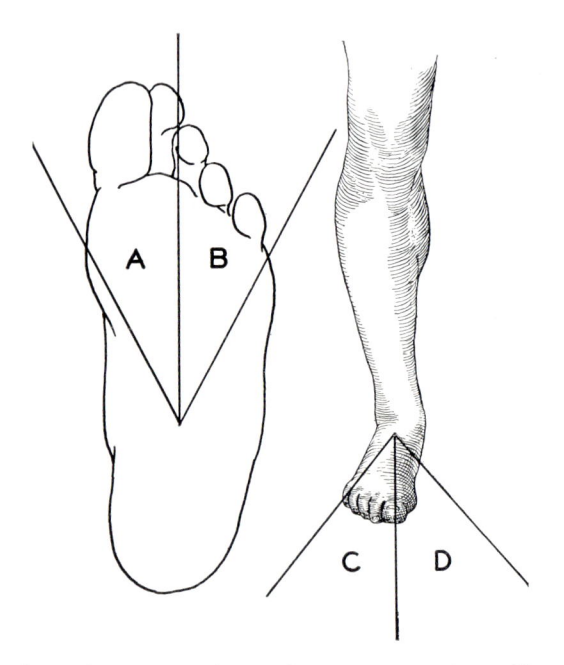

Fig. 239. Terminology of motion in the tarsal joints. **A**, Forefoot adduction; **B**, forefoot abduction; **C**, eversion; **D**, inversion. (After Cave and Roberts.)

FOOT STRAIN

Foot strain is encountered in a large group of patients whose disabilities arise in association with weight-bearing stresses on the foot.

Etiology. Factors which may lead to strain of the foot are incorrect shoes, inadequate muscular and ligamentous support, excessive body weight, and excessive exercise.

Incorrect shoes. Stiff leather shoes with pointed ends distort and compress the toes, making it impossible for the muscles to function normally. Muscle atrophy and loss of supporting power result. There can be little doubt that the modern shoe is the most important cause of many disabilities of the foot, especially in women.

Inadequate muscular and ligamentous support. Inadequate support may follow (1) rapid growth when muscle strength does not keep pace with the growth of the bony framework, and (2) prolonged illness or severe injury of the leg resulting in muscle atrophy and hypotonicity.

Excessive body weight. Obesity often puts so much stress upon the foot on weight bearing that the strength of the supporting ligaments and muscles is exceeded and the arches become abnormally depressed.

Excessive exercise. Too much standing, walking, or running, especially when the individual is not accustomed to such exercise or wears a flexible rubber-soled shoe, is a cause of foot strain.

When the muscles of the leg and foot fail to contribute their support, the body weight must be borne by the ligaments of the foot. Ligamentous tissues function normally as checkrein structures and when subjected to prolonged, unrelieved tension may become painful. Over a period of time gradual stretching of the ligaments may take place, allowing pronation of the foot and loss of the arch.

Clinical picture. Foot strain may be acute or chronic. Both forms affect adults frequently and are rare in childhood. Acute foot strain is manifested by pain and tenderness in the region of the longitudinal arch to such a degree that the patient is scarcely able to bear weight on the foot.

The patient with chronic foot strain complains of fatigue and aching in his feet. The discomfort is felt chiefly in the region of the longitudinal arch but may extend up into the calves. The symptoms are usually worse toward the end of the day; by evening the feet may feel tight and swollen. Often there is a history of recent weight gain, recent illness, or change to an occupation that involves increased walking or standing.

The most important physical finding is localized tenderness beneath the navicular bone at the apex of the longitudinal arch. In some instances pronation of the foot is obvious when the patient stands. This is not always true, for the normal foot and the foot with a high arch are also subject to strain.

Treatment. The immediate problem of foot pain and tenderness responds to local treatment. Hot soaks or contrast soaks may relieve the discomfort. Some form of support for the longitudinal arch should be provided. In the acute case this may be accomplished best by adhesive strapping. In chronic

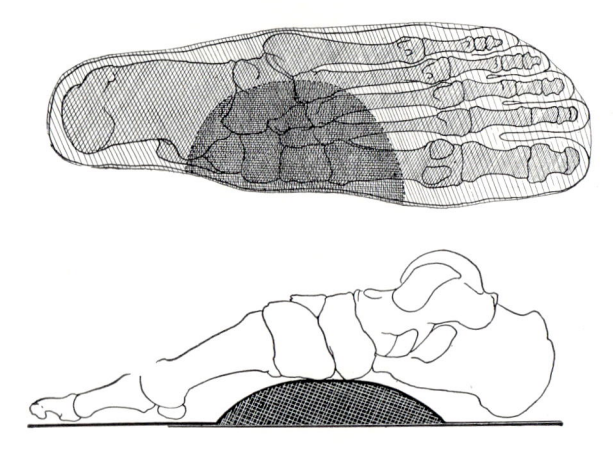

Fig. 240. Longitudinal arch support.

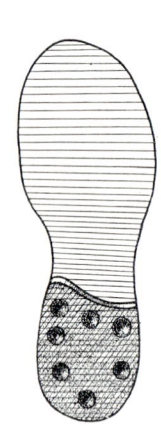

Fig. 241. Thomas or orthopaedic heel. Medial border of the heel is extended forward.

strain the use of a felt or sponge rubber arch pad is helpful (Fig. 240). A shoe with long counter and firm shank will give increased support. To this may be added a Thomas heel, which is extended forward medially to give support beneath the navicular bone (Fig. 241). In addition the medial border of the heel may be raised 3/16 of an inch. Exercises of both long and short muscles of the foot aid in restoring strength. The cause of the foot strain should be investigated and, if possible, treated. Weight reduction may be helpful. Modification of the patient's job is occasionally necessary. With proper treatment most cases of foot strain can be satisfactorily relieved by conservative measures.

FLEXIBLE FLATFOOT (PES PLANUS)

Flexible flatfoot is seen frequently both in children and in adults.

In children

Some eversion of the foot and relaxation of the longitudinal arch are usual in children in the first few years of life. The degree of eversion varies considerably, and it is impossible to make a clear-cut distinction between what should be considered normal and what abnormal. By the age of 5 or 6 years, individuals who are going to acquire a well-developed arch show evidence of it. Many children remain rather flatfooted. Unless the eversion is of severe degree, it is unlikely to lead to discomfort. Rarely does this type of flatfoot cause symptoms in childhood.

The diagnosis of flatfoot in children is usually obvious, but its interpretation may be difficult. When the child stands, absence of the longitudinal arch on the medial side of the foot is apparent. Seen from its posterior aspect, the heel appears everted. Examination of the dorsum shows abduction of the forefoot. The foot is quite mobile and without fixed deformity. There is a normal range of ankle and subtalar motion, and the mobility of the anterior part of the foot may even be increased. Motor power about the foot and ankle is normal. This type of relaxed flatfoot is usually most marked in heavy children; it is often associated with knock-knee. It may be differentiated from paralytic flatfoot by the presence of normal muscle power, from congenital vertical talus and from peroneal spastic flatfoot by the normal mobility and absence of fixed deformity, and from flatfoot associated with a tight heel cord by the normal range of ankle dorsiflexion.

Treatment. In mild cases no treatment is necessary, other than reassurance of the parents. Children with moderate or severe flatfoot are probably best treated by raising the medial border of the heels of their shoes ⅛ inch. A shoe with long counter and Thomas heel may be helpful. It is permissible and probably advisable to allow the child to go barefoot part of the time during the summer. In children, foot exercises are of doubtful value.

In adults

Asymptomatic flatfoot in the adult requires no treatment. Mild or moderate degrees of pronation do not usually cause symptoms. Severe flatfoot in adults, however, with its disturbed mechanical relationships, is likely to result in degenerative articular changes (Fig. 238, C), stiffness, and pain on weight bearing. Moreover, the flat foot, as well as the normal foot, is subject to strain. The treatment of foot strain has been discussed (p. 417).

SPASTIC FLATFOOT

The spastic flatfoot is held in marked eversion by spasm of the peroneal muscles (Fig. 242). The spasm is not caused by an upper motor neuron lesion but is probably of reflex or protective nature associated with irritative changes in one or more of the joints of the foot. The spasm may be relieved and may disappear with rest, only to return when weight bearing is resumed. Spastic flatfoot may be a sequel of an untreated flexible flatfoot and is seen at times in association with obesity or chronic arthritis.

In the early stages the foot is extremely painful. There is often tenderness over the peroneal tendons, and attempts to invert the foot may cause

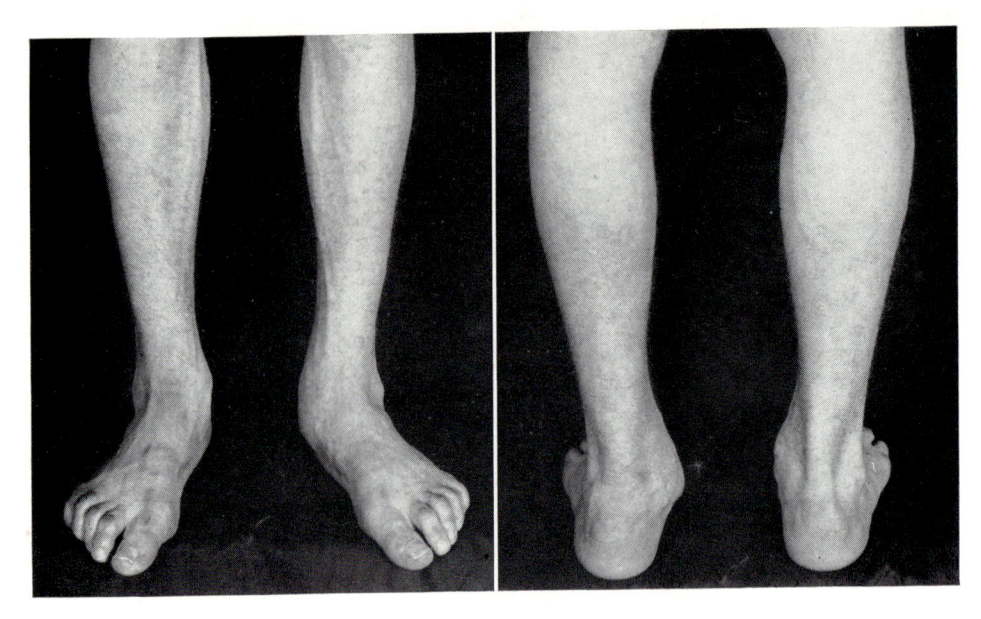

Fig. 242. Left spastic flatfoot in a man 22 years of age. Note severe pronation of left foot, which could not be inverted actively or passively, and atrophy of left calf. The right foot is slightly pronated but showed no joint stiffness and no tightness of the peroneal muscles.

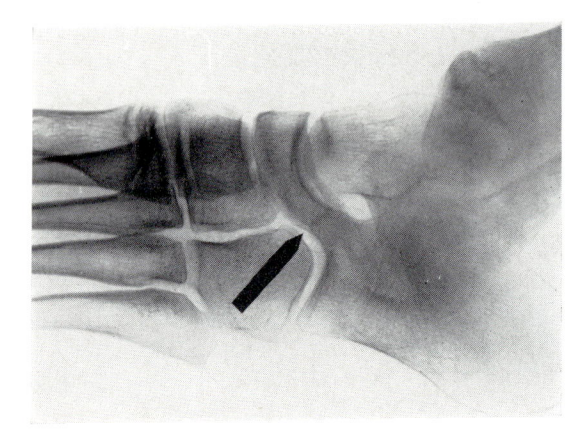

Fig. 243. Oblique roentgenogram of foot of a boy 15 years of age, showing a calcaneonavicular bar. This was bilateral, and a previous diagnosis of spastic flatfeet had been made.

sharp pain. The foot may be swollen, and the extremity may be held in marked external rotation. In acute stages every step is painful and the patient walks with an awkward, shuffling gait. Later the foot may become rigid from the development of secondary bone changes, with proliferation about the joint margins where abnormal pressure and strain are present.

Many rigid, everted flatfeet have a congenital synostosis or synchondrosis between the anterior end of the calcaneus and the navicular bone *(calcaneonavicular bar)*, which may be seen in oblique roentgenograms (Fig. 243). A complete or partial union of the talus and the calcaneus by a bridge of bone situated behind the sustentaculum tali *(talocalcaneal bridge)* may also be found; it can be demonstrated in posterior oblique roentgenograms of the heel. In the presence of either of these anomalies, pain in the partially rigid foot may develop at or shortly before puberty.

Treatment. In the early stages and in the absence of bony abnormalities, correction may be accomplished by the use of casts, which are wedged gradually into inversion. If there is no roentgenographic evidence of bony anomalies, forcible overcorrection under anesthesia, followed by immobilization in plaster, may be helpful. Heat, massage, corrective foot exercises, and a support under the longitudinal arch should then be employed. It is often advisable to allow the patient to walk while the cast holds the foot in the inverted position. Occasionally in severe cases with pain, arthrodesis of the subtalar and mediotarsal joints (triple arthrodesis) is indicated; it is usually followed by complete relief of the pain.

In rigid flatfoot, operations for reshaping the longitudinal arch are seldom to be recommended. The resection of a congenital bony bar or bridge is not followed, as a rule, by increased mobility and is not advised.

SHORTENING OF THE ACHILLES TENDON

Shortening of the Achilles tendon, especially in the weak or everted foot, leads to the development of foot strain. In adults shortening of the Achilles tendon may be due either to a congenital structural change or to reflex muscular spasm from irritation caused by disturbed mechanics of the foot. In the reflex type there is discomfort, which may be associated with tenderness and with sharp pain and spasm on attempting to dorsiflex the foot.

Treatment. In cases of the reflex type, raising the heel of the shoe may lead to relief of the symptoms. In the structural type an attempt should be made to stretch the Achilles tendon by wedged plaster casts or by special stretching exercises. Experience has shown that surgical lengthening of the Achilles tendon weakens this type of foot and should be discouraged. In women pain in the feet is sometimes caused by shortening of the Achilles tendon from wearing shoes with very high heels. In such cases the heels should be gradually lowered and stretching exercises should be carried out. Sudden change from high-heel to low-heel shoes often produces much discomfort in the legs from pull upon the gastrocnemius and soleus muscles and should never be advised.

CLAWFOOT

The typical clawfoot has an abnormally high longitudinal arch, a depression of the metatarsal arch, and dorsal contractures of the toes (Fig. 244). The plantar fascia is contracted, the anterior half of the foot drawn downward and sometimes inward, and the Achilles tendon may be shortened.

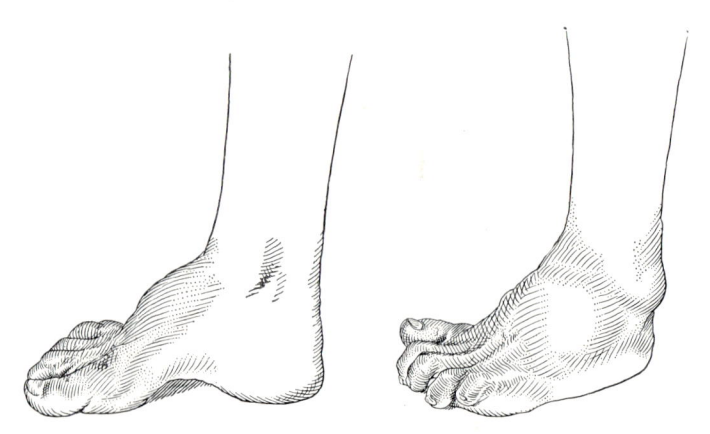

Fig. 244. Clawfoot of moderate degree in young adult. Note high longitudinal arch (cavus), dorsal contracture of the toes, adduction of the forefoot, and slight equinus.

Excessive height of the longitudinal arch is termed *cavus* deformity. It is often seen without other deformities and usually causes few symptoms.

The deformities of clawfoot may be slight or severe. In most instances they show a gradual progression. With the muscular contractures which are associated with clawfoot, there is a loss of the normal elasticity of the arches. Newton Shaffer has applied the term "nondeforming clubfoot" to the type of foot that shows clawing of the toes, a high longitudinal arch, and a short Achilles tendon.

Etiology. In some cases the deformity of clawfoot is the result of an inherited tendency. It may be associated also with the wearing of high heels, which produces a postural equinus, or with excessive use of the leg muscles, as in professional dancers. After poliomyelitis it sometimes develops in the seemingly unparalyzed foot. Imbalance of muscular power in the foot is considered the causative factor in many cases. Clawfoot may occur in the course of progressive lesions of the central nervous system, such as Friedreich's ataxia and peroneal muscular atrophy. Frequently clawfoot has been found in association with spina bifida occulta. It may follow conditions such as cellulitis, fibrositis, rheumatoid arthritis, and the like, and is sometimes seen after compound fractures of the tibia which have been immobilized in poor position or have received inadequate aftercare. Most commonly, however, clawfoot can be ascribed to no specific etiologic factor, and it is then spoken of as "idiopathic clawfoot." Idiopathic clawfoot is a progressive deformity and may be unilateral or bilateral.

Symptoms. Although considerable deformity may be present without causing symptoms, the patient usually complains of early fatigue with exercise and of tender calluses beneath the metatarsal heads and over the proximal interphalangeal joints.

Treatment and prognosis. In mild cases the treatment may consist of simple stretching of the plantar fascia and Achilles tendon and the wearing

Affections of the ankle and foot   423

of proper shoes. The shoes should be fitted with metatarsal pads or bars to relieve strain upon the anterior portion of the foot.

For clawfoot of moderate degree it may be necessary to carry out a plantar fasciotomy and to stretch the foot under anesthesia. Occasionally transplantation of one or more of the extensor tendons of the toes to the distal portion of the metatarsal bones or to the flexor tendons is indicated.

In more severe cases it is sometimes advisable to strip the plantar fascia

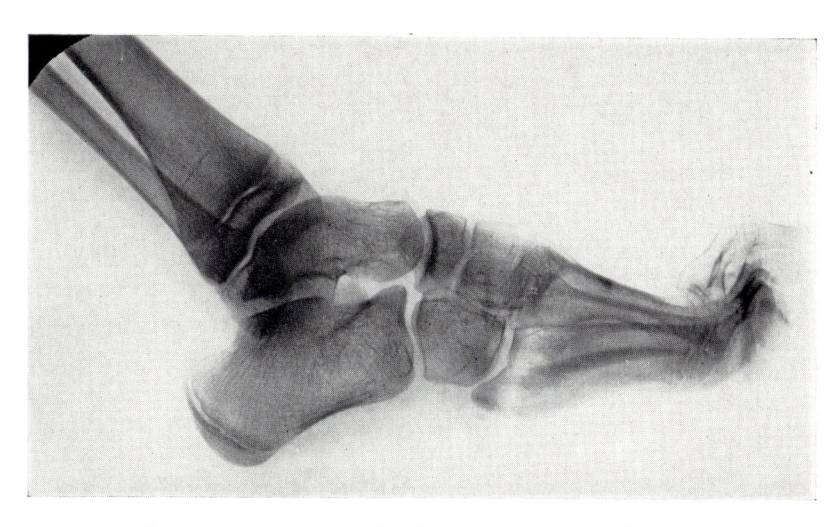

Fig. 245. Lateral roentgenogram of early clawfoot in 11-year-old girl. Note dorsal contracture of toes and plantar flexion of ankle. Both feet were equally involved and became progressively worse despite conservative therapy.

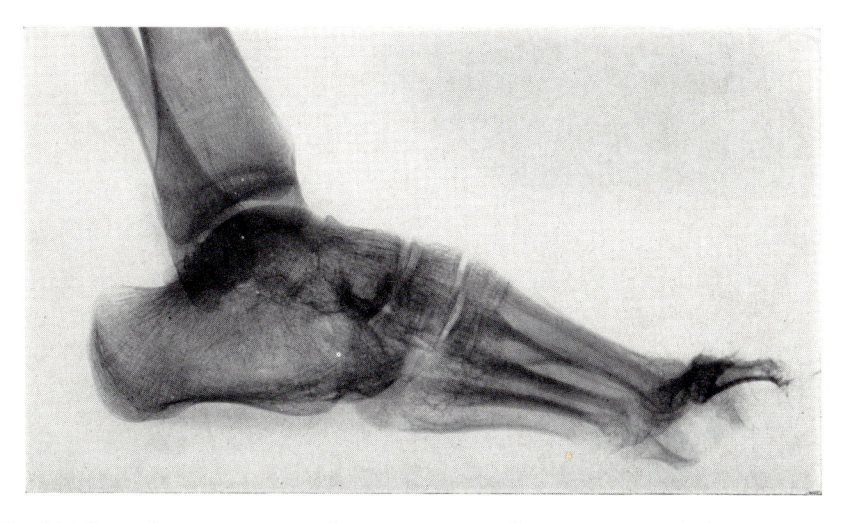

Fig. 246. Lateral roentgenogram of same patient as shown in Fig. 245, three years after mid-tarsal wedge resection and subtalar arthrodesis. Note flattening of the longitudinal arch and improvement in dorsal contracture of the toes. After the surgical treatment the patient was completely asymptomatic.

424 Handbook of orthopaedic surgery

from its attachment to the calcaneus, section the flexor and extensor tendons of the toes, and lengthen the Achilles tendon.

In still more advanced cases dorsal wedge osteotomy combined with subtalar arthrodesis is the only procedure that will effect satisfactory correction of the deformity (Figs. 245 and 246). In extreme cases it may be necessary also to excise the metatarsal heads.

In idiopathic clawfoot the deformity may recur after surgical correction, especially if the operative procedure has involved only tendons and fascia. All of these deformed feet should be fitted with proper shoes and with supports for both the anterior and longitudinal arches. Corrective foot exercises and physical therapy should be started early. The results are often satisfactory when the treatment is properly selected and is followed by observation of the patient over a period of years.

KÖHLER'S DISEASE (AVASCULAR NECROSIS OR OSTEOCHONDRITIS OF THE NAVICULAR BONE)

Osteochondritis of the tarsal navicular bone (Figs. 247 and 248) is an uncommon affection which begins insidiously in childhood, about the fifth or sixth year of age. It causes a variable degree of local discomfort and limping and tends toward gradual spontaneous recovery. The etiology is not established, but the affection seems to fall into the group of localized and self-limited bone diseases of youth that are ascribed to ischemic degenerative changes. Trauma sometimes appears to be a contributing factor. Clinically there are tenderness and slight thickening over the affected navicular bone. The roentgenographic appearance of the navicular is pathognomonic, the bone being small, dense, and of irregular outline and disordered internal structure as though it had been crushed. Microscopic

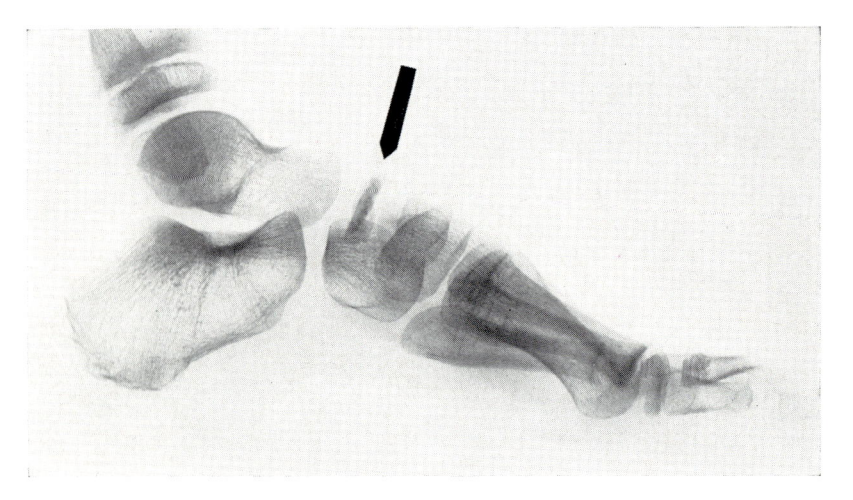

Fig. 247. Lateral roentgenogram showing Köhler's disease (osteochondritis of the navicular bone) in a 6-year-old boy. Note thin navicular of irregular shape and uneven density.

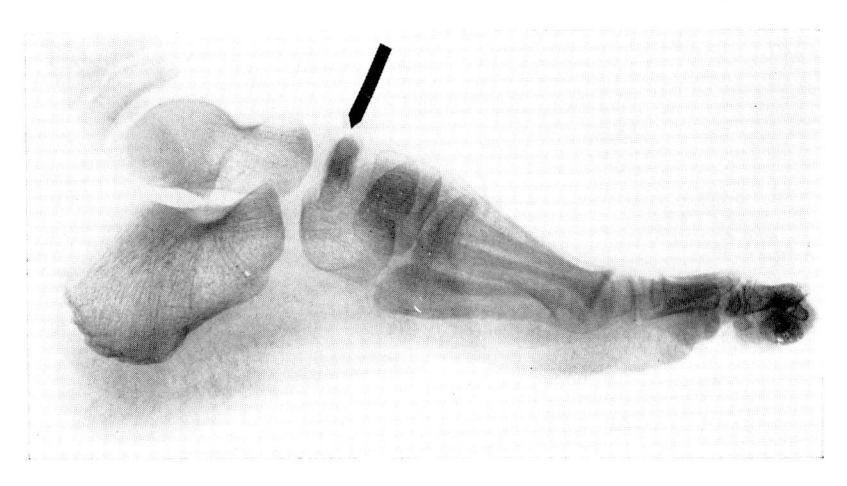

Fig. 248. Lateral roentgenogram of same patient as shown in Fig. 247, five months later. Note improvement in the shape and density of the navicular bone.

sections of such bones have shown massive necrosis, which is followed by organization, resorption of dead bone, and the formation of new bone.

Treatment and prognosis. Protection of the diseased bone from excessive traumatization is important. Support of the longitudinal arch and restriction of activity may suffice. If there is much pain on weight bearing, however, it is preferable to immobilize the foot in slight inversion by means of a plaster cast for a period of six to ten weeks. The results are usually satisfactory, there being little or no permanent disability.

ANTERIOR METATARSALGIA

Etiology. A painful metatarsal arch often occurs in (1) the everted or abducted foot, (2) the foot with a short Achilles tendon, and (3) the foot with a high longitudinal arch, such as the clawfoot. Disturbances of the metatarsal arch are most common in individuals over 30 years of age and occur more often in women than in men. The affection is a result of muscular weakness which allows excessive weight bearing on the middle metatarsal heads. Tight, short, high-heel shoes play an important part in the pathogenesis. A short and tight shoe compresses the anterior part of the foot, elevates the head of the fifth metatarsal bone and throws weight upon the fourth metatarsal, causing pain about its head.

Clinical picture. Often the first symptom is a burning, cramping pain in the anterior part of the foot, usually under the middle metatarsal heads. Occasionally the pain is preceded by the feeling, experienced on standing or walking, that a bone has slipped out of place. Pain on standing and walking may become severe and disabling. At times the pain radiates to the end of the toe, up into the foot, and even into the leg. The pain is seldom experienced with the shoe off. Tenderness is most often found beneath the fourth metatarsal head, although it may be present also beneath the head of the second or third metatarsal. A tender callus frequently develops under the metatarsal heads.

Examination of the foot often shows depression of the metatarsal arch even when the foot is bearing no weight. The most characteristic features, however, are the tenderness and calluses beneath the metatarsal heads. In severe cases there are usually dorsal contracture of the toes and restriction of their motion. It is impossible to flex the toes fully, and any attempt to do so produces pain in the tender areas. Swelling, redness, and increased heat are seldom present. Anterior metatarsalgia may occur in association with hallux valgus or hallux rigidus.

Treatment. The basic objects of treatment are (1) relief of the pain by arch supports and (2) strengthening of the muscles of the foot and ankle by corrective exercises.

The patient should wear a shoe which has a thick sole, adequate width at the toes, a supporting longitudinal arch, and a narrow counter. A small felt or rubber pad, placed immediately behind the metatarsal heads and held in place with circular adhesive strapping, will usually relieve the acute symptoms (Fig. 249). Various types of supports, made of leather, felt, rubber, cork, or metal and designed to elevate the metatarsal arch, may be fitted into the shoe. A transverse bar posterior to the metatarsal heads, made of leather and attached to the outside of the shoe (metatarsal bar, Fig. 250) or placed between the inner and outer soles *(Cook anterior heel)*, will often relieve the symptoms of metatarsal strain. The patient should be instructed regarding hot soaks, contrast baths, massage, and corrective foot exercises. The exercises should be continued for several weeks. With gradual improvement of the muscle strength the affection may be completely relieved.

Occasionally a sensitive plantar wart may be the source of severe pain. Relieving the pressure upon a tender wart by means of proper pads or supports may lead to its disappearance. Curettement, excision, or roentgentherapy may be indicated in selected cases. Manipulation to loosen up adhesions in the anterior part of the foot is occasionally indicated in metatarsalgia. In

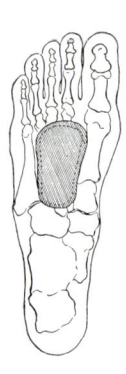

Fig. 249. Metatarsal arch support. Note position just behind the metatarsal heads. (After Lewin.)

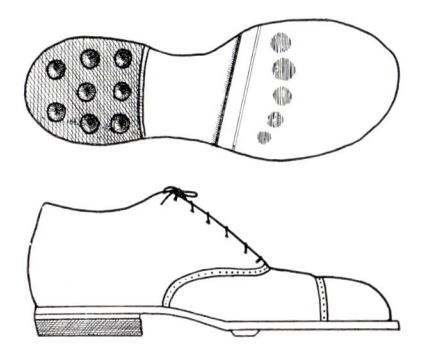

Fig. 250. Shoe with metatarsal bar. Note that bar is fixed to sole just behind the metatarsal heads.

resistant cases associated with malposition of the bones, resection of the metatarsal head in the area of tenderness is occasionally necessary. After such resection it is necessary for the patient to wear a well-fitted support under the metatarsal arch.

MORTON'S TOE (PLANTAR NEUROMA)

In 1876 T. G. Morton described a type of metatarsalgia characterized by sudden attacks of sharp pain usually localized to a single toe. The fourth toe is most commonly involved. The condition is usually unilateral; women are affected more commonly than men. In the early stages there is a burning sensation in the region of the metatarsal head, which may radiate into the toes and be accompanied by paresthesia and numbness. The characteristic pain, however, is sharp and lancinating; it is often so intense as to demand immediate removal of the shoe and manipulation of the toes. After these sudden attacks tenderness may persist for several days and be followed by numbness of the toes.

As a rule the appearance of the foot is normal. A small area of exquisite tenderness may usually be located by firm palpation of the third web space. In late cases it is sometimes possible to elicit crepitation, together with characteristic pain, by careful palpation with one hand while the other squeezes the metatarsal heads together.

In recent years it has been demonstrated that the pain is associated with a localized thickening of the third plantar common digital nerve at its bifurcation in the web space. The enlargement or "neuroma" is presumably a result of repeated traumatization of the nerve trunk by the metatarsal heads. Microscopically it shows proliferation of neurilemma cells and interstitial fibrosis.

Treatment. The symptoms can sometimes be relieved by a metatarsal arch support. Excision of the enlarged segment of the digital nerve is a safe and effective procedure, produces little loss of sensation, and is the treatment of choice in most cases. Sometimes exploration discloses a bursa which also should be excised.

STRESS FRACTURE OF A METATARSAL BONE (MARCH OR FATIGUE FRACTURE)

Fracture of a metatarsal shaft, usually the second or third, may result from the stress associated with weight bearing after prolonged walking has exhausted the muscular and tendinous support of the foot. A congenital shortening of the first metatarsal bone, *metatarsus atavicus*, which throws an increased leverage on the shaft of the second metatarsal, may be a predisposing factor. Symptoms may be completely absent at the instant of fracture, beginning a week or more later as exuberant callus forms. The pain and swelling which appear at this time may lead to an erroneous diagnosis of malignant tumor. On the other hand, the onset of pain may precede the appearance of roentgenographic changes by one or two weeks, causing the patient to be unjustly suspected of malingering. Stress fractures are especially common in army recruits during their basic training. In a reported series these fractures were found most frequently during the tenth week of training and were seldom observed in the Negro recruit. Stress fractures have been reported as occurring in the femur, inferior pubic ramus, and many other bones.

Treatment. Extensive experience in the Armed Forces has demonstrated that rest, adhesive strapping, and the use of an anterior arch pad constitute the most effective form of treatment. Sometimes, however, a plaster cast is advisable for a period of from three to four weeks. After the cast has been removed, the patient's shoe should be fitted with an anterior arch pad or a metatarsal bar and he should not engage in excessive walking for several months.

FREIBERG'S DISEASE (AVASCULAR NECROSIS OR OSTEOCHONDRITIS OF A METATARSAL HEAD)

Freiberg's disease is characterized by the gradual development of degenerative changes in the head of the second metatarsal bone (Fig. 251) or, rarely, in other metatarsal heads. The affection is uncommon; it occurs usually in adolescent children but is often seen in adults. The etiology is believed to be a disturbance of the circulation which results in a localized ischemic necrosis. Trauma is possibly a contributing factor. The roentgenograms show bone absorption and deformation, with thickening of the distal portion of the affected bone. Clinically there are pain on weight bearing and thickening and tenderness of the affected metatarsal head.

Treatment. In the acute stage of the affection, treatment by means of a plaster boot or anterior arch pad is usually sufficient. Occasionally in late cases it is necessary to resect the excess bone or to excise the deformed metatarsal head in order to relieve the pain and discomfort. After such operations the use of an anterior arch support is advisable.

HALLUX VALGUS

Hallux valgus is a lateral angulation of the great toe at its metatarsophalangeal joint. There is usually an associated enlargement of the medial

Affections of the ankle and foot 429

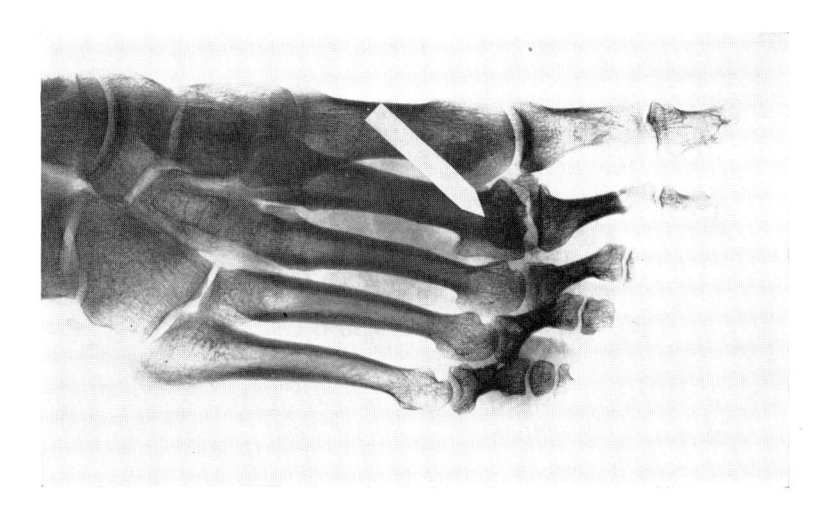

Fig. 251. Oblique roentgenogram showing Freiberg's disease (osteochondritis of head of second metatarsal bone). Note the flattening, irregularity, and bone production about the head of the second metatarsal. The patient was 40 years of age.

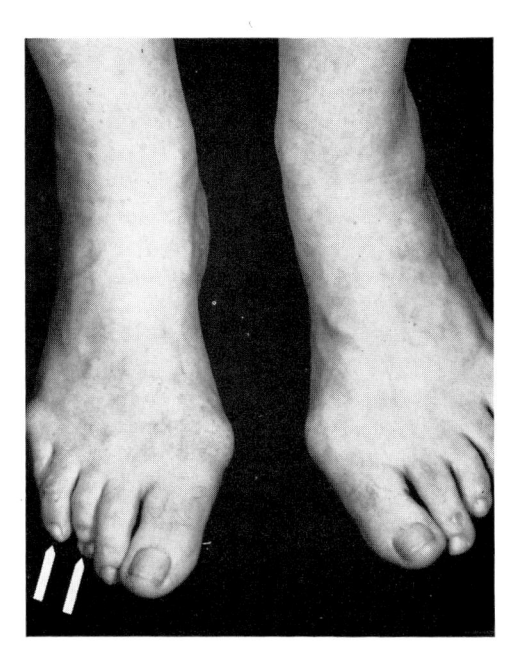

Fig 252. Bilateral hallux valgus and bunion in adult. Note also that right third and fourth toes show hammer-toe deformity.

side of the head of the first metatarsal bone, together with the formation of a bursa and callus over this area (Fig. 252). The bony prominence and its overlying bursa constitute the so-called "bunion."

Etiology and pathology. Hallux valgus is frequently familial. It is much more common in women than in men. Adduction of the first metatarsal bone may initiate the deforming changes; narrow, pointed, and short shoes doubtless aggravate them. Adduction or varus deviation of the first metatarsal is accompanied by abduction of the great toe; in extreme cases all of the metatarsals may be adducted and all of the toes abducted. The anterior part of the foot is widened and the anterior arch depressed. Contracture of the flexor and extensor hallucis longus muscles is associated with a lateral displacement of the extensor tendons. As the great toe deviates laterally the second toe may be forced to ride up over it, which often results in a painful callus from friction against the shoe. Occasionally the malalignment and the symptoms are aggravated by degenerative arthritic changes. Atrophy of articular cartilage may be extensive. The pain of hallux valgus may be caused by traumatic arthritis, pressure upon digital nerves, and compression and inflammation of the bursa overlying the metatarsal exostosis.

Treatment and prognosis. In mild cases, properly fitting shoes and repeated overcorrection by stretching may prevent progression of the deformity and afford relief of the discomfort. The patient should sleep with a pad or special toe separator between the first and second toes. The depression of the metatarsal arch should be corrected by a supportive pad and exercises. In acute infection of the bursa, rest and hot compresses are indicated.

When considerable deformity is accompanied by disabling pain, surgical treatment is indicated. It is the only available method of correcting the deformity and so relieving the pain. Many different operative procedures for the treatment of hallux valgus have been described. The simplest of these is removal of the exostosis and the bursa. In addition, the ligaments on the medial side may be reefed, the capsule on the opposite side divided, and the extensor hallucis longus tendon sectioned or lengthened *(Silver operation).* Transplantation of the adductor hallucis tendon from phalanx to metatarsal, as described by McBride, is frequently advisable.

Resection of the proximal half of the first phalanx *(Keller* or *Schanz operation)* is often the procedure of choice for the correction of severe deformity. In the absence of arthritic changes, a wedge osteotomy of the proximal end of the first metatarsal bone, after removal of the exostosis and bursa, may be the operation of choice; it corrects the varus deformity of the first metatarsal bone, which is an important contributing factor in hallux valgus. Many other surgical procedures for hallux valgus have been described. The choice of procedure depends upon the individual case.

After all operations for hallux valgus, the great toe should be held in an overcorrected position, either by a splint or by a soft cushion pad placed between the first and second toes, until it is unlikely that the deformity will recur. Hot soaks, massage, and corrective foot exercises should be employed as long as tenderness and stiffness persist. Some patients recover rapidly from operations for hallux valgus and are permanently relieved of pain, especially those who have had the minimum of surgery performed and who can be relatively inactive in their occupations. Others experience pain for several months afterward. The patient should be observed periodically in an effort to forestall recurrence of the deformity. Hallux valgus operations on military personnel in World War II seldom resulted in return to full active duty.

HALLUX VARUS

Hallux varus, in contrast to hallux valgus, is a medial angulation of the great toe at the metatarsophalangeal joint. This deformity usually is congenital in origin; however, trauma, infection, muscle imbalance from paralysis of the adductor hallucis, or a bunion operation in which the outer capsule and insertion of the adductor hallucis tendon have been severed, may also be responsible for hallux varus.

Treatment. Mild cases can be corrected surgically by releasing the contracted structures on the medial side of the toe and plicating the lateral part of the joint capsule. Greater degrees of deformity may require additional measures such as osteotomy of the metatarsal head and use of the sectioned extensor hallucis brevis tendon as a tenodesis to maintain the corrected alignment.

HALLUX RIGIDUS

Hallux rigidus is characterized by restriction of motion in the first metatarsophalangeal joint, occasioned usually by trauma, osteoarthritis, or disuse associated with chronic foot strain. Burning and throbbing pain occur in the affected part of the foot after standing or walking. Since dorsiflexion of the toe is limited, pain is especially marked in the latter part of the stance phase of walking, as the patient comes up on the ball of his foot.

Treatment. In mild cases the treatment consists of (1) wearing a thick, inflexible sole on the shoe or (2) having a long steel strip inserted between inner and outer soles of the shoe in order to restrict motion in the affected metatarsophalangeal joint. The use of a metatarsal bar on the shoe is sometimes helpful. Occasionally slight elevation of the medial side of the sole of the shoe will abolish the pain. If the symptoms cannot be relieved in such ways, surgical removal of the proximal half of the first phalanx is helpful. An alternative procedure, often followed by complete relief of pain, is arthrodesis of the first metatarsophalangeal joint.

HAMMER TOE

Hammer toe is characterized by dorsiflexion of the metatarsophalangeal joint and plantar flexion contracture of the proximal interphalangeal joint (Fig. 253). Although any toe may be so affected, the second is most frequently involved. Tender corns and calluses are usually present on the toe.

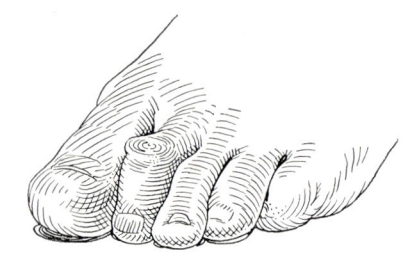

Fig. 253. Hammer toe.

The deformity may be due to the pressure of a short, narrow shoe upon the end of a long toe. The deformities may begin in early childhood, however, and are often found in association with hallux valgus. Accordingly there may be a familial influence in the etiology.

Treatment. In early cases simple manipulation and splinting of the affected toe may suffice to relieve the moderate discomfort. In older cases arthrodesis of the proximal interphalangeal joint in extension is indicated. Sometimes complete excision of the proximal phalanx yields a very satisfactory result. Hammer-toe deformity of the second toe associated with hallux valgus has often been wrongly treated by amputation of the second toe, which results in an increase of the hallux valgus.

OVERLAPPING OR DORSAL DISPLACEMENT OF THE TOES

Overlapping most often involves the little toe. It may be of developmental origin or may arise from wearing tight shoes. The toe may become very painful because of corns or callus formation.

Treatment. In infants and younger children manipulation and splinting of the toe may correct the deformity. Tenotomy or transplantation of the extensor tendon may be necessary. When this treatment fails to produce satisfactory relief of the symptoms, resection of the proximal phalanx or amputation of the toe may be indicated.

PIGEON-TOE

Pigeon-toe is habitual turning in of the feet on walking and may be encountered in association with flexible flatfoot in small children. It is a physical sign rather than a disease entity and is often found together with hallux varus, metatarsus varus, bowlegs, medial torsion of the tibia, congenital contracture of the internal rotators of the hip, increased anteversion of the femoral neck, or relapsed clubfoot. Some observers believe that medial torsion of the tibia is the most common cause.

Treatment. Infants and young children should not be allowed to spend too much time in sleeping and sitting positions in which the lower limbs are internally rotated. The deformity is usually corrected spontaneously as the child grows older. Raising the outer border of the soles of the shoes ⅛ to ¼ inch may hasten the improvement. The child should be instructed to walk with the toes pointed out. If torsion is present in the tibia or the femur, the use of a Denis Browne night splint to hold the lower extremities in wide external rotation may be very helpful. For older children, roller skating provides excellent corrective exercise.

AFFECTIONS OF THE HEEL

Affections of the heel include the results of inflammation and injury either (1) about the insertion of the Achilles tendon or (2) under the calcaneus on weight bearing.

Inflammation and injury about the insertion of the Achilles tendon

Pain in the back of the heel is the outstanding symptom of these locally disabling affections.

Tenosynovitis

Swelling is usually noticeable in the region of the Achilles tendon, and fine crepitus on motion is often unmistakable. The affection is usually marked by acute local tenderness and considerable disability. The treatment consists of rest, avoidance of pressure, and the application of heat to the tender area. When it is necessary for the patient to walk, a pad should be placed in the shoe to elevate the heel and so lessen the excursion of the tendon. In chronic Achilles tenosynovitis, rest, contrast baths, and massage are indicated.

Bursitis

Inflammation of the retrocalcaneal bursa, which is situated between the Achilles tendon and the calcaneus, causes local tenderness and pain upon motion. The disorder is treated by rest, heat, and elevation of the heel by means of a pad. If the symptoms do not subside with this type of therapy, the bursa may be excised. The irritation of a tight shoe sometimes causes a bursa (the *superficial calcaneal or posterior Achilles bursa*) to form between the Achilles tendon and the skin. In inflammation of this bursa, relief of pressure and application of heat are indicated. Occasionally, when the bursa becomes frankly infected, it should be incised or resected.

Periostitis

Discomfort may sometimes be caused by inflammation of the periosteum at the attachment of the Achilles tendon. The treatment is similar to that of bursitis.

Calcaneal apophysitis or epiphysitis

Sometimes called *Haglund's disease*, this condition is a somewhat uncommon affection of children, occurring most often in boys between 9 and 14 years of age. Calcaneal epiphysitis is a low-grade inflammatory reaction, occurring in the posterior calcaneal epiphysis, accompanied by pain and swelling, and ascribed to chronic pressure or strain. Roentgenograms may show the epiphysis to be irregular or segmented with areas of increased density. However, in children many roentgenograms of the calcaneus show such changes in the absence of symptoms. The affection is treated by relieving the local strain and pressure. Raising the heel of the shoe ½ inch for several months usually proves effective. It is occasionally advisable to apply a plaster cast in order to secure complete rest of the affected area.

Partial or complete rupture of the Achilles or plantaris tendon

Incomplete rupture of the Achilles tendon may be followed by the formation of small irregular masses of fibrous consistency. Occasionally calcification similar to that of myositis ossificans occurs in these masses; when pain is persistent in such cases, the calcified area should be excised. Complete rupture of the Achilles tendon by indirect violence is occasionally seen; as a rule it occurs in athletic individuals of stocky build. The power of voluntary plantar flexion is greatly diminished, and the rupture is evident on palpation. Recent ruptures should be treated by immediate exploration and suture. Rupture of the plantaris tendon, evidenced by a sudden sharp pain like the sting of a whip, may occur frequently, but clinical differentiation from incomplete rupture of the Achilles tendon is often questionable. The treatment consists of rest, adhesive strapping, and support of the heel. Ruptures of other tendons of the ankle and foot are quite rare.

Inflammation and injury under the calcaneus

Localized tenderness beneath the heel, which may cause sharp pain on standing and walking, is frequently found in middle-aged men and less commonly in women. The patient may be severely disabled by heel tenderness, especially if it is bilateral. In some instances the onset of symptoms can be related to an occupation requiring prolonged standing or to an excessive gain in weight. The exact cause, however, and pathologic nature are unknown. The skin and subcutaneous fat of the weight-bearing surface of the heel are specialized structures designed to withstand the tremendous stresses of everyday walking; they may be affected by trauma or inflammation. In the past a low-grade periostitis, fascitis, or bursitis has been postulated. Frequently, ossification at the attachment of plantar fascia to calcaneus appears in the lateral roentgenogram as a calcaneal spur. Whether the spur is related to the pain in most cases is doubtful.

Treatment. In mild cases complete relief can often be obtained by the use of (1) a soft rubber heel pad with a hole cut in its center to relieve pressure upon the tender area, (2) a cupped metal plate to eliminate pressure in this area, (3) a special heel which is shaped to bear all the weight at its posterior margin, or (4) a high longitudinal arch pad. Rest, hot applications, and massage should also be used. An injection of procaine into the tender area may be followed by relief of the symptoms. Weight reduction and change to sedentary occupation may be helpful. With time the symptoms usually subside. When the pain persists, surgical excision of a thin slice of cortical bone from the inferior surface of the calcaneus should be considered. Even after such operation, however, the resumption of weight bearing is sometimes followed by recurrence of the symptoms.

EXOSTOSES OF THE BONES OF THE FOOT

There are certain points in the foot at which pressure from shoes is likely to cause chronic irritation and the resultant formation of exostoses and bursae. The lateral side of the fifth metatarsal head sometimes develops such changes, which are similar to those of a bunion and have been called a "bunionette." Other sites are the medial and upper aspects of the navicular bone, the dorsum of the first cuneiform, the plantar aspect of the calcaneus, and the posterior surface of the calcaneus at or above the attachment of the Achilles tendon. Occasionally an exostosis forms beneath a toenail; such localized proliferation is termed a *subungual exostosis,* is seen most frequently in the great toe, and may cause acute tenderness.

Treatment. If removal of the causative pressure cannot be accomplished satisfactorily, the exostosis and bursa should be excised. Subungual exostosis is treated by excision of the nail, when necessary, and of the underlying phalangeal exostosis.

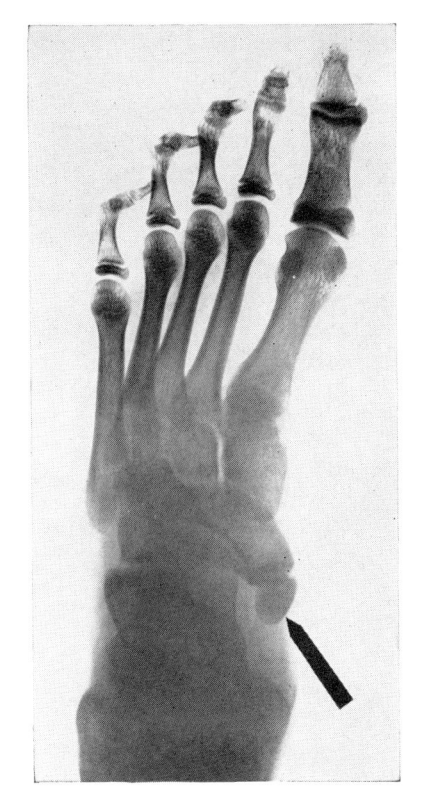

Fig. 254. Roentgenogram showing accessory navicular bone (os tibiale externum). Note well-demarcated, small bone adjacent to medial border of navicular.

ACCESSORY BONES OF THE FOOT

Twenty-one accessory bones of the foot have been described. This number includes the *sesamoid bones,* which are embedded in tendons. Two sesamoid bones are found constantly under the base of the great toe. Sometimes these bones are the site of pain and tenderness following local trauma. In such cases the symptoms may be completely relieved by excision of the sesamoids. These small bones are sometimes bipartite, and this developmental variation must be distinguished from fracture. Painful bursae which sometimes occur in association with the sesamoid bones may require excision. Approximately 25% of the feet of adults and 22% of the feet of children under 16 years of age have roentgenographic evidence of one or more accessory bones in addition to the sesamoid bones.

The most common of the abnormal accessory bones in adults are the *os trigonum,* which is found posterior to the talus; the *os tibiale externum* or *accessory navicular,* located at the medial aspect of the navicular bone (Fig. 254); and the *os peroneale,* lying in the peroneal tendons on the lateral side of the foot. In children the following three accessory bones are observed most frequently, in this order: *accessory navicular, os Vesalianum* (located near the tuberosity of the fifth metatarsal), and *os trigonum*. These bones are often mistaken for fracture fragments and in obscure injuries of the foot should be carefully differentiated. They can usually be recognized without difficulty because of their typical size, shape, position, and smoothly rounded outline. A large accessory navicular bone may be associated with local tenderness from pressure of the shoe and with pain and weakness in the longitudinal arch; in such cases excision of the accessory navicular and fixation of the posterior tibial tendon into a groove well beneath the navicular bone *(Kidner operation)* is frequently indicated. The results of this procedure are usually good.

DISPLACEMENT OF THE PERONEAL TENDONS

Occasionally an abnormal mobility of the tendon sheaths and laxity of the ligaments behind the lateral malleolus allow one or both of the peroneal tendons to become displaced from their groove and to slip anteriorly over the malleolus. The displacement usually occurs on active dorsiflexion and eversion; it is sometimes accompanied by severe pain. Occasionally this affection is of developmental origin; more commonly it is a sequel of trauma.

Treatment. If the diagnosis is made immediately after the displacement has occurred, manipulative replacement and immobilization by means of a plaster boot may effect a cure. Increasing the height of the heel will help to prevent recurrence of the displacement. In some cases the displacement will recur unless a brace is worn to prevent inversion and active eversion of the foot. In chronic recurrent cases operation yields the most satisfactory results, since it affords permanent cure. The tendon sheaths may be sutured firmly into their normal position, the depth of the peroneal groove may be increased, or a strip of the Achilles tendon may be used to form a stabilizing loop.

CHAPTER 21

Affections of the neck, shoulder, and jaw

Deformities and disabilities of the neck and the shoulder are common; their diagnosis and treatment form an important part of orthopaedic surgery. The differentiation of certain neck and shoulder entities as the cause of upper extremity pain in the individual patient often requires experience and judgment. Temporomandibular joint disabilities of orthopaedic interest are seen less commonly; they include derangements of the articular disk, luxations, and ankylosis.

Affections of the neck
TORTICOLLIS (WRY NECK)

Torticollis is a deformity of the neck which, as a rule, includes elements both of rotation and of flexion. In most cases one sternocleidomastoid muscle is shortened. This shortening results in flexion of the neck or tilting of the head toward the affected side and rotation of the chin toward the opposite side. Torticollis may be congenital or acquired.

Congenital torticollis

Etiology and pathology. The term "congenital torticollis" includes all cases in which the deformity is evident at birth. Many causes have been adduced, such as abnormal position of the head in utero; prenatal injury and interference with the vascular supply to the sternocleidomastoid muscle; a fibroma of prenatal origin in this muscle; rupture of many of the sternocleidomastoid muscle fibers during birth, with hematoma and scar tissue formation; and a primary congenital defect in the vertebrae of the cervical spine. Congenital torticollis is seen with relative frequency after difficult deliveries, with abnormal presentations, and in primiparas.

A nontender, cylindrical enlargement of the sternocleidomastoid muscle is sometimes observed in the newborn infant; it usually regresses slowly in from three to six months. Incomplete regression may be followed by the development of a permanent contracture of the sternocleidomastoid muscle. The shortening of the sternocleidomastoid muscle is associated with an increased amount of fibrous tissue in its substance. A secondary contracture develops in the adjacent tissues of the neck.

Clinical picture. Congenital torticollis is seen more commonly in females than in males. At first the deformity may be slight. It may not be noticed until the child is able to sit or stand, although a mass may be felt in the muscle in the first few weeks of life. In other cases, however, the deformity is severe, with a characteristic flattening and shortening of the face on the side to which the head is tilted. The facial asymmetry begins to develop within the first three months and is thought to result from impaired blood supply to the depressed side of the head. When correction of the torticollis is accomplished in early years, a gradual decrease of the asymmetry will take place. The chin is rotated away from the side of the shortened muscle, and the head is displaced and tilted toward the side of the shortening (Figs. 255 to 257). The shoulder on the affected side may be elevated. Rotation and lateral bending of the neck are restricted, whereas flexion and extension are usually of normal range. Attempts to correct the deformity cause the affected muscle to tighten. There is often an associated cervicodorsal scoliosis. Eyestrain may occur from ocular imbalance secondary to the deformity. In the rare affection of double torticollis the chin is elevated in the midline.

Diagnosis. Tuberculosis of the cervical spine presents the greatest difficulty in differential diagnosis; in tuberculosis, however, the chin usually points toward the tight sternocleidomastoid muscle instead of away from it. Dislocations and fractures are to be differentiated, as well as osteo-

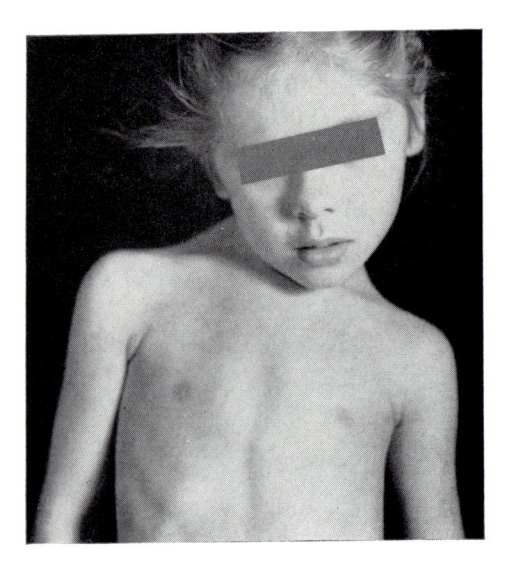

Fig. 255. Congenital torticollis in 5-year-old girl. Note flexion of head and neck to the right, pointing of chin to the left, flattening of right side of face, and high right shoulder.

Affections of the neck, shoulder, and jaw 439

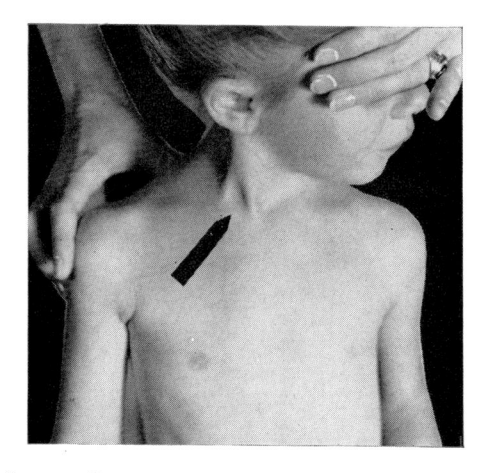

Fig. 256. Congenital torticollis in 5-year-old girl (same patient as shown in Fig. 255). Note prominence of sternal and clavicular heads of right sternocleidomastoid muscle when it is tightened by correcting the lateral flexion.

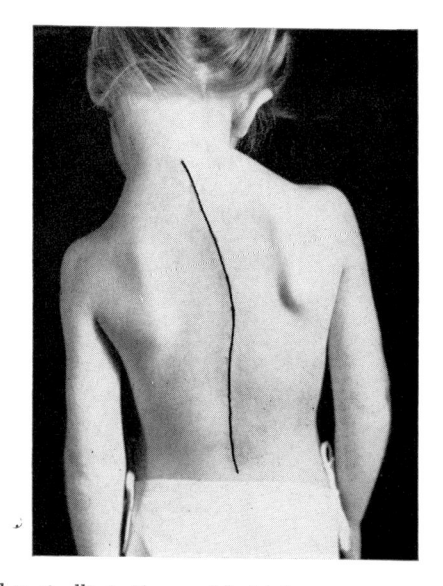

Fig. 257. Congenital torticollis in 5-year-old girl (same patient as shown in Figs. 255 and 256). Note elevation of right shoulder, right thoracic scoliosis, and flexion of trunk to the left.

myelitis, acute myositis, and lymphadenitis. Acute ocular and oral diseases sometimes cause a similar deformity. Of great differential value is the history of painless deformity since birth. The clinical diagnosis should always be supplemented by roentgenographic examination of the cervical spine.

Prognosis. There is little hope of improvement without treatment. Proper treatment in infants and children often results in complete cure. Following correction of the torticollis, the asymmetry of the face gradually becomes less noticeable. In cases corrected before the age of 3 or 4 years, the facial deformity may completely disappear.

Treatment. The fundamental principle of treatment is overcorrection of the shortened sternocleidomastoid muscle. The treatment should be started as soon as the deformity is recognized.

Nonsurgical treatment. Early cases with slight deformity may often be corrected by simple stretching of the head and neck into the overcorrected position and by exercises to strengthen the weak muscles. Rarely it may be wise to stretch the contracted structures under anesthesia and to follow this by fixation in a special brace or plaster cast. Continued observation is most important. In the milder cases the results of nonsurgical methods are good.

Surgical treatment. Cases of moderate or severe deformity and all late cases require operative treatment, which in brief consists of section of the sternocleidomastoid muscle; maintenance of overcorrection of the deformity, which may be accomplished by means of plaster cast, brace, or traction; and finally a program of exercises for securing muscle balance to maintain the correction permanently. If a tumor is present in the muscle, some orthopaedic surgeons believe that it should be excised very early, i.e., in the first few months of life. In some clinics good results have been reported without the use of a postoperative support. The procedure used most commonly is open section of the sternocleidomastoid muscle near its origin from sternum and clavicle. All tight fascial structures, which may include the platysma muscle, should also be sectioned. After operation corrective exercises should be started and continued until there is no tendency toward recurrence, which may be for as long as six months. Many surgeons prefer to use a corrective brace during this period. There is always danger of a recurrence of the deformity; this should be explained to the parents before treatment is started. When the sternocleidomastoid muscle is extremely contracted and fibrotic, its complete excision may be preferable to myotomy.

Acquired torticollis

Most cases of acquired torticollis occur in the first ten years of life. Acquired torticollis, unlike congenital torticollis, is often accompanied by pain.

The following types of acquired torticollis are most frequently observed:
1. *Acute,* caused by direct irritation of the muscles from injury or by an inflammatory reaction of the muscles (myositis) or of the cervical lymph nodes (lymphadenitis).
2. *Spasmodic,* in which rhythmic convulsive spasms of the muscles take place as a result of an organic disorder of the central nervous system. This will be discussed separately.
3. *Hysterical,* due to psychogenic inability of the patient to control the muscles of the neck.

In addition, torticollis may be associated with tuberculosis, osteomyelitis, arthritis, and injuries of the cervical spine; with contracture of scar tissue in the neck following a burn; with paralysis of the sternocleidomastoid muscle; with scoliosis of the cervical spine; and with meningitis and ocular defects.

Treatment. The treatment of acquired torticollis should be directed toward the removal of local and general causes. Acute traumatic or inflammatory torticollis is sometimes relieved by hot applications and gentle massage and stretching of the neck. If severe contractures of the sternocleidomastoid muscle and the surrounding tissues persist after the causative process has subsided, they should be divided and aftercare as described for congenital torticollis should be given.

Spasmodic torticollis

Etiology. The cause of spasmodic torticollis is thought to be either (1) an organic lesion of the central nervous system or (2) reflex contractions from irritation of the cervical nerve roots by arthritic changes. It seems to occur most often, however, in individuals with a psychoneurotic tendency or a history of periods of stress, overwork, and anxiety.

Clinical picture. The deformity comes on gradually in adult life. The first symptoms are usually stiffness and discomfort of the muscles of one side of the neck. These are followed by a drawing sensation and a momentary twitching or slight contraction that pulls the head toward the affected side. The symptoms slowly become more marked until a convulsive spasm of the muscles develops and draws the head forcibly to one side. The spasm may exhibit either an irregular or a regular rhythm; it is independent of voluntary control and becomes especially marked when the patient grows excited. It may be associated with severe neuralgic pain throughout the head and neck. It is interesting to note that often the convulsive spasms can be inhibited by the light pressure of a finger against the head.

Prognosis. There is little tendency toward spontaneous recovery. The results of surgical treatment are sometimes good.

Treatment. Occasionally conservative methods, consisting of psychotherapy, muscle training, and prolonged mechanical support of the neck with a well-fitting brace or plaster cast, lead to relief. Operative measures, however, may be necessary. A resection of the spinal accessory nerve may relieve the spasmodic jerkings, or it may be necessary to remove the posterior branches of the upper cervical nerve roots as well as to divide the affected rami.

CERVICAL ROOT SYNDROME

The term "cervical root syndrome" is used to describe the symptoms and signs produced by compression or irritation of cervical nerve roots in or about intervertebral foramina before they divide into anterior and posterior rami.

Etiology. Among the causes of the cervical root syndrome are (1) degenerative disk disease without trauma, (2) neck sprains in traffic accidents,

(3) neck injuries in contact athletics, (4) twisting of the neck in sleep or while anesthetized, and (5) certain postural abnormalities.

Posterior subluxations of the cervical vertebrae produced by hyperextension of the cervical spine may compress the nerve roots by narrowing the vertical diameter of the foramina anteriorly. Flexing the neck increases the vertical diameter of the foramina and does not result in nerve compression. Subluxations are most likely to occur when the supporting ligaments and capsular structures are relaxed.

Hypertrophic spurring in the cervical spine develops over a considerable period of time, allowing ample opportunity for the roots to become adjusted to the new relationships. When subluxation occurs, it causes compression more readily if spurs are present. Hypertrophic changes are frequently found around the lateral synovial intervertebral joints and the posterior joints. Spurring most often occurs at the levels of greatest motion and stress, namely, between the fourth and fifth cervical vertebrae and between the fifth and sixth.

Oblique roentgenograms of the cervical spine best reveal fractures in the region of the foramina. Hemorrhage, edema, and local inflammation cause root irritation, which may be superimposed on compression occasioned by displacement at the time of fracture.

Dissections of cervical spines have shown that posterior herniation of the nucleus pulposus is unlikely to compress the cervical roots. Posterior herniation causes a central protrusion below the exit of the roots, producing pressure on the spinal cord. Thus the diagnosis of posterior herniation is suggested when signs of cord compression are aggravated by flexion of the neck.

The predisposing causes of cervical root irritation include swelling of the roots after traumatic intervertebral compression, congenital fusion anomalies which alter normal stress patterns, postinflammatory adhesions, and rheumatoid arthritis. Occasionally, a calcified vertebral artery may press on the nerve roots during hyperextension.

Persistent irritation of the cervical roots may produce reflex stimulation of the cervical sympathetic system, causing symptoms such as blurring of vision, dilation of the pupils, loss of balance, headache, swelling and stiffness of the fingers, tendinitis, and capsulitis.

Clinical picture. Pain, usually in the neck and arm, is the presenting complaint. The pain is increased by neck motion and often aggravated by coughing and sneezing. It may radiate to the finger tips and is frequently associated with paresthesias in the dermatome of the involved root. Headache, usually occipital, is a common complaint. Other areas of pain radiation include the upper dorsal and scapular regions and occasionally the chest. Weakness of grip or of arm function may be a complaint. Occasionally patients are disturbed by vertigo or blurring of vision, which has been attributed by some observers to spasm or compression of the vertebral artery.

The physical findings include painful limitation of neck motion, tenderness over the cervical spine, and neurologic changes in the upper extremity. The patient frequently holds his neck stiff and tilted slightly to one side. The cervical muscles may feel tense. With the patient sitting and his neck slightly hyperextended, pressure on top of the head usually reproduces the pain. Neurologic changes include muscle weakness and atrophy, diminished reflexes, and sensory disturbances corresponding to the level of root irritation.

It will be remembered that in the cervical spine the root emerges above the vertebra of corresponding number. If the sixth root is involved, hypesthesia of the thumb and radial side of the hand, weakness of the biceps muscle, and decrease in the deep tendon reflexes of the biceps and brachioradialis may be noted. Seventh root involvement may be manifested by triceps weakness, diminished triceps reflex, and sensory changes in the middle and ring fingers.

Roentgenographic picture. Upright, lateral roentgenograms may be made with the neck (1) in neutral position, (2) in flexion, and (3) in hyperextension. Most patients show loss of the normal lordosis of the cervical spine. Some have a reverse curve in three or four segments. The apex of the reverse curve is frequently the site of maximal irritation.

When the lateral views show a persistent anterior subluxation of a vertebra, oblique flexion views may disclose a fracture of its neural arch. Minor subluxations are present in many cases; they are considered normal by some observers, pathologic by others.

Anteroposterior views may be taken with the tube tilted upward from 25 to 30 degrees in order that the central rays pass through the intervertebral spaces and demonstrate the upward projections at the sides of the superior surfaces of the vertebrae. Fractures of the odontoid process, or atlantoaxial subluxation, may be found on open mouth views.

Myelography may be indicated if thorough conservative therapy has failed and the symptoms and signs strongly suggest a cervical disk lesion.

Differential diagnosis. The cervical root syndrome must be differentiated from frank cervical disk protrusion; spinal cord tumor; peripheral nerve irritation; reflex pain from somatic or visceral sources; and traumatic subluxations, dislocations, and fractures.

Treatment. It should be explained to the patient that as a rule the outlook for recovery is excellent.

Heat frequently relieves root irritation pain, and massage may be helpful. Sharply localized areas of tenderness may be injected with procaine. Intermittent traction of 15 to 25 pounds with a head halter or the Sayre suspension apparatus may relieve the pain. Some patients require bed rest with continuous neck traction. A Thomas collar for immobilization of the neck may be indicated; if used it should not place the neck in hyperextension. The collar should be worn until pain on motion of the neck has subsided.

Postural exercises may be indicated. For sleeping, a cylindrical pillow that maintains the neck in a neutral position may be helpful. Analgesics

444   Handbook of orthopaedic surgery

and mild sedatives may be needed; habit-forming drugs should be avoided.

In severe cases, when the symptoms and signs have persisted despite prolonged conservative therapy, surgical treatment in the form of foraminotomy, disk excision, or localized arthrodesis may be advisable.

CERVICAL RIB AND THE SCALENUS SYNDROME

Cervical ribs are congenital anomalies consisting of supernumerary, independent units of growth similar to the first dorsal ribs. The extra ribs are attached most often to the seventh cervical vertebra but may be attached to the sixth. Cervical ribs are usually bilateral; when this is the case, one rib is always higher and presents a more advanced stage of development than the other.

Four types of cervical rib are found:
1. An exaggeration of the transverse process of the seventh cervical vertebra, with a fibrous band connecting it with the first rib (Fig. 258).
2. An incomplete rib attached to the seventh cervical vertebra with a band running to the first rib.
3. A complete rib which articulates with the first rib (Fig. 258).
4. A complete rib which is fused with the first rib anteriorly.

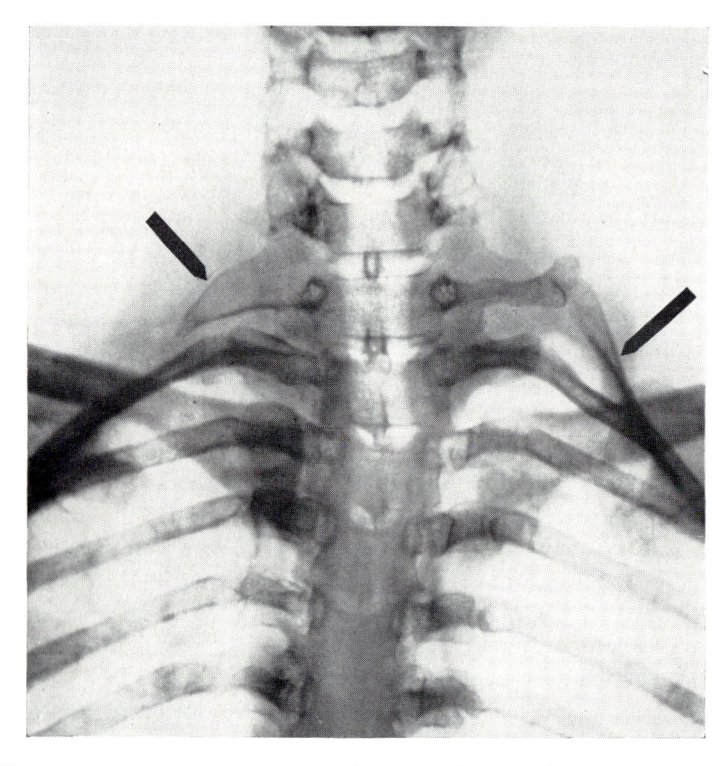

Fig. 258. Anteroposterior roentgenogram showing left cervical rib and enlarged right transverse process of seventh cervical vertebra.

The lower roots of the brachial plexus are in close approximation to the anomalous ribs. The seventh cervical trunk crosses over the transverse process of the seventh cervical vertebra, and the eighth cervical trunk crosses over either the extra rib or the fibrous band. The subclavian vessels also are quite close. The artery lies in front of the rib and often presents at this point a localized dilatation that causes an increased pulsation in the neck. The subclavian vein lies a considerable distance below and in front of the artery and is seldom pressed upon or affected by the cervical rib. The scalenus anterior muscle is attached to the first rib in front of the inferior and middle trunks of the brachial plexus and the subclavian artery.

Clinical picture. Although cervical ribs may be present without causing symptoms, a characteristic clinical picture frequently develops. The symptoms usually appear in adult life, most often at the age of about 30 years. They occur much more commonly in women than in men.

Locally there may be a tumor in the neck, which may be both palpable and visible. It is most frequently found as a firm, rounded, immovable mass, 2 to 3 cm. above the middle of the clavicle. Above this there is usually a palpable pulsation that is caused by the subclavian artery. About this area lies the brachial plexus. As postural changes result in gradual stretching of the middle and lower portions of the brachial plexus over the rib, friction takes place with use of the shoulder and arm. At first there is no pain, but repeated trauma finally produces a definite brachial neuritis. This may be followed by weakness and atrophy, starting in the intrinsic muscles of the hand and involving finally the entire extremity. Occasionally a clawhand deformity develops (Fig. 147). Paresthesia of the arm and forearm, especially of the part supplied by the ulnar nerve, is sometimes present and may be accompanied by radiating pain. Tingling and numbness are often the first symptoms, but later, as the pressure becomes more severe, anesthesia and paralysis may develop. At first, relief can be secured by changing the position of the arm. As the condition progresses, however, change of position no longer relieves the pain. Pallor, coldness, and cyanosis may appear in the fingers. There may be diminution of the volume of the radial pulse, especially when the shoulder is pushed back and down or when the arm is elevated over the head. Some observers believe that these changes result from the action of the affected sympathetic nerve fibers in the lower part of the brachial plexus, whereas others believe that they are caused by direct mechanical pressure upon the subclavian artery. In advanced cases thrombosis of the subclavian artery may take place, giving rise to gangrene, which starts in the fingers. Gradually a collateral circulation may be established, however, which will compensate for the circulatory impairment. Occasionally the patient presents a scoliosis of the cervical spine with its convexity toward the side of the cervical rib.

Clinical manifestations similar to those of cervical ribs are sometimes encountered in the absence of demonstrable bony abnormality at the base of the neck. In such patients compression of the brachial plexus and the subclavian artery may be caused by spasm of the scalenus anterior muscle, the nerves and artery being pressed against the first rib by the tense muscle. This condition has been called the *scalenus syndrome*. Some observers believe that even in the presence of a cervical rib, spasm of the scalenus anterior muscle may be entirely responsible for the clinical picture by compressing the brachial plexus and subclavian artery against the extra rib.

Differential diagnosis. Because of the weakness and atrophy of the smaller muscles of the hand, the presence of a cervical rib is sometimes confused with syringomyelia, progressive muscular atrophy, injury of the spinal cord, and ulnar palsy. The factor of pain down the arm may confuse the diagnosis with that of arthritis of the cervical spine or peripheral neuritis. Subacromial bursitis must occasionally be excluded. Occupational neuroses that give similar neuralgic symptoms must be differentiated. Rupture and protrusion of a cervical intervertebral disk must be considered; it can often be differentiated by the localization of symptoms and signs to a single nerve root, which is most often the sixth or seventh. Any patient whose symptoms fail to respond to conservative orthopaedic measures, however, should receive neurosurgical consultation concerning the possibility of a cervical disk protrusion.

Treatment. Conservative measures should be tried, especially in cases which seem to be improved by rest. As a psychogenic factor is often present, psychotherapy should be considered. Injection of procaine into the scalenus anterior muscle often produces temporary relief, as may injection of procaine into the stellate ganglion. To relieve the strain upon the lower brachial plexus and roots, the shoulder should be brought upward and backward with the use of a sling or brace. Hot baths, massage, and active exercises for the shoulder and arm should be given. Emphasis should be placed upon exercises for strengthening the trapezius and levator scapulae muscles. In some cases change to an occupation which does not put a strain upon the shoulder or arm will result in complete relief of the symptoms.

When the response to conservative treatment is unsatisfactory, surgical removal of the cervical rib may be indicated and may be followed by complete relief of the symptoms. However, the symptoms can often be cured by tenotomy of the scalenus anterior muscle, which may be compressing the subclavian artery and irritating the inferior and middle trunks of the brachial plexus. Tenotomy of the scalenus anterior, because of its technical ease and safety, is the operation of choice and always should be done before excising a cervical rib. At the time of such a tenotomy, all other tight fascial and muscle structures compressing the neurovascular bundle should be freed and incised. Occasionally in severe obliterative vascular conditions, a portion of the clavicle may have to be removed to provide relief.

Affections of the shoulder

The shoulder possesses less stability and less mechanical protection than any other large joint of the body. The glenoid fossa of the scapula is shallow, presenting only a slight concavity for the large globe of the humeral head.

Affections of the neck, shoulder, and jaw 447

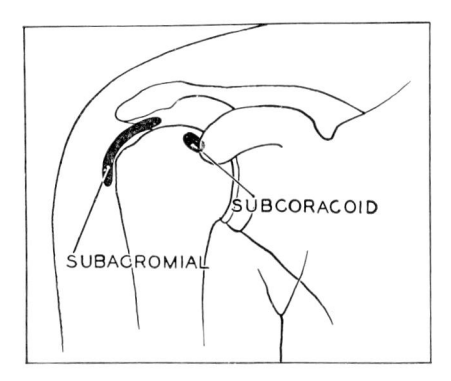

Fig. 259. Most commonly affected bursae about the shoulder.

The concavity is disposed vertically, moreover, and gravity, instead of increasing joint stability as in the case of hip or knee, exerts through the entire weight of the arm a constant force tending to produce a shearing strain. Not only does the bony configuration of the shoulder joint afford little stability, but the capsular ligaments, necessarily long and loose to permit the wide range of shoulder motion, oppose little strength to any force tending to cause a subluxation. It is therefore to be expected that the muscles and tendons about the shoulders play a relatively important part in maintaining joint stability. They form, in fact, a flexible but strong protective covering closely investing the entire joint, and in part the tendons are actually fused with the capsule. To provide for motion with a minimum of friction, the shoulder bursae (Fig. 259) are important, and these structures are in close relationship with the tendons and with the capsule.

These anatomic considerations are of significance in the interpretation of common clinical findings in affections of the shoulder. The intimate association of synovial membrane, ligaments, tendons, and bursae makes multiple involvement likely when the shoulder is injured, renders specific diagnostic analysis difficult, and leads to a confused terminology of shoulder affections. That any acute injury of the shoulder is likely to clear up slowly and incompletely, leading to symptoms of chronic nature, is a common clinical observation. Increasing the likelihood of a chronic disability are the constant drag of the unsupported arm on the shoulder joint and also the fact that in adduction, the position in which the injured joint is most conveniently held, contractures and atrophy quickly develop and decrease the range of painless motion.

MINOR INJURIES: TRAUMATIC SYNOVITIS, SPRAIN, AND STRAIN

Clinical picture. After most shoulder injuries pain is severe; it is sometimes felt not only about the joint itself but throughout the arm, particularly on its lateral aspect about the insertion of the deltoid muscle. Tenderness also may be generalized. There is usually pain on motion, especially on abduction or external rotation, which results in the arm's being held closely against the side of the thorax. If the arm is allowed to remain in this position, a vicious circle is set up: adhesions, contractures, and atrophy develop and further increase the disability.

Differentiation of the various types of injury at the shoulder is important to treatment. *Acute traumatic synovitis* undoubtedly is of common occurrence but is relatively of less importance than in the weight-bearing joints; it is associated usually with injury of one or more of the surrounding structures. Shoulder *sprain,* or stretching or slight tearing of the capsular ligaments, accompanied by extravasation of blood, is a common athletic injury characterized clinically by tenderness over the joint capsule, pain on motion, and slow recovery. Muscular *strain* about the shoulder is suspected when particular pain is elicited by contraction of a specific muscle against resistance and when localized tenderness is present over the muscle or its tendon.

Treatment. The first essential in the treatment of any acute injury of the shoulder is rest. This may be facilitated by the use of a sling, often in conjunction with a shoulder cap of adhesive plaster. In the more severe cases it may be preferable to support the joint in abduction, which is the position of physiologic rest and the one in which adhesions and contractures are least likely to occur. If the shoulder is seen within the first few hours after injury, application of cold by means of an ice cap may retard extravasation of blood. Afterward heat is applied constantly to relieve pain and to hasten absorption of the extravasated blood. However, rest must not be continued for too long a time. Massage, followed by gradually increasing active exercise, should be started as soon as the acute symptoms have begun definitely to subside.

SUBACROMIAL BURSITIS

The subacromial or subdeltoid bursa is a large, flat, thin-walled sac covering laterally the upper end of the humerus and the shoulder joint (Fig. 259). It consists of an upper or subacromial portion, which overlies the tendon insertions into the shoulder capsule and the greater tubercle of the humerus and which is in turn covered by the acromion, and a lower or subdeltoid portion, which overlies the humeral tubercle and is covered by the deltoid muscle. The two portions are occasionally separated by a thin membrane; they never communicate with the cavity of the shoulder joint. In opening the normal shoulder the bursa is scarcely recognizable as a definite structure, but in common inflammatory states it may be so distended and thickened as to be palpable even through the deltoid muscle.

Subacromial bursitis is commonly accepted as a disease entity, although clinically it often cannot be differentiated with certainty from lesions of other closely related structures about the shoulder joint. Its usual cause is presumably degenerative or minor traumatic changes in the musculotendinous cuff, to which the bursal floor is closely adherent. Pyogenic infection of the subacromial bursa is a relatively rare entity.

Clinical picture. Subacromial bursitis is seen most often in patients between 40 and 50 years of age, is more common in women than in men, and occurs with relatively high frequency in sedentary individuals. The patient with acute bursitis experiences severe pain in the shoulder, sometimes referred down the entire extremity as well. This pain may permit the arm to be swung in the sagittal plane but sharply limits any rotation or abduction. Often when abduction is carried out passively an angle can be identified at which pressure of the inflamed sac beneath the acromion causes a sudden increase in the intensity of the pain. Tenderness may be generalized over the shoulder joint but is often most marked over the central portion of the bursa just beneath the acromion. In more chronic cases the signs are much less definite, and, since in such cases there must almost surely be associated pathologic changes in other structures about the joint and contiguous to the bursa, the term "periarthritis" is often applied to them (p. 452). In chronic bursitis an old tear of the musculotendinous cuff of the shoulder joint or degenerative changes in the tendon of the long head of the biceps may be present. Long-standing cases frequently present disabling adduction contracture, limitation of rotation, and muscle weakness and atrophy. Roentgenograms are indicated to investigate the possible presence of calcification in the bursa or the rotator cuff (Fig. 260), and of arthritic changes in the shoulder joint.

Treatment. The first essential in the treatment of *acute bursitis* is rest

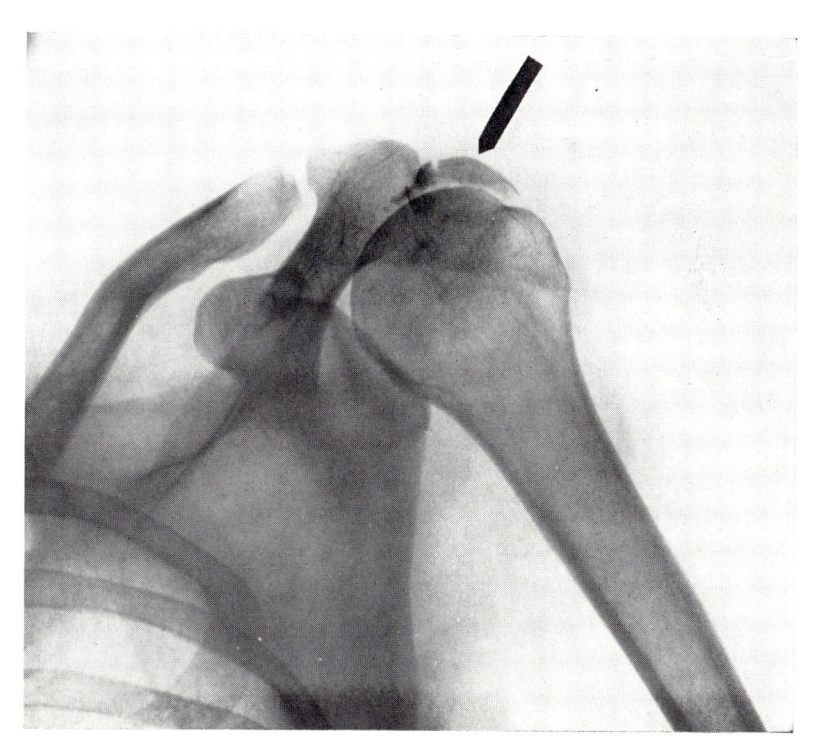

Fig. 260. Roentgenogram of shoulder showing extensive calcification in subacromial bursa.

and support, preferably in bed and with the arm in as much abduction as can be secured. Pillows or splints may be used. A simple Velpeau dressing may give sufficient immobilization to relieve the pain, but the position of adduction must not be long maintained. Frequently, light adhesive traction gives the best combination of immobilization, support, and gentle corrective force. Heat is indicated and may afford full relief of the pain. It is best applied by the use of compresses or electric pad. Diathermy treatments are sometimes effective in relieving the acute symptoms. Ultrasonic therapy has also been considered helpful. In some cases, particularly those in which heat seems to aggravate the pain, the application of ice packs is very effective. Procaine block of the suprascapular nerve, which carries a large part of the sensory supply of the shoulder joint, is often most helpful. Injection of a weak solution of procaine into the inflamed bursal sac sometimes leads to instant relief of the pain. If this form of therapy is employed, the bursa should be punctured by numerous needle holes from different directions. Sometimes it is possible to irrigate the bursa with normal saline by placing two needles from different angles into the sac. Part or all of a calcific deposit may at times be removed in this manner. Injection of hydrocortisone into the bursa may decrease the inflammatory reaction. Roentgentherapy often affords satisfactory relief, especially when calcification is present. Phenylbutazone has been reported to give effective relief in twenty-four to forty-eight hours. If the severe pain of an acute bursitis fails to respond satisfactorily to these measures, excision of the bursa and of any calcific material in the rotator cuff may be indicated.

As the discomfort and tenderness become less acute, massage and exercise of the shoulder should be started. Full range-of-motion exercises should be done briefly each day as soon as the decreasing pain will allow; they should be continued for at least six weeks. When full mobility is not regained with abduction traction and exercises, gentle manipulation of the shoulder under anesthesia is occasionally indicated. Manipulation must always be carried out with the greatest caution in order to avoid fracture of the atrophic humerus at its surgical neck. It should never be done in the presence of active arthritis. It should be followed by physical therapy including active exercises to develop the abductors of the shoulder. An abduction splint is sometimes indicated.

In chronic or recurrent cases irrigation of the subacromial bursa sometimes relieves the pain. Excision of the bursa often affords complete relief. Operation is inadvisable unless more conservative measures have failed to alleviate the symptoms.

Excision of the small calcified bodies or soft calcareous materials which in the roentgenogram are sometimes visible near the floor of the bursa (Fig. 260) may be carried out when their presence is associated with obstinate pain and tenderness. Otherwise their removal is not indicated, since they have frequently been observed to undergo resorption under roentgentherapy or diathermy treatment or after needling, or even to disappear spontaneously.

SUBCORACOID BURSITIS

Inflammation of the subcoracoid bursa, which lies between the capsule of the shoulder joint and the coracoid process of the scapula (Fig. 259), arises when the shoulder is allowed to droop forward, causing the lesser tubercle of the humerus to impinge against the coracoid process. The pain is always well localized and accompanied by a limitation of rotation and abduction of the shoulder. Subcoracoid bursitis is sometimes difficult or impossible to differentiate from bicipital tenosynovitis or a partial tear of the capsule of the shoulder joint.

Treatment. The treatment is similar to that of subacromial bursitis, and, in addition, postural exercises to correct the shoulder girdle deformity are useful.

BICIPITAL TENOSYNOVITIS

Bicipital tenosynovitis is a frequently observed affection causing pain and stiffness in the shoulder joint; it is an inflammation of the tendon-tendon sheath gliding mechanism of the long head of the biceps muscle, which results in adhesions that bind the tendon to the bicipital groove and inner surface of the rotator cuff. It may be bilateral. It occurs most commonly in women in their early forties. In older individuals bicipital tenosynovitis tends to persist longer than in young adults and to lead to partial stiffness of the shoulder.

Etiology. Anomalies such as inadequate depth of the bicipital groove, or abnormal ridges that develop in association with certain occupations requiring excessive use of the arms, may produce trauma to the tendon and an inflammatory reaction. These factors in addition to normal physiologic wear and tear are responsible for degenerative changes, which increase in severity with each successive decade. Such changes include fraying, shredding, and fasciculation of the tendon and roughening of the bicipital groove. Adhesions may be formed in the tendon sheath. Tenosynovitis is a common sequel of fractures and fracture-dislocations involving the bicipital groove.

Clinical picture. The pain may have an insidious onset or be precipitated by strenuous activity, such as shoveling snow or playing tennis. The pain is located first over the anterior and medial region of the shoulder and then may radiate to the belly of the biceps muscle and flexor surface of the forearm. Pain also may occur at the insertion of the deltoid muscle, inferior angle of the scapula, and even in the base of the neck. Pain may first be noticed on putting the arm back of the body or head. On palpation, exquisite tenderness may be elicited over the intertubercular sulcus or on rolling the biceps tendon with the examining fingers.

Treatment. The early treatment of bicipital tenosynovitis is conservative, consisting of rest, moist heat, and voluntary elimination of the painful arcs of motion. Procaine and hydrocortisone injection of the tender area, done with strict aseptic precautions, may give prompt relief. When conservative management does not relieve the pain and disability and the recurrences are frequent, surgical treatment is indicated. The tendon of the long head of the biceps may be sectioned and reattached to the humerus below the bicipital groove, or to the coracoid process.

FROZEN SHOULDER
(ADHESIVE CAPSULITIS, PERIARTHRITIS)

The term "frozen shoulder" has been used to designate a shoulder showing severe limitation of motion as a result of degenerative changes involving to a varying degree the musculotendinous cuff, synovial membrane, articular cartilage, bicipital tendon and tendon sheath, and surrounding structures.

These changes consist of edema, fibrosis, and round cell infiltration indicating a low-grade inflammatory process. This results in loss of elasticity of the periarticular tissues, which become shortened and fibrotic, thereby firmly fixing the humeral head in the glenoid cavity. Muscle atrophy becomes pronounced. The contracted coracohumeral ligament and subscapularis tendon prevent external rotation of the head of the humerus.

This condition, occurring most frequently after middle life, may be initiated by muscular inactivity in the presence of a degenerative alteration such as bicipital tenosynovitis or changes in the musculotendinous cuff. It may sometimes be a part of the shoulder-hand syndrome (p. 455).

Clinical picture. The condition may have an insidious onset, follow direct or indirect local trauma, or be a sequel to injuries of the distal part of the extremity. It also may follow cerebrovascular accidents or come about as the result of referred shoulder pain from cardiac or cervical nerve root affections. It frequently follows subacromial bursitis, calcific tendinitis, and tenosynovitis of the long head of the biceps. Because degenerative changes in the rotator cuff and long head of the biceps are present in most individuals beyond the age of 40 years, any painful affliction of the upper extremity which causes a person of this age to keep his arm in an adducted, internally rotated position may trigger pathologic changes leading to a frozen shoulder. The pain is accentuated by attempts at scapulohumeral joint motion, particularly abduction, external rotation, and extension. The pain may radiate, as in bicipital tenosynovitis, to the anterolateral aspect of the shoulder region, biceps muscle belly, flexor surface of the forearm, and inferior angle of the scapula. Tenderness may be elicited over the intertubercular sulcus and the tendon of the biceps. The pain is often most severe at night. The stiffness may progress to almost complete limitation of scapulohumeral motion.

The clinical course of the frozen shoulder is variable. After periods of pain and dysfunction, the inflammatory process may subside, with resolution of the adhesions, disappearance of pain, and restoration of muscle activity and circulation. On the other hand, in a minority of the cases the pathologic changes remain static for very long periods with persistent pain and dysfunction.

Muscle activity, which is essential to normal tissue metabolism, is necessary to abort or reverse the pathologic processes responsible for frozen shoulder; however, the extent of normal muscle action is limited by the intensity of the pain.

Treatment. The initial treatment of the frozen shoulder syndrome is conservative, consisting of the use of moist heat, gravity-free exercises within painless arcs of motion, and sedation. Later, antigravity exercises such as finger tip wall-climbing should be instituted. Procaine blocks of the sympathetic ganglia may relieve the pain. Adhesive traction with the shoulder abducted may be most helpful. Manipulation is contraindicated if any active inflammation remains or if the process is of long duration. It may be possible to help some of these patients in the late stage by surgical measures such as exploration of the subacromial bursa and biceps tendon or *acromioplasty* (partial resection of the acromion).

RUPTURE OF THE SUPRASPINATUS TENDON AND TEARS OF THE MUSCULOTENDINOUS CUFF

Rupture of the supraspinatus tendon is a common and important cause of shoulder disability. In severe cases the tear may be extensive, involving not only the supraspinatus tendon but also nearly the entire musculotendinous cuff of the shoulder.

Pathology. The flattened tendon of the supraspinatus muscle, after blending intimately with the adjacent infraspinatus tendon and the capsule of the shoulder joint, inserts into the highest facet of the greater tubercle of the humerus. The supraspinatus tendon thus forms both the roof of the shoulder joint and the floor of the subacromial bursa.

Rupture of the supraspinatus tendon usually occurs near its insertion (Fig. 261). Retraction of the muscle after extensive tears leaves a direct opening between the subacromial bursa and the shoulder joint. This communication may be demonstrated by arthrography, or roentgenograms taken

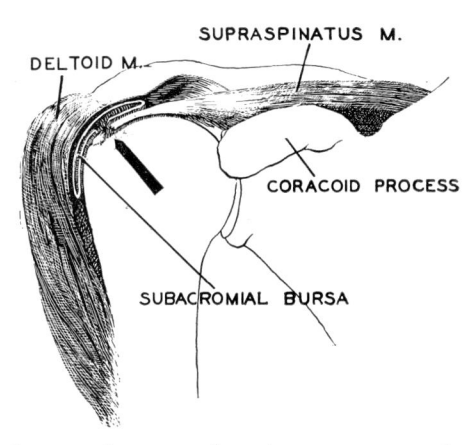

Fig. 261. Rupture of supraspinatus tendon. Arrow points to the rupture. Note that shoulder joint communicates with the subacromial bursa through the rupture.

after the injection of a radiopaque dye into the shoulder joint. Minor lacerations are probably common in later adult years and have been found in a large percentage of routine postmortem examinations. At times a small fragment of the greater tubercle of the humerus is torn away, together with avulsion of the tendon near its insertion.

With time the pathologic changes accompanying complete rupture become more pronounced. Progressive retraction of the muscle widens the rent in the joint capsule. The distal stub of the tendon, at first a sharply outlined mass, becomes atrophic and may disappear, while the edge of the tubercle gradually becomes rounded and smooth.

Etiology. There is almost always a history of trauma, and at times the rupture accompanies an anterior dislocation of the shoulder. The mechanism is presumably an indirect violence associated with sudden powerful elevation of the arm in an attempt to regain balance or to cushion a fall. The presence of a heavy object in the hand increases the likelihood of rupture. Degenerative changes in the cuff predispose to and generally precede rupture.

Clinical picture. Rupture of the supraspinatus tendon is most common in laborers past the age of 40 years. The rupture is accompanied by a transient sharp pain in the shoulder, and a few hours later there begins a steady ache that may last for several days.

Examination with the humerus adducted discloses a tender point below the acromion, and a sulcus between acromion and tendon insertion may be palpable. As a rule, the ability to initiate and maintain abduction of the shoulder is not lost when the supraspinatus tendon alone is ruptured, but is absent in complete or massive avulsions of the cuff.

When the arm is carried into abduction, there is transient pain and slight crepitus as the torn insertion of the tendon passes under the edge of the acromion; the same pain is felt at the corresponding angle as the arm is again lowered.

Subsequently the patient may experience severe shoulder pain for months. This is often most marked at night and is so aggravated after exertion during the day that any type of active work becomes impossible. In late cases atrophy of the supraspinatus and infraspinatus muscles is a constant sign.

Treatment. For complete rupture of the supraspinatus tendon and extensive tears of the musculotendinous cuff, early surgical repair is indicated. When the diagnosis is in doubt, exploration may be carried out through a short vertical incision. For the repair a wide exposure is necessary and may be gained by extending the incision posteriorly with osteotomy of the acromion, exposing the whole roof of the shoulder joint. It is often advisable to divide the coracoacromial ligament. Temporary use of an abduction brace after operation is sometimes helpful. Chief reliance, however, is placed upon active exercises of the shoulder. These are started two weeks after operation, increased gradually, and continued until maximum function has been regained.

THE SHOULDER-HAND SYNDROME

The shoulder-hand syndrome is a painful shoulder disability with swelling and pain in the homolateral hand. The shoulder changes are identical with those seen in some forms of frozen shoulder.

Etiology. This syndrome, which is thought to be a manifestation of reflex sympathetic dystrophy, may follow any painful shoulder lesion, rheumatic or traumatic. It may be a sequel to myocardial infarction, pleurisy, other painful intrathoracic lesions, cerebrovascular accidents, trauma, rupture of a cervical disk, or cervical arthritis. In all of these affections the patient tends to keep the painful shoulder immobilized. The shoulder-hand syndrome may also arise without known predisposing cause.

Clinical picture. Pain and stiffness of the shoulder with diffuse, nonpitting edema and stiffness and pain in the hand develop acutely or over several months. Symptoms in shoulder and hand may develop together, or either the shoulder or the hand may be affected initially. After three to six months there is gradual relief, but atrophy and stiffness of the hand, with flexion deformity of the fingers and extension contractures of the metacarpophalangeal joints, become more pronounced as the swelling recedes. Recovery occurs by slow stages. Shoulder symptoms and hand swelling require about a year to resolve; trophic changes may disappear in two to four years. Residual stiffness of the metacarpophalangeal joints may be permanent.

Roentgenographic picture. The bones become osteoporotic; the joints show little roentgenographic change.

Differential diagnosis. The differential diagnosis should include rheumatoid arthritis, scalenus syndrome, scleroderma, postinfarction sclerodactyly, causalgia, and Sudeck's atrophy limited to the hand. Diagnosis depends on the following findings: a painful, stiff shoulder, uniform swelling of the hand, and a limitation of motion of all finger joints. There is no true joint swelling, and the sedimentation rate is normal.

Treatment. The treatment is conservative. Daily range-of-motion exercises improve shoulder function. Active and passive exercises of the hands should be continued indefinitely. Heat or cold may give relief. Procaine blocks of the brachial plexus or stellate ganglion are of value early in the course of the disease, as is cortisone to a lesser extent. The oral use of sympathetic blocking drugs may also be of help.

Prognosis. The prognosis is usually good, but some patients show permanent stiffness of the shoulder or fingers. Psychologic factors influence the prognosis in that the neurasthenic patient may refuse to exercise the shoulder and the fingers in the presence of pain.

RUPTURE OF THE BICEPS BRACHII

Rupture of the biceps brachii is of infrequent occurrence. The long head may rupture at or near its origin from the glenoid tubercle, at some point within the bicipital groove, or at the musculotendinous junction.

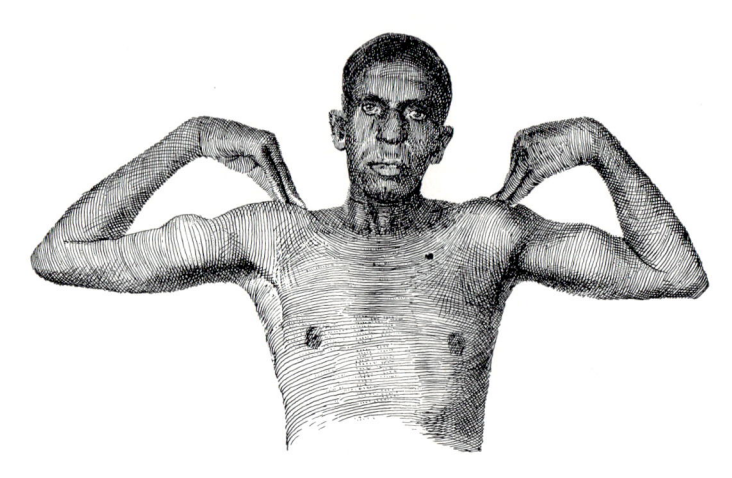

Fig. 262. Rupture of the long head of the right biceps muscle. Note localized bulge in right arm. (After Conwell.)

Rupture may also occur within the muscle belly of one or both heads, or at their insertion into the tuberosity of the radius.

Etiology. Rupture of the biceps is ordinarily a result of sudden indirect violence, usually without direct injury of the overlying tissues. Rupture of the long head as it traverses the bicipital groove is said to be associated always with a previous weakening of the tendon by degenerative changes. In older individuals such ruptures may follow violence of trivial degree.

Clinical picture. At the moment of rupture there is usually sharp pain and occasionally an audible snap. The most characteristic physical finding is a sharply convex bulge near the middle of the arm (Fig. 262). There may be slight local tenderness and weakness of flexion of the elbow and supination of the forearm as compared with these motions in the normal arm. The roentgenogram sometimes shows a small avulsion fracture of the glenoid rim. Rupture of the long head is sometimes difficult to differentiate clinically from dislocation of this tendon out of the bicipital groove.

Treatment. Early cases should be treated by immediate exploration and suture. When separation from the glenoid tubercle or rupture of the tendon of the long head has occurred, the proximal portion of the tendon may be excised and its distal portion fixed to the coracoid process or into the floor of the bicipital groove. Adequate postoperative immobilization should be followed by a program of graded exercise. In older or inactive individuals rupture of the long head, in contrast to rupture near the radial tuberosity, causes little disability and may not require operation.

SNAPPING SHOULDER

A shoulder in which an audible click or snap can be elicited by appropriate muscular contractions is occasionally observed. This condition is known as snapping shoulder and sometimes becomes habitual or involuntary, especially if the patient learns how to cause the snap and elicits it repeatedly. The sound is produced by an incomplete luxation of the joint or by the slipping of a taut tendon over a bony prominence. Rarely a structural change, such as the presence of an anomalous group of muscle fibers, has been demonstrated at exploratory operation. As a rule the symptoms are trivial and no treatment is required.

RECURRENT DISLOCATION OF THE SHOULDER

Traumatic anterior dislocation of the shoulder joint, even when treated according to accepted principles, is sometimes followed by repeated dislocations. In two reported series the percentages of recurrence were 50 and 57, respectively, by far the highest percentage being in persons under 20 years of age. The incidence of recurrence is somewhat less in patients whose first dislocation has been immobilized for at least three weeks. Cases of recurrent dislocation are common enough to form an important clinical entity, especially in the military services. Recurrent posterior dislocation is rarely encountered.

Etiology and pathology. Factors which may facilitate repeated dislocation are incompletely healed tears or relaxation of the capsular ligaments, weakness of the surrounding musculature, and congenital or acquired changes in the contour of the humeral head or of the glenoid fossa. In most cases, however, avulsion of the glenoid labrum from the anterior rim of the glenoid cavity seems to be of chief importance, together with erosion of the glenoid rim and a defect of the posterolateral aspect of the head of the humerus.

Clinical picture. The majority of patients are young adults. The condition is seen with especial frequency in athletes and in persons subject to the trauma of epileptic seizures. At first the dislocation occurs only after severe trauma, but successive recurrences require less and less causative force, and finally dislocation may follow any movement, however trivial, which involves abduction of the shoulder. With successive recurrences, reduction of the displacement becomes correspondingly easier. The pain attending dislocation similarly decreases, but the disability remains extreme, and the patient may feel a constant dread of impending displacement. Atrophy of the muscles of the shoulder girdle sometimes occurs, and rarely signs of involvement of the brachial plexus develop.

Treatment. The nonsurgical treatment of recurrent dislocation consists of (1) preventing the displacement by limiting abduction of the arm and (2) carrying out resistive exercises to strengthen the muscles which internally rotate the shoulder. The displacement may be prevented by strapping the arm to the thorax, by pinning the sleeve to the coat, or by applying a chest belt and an arm band connected by a short flexible strap. Such devices are inconvenient and annoying.

The treatment of choice is surgical. Many procedures have been devised. Bankart's suture of the capsule to the glenoid rim, a difficult but highly effective procedure, is the operation of choice of many surgeons. In the Nicola operation the tendon of the long head of the biceps, sometimes reinforced by a strip of the joint capsule, is placed in a tunnel through the humeral head to act as a suspensory ligament. This operation has been popular but not always successful in preventing redislocation. The Putti-Platt operation, the principle of which is to limit external rotation of the shoulder, is used in many clinics. In this operation the subscapularis tendon and the capsule are divided 1 inch from their humeral attachment, the cut end of the lateral portion is sutured to the anterior rim of the glenoid fossa, and the cut end of the medial portion is attached to the tendinous cuff over the greater tubercle of the humerus; thus, the medial portion of the tendon overlaps the lateral. There have been many modifications of these procedures.

After all operations for recurrent dislocation of the shoulder, carefully graded exercises should be carried out for many months, with precautions against strenuous exercise requiring abduction of the shoulder.

OLD DISLOCATION OF THE SHOULDER

Cases of unreduced shoulder dislocation of long duration are occasionally seen and present a difficult therapeutic problem. The patients show an obvious deformity and on attempting to use the affected shoulder may have considerable pain and disability. The nerves of the brachial plexus are sometimes affected (p. 250).

Pathology. When the humeral head remains displaced from the glenoid cavity a series of pathologic changes makes reduction more and more difficult as time goes on. The glenoid cavity fills with granulation tissue, and the torn capsule contracts. The head of the humerus becomes bound down by scar tissue, and the muscles about the joint become shortened and fibrotic. Atrophy of the humerus develops rapidly and may constitute a formidable obstacle to manipulation.

Treatment. If the dislocation has been present for not more than eight weeks it can occasionally be reduced by closed manipulation. In order to provide adequate relaxation, the anesthetic agent may be supplemented with a muscle-relaxant drug given intravenously. Care must be taken not to employ sudden or excessive force that might injure the brachial plexus, rupture the axillary vessels, or fracture the humerus at its surgical neck. After reduction the arm may be bandaged to the side or may be immobilized in plaster in slight abduction and flexion. Two weeks later a program of daily physical therapy, including active exercise, is started.

For older dislocations and those which previously have failed to be reduced by closed manipulation, operation may be indicated. A wide exposure is necessary. After reduction the arm is immobilized at the side by a plaster or adhesive dressing. Again the aftertreatment consists of the prolonged use of daily physical therapy.

Occasionally it is advisable to excise the head of the humerus. The functional result is sometimes satisfactory. In some cases, because of the patient's age or poor general condition, the long duration of the dislocation, or the absence of significant pain or limitation of motion, strenuous efforts to effect replacement are not to be advised.

OLD ACROMIOCLAVICULAR DISLOCATION

Dislocation of the acromioclavicular joint is a common injury. It occurs frequently in football players as a consequence of falls or blows upon the point of the shoulder, and the resulting disability when the arm is elevated makes it impossible to pass the ball effectively. The diagnosis is usually evident upon inspection and palpation but should be supported by roentgenographic examination to exclude the possibility of fracture of the acromial end of the clavicle. The roentgenogram should always be taken with the patient standing and the arm unsupported or carrying a weight, because often in the supine position the dislocation becomes spontaneously reduced and the instability will not be evident. Unless carefully treated, acromioclavicular dislocations are likely to become chronic, since the weight of the dependent extremity tends to maintain the dislocation.

Pathology. The usual displacement is a dropping of the acromion downward and forward because of the weight of the arm; the acromial end of the clavicle thereby acquires undue upward prominence and mobility. More important than the tearing of the articular capsule and rupture of the acromioclavicular ligaments is rupture of the powerful coracoclavicular ligaments that normally prevent upward displacement of the lateral end of the clavicle.

Treatment and prognosis. In many cases of old acromioclavicular dislocation the disability is negligible and no treatment is indicated other than a program of active exercises for the shoulder. If the symptoms are disabling, however, they can be satisfactorily relieved by operation, although a slight prominence of the lateral end of the clavicle frequently recurs. The strongest repair is secured by tying the clavicle down to the coracoid process as well as to the acromion; this may be done effectively by constructing new coracoclavicular and acromioclavicular ligaments of fascia lata. After operation the position of reduction must be maintained for eight weeks by means of temporary internal fixation with wires or pins through the acromion into the clavicle, an ample adhesive dressing, or a plaster jacket incorporating support of the arm. Lifting of heavy objects should be avoided for an additional eight weeks.

An alternative procedure, consisting of excision of the lateral end of the clavicle, apparently produces satisfactory functional results. Fusion of the acromioclavicular joint limits mobility of the shoulder and is therefore inadvisable.

OLD STERNOCLAVICULAR DISLOCATION

Dislocation of the sternal end of the clavicle occurs much less frequently than acromioclavicular dislocation. Sternoclavicular dislocation may result from a violent fall or blow upon the shoulder, in which case the sternoclavicular ligaments are ruptured and the intra-articular fibrocartilage remains attached usually to the clavicle. The displacement tends to persist unless corrected by treatment. In debilitated individuals chronic or recurrent dislocation is sometimes found without history of acute trauma. The dislocation also may develop gradually when there is a paralysis of the pectoral muscles. In sternoclavicular dislocation the end of the clavicle is ordinarily displaced anteriorly, and the deformity is usually evident upon inspection and palpation.

Treatment. Surgical treatment is indicated only if the deformity is accompanied by pain. The most effective treatment is to suture the end of the clavicle to the sternum or the first rib with fascia lata. After operation the corrected position must be maintained for six to eight weeks by means of a pressure pad and a strong adhesive dressing. The lifting of heavy objects should be avoided for an additional period of several weeks.

Affections of the jaw

Disability of the temporomandibular joint, while forming a relatively uncommon condition in orthopaedic surgery, may nevertheless represent to the individual patient an affliction of peculiarly distressing nature. Two clinical entities of fairly frequent occurrence, snapping jaw and ankylosis of the jaw, can be efficiently relieved by resort to the methods of joint surgery.

SNAPPING JAW

The term "snapping jaw" is applied to a common clinical condition which is characterized by a clicking sensation in the temporomandibular joint on opening and closing the mouth. Usually the symptoms are trivial, but a few patients experience severe pain or locking of the jaw and require careful investigation and treatment.

Pathology. Except for an occasional case attributable to malocclusion of the teeth, intractable snapping of the jaw is caused by one of two distinct pathologic entities: (1) mechanical derangement of the articular disk or (2) recurrent dislocation of the temporomandibular joint, with irregularity of the joint surfaces. In the etiology both developmental and traumatic factors are presumably concerned. Derangements of the articular disk are in some respects analogous to disorders of the semilunar cartilages of the knee. In dislocation of the jaw the condyle of the mandible, which slips forward when the mouth is opened, reaches a position anterior to the articular tubercle of the temporal bone.

Clinical picture. The condition of snapping jaw is usually of gradual onset during adolescence or early adult life, occurring most commonly in young women. The slipping may at first take place only when the mouth is opened widely, as in yawning, but often becomes increasingly frequent and troublesome and in some cases leads to intense discomfort. The diagnosis may be evident from the history and physical findings but should be further investigated with roentgenograms of the temporomandibular joints taken with the mouth in open and in closed positions.

Treatment. Early cases may be treated with heat and massage daily over a period of several weeks, combined with a soft diet and avoidance of any unnecessary motion of the jaw in talking. Dental consultation concerning the occlusion may be advisable. Partial rest secured by the use of a Barton bandage or Thomas collar may be helpful. Complete rest of the jaws, obtained by wiring the teeth for several weeks, is often curative. In some cases, however, operation becomes necessary, the type of procedure depending upon the pathologic changes demonstrated at exploration. For lesions of the fibrocartilage, simple excision of the disk has given satisfactory results. Reefing of the joint capsule is sometimes indicated. Recurrent dislocation may be treated effectively by the creation of a bone block, as described by Mayer.

ANKYLOSIS OF THE JAW

Loss of motion in the temporomandibular joint constitutes a deforming and extremely disabling affection which can be relieved by surgical measures.

Etiology. Ankylosis of the jaw is most frequently seen as the late result of a local traumatic lesion. It is at times a sequel of osteomyelitis of the temporal bone following infection of the middle ear. In other cases the ankylosis may result from rheumatoid arthritis of the temporomandibular joint.

Treatment. The operation of choice is an arthroplastic procedure in which the head of the mandible and the upper portion of the ramus are resected. A layer of fascia or fat may be placed around the end of the ramus but is not essential to a good clinical result.

CHAPTER 22

Affections of the elbow, wrist, and hand

IN MANY INSTANCES affections of the elbow, wrist, and hand may lead to serious functional and economic loss. Accordingly their prompt recognition and careful treatment are of the greatest importance.

Affections of the elbow

The elbow is a hinge joint with a range of motion of from zero to 150 degrees of flexion. Pronation and supination are made possible by rotation of the head of the radius on the capitellum of the humerus. Despite the wide extent of elbow motion, stability is well maintained by the fitting of the trochlea of the humerus deeply into the trochlear notch of the ulna, by powerful muscular and tendinous supports, and by strong collateral ligaments. Stability of the radiohumeral joint is not due to bony configuration, since the head of the radius presents only a shallow concavity for articulation with the capitellum, but rather to the strong annular ligament that holds the radial head in approximation with the radial notch of the ulna.

The wide range of motion in the elbow region renders its structures peculiarly liable to strains and sprains. Because of its tendinous investment and its exposed position, the elbow may suffer attacks of bursitis, and, because of the proximity of important structures on its anterior aspect, injuries of the elbow occasionally lead to important circulatory and neurologic complications.

STRAINS AND SPRAINS

Muscular strains about the elbow are common results of isolated episodes of slight trauma or of unaccustomed repeated trauma of minor degree.

Diagnosis. An effort should always be made to allocate the lesion to one muscle or muscle group; this is best done by careful localization of the maximum pain and tenderness and by analysis of the type of resisted active motion which causes most discomfort. In differential diagnosis ligamentous sprain, bursitis, and minor fractures must be kept in mind. In youth epiphyseal separations in the elbow region are particularly important be-

Affections of the elbow, wrist, and hand 463

cause of the large number of epiphyses and the wide range in the time of their consolidation; the first of these epiphyses makes its roentgenographic appearance at 17 months, and the last union is not complete until the age of 20 years. It is advisable to examine the elbow roentgenographically after any considerable injury, and in children a film of the normal elbow is valuable for detailed comparison with the traumatized area.

Treatment. Strain is treated by temporary immobilization of the affected muscle in a position of relaxation by means of removable plaster splints, adhesive plaster, or sling. Physical therapy consisting of heat and massage is started at once and is followed by graded active exercise.

Ligamentous sprain, while resembling muscle strain in causation, symptomatology, and treatment, may be slower in subsiding. Sprain of the radial collateral ligament occurs fairly commonly among baseball, tennis, and golf players.

OLECRANON BURSITIS

About the elbow joint as many as ten bursae have been described, but most of these are inconstant and of little clinical significance. The *olecranon bursa* (Fig. 263), situated between the tip of the olecranon and the skin, is frequently involved by inflammatory changes. A single episode of local injury may produce olecranon bursitis, but continued traumatization of slight degree is a more common cause. The diagnosis is usually evident from the history of injury; from the localization of pain, swelling, and tenderness posteriorly only; and from the slight restriction of flexion by pain as the inflamed structure is placed under tension.

Treatment. The type of therapy varies with the acuteness of the individual case. Purulent bursitis is uncommon; its treatment includes rest, heat, aspirations, antibiotics, and sometimes incision and drainage. The more frequent nonspecific inflammation may usually be cured by aspiration

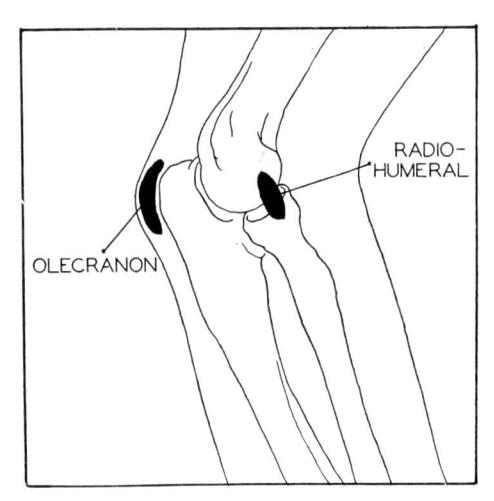

Fig. 263. Most commonly affected bursae about the elbow.

of the fluid, application of a compression bandage and local heat, and care to prevent repetition of the causative trauma. In chronic cases the bursal sac may become greatly thickened; this condition is sometimes called *miner's elbow*. The sac sometimes contains many small loose bodies. Such chronic changes are indications for excision of the bursa. It is occasionally necessary to remove in addition to the bursa a small bony spur which may lie at the tip of the olecranon and may extend for a short distance into the triceps tendon.

RADIOHUMERAL BURSITIS
(TENNIS ELBOW, EPICONDYLITIS)

The common disorder called tennis elbow exhibits typical clinical characteristics; its cause, however, has not been established. In some instances irritation of bursal tissue overlying the radiohumeral joint capsule (Fig. 263) seems to be responsible. However, at operation a definite bursal sac is seldom found. Many observers believe that the usual lesion is a partial rupture of the origin of the extensor muscles with a secondary traumatic periostitis at the lateral epicondyle. Other observers believe that the lesion is a radiohumeral synovitis due to pinching of synovial tissue between radial head and capitellum.

Clinical picture. The usual onset is a gradually increasing discomfort following continued slight traumatization in the region of the radiohumeral joint. Tennis playing, which requires repeated pronation and supination of the forearm with extension of the elbow, is a common cause. The condition may begin following forceful supination, such as is required in using a screwdriver, particularly in persons unaccustomed to such activity. The disorder is frequent among athletes, butchers, carpenters, and the like. Pain is experienced in the lateral aspect of the elbow, particularly when the patient reaches forward to pick up an object or to turn a doorknob, and the discomfort may spread down the entire forearm; it may be very persistent and annoying. Examination shows a small area of tenderness over the lateral condyle of the humerus and the radiohumeral joint. The grip may be weak. Passive motion of the elbow is unaffected, but active extension against resistance may cause intense discomfort. Roentgenograms are usually negative.

Treatment. Radiohumeral bursitis may be treated nonsurgically or surgically. Temporary immobilization of the elbow with a sling, adhesive dressing, or plaster cast and the use of heat and massage will usually produce relief. The application of a dorsiflexion splint to the wrist, which relaxes the extensor tendons, is often helpful. The tender area may be injected with procaine or hydrocortisone. Excellent results from manipulation of the elbow with or without anesthesia have been reported. In cases which fail to respond to these measures, operation is indicated. The common extensor origin should be released from the epicondyle; any bursal tissue found between the common extensor tendon and the joint capsule should be excised.

BICIPITORADIAL BURSITIS

Occasionally discomfort and tenderness in the region of the bicipitoradial bursa, together with increased antecubital pain on resisted flexion-supination of the elbow, follow violent use of the biceps with the forearm pronated, as in the pitching of a baseball. Treatment consisting of rest, heat, and massage is indicated.

RADIOHUMERAL SUBLUXATION IN CHILDREN

A common and sometimes unrecognized occurrence in children, usually between 2 and 5 years of age, is subluxation of the proximal end of the radius on the capitellum of the humerus. This condition has been termed "nursemaid's elbow" or "pull syndrome" because of the mechanism by which it is produced: a sudden, direct pull on the elevated extremity with the elbow extended and the forearm pronated. This may occur when a child falls while his hand is being held by an adult. The diagnosis is made on the history, together with characteristic physical findings. The child refuses to use the arm, and the elbow is held slightly flexed. Because of failure to use the arm the condition may be mistaken for a paralysis, such as that caused by a brachial plexus injury. All movements are of essentially normal range except supination. The forearm is held in neutral position as regards rotation, and attempts to supinate cause pain and a sensation of mechanical blocking.

Treatment. A very brief manipulation without anesthesia is indicated. With the child's elbow flexed to a right angle, the forearm is supinated quickly while pressure is exerted on the radial head by the operator's thumb. As the point of obstruction is passed, a definite click is usually felt; following this the child almost immediately resumes use of the arm. If for any reason prompt reduction is not carried out, the subluxation will generally undergo spontaneous reduction in a few days.

OLD DISLOCATION OF THE ELBOW

Old unreduced posterior dislocation of the radius and ulna on the humerus is occasionally encountered and presents a characteristic clinical picture. The deformity is usually obvious to inspection and palpation, the olecranon and the triceps tendon appearing abnormally prominent posteriorly. There may be severe pain on resisted motion, and the mobility is much restricted, particularly flexion.

Treatment. When the dislocation has been present for as long as two or three weeks, an open reduction is usually necessary, since forced manipulation is likely to damage the soft tissues or to fracture the humeral condyles. A wide operative exposure is essential and is often gained by the posterior route with division of the triceps tendon. Care must be exercised to avoid injury of the ulnar nerve. After reduction, suture of the triceps tendon, and closure, the elbow is immobilized in flexion. In the aftertreatment physical therapy is of value but must be carefully supervised and should not include passive stretching.

VOLKMANN'S ISCHEMIC CONTRACTURE

The very disabling contracture of fingers and wrist first described in 1875 by von Volkmann is an occasional complication of injuries of the upper extremities and particularly of supracondylar fractures of the humerus. An analogous condition is sometimes observed in the lower extremities, where it has been known to follow the use of Bryant's overhead traction for fractures of the femur. The muscles of the forearm are indurated and rigid, the joints present unsightly contracture deformities, and the hand may become almost completely useless. Except in the mildest cases, one or more of the major nerve trunks may be involved as well as the muscles. The condition is seen much more often in children (Fig. 264) than in adults.

Etiology and pathology. The cause of the contracture is thought to be a severe ischemia resulting from spasm of the brachial artery an inch above its bifurcation, with reflex spasm of the collateral vessels. Early exploration at the site of injury may show a severe segmental spasm of the brachial artery, extending down into the radial and ulnar branches, narrowing them to the size of a string and obliterating their lumina. A visible lesion of the vessel itself may or may not be present.

The muscle bellies, which require a great deal of blood, are rapidly and profoundly affected by the ischemia. Microscopically, evidence of widespread degeneration and necrosis of the muscle fibers is quickly followed by round cell infiltration and by the extensive formation of fibrous tissue which later undergoes progressive contraction. Nerves to the forearm and hand may be damaged by the original injury or by the subsequent ischemia.

Clinical picture. Ischemic contracture occurs most commonly after fracture of the lower end of the humerus. Severe pain should at once suggest

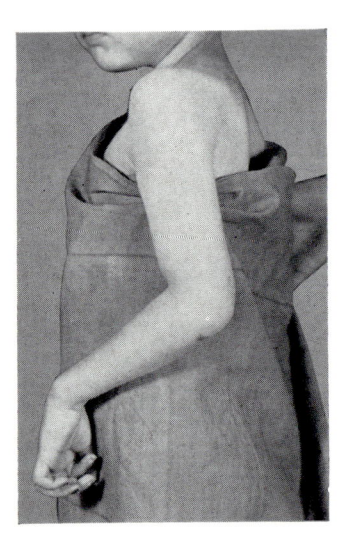

Fig. 264. Volkmann's ischemic contracture in 6-year-old boy, following supracondylar fracture of left humerus. Note deforming contractures of wrist and fingers with atrophy of the forearm.

the onset of this complication, but pain is not always present. The most important clinical sign is absence of the radial pulse. The hand may quickly become cyanotic, slightly swollen, and cold, and the fingers may be insensitive and powerless. Ischemia of forty-eight hours' duration usually results ultimately in a severe degree of contracture. As fibrosis proceeds, the forearm becomes hardened and shrunken, and the hand develops severe claw deformity (Fig. 264) and extreme disability. Flexion of the interphalangeal joints in the clawhand increases with attempts to extend the wrist. In severe cases, there may be fixed flexion of the elbow and pronation of the forearm. Examination may show also a paralysis that has resulted from damage of one or more nerve trunks.

Treatment. The early treatment of Volkmann's contracture is exceedingly important and in each case should be instituted as soon as possible. Prophylactic treatment should begin immediately after the original injury, as ischemia lasting six hours will cause a contracture. If there are no signs of circulatory embarrassment in the forearm and hand, reduction of the fracture may be carried out at once or may be started by elevation in skin traction. If reduction by manipulation is elected, several precautions are to be observed. Flexion should never be forced against resistance and must never be carried to the point of decreasing the strength of the radial pulse. When at the original manipulation sufficient flexion cannot be obtained to maintain satisfactory alignment, a second or third closed reduction can usually be carried out with safety in the following few days, the elbow being splinted in increasing flexion as the edema and hemorrhage in the antecubital fossa subside. After gentle manipulation, immobilization is secured by a posterior splint of plaster applied with care to avoid constriction. Observation during the next few days must be frequent and critical, and if severe pain or the signs of circulatory obstruction appear, immediate loosening or removal of the bandages is obligatory.

In borderline cases in which ischemia appears imminent, the safest treatment is to regard the fracture as of decidedly secondary importance and to concentrate all efforts upon improving the circulation. Procaine block of the brachial plexus may avert a catastrophe. Sympatholytic drugs, which produce vasodilation, may prove useful. Elevation of the arm by means of traction, with the elbow in partial flexion, and the application of cold are indicated until there is sufficient circulatory improvement to permit of a closed reduction. Skeletal traction by means of a Kirschner wire inserted through the olecranon may be used, but skin traction is usually adequate.

When the signs of acute severe ischemia are manifest, immediate surgical intervention is indicated. The hematoma should be evacuated through an anterior incision, and distended fascial compartments of the forearm opened. The artery must be exposed at the level of injury, care being taken to avoid damage of any of its branches. If warm saline applications, gentle massage of the vessel, and the intravenous injection of papaverine fail to restore the radial pulse, or if a lesion of the arterial wall is manifest, the constricted segment should be resected between ligatures. Collateral vessels, thus freed of reflex spasm, will in most cases maintain an adequate circulation. The fracture may be reduced gently before the wound is closed. In the next few days, repeated procaine block of the brachial plexus or the stellate and cervical sympathetic ganglia may be indicated. A sympatholytic drug may be used. The wrist and fingers should be splinted in functional position to forestall contractures.

Treatment of the late case is frequently unsatisfactory. Moderate improvement of the deformity and recovery of power often follow gradual stretching of the contracted muscles. This may be accomplished by means of a banjo splint fitted with elastic finger traction and hinged for progressive extension of the wrist or by the gradual wedging of a well-molded plaster cast. Intensive physical therapy is essential. When conservative measures prove ineffective, surgery is indicated. Many of the earlier operative procedures have not proved worth while and have been abandoned. Tendon lengthening is occasionally necessary. The muscle-sliding operation of Page, in which the attachment of the flexor muscles at the elbow is cut and pulled distally by hyperextension of the fingers and wrist, has in some hands produced good results. Good results in old cases have recently been reported following an extensive resection of the necrotic muscle and scar tissue, accompanied by muscle and tendon lengthening and transplantation if indicated. Arthrodesis of the wrist is occasionally indicated. When there is definite involvement of a nerve trunk, exploration for the purpose of freeing and repairing the nerve may be of benefit. Occasionally a nerve graft may be indicated.

TRAUMATIC MYOSITIS OSSIFICANS

Another important complication of injuries about the elbow, seen also in other parts of the body, is the formation of excessive amounts of new bone which may restrict the range of joint motion. Such new bone may be the result of any of several related pathologic processes. Excessive bone formation resulting simply from an active healing process and limited in area to the actual site of bony or periosteal injury is called *exuberant callus*. Bone produced by the organization and ossification of a hematoma, a process directly analogous to callus formation, may be found beneath the periosteum or extending out into the muscle or other soft tissues and is called *ossifying hematoma*. Intramuscular ossification following local injury is known as traumatic myositis ossificans. It is not to be confused with *progressive myositis ossificans,* a rare systemic disease described on p. 119.

Traumatic myositis ossificans may result either from repeated slight injuries or from a single episode of more severe trauma. Examples of the chronic type are the *rider's bone,* which forms within the thigh adductors of horsemen, and the ossification within the pectoralis major which in soldiers sometimes follows the habitual firing of a rifle. Intramuscular ossification following a single injury may occur in various regions of the body but is most frequent in the thigh, in the upper part of the arm, and

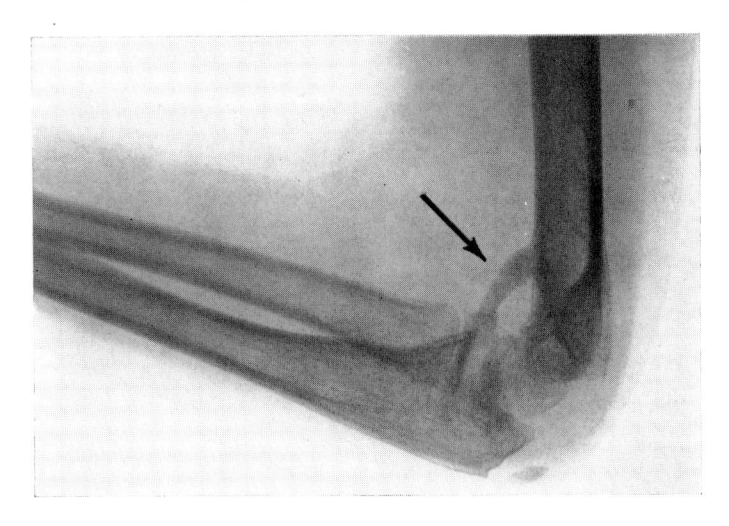

Fig. 265. Roentgenogram of traumatic myositis ossificans in elbow of 11-year-old boy. Note bony projection anterior to distal end of humerus. Eleven weeks previously the medial epicondyle of the humerus had been fractured.

about the elbow joint. Ossification in and about the elbow (Fig. 265) is of particular importance because it may cause a serious limitation of joint motion.

Etiology and pathology. The exact genesis of the new bone is uncertain. Osteoblasts from nearby injured periosteum may play a part, whereas in many cases a metaplasia of local connective tissue cells into bone-forming cells seems to take place. Some observers have attributed importance to a constitutional factor predisposing to ossification.

The new bone forms commonly in the lower portion of the belly of the brachialis muscle, anterior to the elbow joint. It may appear first as minute osteocartilaginous spicules which lie parallel to the muscle fibers; these later coalesce, forming an irregular bony mass that gradually becomes more rounded, homogeneous, and dense. Rarely a complete bridge of bone may develop, forming an extra-articular ankylosis. Usually the bone formation ceases within three to six months. The bony mass may be connected to the shaft by an osseous pedicle or a fibrous septum or may lie entirely separate from it. Spontaneous regression of the mass occurs frequently and may result in its complete disappearance.

Clinical picture. Traumatic myositis ossificans is seen most frequently in patients between the ages of 15 and 30 years. In the case of the elbow joint, the antecedent injury is most often a posterior dislocation or a fracture of the lower end of the humerus, but the condition may follow an uncomplicated strain or contusion. The diagnosis is to be suspected when tenderness, swelling, limitation of elbow motion, or pain on motion fails to clear up within the usual period, or when after an initial improvement these signs begin to become more marked. The area of ossification is usually palpable and is demonstrable in the roentgenogram after three or four weeks. Early osteogenic sarcoma must be considered in the differential diagnosis but can as a rule be definitely excluded by the roentgenogram.

Treatment. The stage at which the process is encountered determines the treatment. Since vigorous physical therapy is believed to stimulate the ossification, massage and strenuous exercise are to be avoided after elbow injuries; this is not likely to lead to contractures, since in the elbow—and particularly in young individuals—motion may be readily regained after immobilization. When a diagnosis of myositis ossificans in the region of the elbow has been made, prolonged rest of the elbow is indicated. Although guarded active motion may do no harm, the most certain method of treatment is immobilization. This is best obtained by means of a light, well-fitting plaster cast, extending from the upper arm to the metacarpal heads, with the elbow at an angle of from 80 to 90 degrees of flexion and the forearm in a mid-position of rotation. Immobilization should be continued until arrest of the process of ossification is definitely demonstrable in the roentgenograms. Active motion may then be gradually restored, but massage and passive stretching should be avoided.

Operation is contraindicated in the early stages of the ossification, as additional trauma will usually be followed by an increased formation of bone. When, despite an adequate period of waiting, which should be at least six to twelve months, the bony tumor has failed to be absorbed and is causing either limitation of joint motion or serious discomfort, surgical intervention is indicated. Complete excision of the bony mass should be carried out with care to avoid unnecessary trauma and to control carefully all hemorrhage. Immobilization for a period of two weeks after operation is advisable.

Traumatic myositis ossificans in other parts of the body presents essentially the same clinical picture and is treated in the same way.

Affections of the wrist and hand

The importance of the wrist and hand as compared with other parts of the extremity cannot be overemphasized. The more proximal portions of the upper extremity subserve primarily the purpose of putting the hand in positions where it can best carry out its functions.

Disabilities of the wrist and hand are extremely common. They fall largely into two major groups: (1) traumatic lesions and (2) infections. Many of the traumatic disorders are important not so much because of their immediate symptomatology as because of their disabling sequelae. Acute infections and injuries of the hand require surgical treatment based upon detailed anatomic and clinical study; for reference the works of Kanavel and of Bunnell are excellent. In addition to frank traumatic and infectious lesions, the wrist and hand are subject to a number of affections of chronic type, the causes of which are less well known. With the numerous and well-planned technics for treating injuries and diseases of the hand that were developed during and since World War II, hand surgery has become a large subject in itself. This has resulted in better care of affections of the hand and improved functional results.

Anatomy. The wrist joint is of double-hinge type, permitting approximately 180 degrees of motion in the anteroposterior plane and approximately 80 degrees in the lateral. A small part of the anteroposterior motion takes place in the intercarpal joints, but they do not contribute to lateral movement. The stability of the wrist is maintained not by bony configuration but by ligaments and the numerous tough, fibrous tendon sheaths that closely invest them.

On their volar surface the wrist bones form a concave arch which is converted into a tunnel by the transverse carpal ligament. Through this carpal tunnel pass the tendons of the flexor digitorum sublimis and profundus, the median nerve, and the flexor pollicis longus tendon. In this snug compartment, swelling from any of several causes may compress the median nerve and produce the *carpal tunnel syndrome* (p. 254). Where long flexor tendons must pull at an angle, such as in the wrist, distal palm, and digits, they are invested in a double-layered synovial sac or tendon sheath. This delicate membrane facilitates the smooth gliding of the tendon. To prevent the flexor tendons from bowstringing in the distal palm and fingers, the tendons and their synovial sheaths are encased in ligamentous tunnels. In these narrow passages, the "'no man's land" of Bunnell, fibrous adhesions of the tendon, sheath, and tunnel wall may immobilize the tendon and destroy its function. Within the digital tunnel the sublimis tendon, which proximally lies superficial to the profundus tendon, splits and passes to the dorsal side of the profundus to insert near the base of the middle phalanx. The profundus continues distally to insert on the base of the distal phalanx. The long extensor tendons on the dorsum of the hand do not traverse such tight compartments but rather fan out flatly over the dorsum of each metacarpophalangeal joint to form complex dorsal hoods. The central slip of a hood inserts on the base of the middle phalanx while the lateral bands, to either side of the central slip, continue distally to insert on the dorsum of the base of the distal phalanx. The long extensor muscles are primarily extensors of the metacarpophalangeal, or proximal, joints. The dorsal hoods are joined, just distal to the metacarpophalangeal joints, by the lumbricales and interossei. These intrinsic muscles act as flexors of the proximal and extensors of the middle and distal joints of the fingers.

Physical examination. Examination of the hand is essentially the clinical application of a good working knowledge of its anatomy. The origin, insertion, innervation, and function of each of the muscles which control the hand must be known before the clinician can appreciate the effects of lesions involving these structures.

AFFECTIONS OF TENDONS AND TENDON SHEATHS
Tendon lacerations

Tendon lacerations are common, serious problems. They frequently cause substantial disability of the digit or the entire hand and, as industrial injuries, result in the loss of many man-hours of work. In most instances early diagnosis and proper care of tendon injuries will yield good or excellent results. Failure to make the diagnosis or inadequate treatment may lead to permanent disability.

Tendon lacerations may be caused by any sharp instrument which penetrates the skin over the course of the tendon. They frequently result from accidents, such as grasping a sharp blade in the hand or falling on pieces of glass, or from the careless use of a power tool. The skin opening may be small and clean-cut or an extensive, jagged wound; in either case there may be associated injury of neurovascular and bony structures. Tendon injury should be suspected in the presence of every laceration of wrist, hand, or digits. The diagnosis is strengthened by demonstration of the patient's inability to move the joint served by the tendon in question. This test may be difficult in the case of the severely injured hand, but with careful, gentle examination the diagnosis can usually be made. In the case of a volar laceration near the proximal finger crease, only the sublimis may be severed and the diagnosis may not be obvious, since the profundus will flex both the middle and the distal joint. Examination will show, however, that the patient is unable to flex the middle joint against resistance while keeping the distal joint extended. The diagnosis of tendon laceration is confirmed at operation when the wound is treated.

Treatment. The treatment is based on knowledge of the detailed anatomy of the hand and of the physiology of tendon healing. In the case of fresh, clean lacerations primary repair of the tendon may be carried out, provided that it has not been severed in the region of the tight flexor tunnels, i.e., between the distal palmar crease and the middle phalanx ("no man's land"). For lacerations in the latter area, simple closure of the skin wound followed by a delayed tendon graft is advisable.

Tendon ruptures

Rupture may occur in almost any tendon of the hand. Ruptures are more common in extensor than in flexor tendons. As a rule, ruptures of flexor tendons occur at their site of insertion. Ruptures within the tendon are usually the result of local changes from disease or injury, rheumatoid arthritis and tenosynovitis being common offenders.

Rupture of the extensor pollicis longus tendon

The tendon of the extensor pollicis longus muscle is occasionally ruptured as a late effect of either of two conditions: (1) occupational trauma, as frequently observed in kettledrummers, and (2) fracture of the lower end of the radius. In either case the rupture is preceded by chronic degenerative changes in the tendon; these may result from friction against irregularities in the groove in the radius, from impairment of the blood supply, or from direct laceration of the tendon itself.

Clinical picture. Unlike the rupture of a normal tendon, the separation may occur without pain or sensation of snapping. Following fracture of the radius, the rupture often takes place on exertion from one to three months after the original trauma. The diagnostic signs are inability to extend the distal phalanx of the thumb against resistance and absence of the subcutaneous bowstring formed by the normal tendon when the thumb is actively extended.

Treatment. Exploration, followed by tendon suture, graft, or transference, is indicated. Cautious early mobilization is to be employed postoperatively.

Rupture of the central extensor slip

Rupture of the central extensor slip near its insertion into the base of the middle phalanx causes a flexion deformity of the proximal interphalangeal joint. The lateral bands to either side of the central slip gradually subluxate to the sides of the joint. They continue to exert force on the distal joint, which becomes hyperextended. This tendon lesion and finger attitude are known as a boutonniere (or buttonhole) deformity. The treatment consists of suturing the central slip and repositioning the lateral bands.

Mallet finger (baseball or dropped finger)

Sudden forcible flexion of a distal phalanx may cause an avulsion of the extensor tendon at its insertion. A small portion of the posterior lip of the phalangeal base is often torn away with the tendon. The injury is common among athletes and has been called *mallet, baseball,* or *dropped finger*.

Clinical picture. The history of injury together with inability to extend actively the distal phalanx is diagnostic. In early cases swelling and tender-

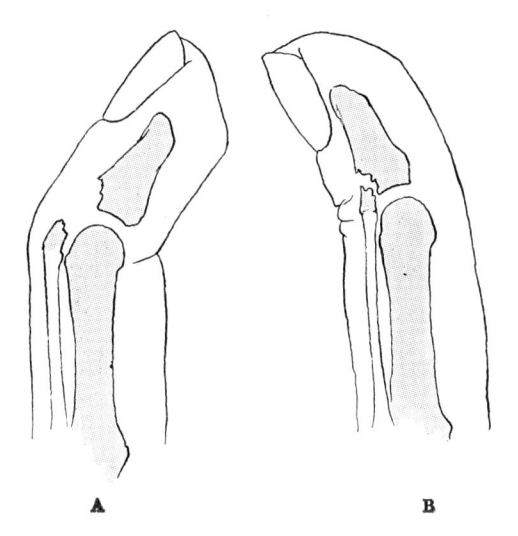

Fig. 266. Mallet finger. **A,** Typical deformity due to avulsion of tendon together with a small fragment of bone. **B,** Position of reduction. Whereas in treatment the distal joint of the finger is immobilized in hyperextension, the middle and proximal joints should be held in the better functional position of flexion.

ness may obscure the loss of power in the finger. Roentgenographic examination should always be made.

Treatment. The distal interphalangeal joint should be held constantly in hyperextension (Fig. 266) for from four to six weeks while the proximal interphalangeal joint is held flexed. This can be done with a plaster splint or a small metal splint bent to fit the finger. The insertion of a small wire or pin through the distal phalanx, across the hyperextended distal phalangeal joint, and into the middle phalanx has proved at times to be an effective method. The results of adequate treatment are usually good. In late cases one may resort to suture of the tendon or of the bone fragment to the phalanx, but the results are often unsatisfactory.

Tenosynovitis

Tenosynovitis is an inflammation of the synovial sheaths covering the tendons. It may be traumatic or infectious in origin.

Traumatic tenosynovitis

Traumatic tenosynovitis is a frequent clinical entity following minor occupational injury of the wrist region. It also occurs frequently in the sheaths of the anterior and posterior tibial and the Achilles tendons.

Etiology and pathology. Traumatic tenosynovitis is usually a result of strenuous, oft-repeated, or unaccustomed use of the adjacent joint. Serous or fibrinous fluid may accumulate in the affected tendon sheath, sometimes resulting later in chronic sclerosing changes and stenosis.

Clinical picture. Pain or motion of the affected tendon is the presenting symptom. Swelling usually occurs but may not be conspicuous, and redness is usually absent. Tenderness on pressure over the tendon sheath is a constant finding. On motion of the affected tendon unmistakable crepitation can usually be elicited. Disability of marked degree may develop rapidly.

Diagnosis. In differential diagnosis other lesions resulting from minor trauma in the affected region must be excluded. *Muscular strain* and *ligamentous sprain* are usually preceded by a single traumatic episode and are accompanied by pain and tenderness limited to the structure involved. At the wrist, fractures with little displacement are common, and, when the history is at all suggestive, fracture must be ruled out by roentgenographic examination, including oblique projections to visualize the scaphoid bone.

Treatment. Acute traumatic tenosynovitis often responds quickly to complete immobilization. In the wrist and forearm an elastic bandage, adhesive strapping, or a leather cuff may be used, but in most cases it is preferable to begin the treatment with the more effective support of well-fitting anterior and posterior plaster splints. In the ankle and lower leg, strapping or plaster immobilization is usually indicated. The application of heat is often a helpful adjunct. Immobilization should be continued until all tenderness has subsided, when carefully graded activity is to be resumed. Hydrocortisone injected into the tendon sheath space is sometimes effective in relieving the pain.

Stenosing tenosynovitis

First described by de Quervain in 1895 and sometimes called *de Quervain's tenovaginitis,* stenosing tenosynovitis commonly involves the abductor pollicis longus and extensor pollicis brevis, producing a stenosis of their sheaths in their common osseofibrous canal. The condition is most common in middle-aged and elderly women. The patient complains of disabling pain which is most severe near the styloid process of the radius. There may be local swelling. Pain is present on moving the wrist and thumb, especially with ulnar deviation and opposition of the thumb to the little finger *(Finkelstein test).* The pain may shoot into the thumb or up into the wrist and forearm. The thickened tendon sheath can sometimes be palpated as a hard, tender nodule over the styloid process of the radius. The involvement is frequently bilateral. Splinting of the wrist and thumb by means of a light plaster cast and injection of hydrocortisone into the tendon sheath may relieve the symptoms. Recurrence following conservative therapy is common. Release of the constriction by longitudinal incision or by partial resection of the sheath is usually curative. The operation should include search for anomalous tendons, which are common in this region.

Snapping finger or thumb

Occasionally a finger or thumb is seen which, at a single constant angle, shows a partial obstruction of the movement of flexion or of extension. Motion past the angle of obstruction, which often must be accomplished passively, may be accompanied by a definite sensation of snapping. This affection, called snapping finger or *trigger finger,* is usually of gradual and painless development. Its cause is unknown; however, trauma may be a contributing factor. The pathologic changes consist of a localized stenosis of the flexor tendon sheath, located usually near the metacarpophalangeal joint, and a nodular thickening of the tendon. Usually a small mass is palpable clinically. When this condition is found in young children, it is thought to be congenital in origin. Several members of the same family may be affected. In some instances the finger or thumb remains contracted and cannot be forcibly extended.

Treatment. A trial of nonsurgical treatment, consisting of immobilizing the digit by means of a plaster cast for several weeks, may be made. If conservative treatment fails, operation is usually indicated; the skin incision should be transverse. Sometimes simple longitudinal section of the fibrous sheath at the point of constriction will afford complete relief, but resection of a small portion of the sheath is advisable. After operation active motion should be started at once.

Acute suppurative tenosynovitis

Acute suppurative tenosynovitis results from an infection by staphylococci or streptococci commonly introduced into the tendon sheath through a puncture wound. The puncture is usually on the volar surface, the most vulnerable areas being the volar digital creases where the sheaths are unprotected by subcutaneous tissue. Occasionally an infection of the pulp space of the finger tip, or *felon* (possibly secondary to a phalangeal osteomyelitis, or *bone felon*), may extend into the synovial sheath. The rapid accumulation of pus under pressure distends the sheath; if allowed to continue it ultimately cuts off the blood supply to the tendon, causing necrosis and sloughing. In the middle and ring fingers the infection may break into the midpalmar space and thence extend through the lumbrical canals to the dorsum of the hand. The tendon sheath of the thumb is continuous with the radial bursa at the wrist, and that of the small finger is usually continuous with the ulnar bursa. Therefore involvement of these digits is especially serious, since rapid proximal spread of infection may take place.

Clinical picture. When the infection is limited to a single tendon sheath the patient presents a painful, swollen, tense finger held in a partially flexed position. There is acute tenderness over the course of the tendon sheath, and any attempt to extend the finger is extremely painful. The patient usually has a leukocytosis and moderate fever. He may experience some relief of pain as the infection breaks out of the sheath to spread to a palmar space or to the forearm. If untreated, an extensive infection may result in a totally useless hand.

Treatment. The treatment must be instituted early if satisfactory results are to be obtained. The most important measure is immediate and adequate drainage of the involved tendon sheath and other, secondarily infected spaces. Antibiotic treatment is important but unless instituted in the earliest phase of the disease cannot alone be expected to control the infection. The meager blood supply of the tendon, which may be completely compromised by the infection, limits the effectiveness of antibiotics. Careful splinting in functional position is important. If the hand infection progresses to the point of necrosis and sloughing of the tendon, the prognosis for future function is unfavorable.

Tuberculous tenosynovitis

Tuberculous tenosynovitis is encountered as a diffuse granulomatous, and often purulent, involvement of the tendon sheath or as a cystic expansion of the sheath containing particles of fibrin known as *rice bodies;* its treatment varies with the individual case but in general consists of excision of the pathologic tissue and temporary immobilization of the wrist. The postoperative result is usually satisfactory. Streptomycin and isoniazid are important adjuvants to surgery, and in some cases excellent results have been reported from their use alone. The streptomycin should be accompanied by para-aminosalicylic acid to decrease the likelihood that the organisms will become streptomycin-resistant.

Acute calcific tendinitis

Calcium deposits may occur in the tendons of the wrist and hand and present a problem similar to that seen at the shoulder. The most common site is in the flexor carpi ulnaris tendon near the pisiform bone. The onset of symptoms is usually sudden and the pain intense. Occasionally there is a history of acute or chronic trauma. Swelling and localized tenderness, as well as pain on motion of the involved tendon, are usual findings. Roentgenograms show a minute deposit of calcium in the affected area. The condition is usually self-limited; the duration of the symptoms may be shortened by injecting a small amount of local anesthetic into the tender area. Hydrocortisone may also be injected.

Ganglion

The wrist is the commonest site of the ganglion of joint or tendon sheath, a frequently seen but little understood lesion of benign character.

Pathology and etiology. The typical ganglion is a small, smooth, cystic structure containing a thick, clear, mucinous fluid. It is usually connected to the capsule of an adjacent joint or to a tendon sheath by a narrow pedicle without a lumen; sometimes no pedicle is demonstrable. Ganglia may reach considerable dimensions and may be multilocular or multiple.

The etiology is obscure. It was formerly thought that these cysts result from herniation of the lining membrane of a joint or tendon sheath. Recent observations have led to the belief that they are produced by a colloid degeneration, which occurs locally in the connective tissue and which may be related to ischemic changes. It has also been suggested that the cyst formation is possibly analogous to the developmental process that leads, in tissue of similar origin, to the formation of the normal joint cavities.

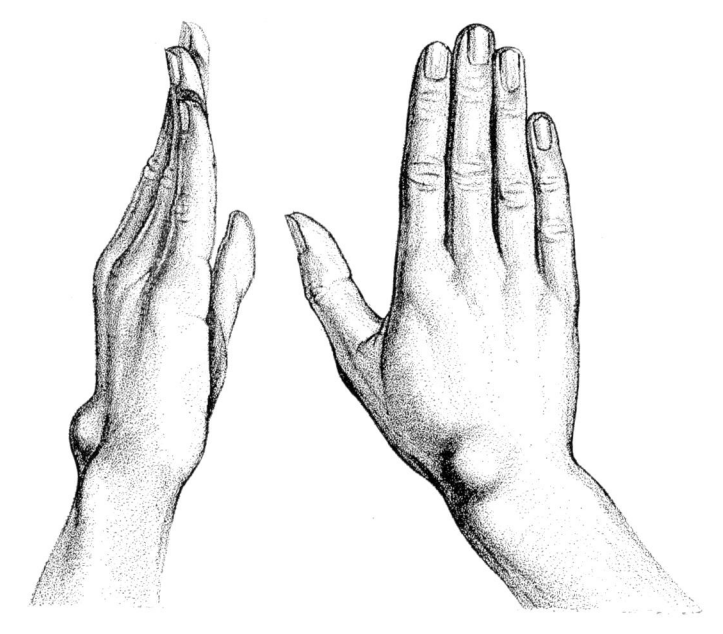

Fig. 267. Ganglion of wrist. Note smooth, well-demarcated swelling on dorsolateral aspect of the wrist.

Clinical picture. Ganglia occur most commonly in patients between the ages of 15 and 35 years. At the wrist they are most frequent on the dorsum (Fig. 267) but are found also on the volar aspect. Small ganglia near the joints of the fingers are common. About the knee, ganglia may appear in the popliteal space, laterally in front of the tendon of the biceps, or anteriorly beneath the patellar ligament. The front of the ankle and dorsum of the foot are other common sites.

The swelling is of slow growth and causes few symptoms. Occasionally there is discomfort in the adjacent joint or tendons, particularly after overuse or strain. The swelling is tense or fluctuant, rounded, nontender, and not fixed to the skin. It often varies in prominence with motion of the adjacent joint. Ganglia frequently regress or disappear spontaneously. In differential diagnosis ganglia must be distinguished from benign soft tissue tumors such as fibromas and lipomas, from bursitis, and from tuberculous tenosynovitis.

Treatment. The old treatment of rupturing the cyst by trauma or pressure is painful and likely to be followed by recurrence. The combination of aspiration, chemical cauterization, and application of a pressure bandage is sometimes employed. The most successful results, however, are obtained from surgical excision, although the recurrence rate has been reported to be high. The operation must be planned with the realization that the ganglion may be found to arise not from a superficial structure but from the articular capsule.

CONTRACTURES OF THE WRIST AND HAND

Contractures are the result of shortening of the soft tissues. The shortening may involve skin, muscle, or ligament and is usually the result of replacement of a part of these tissues by scar. Contractures in the hand limit its mobility and function. The principal causes of hand contractures are trauma, infection, nonspecific inflammatory processes, nerve lesions, ischemia, and congenital changes.

Skin contractures

The most common causes of skin contractures are scars secondary to lacerations, poorly placed surgical incisions, keloids, and burns. A laceration that crosses perpendicularly a skin crease in the wrist, hand, or finger will result in a scar, which gradually hypertrophies, contracts, and pulls the underlying joint into deformity. Surgical incisions should avoid skin folds.

Treatment. The treatment of skin contractures involves revision of the scar by technics such as Z-plasty. When the scar is extensive, its replacement by a free or pedicle skin graft is often necessary.

Metacarpophalangeal and interphalangeal contractures

Metacarpophalangeal joint contractures are frequent complications of injuries to the upper extremity and of injudicious immobilization. Extension contracture of these joints is the result of shortening of their collateral ligaments. These ligaments are eccentrically attached in such a way that they are relaxed when the joint is extended and are tight in flexion. Thus abduction and adduction are possible in the extended position but quite limited when the metacarpophalangeal joints are flexed. A cast or splint extending beyond the distal palmar crease may immobilize these joints in extension. If the collateral ligaments are allowed to shorten in this position, flexion will no longer be possible. Only in rare instances should the metacarpophalangeal or other finger joints be immobilized in extension, and then only for the shortest possible time. The use of the straight tongue depressor as a splint for injured fingers is to be condemned, for it has frequently led to a permanently straight, stiff finger.

Treatment. Since a primary cause of extension contracture of the finger joints is immobilization in the extended position, the treatment is first prophylactic. Careful attention to the details of splinting in functional position, and early, active flexion exercises are important. Established contractures are difficult to eradicate. Active flexion exercises and the use of knuckle-bender elastic splints are usually indicated. Surgical release is occasionally helpful.

Intrinsic contracture of the hand

Intrinsic contracture of the hand is the result of a shortening of the small muscles of the hand, usually secondary to trauma, ischemia, or rheumatoid arthritis. Contracture of the lumbrical and interosseous muscles results in a flexion deformity of the metacarpophalangeal joints and hyperextension of the proximal interphalangeal joints. The distal joints may become flexed because of pull from the profundus. Involvement of the thumb muscles results in an adduction deformity with flexion of the proximal joint and extension of the distal. This combination of deformities is referred to as an *intrinsic plus hand*. It is the opposite of the clawhand seen after combined median and ulnar nerve injuries, the *intrinsic minus hand,* in which the metacarpophalangeal joints are hyperextended and the interphalangeal joints flexed. The clinical test for intrinsic contracture is carried out by flexing fully the metacarpophalangeal joints to relax the tight lumbricales and interossei. This will permit flexion of the interphalangeal joints. When the metacarpophalangeal joints are extended, which tightens the intrinsic muscles, it is impossible to flex the interphalangeal joints.

Treatment. The treatment of intrinsic contracture consists of gradual stretching with elastic splints, supplemented by surgical release of the extensor components of the intrinsic muscle mechanisms.

Dupuytren's contracture

The common affection first analyzed and described by Dupuytren in 1832 is a slowly progressive contracture of the palmar fascia, occurring most often in men between 55 and 75 years of age. When it occurs in women, it is nearly always in a younger group. As a rule, the changes involve the ring finger, little finger, or both (Fig. 268). Dupuytren's contracture is usually

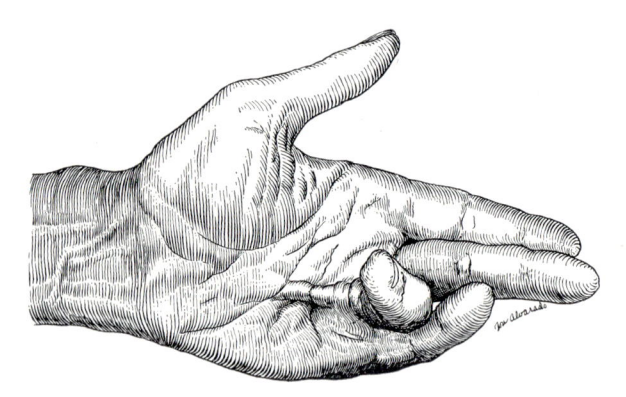

Fig. 268. Dupuytren's contracture of ring finger. Note flexion deformity of ring finger and prominent band caused by localized contracture of the palmar fascia. (After Colonna.)

bilateral; when unilateral, it is found more frequently in the right hand. It is found in 2 to 3% of the older population and is uncommon in the Negro race.

Pathology. The essential morbid process is a chronic inflammation of the palmar fascia, with progressive fibrosis and contracture, principally of the pretendinous bands of the palmar aponeurosis to the fingers. In advanced cases the skin is secondarily involved. Changes in flexor tendons and digital joints are slight and occur only in late and extreme cases.

Etiology. The cause is unknown. The possible etiologic role of chronic trauma has not been established by analysis of statistics. In some cases there is a hereditary factor.

Clinical picture. The contracture is first evidenced by the appearance of a small nodular, painless thickening in the palmar fascia overlying a flexor tendon in the region of a metacarpophalangeal joint, often associated with a dimpling of the skin at this point. A thickened longitudinal band is gradually formed, and flexion contracture of the finger progressively increases. The metacarpophalangeal and adjacent interphalangeal joints become flexed, while the distal interphalangeal joint, controlled by no prolongations of the palmar fascia, retains a normal range of extension. In extreme cases the tip of the finger may be drawn into constant contact with the palm. As a rule there is little pain or tenderness. Frequently both hands are involved; usually the affection appears much earlier, however, in one hand than in the other. In some cases the plantar fascia shows small nodular thickenings similar to those in the palmar fascia.

Differential diagnosis. Flexion contractures secondary to congenital malformation, spasticity, trauma, and infection must be excluded. The insidious and painless onset, the presence of flexion at the metacarpophalangeal level, and the inability to extend the proximal interphalangeal joint even when the wrist is flexed are characteristic of Dupuytren's contracture. It should be remembered that in some instances the microscopic appearance of the lesion in its early stage may simulate that of fibrosarcoma.

Treatment. In the earliest cases frequent forced extension may be of some value. For all other cases the only effective treatment is surgical. Frequently the procedure of choice is a careful and thorough excision of the abnormal palmar fascia. Postoperatively a splint is worn for a few days, but active and passive motion must be begun as soon as healing of the skin permits. Excision of the fascia obviates, as a rule, the danger of recurrence. However, it is a major procedure. The simple operation of multiple subcutaneous divisions of contracted fascial bands with a tenotomy knife is sometimes preferred, particularly for cases in which the contracture is well localized. For satisfactory results all of the constricting bands must be divided, and the postoperative treatment, including the use of an extension splint at night in addition to exercises, must be prolonged in an effort to prevent recurrence of the contracture.

AFFECTIONS OF THE BONES OF THE WRIST AND HAND
Avascular necrosis of the carpal bones

Avascular necrosis, a rare and little understood affection of one or more of the bones of the carpus, is characterized by the gradual development of pain and disability in the wrist, associated with typical roentgenographic changes. A history of antecedent injury is often obtainable, and the condition is sometimes termed *traumatic osteitis* or *osteoporosis*. The etiologic mechanism is usually considered to be a local nutritive disturbance dependent upon circulatory changes induced by trauma. The pathologic changes are those of avascular necrosis. Involvement of the lunate bone is often known as *Kienböck's disease*, and of the scaphoid bone as *Preiser's disease*.

Clinical picture. The majority of patients are men between the ages of 20 and 40 years. The initial trauma may be trivial or severe and may cause pain and swelling that persist for several days or weeks. A period of months or even years then elapses in which no symptoms are present. Thereafter a gradual development of aching pain takes place, at first felt only on jarring or on exertion but later persistent and severe. Local swelling and tenderness appear, dorsiflexion becomes limited, and the disability may become extreme. When the lunate bone is severely affected, the head of the third metacarpal may lose its normal dorsal prominence because of a proximal displacement of the entire bone, and longitudinal thrusts upon the metacarpal in a proximal direction will cause pain. The range of wrist motion often becomes restricted.

Roentgenographic picture. In early films there may be no definite changes, but as the condition advances characteristic alterations of the affected bone appear. It becomes flattened and may be abnormally dense. In some cases irregular areas of rarefaction are conspicuous, suggesting fragmentation. In adjacent bones, the changes of an early traumatic arthritis often develop.

Treatment. Nonsurgical treatment is usually indicated. The wrist is immobilized in a short dorsiflexion splint, which may be removed daily for gentle underwater exercises. If after several months the improvement is found to be unsatisfactory, excision of the affected bone or bones may be advisable; postoperatively the wrist should be immobilized for one month, after which exercise is gradually resumed. In late cases with pain and advanced arthritic changes, arthrodesis of the wrist is sometimes indicated.

Old dislocation of the lunate bone

Two lesions of the carpus are frequently seen following episodes of moderate or severe trauma: (1) fracture of the scaphoid bone and (2) anterior dislocation of the lunate bone. Cases of neglected scaphoid injuries are discussed on p. 302, in the chapter on fracture deformities. Unreduced dislocation of the lunate bone is an important entity, since it results in severe disability of the hand.

Pathology. When, by a fall upon the hyperextended hand, the lunate bone has been squeezed from its position between the radius and the capitate, it lies anteriorly, with its concave distal surface rotated forward (Fig. 269). In this position the lunate is located immediately beneath the structures crossing the volar aspect of the wrist and is likely to cause involvement of the flexor tendons by friction and of the median nerve by pressure.

Clinical picture. Enlargement of the anterior aspect of the wrist is usually obvious, and in some cases the displaced bone is palpable. There may be noticeable atrophy of the muscles of the hand. The wrist and fingers are held slightly flexed, extension is limited and painful, and the grip is markedly weakened. In a large proportion of the cases the characteristic anesthesia and paralysis that result from involvement of the median nerve will be found.

Treatment. In late cases the displaced lunate bone should be excised, and following its removal a plaster splint or cast should be applied for immobilization. Physical therapy is begun after a week and must usually be employed daily for an extended period.

Old posterior dislocation of the lunate bone is seen only rarely; the treatment, like that of unreduced anterior dislocation, is excision of the lunate followed by splinting and physical therapy.

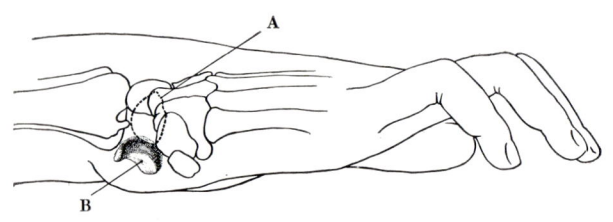

Fig. 269. Anterior dislocation of the lunate bone. **A,** Normal position of lunate bone; **B,** position after dislocation. (Drawing from roentgenogram.)

Accessory bones of the wrist and hand

According to the findings of comparative anatomy and embryology, a large variety of accessory or supernumerary bones may occur in the carpal region. Clinically, however, accessory bones of the hand are much less frequent and less important than those of the foot.

Of chief diagnostic significance is the rare *divided scaphoid*, resulting from failure of radial and ulnar anlagen of the scaphoid bone to fuse. Roentgenographically this condition resembles an ununited fracture, but most authorities agree that it is of purely developmental origin. It is possible that imperfect fusion is a predisposing factor in traumatic fractures of the scaphoid. The hamulus of the hamate bone may develop separately, and the ulnar styloid process may fail to unite with the distal end of the ulna. In differential diagnosis it must be remembered, however, that these developmental variations are extremely uncommon.

Developmental fusion of one or more adjacent carpals sometimes occurs. An accessory epiphysis is rarely seen at the proximal end of the second or fifth metacarpal bone.

Madelung's deformity

Madelung's deformity is an uncommon affection of the wrist, characterized by dorsal prominence of the lower end of the ulna, instability of the distal radioulnar articulation, and local changes in the conformation of the radius and ulna (Fig. 270).

Etiology. The cause has not been definitely established but is apparently a local nutritional or growth disturbance resulting from changes secondary to congenital abnormality or occupational trauma. In some instances there is a hereditary factor.

Clinical picture. The condition is usually seen in adolescents and is not infrequently bilateral. The patient complains of deformity of the wrist and of a feeling of weakness and insecurity. The wrist may appear enlarged, and on palpation there may be demonstrable instability of the radioulnar joint. The end of the radius is displaced anteriorly, carrying with it the carpus and hand. There are a resulting dorsal prominence of the lower end of the

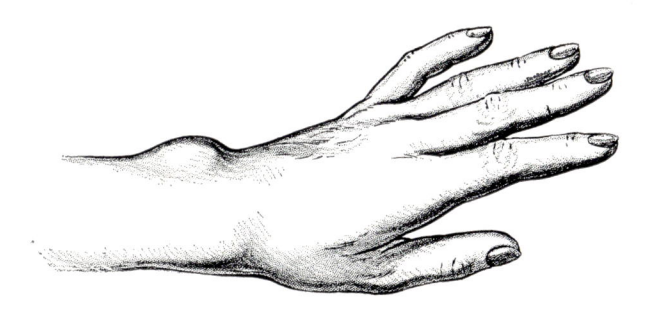

Fig. 270. Madelung's deformity. Note dorsal prominence caused by posterior subluxation of distal end of ulna.

ulna and an abnormal limitation of dorsiflexion. In severe cases the range of supination and pronation may be decreased.

Treatment. In all except the most advanced cases a trial of nonsurgical treatment is indicated. The wrist is immobilized by a dressing that incorporates a short dorsiflexion splint and a pressure pad over the prominent distal end of the ulna. Graded exercises may be given to strengthen the local musculature. Excision of the distal end of the ulna is sometimes helpful. In advanced cases it may be advisable to reinforce surgically the ligaments at the distal radioulnar joint. In severe late lesions osteotomy of the radius or ulna may be necessary in order to correct the deformity.

APPENDIX

Fracture principles

SINCE FRACTURES are an essential part of orthopaedic surgery and since the medical student often starts his study of orthopaedic diseases and fractures simultaneously, a brief presentation of the nomenclature and principles of fracture management may prove useful. Of the many excellent fracture texts, of either introductory or reference type, a number are listed in the bibliography (p. 570).

Definitions

Certain terms are in common usage in the description of bone injuries. A *fracture* is defined as any break in the continuity of bone. The term *fractured bone* is generally used interchangeably with *broken bone*. A strong distinction is made between a fracture in which there is communication between the bone and the outside, an *open* or *compound fracture*, and a fracture in which there is no such communication, a *closed* or *simple fracture*. In the case of the open injury, infection, osteomyelitis, delayed union, and even nonunion of the fracture are frequent complications. *Pathologic fractures* occur in bones weakened by pre-existing disease such as tumors, cysts, osteomyelitis, or osteoporosis.

Certain terms used to describe the configuration of fractures are of more than academic interest because they often convey information on the mechanism of injury and carry implications affecting the choice of treatment. Fractures are described as *transverse, oblique,* or *spiral* according to the direction taken by the line of breakage. *Transverse fractures* are usually caused by simple angulatory forces, while *spiral fractures* result from torsion. A fracture is said to be *comminuted* when the bone is broken into three or more fragments. Spiral, oblique, and comminuted fractures are often unstable; frequently their reduction cannot be maintained by simple cast fixation without danger of overriding of the fragments and shortening of the extremity.

Diagnosis

Establishing the diagnosis is the first step in the care of fractures. The ease of diagnosis varies with the severity and location of the fracture and with the degree of displacement and deformity. The presence of other serious injuries may obscure the fracture and make diagnosis more difficult. The clinician's awareness that certain types of injuries are likely to cause certain fractures and that some fractures may show little external evidence of deformity facilitates diagnosis. The diagnosis is based on data obtained from the history, physical examination, and roentgenograms.

History. A thorough history is important. Although difficult or impossible to obtain from a seriously injured patient, certain points in the history should always be sought. Details of the injury or accident should be carefully recorded, since they may give helpful information regarding the severity and type of forces involved. A record of the time and place of the injury should be made. The age of the patient is important, since certain fractures predominate in particular age groups. A history of pain or deformity preceding fracture may be the first clue to the diagnosis of a pathologic fracture. In the case of open fractures it is important to learn whether the patient has had immunization to tetanus. Since the treatment of many fractures requires general anesthesia, one must often learn the time of the patient's last meal and what was eaten. A history of recent respiratory infection or of cardiac or renal difficulties may modify the treatment. Inquiry concerning allergies, particularly to medications used in connection with anesthesia and to antibiotics and antitoxins, is essential.

Physical examination. Immediate attention should be given to the patient's general condition. In *severely injured patients* the three most serious problems are (1) respiratory difficulties, (2) acute hemorrhage, and (3) shock. If any or all of these problems exist, they must be dealt with immediately.

Respiratory difficulties include obstruction due to edema from soft tissue injury about the face and neck, foreign bodies, and accumulated secretions in the respiratory tract. Emergency tracheotomy may be necessary. Tension pneumothorax, open wounds of the chest, and an unstable or flail chest are other acute respiratory problems requiring immediate attention.

Acute hemorrhage is obvious if external. Venous bleeding from a large wound can usually be controlled by direct pressure through a sterile dressing placed in the wound. Mild arterial bleeding can be controlled in a similar manner, but a bleeding larger artery may require direct clamping in the emergency room. Digital pressure over the arterial supply proximal to the bleeding area may be effective as a temporary expedient. Rarely is the use of a tourniquet to control hemorrhage warranted. If a tourniquet is used, the person applying it should be in constant attendance and responsible for release of the tourniquet within one half to one hour after its application. Internal hemorrhage within pleural, pericardial, or abdominal cavities may not be obvious. It should be suspected when shock persists despite adequate transfusion, and in the presence of injuries to chest or abdomen.

Shock, manifested by cold and clammy skin, rapid and thready pulse, and lowered blood pressure, is usually the result of blood loss. The amount of blood lost by a patient is difficult to determine and is frequently underestimated. A great deal of bleeding may have occurred from the relatively small wound of an open fracture or from small scalp lacerations, but if the bleeding has ceased when the patient reaches the emergency room extensive blood loss may not be suspected. A closed fracture of the femur in a large person may be followed by loss of a great quantity of blood in the soft tissues of the thigh. Intrapleural bleeding, or intra-abdominal bleeding from rupture of liver or spleen, may result in shock. Hemorrhagic shock is most effectively treated by whole blood transfusion. When compatible blood is not immediately available, the blood pressure may be temporarily sustained by giving intravenous dextrose in saline, or by giving plasma or a plasma expander such as dextran. Shock may result also from cardiorespiratory embarrassment with decreased oxygen supply to the tissues, vasodilatation, and circulatory collapse. Additional causes of shock include burns, crush injuries, overwhelming bacterial infections, and toxic conditions such as gas gangrene. Common to all forms of shock is a deficiency in the volume of circulating blood with respect to the effective capacity of the cardiovascular system. If the deficiency persists or increases, the outlook for survival is poor. In addition to causing shock, crush injuries result in severe soft tissue damage and necrosis and may be associated with acute renal failure.

If none of these three grave emergencies exists, or after their treatment has been started, one may proceed with a more detailed physical examination. This is best carried out with the patient completely undressed. Some of the clothing may have to be cut away. Much of the examination can be done with the patient supine on a table or stretcher. Observation of the entire body for lacerations, abrasions, swelling, or deformity can be carried out in seconds; unless this simple process of *looking* is done in a routine head-to-toe manner, it is surprising how many injuries may be overlooked. The second step in the examination is palpation of the entire skeletal system. Any tenderness, induration, or deformity is sought. Again, in a matter of a minute or two, every major bone in the body can be felt, the patient being moved very little during the process. The skull and jaw are palpated, the cervical spine next—and gently—and then the clavicles, sternoclavicular and acromioclavicular joints, shoulder, humerus, and elbow. The medial and lateral epicondyles, as well as the olecranon and radial head are easily located. Palpation continues down the forearm to the small bones of the wrist and hand. Next the rib cage and sternum are carefully examined. The patient is then turned very slightly to enable the examiner to get his hand under the patient's back. Thoracic and lumbar spinous processes are palpated, as well as the sacrum, sacroiliac joints, and ischial tuberosities. The skin of the back and buttocks may be inspected at this time. Palpation is continued anteriorly over the iliac crests, trochanters, pubis, thigh, patella, knee, tibia, ankle, foot, and toes. The circulation in the extremities is evaluated by noting temperature, color changes, and pulses. Sensation in the extremities may be briefly tested at this time. The patient is then asked to move fingers and toes.

A brief survey of the patient's cranial nerve function is followed by inspection of mouth, ears, and eyes. Auscultation of the chest and palpation of the abdomen may be done next.

The entire examination is a quick but careful survey that can be carried out rapidly with little disturbance to the patient. It will be modified by positive findings; more detailed neurologic evaluation, for example, would be given a patient with evidence of head or spinal cord injury.

After this brief survey, attention is focused on the *injured area*. Other than distortion from swelling, there are three types of deformity which may be associated with fracture of a long bone: *angulation, shortening,* and *rotation.* Obvious angulation indicates fracture. One should be cautious, however, and by gentle, careful palpation seek possible associated fractures or dislocations above and below the angulation. When tenderness is not accompanied by deformity, the examiner may cautiously apply a slight bending force to the long bone, grasping it above and below the level of tenderness; if pain in the tender area results, a fracture is to be strongly suspected. Joint motion should be tested with the extremity well-supported by the examiner's hands and need not be carried beyond the point of pain.

When a fracture is suspected, the circulation and nerve supply distal to the injury should be carefully evaluated. In the lower extremity, simple tests for peroneal, tibial, and femoral nerve function should be done. Injuries to the blood supply manifest themselves by coolness, blanching or cyanosis, decreased sensation and motor function, and diminished or absent pulses distal to the injury. Vascular injuries are particularly common following elbow fractures; they demand immediate treatment. To evaluate possible nerve injury in the upper extremity the simple tests for radial, median, and ulnar function are quickly carried out (see Chapter 12). Where there is severe injury to the wrist or hand these tests may be difficult, but with diligence a satisfactory evaluation can be made.

It should be noted that in emergency situations a thorough physical examination can be carried out in a very few minutes and that no equipment is required other than the hands and eyes of the examining physician.

When a fracture is suspected, the injured part should be splinted before the patient is moved to another location. Excessive motion at the fracture site not only is painful but also may increase soft tissue damage, injure blood supply and nerves, and even cause sharp fracture fragments to penetrate the skin, converting a closed injury into an open fracture. For ankle fractures an ordinary pillow wrapped about the leg and ankle and supported on the stretcher is quite effective. In the case of the humerus, having the patient hold the arm close to his body may be effective enough. Padded board splints are useful for forearm fractures. Prefabricated metal splints in common use for the leg and thigh require careful padding to prevent pressure sores about the heel, malleoli, and fibular head. For serious fractures of the leg, knee, and femur, the Thomas splint (Fig. 271), which facilitates traction, remains an effective device; it should be available in every emergency room, and every physician should know how to use it.

Roentgenographic examination. After emergency treatment, physical ex-

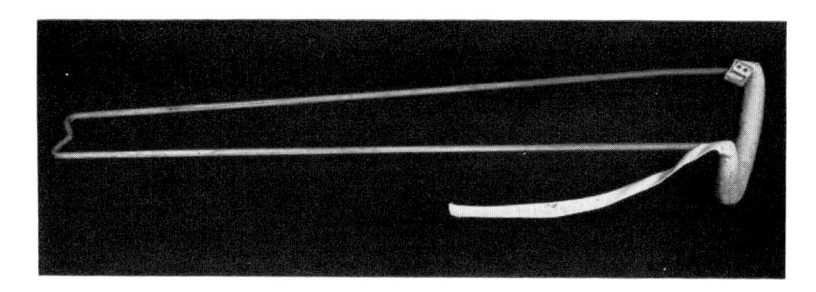

Fig. 271. The Thomas half-ring splint, which is used to provide support and traction for either upper or lower limb.

amination, and splinting, roentgenograms of the fracture should be made; they should be considered an integral part of the examination. The attending physician who has examined the patient can best tell the x-ray technician what views need be taken and where the x-ray tube should be centered. In severe injuries it is wise for the physician to accompany his patient and to aid in the taking of the films. He is best able to protect the injured area during x-ray positioning, and he will be assured that indicated views will be taken. In less severe injuries, adequate instructions should accompany the patient. A small mark on the patient's skin at the area of suspected fracture will often aid the technician in proper centering. Views of suspected areas should always be made in at least two planes, perpendicular to each other; additional oblique views are sometimes necessary. The fracture may be apparent on only one of several views. All necessary exposures should be made at the initial examination, any suspected areas being included. For early roentgenograms large films are best; many a fracture or dislocation has been overlooked by not being included on a small film.

Principles of fracture treatment

Following interpretation of the roentgenograms, the optimal treatment must be chosen. This will depend upon many factors, including the general condition of the patient, the presence of associated injuries, whether or not the fracture is open, and the location and displacement of the fracture. Fracture treatment includes three basic objectives:

1. *Reduction,* or replacement of the bone fragments to as near anatomic position as possible
2. *Maintenance of reduction* until healing is sufficient to prevent displacement
3. *Restoration of function* of the muscles, joints, and tendons

Reduction. Many fractures with little or no displacement require no reduction, only maintenance of position. Fractures with displacement may be reduced in several ways. Since reduction is painful and involves counteracting strong muscle pulls, general or regional anesthesia is usually necessary. Reduction by *manipulation* is the most common method of restoring the alignment of fractured long bones. It may involve longitudinal traction to restore length, angulation to allow locked fragments to disengage and slide past one another, and manual pressure of the bone fragments into proper position. The details of manipulation vary with the individual fracture and the displacement of the fragments. A second method of fracture reduction is *traction* applied over a period of several hours or days. Reduction by sustained traction is generally used when the traction will also maintain reduction. It is used most commonly in the treatment of femoral shaft fractures and cervical spine injuries. A third method of fracture reduction is *open surgery*. Occasionally the fragments may be caught within the soft tissues in such a manner that reduction by manipulation or traction is either impossible or dangerous. In such instances reduction under direct vision is advisable. More frequently, however, open reduction is utilized because internal fixation is contemplated for maintenance of the reduction. It must always be remembered that open reduction is a hazardous procedure. It converts a closed fracture into an open one, and if unsuccessful or complicated by infection it may result in a much more serious situation than was present before operation. In children, with the exception of certain specific fractures about the elbow and hip, it is extremely rare that open reduction need be undertaken.

Maintenance of reduction. After a fracture has been reduced, the corrected alignment must be maintained until bone healing is well advanced. The three common methods by which fractures are held in position during the healing phase are (1) *external fixation* by means of cast or splint, (2) *traction*, and (3) *internal fixation* by nail, plate, or screws. In many fractures the indication for one of these methods is fairly clear-cut and it is used practically to the exclusion of the others. For example, in maintaining the reduction of fractures of the femoral neck, internal fixation has so many advantages that traction or external fixation is rarely used. On the other hand, many fractures may be treated satisfactorily by any of several methods.

1. *External fixation:* External fixation is the most common method of maintaining reduction. It may be accomplished by means of a plaster cast or by splints of metal or wood. Splints are of limited value, since it is difficult to make them conform to the contour of the individual patient, and unless carefully applied with adequate padding they cause pressure sores over bony prominences. Plastic materials have also been used for external fixation, but to date nothing else has been found quite so satisfactory as the plaster-of-Paris bandage first introduced by Mathijsen in 1852. Plaster of Paris is anhydrous calcium sulfate. In powder form it is incorporated in rolls of crinoline bandage which are dipped in water and then wrapped about the extremity. The fact that this wet bandage can be molded to the contour of the extremity and to the requirements of the individual fracture accounts chiefly for its superiority over other methods of external fixation. Plaster of Paris sets in a matter of minutes and forms a strong and durable support for the injured extremity. Plaster cast fixation is especially applicable where bones are close to the surface and can be held efficiently by

the cast, as in fractures about the wrist, ankle, and tibia. Casts are less effective for immobilizing fractured bones that lie deep in muscle, such as the femur. In fractures of the long bones, casts are effective in controlling angulation and rotation, but another type of fixation is required when shortening is likely, as in oblique or comminuted fractures. Plaster cast fixation is used for most children's fractures.

Although the use of plaster of Paris is relatively simple, certain precautions must be observed. Since the hardened cast is quite rigid, bony prominences must be protected by adequate padding. Otherwise pressure sores may develop. Where major nerves pass between bone and skin, such as the ulnar nerve at the elbow and the common peroneal nerve around the neck of the fibula, protective padding is especially important. A common cause of foot drop is peroneal nerve injury from an improperly applied cast. It must be kept in mind that after the plaster has set a circular cast cannot expand. If post-injury swelling takes place within a tight cast, circulatory embarrassment may produce serious consequences. Whenever there is doubt of the adequacy of the circulation in a casted extremity, the cast should be split and spread immediately.

2. *Traction:* For fractures that cannot be immobilized efficiently by casts, maintenance of reduction by means of traction may be advisable. When traction is applied to an acutely injured extremity, the muscles act as an internal splint to protect the fracture, and the patient usually experiences

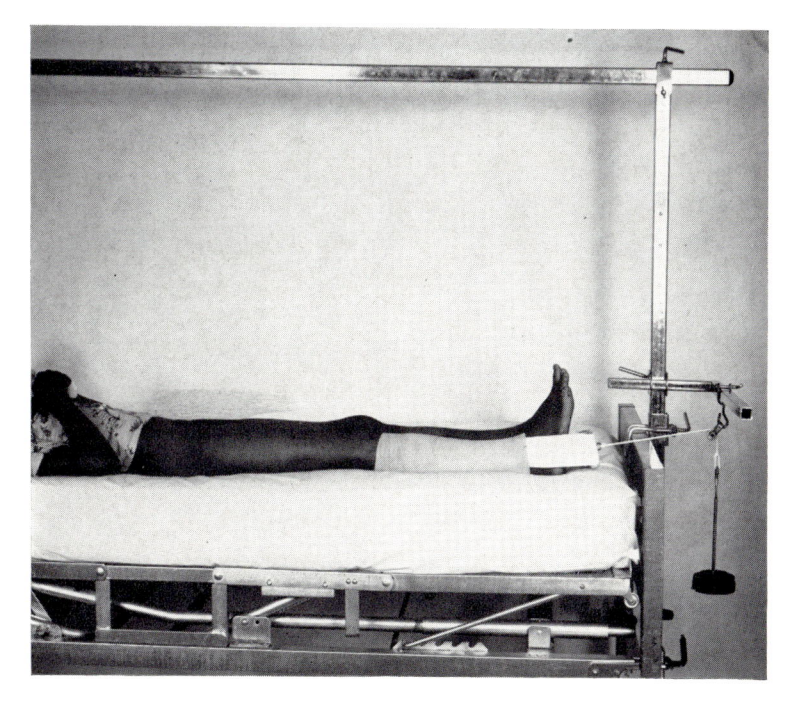

Fig. 272. Buck's extension, used to exert traction in the long axis of the lower limb with knee and hip in neutral position.

relief of pain. The principal disadvantage of treatment by traction is that it requires the patient to remain in bed and in hospital.

Traction may be applied in several ways. *Skin traction,* usually applied by means of an adhesive, cloth strips, and an encircling elastic bandage, may be used when not more than 5 or 6 pounds of pull is required. It is frequently used for longitudinal pull on the leg, as in *Buck's extension* (Fig. 272). When used as *Bryant's traction* (Fig. 273) in the treatment of femoral shaft fractures in children under the age of 3 years, great care must be taken to watch for ischemia. Older children with femoral fractures are often treated by *Russell's traction* (Fig. 274). Traction may be applied to the neck by means of a cloth head halter, and to the pelvis by a canvas girdle.

Skeletal traction, applied by drilling a wire or pin transversely through a bone, has several advantages over skin traction. It makes possible the stronger traction required in many cases. For example, a femoral shaft fracture in a muscular adult may need as much as 20 to 40 pounds of pull for reduction. Skeletal traction can be applied to distal areas, such as the ankle, where skin traction cannot be used. Abrasions, blisters, and reaction to adhesives, often troublesome with skin traction, are avoided by skeletal traction. In general, skeletal traction is comfortable and well tolerated by the patient.

Skeletal traction is most commonly applied through the proximal part

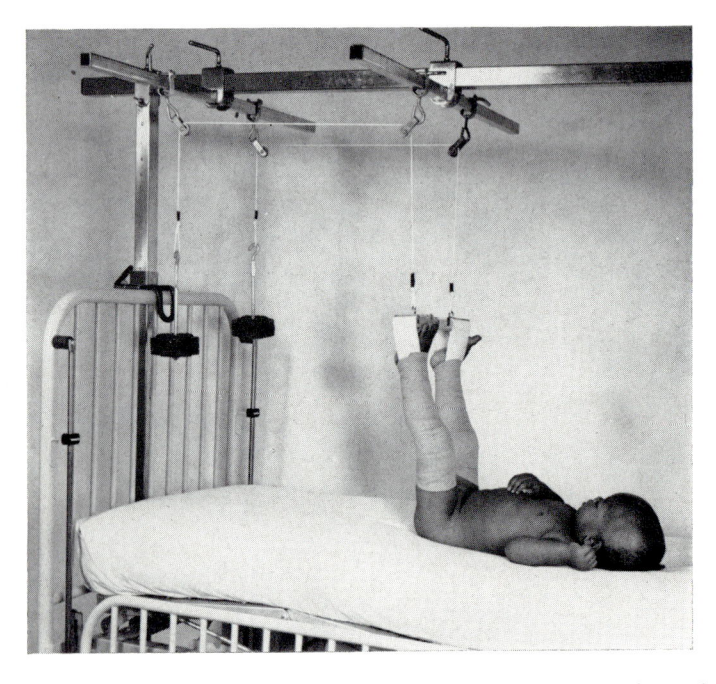

Fig. 273. Bryant's traction, used for fracture of a femoral shaft in an infant. The flexed-hip position facilitates countertraction by the body weight, placement in the crib, and the nursing care. The feet must be observed several times daily for any sign of circulatory impairment.

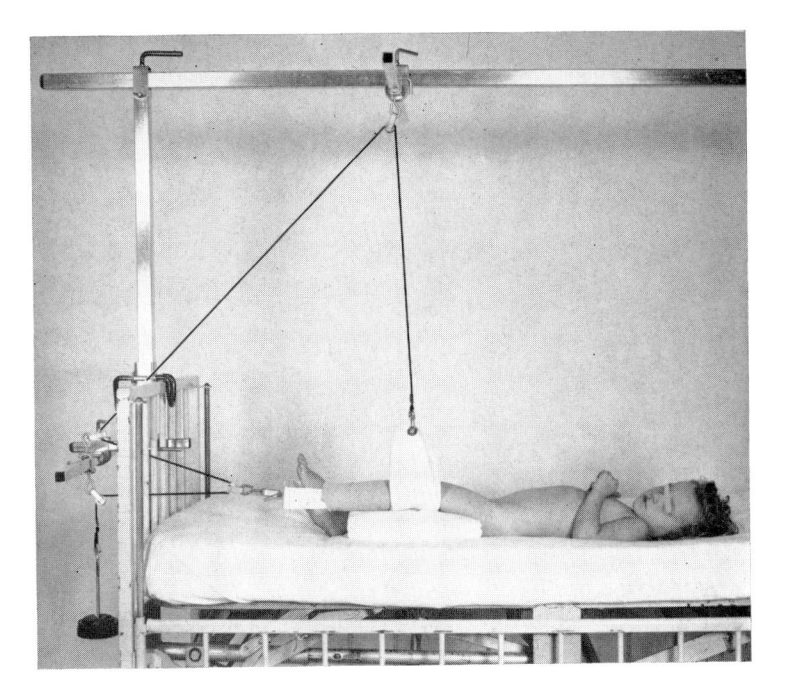

Fig. 274. Russell's traction, applied for a fracture of the left femoral shaft in a girl 5 years of age. This rope-and-pulley arrangement results in a traction force acting in the long axis of the femur that is approximately twice as great as the force which suspends the knee. This type of skin traction is especially useful for children over the age of 3 years and for adolescents.

of the tibia, just distal to the tibial tubercle, in the treatment of femoral fractures. Other areas that may be used are the distal part of the femur or tibia, the calcaneus, and, in the upper extremity, the olecranon. Since the application of skeletal traction introduces the possibility of infecting the bone through which the wire is inserted, strict aseptic technic is obligatory.

Skeletal traction is usually applied by means of a *Steinmann pin* or *Kirschner wire*. The Steinmann pin, with a diameter of ⅛ inch or more, is relatively rigid and may be attached by a simple yoke to the rope and pulleys. The Kirschner wire has a much smaller diameter, is quite flexible, and must be supported by a special spreader which bowstrings the wire tightly to prevent bending. It has the advantage of requiring only a small opening in skin and bone. On the other hand, the Kirschner wire is so thin that it may cut through osteoporotic bone.

The most frequent use of skeletal traction is in treating fractures of the femoral shaft in adults. While in traction, the extremity may be supported in a Thomas splint. A *Pearson attachment,* clamped to the splint, allows knee flexion. Since the patient is to remain in this apparatus for weeks or months, he must be allowed some mobility for change of position in bed, but during such movements the pull upon his fractured femur must remain

494   *Handbook of orthopaedic surgery*

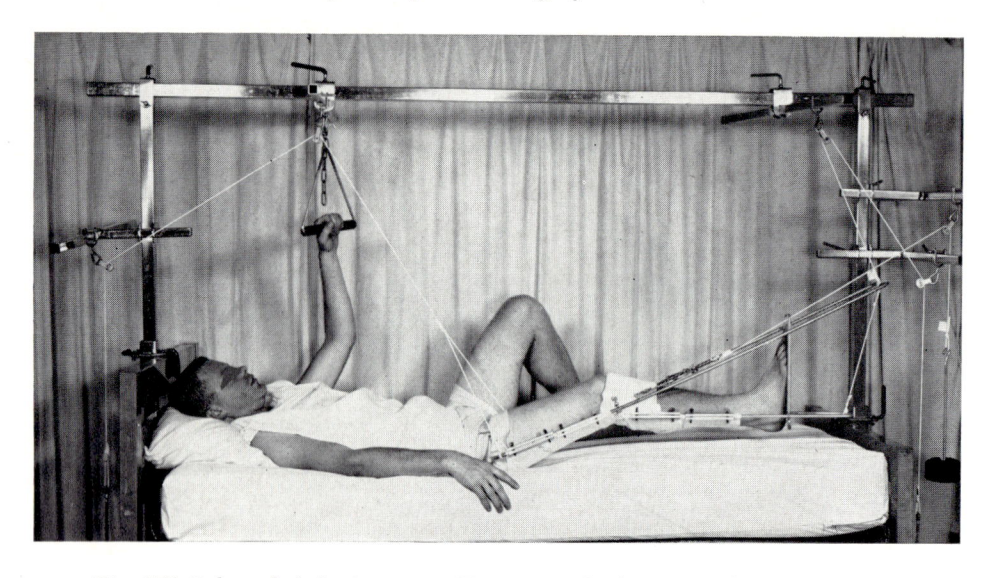

Fig. 275. Balanced skeletal traction. Traction in the long axis of the right thigh is applied by means of a Kirschner wire through the proximal portion of the tibia. The limb is supported by a Thomas splint beneath the thigh and a Pearson attachment beneath the leg. An additional attachment prevents foot drop. Weights apply countertraction to the upper end of the Thomas splint and suspend its lower end. By using his left limbs as shown, the patient can shift the position of his hips without change in the amount of the traction.

undisturbed. This is accomplished by so balancing the suspended Thomas splint by means of weights and pulleys that it will move up or down with the patient without disturbing the fracture. Such traction is a form of *balanced traction* (Fig. 275). Countertraction is provided by the splint and by the weight of the patient's trunk; when necessary the countertraction may be increased by elevating the foot of the bed on blocks.

Skeletal traction is also used frequently in the treatment of dislocations and fractures of the cervical spine, being applied through the outer table of the skull. The most commonly used devices are *Crutchfield* or *Barton* tongs. Both are comfortable and well tolerated; they allow use of the strong traction (30 to 40 pounds) that is sometimes required for reducing dislocations of the cervical vertebrae.

Proper use of traction in the treatment of certain fractures yields excellent results, often superior to those of other methods. Skillful care and patience, however, are required. Traction apparatus must be inspected at least twice a day. Too little traction allows overriding of the fragments and shortening. Too much traction is worse; it separates the fragments and may result in delayed union or nonunion. Traction may be used throughout the period of fracture healing. More frequently, however, it is discontinued when union becomes strong enough to prevent angulation within a plaster cast. After the cast has been applied the patient may be discharged from hospital.

3. *Internal fixation:* Internal fixation is the third method of maintaining the reduction of a fracture. It is usually effected by means of metal plates, rods, or screws. It is used when other methods of maintaining reduction are impracticable or unreliable. Among the disadvantages of internal fixation is the fact that it converts a closed fracture into an open one. Infection resulting from the surgical treatment of a closed fracture may be a major tragedy.

Although metallic implants had been used previously, it was not until early in the twentieth century that reasonably good results were obtained. A scrupulous "no-touch" technic developed by Sir Arbuthnot Lane lessened the danger of bacterial contamination during the insertion of metal plates. His success with metallic internal fixation stimulated its wider use by surgeons perhaps less skillful than Lane, however, with the result that many cases of osteomyelitis and nonunion occurred. It became apparent that some of the failures resulted from an unfavorable tissue reaction to the metal. In 1937 Venable and Stuck called attention to the electrolysis of metallic implants. They found that an alloy of cobalt, chromium, and molybdenum (Vitallium) was well tolerated by the tissues. With the development of Vitallium and certain stainless steels, the feasibility of internal fixation increased. Attention then became focused on the design of devices for use in various types of fractures.

One of the simplest forms of internal fixation is the *transfixation screw.* This is applicable to oblique fractures, especially those of the tibial shaft. Fixation with transverse screws alone is not strong enough to maintain reduction. With the external support of a cast, however, transfixation screws can preserve the reduction of an oblique fracture that would override and shorten if treated by cast alone.

Another common method of internal fixation is the use of a *bone plate.* A metal plate is fastened to the surface of the fragments by at least two screws above and two below the fracture; the screws should be long enough to traverse both sides of the cortex. Plate fixation usually requires the additional support of a cast. Application of the plate involves periosteal stripping, which may tend to delay union by compromising the already impaired blood supply of the fragments. Some bone plates may also delay union by holding the fragments apart after slight resorption of the fractured surfaces has taken place early in the healing process. Fractures heal most readily when the pressure of contact between the injured surfaces is physiologic. Eggers has stressed the importance of contact-compression in fracture healing and has designed slotted plates which, affixed loosely to shaft fragments by screws, both maintain alignment and allow physiologic adjustment of the contact between the fractured surfaces.

A third type of internal fixation now in common use is the *intramedullary rod* (Fig. 276). The fixation of femoral shaft fractures by inserting a long, inflexible rod down the medullary cavity was popularized in Germany by Küntscher during World War II. Treatment by this method provides excellent fixation of certain fractures, promotes contact-compression, obviates immobilization of the joints, and enables the patient to walk with

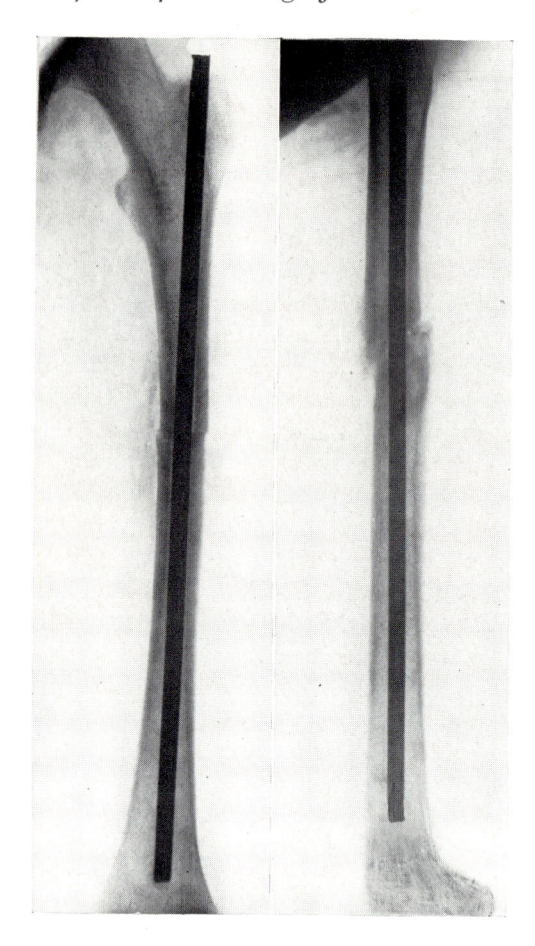

Fig. 276. Anteroposterior and lateral roentgenograms of Küntscher intramedullary rod, or nail, used to fix the fragments of a fracture of the middle third of the femoral shaft in an adult.

crutches soon after the injury. Intramedullary fixation is also used for certain fractures of the shafts of other long bones.

One fracture deserves particular mention in connection with internal fixation. This is the hip fracture, or fracture of the femoral neck. Because of the strong shearing force across the fracture line caused by muscle pull and because the circulation to the femoral head is most precarious, fractures of the femoral neck frequently fail to unite. In fact, at one time it was thought that these hip fractures never united. Royal Whitman demonstrated early in the twentieth century that many of these fractures united if held in abduction and internal rotation by a cast. However, since the old people who most often sustain this fracture tolerate prolonged immobilization poorly, the cast treatment left much to be desired. Internal fixation of femoral neck fractures by means of a three-flanged nail inserted just below the greater trochanter, up the femoral neck, and into the head (Fig. 277),

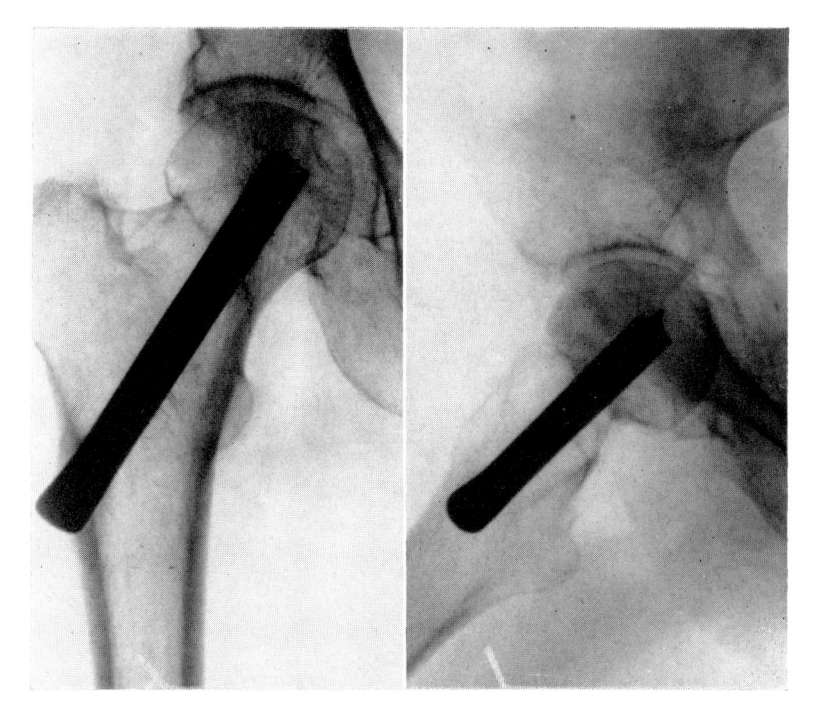

Fig. 277. Anteroposterior and lateral roentgenograms of a Smith-Petersen three-flanged nail used to fix the fragments of a fracture of the femoral neck.

which was introduced by Smith-Petersen about thirty years ago, enables these older patients to be up in a chair within a day or two after operation and has also resulted in a much higher rate of union. Instead of the nail, any of several other internal fixation devices, such as multiple pins, may be used. For hip fractures, early reduction and surgical fixation is the least hazardous method, since the mortality rate is lower than that in cases treated by cast immobilization or by traction.

Restoration of function. After adequate reduction and immobilization, most fractures progress to solid bony healing. In most instances, especially following cast immobilization, the patient develops some joint stiffness and muscle atrophy by the time the fracture has healed. The degree of stiffness and atrophy varies with many factors. A child develops little stiffness, even after long immobilization, and it usually clears up rapidly, whereas in older people some limitation of joint motion after fracture and immobilization may be permanent. The longer the period of immobilization, the more severe the stiffness. The surgeon has the constant problem of being sure that immobilization is continued long enough for firm healing of the fracture but discontinued as soon as joint motion can be resumed safely. Another important cause of joint stiffness is soft tissue damage at the time of fracture, since torn muscles and ligaments are replaced in part by inelastic scar tissue. Infection also leads to scarring and loss of elasticity; an open fracture which becomes infected is likely to be followed by considerable stiffness in adjacent joints. Fractures near joints, and particularly fractures involving the articular surfaces, may not only disrupt the mechanics of joint function but may also lead to fibrous adhesions within the joint. Pre-existing joint disease increases the tendency to stiffness after immobilization. A patient with chronic arthritis who sustains a fracture may develop ankylosis after a long period in a cast.

Measures to prevent or minimize joint stiffness should be started early in the period of fracture healing. Active movement of the joints above and below the cast should be carried out at frequent intervals. An exercise program is especially important in treatment of the common Colles' fracture of the distal end of the radius. This fracture, often seen in older people, may be followed by serious stiffness in the fingers and shoulder, but this can be prevented by seeing that the patient carries out a program of finger and shoulder exercises during the immobilization period. Setting or isometric exercises of the muscles covered by the cast can usually be started by the patient a day or two after application of the cast and increased as the fracture stabilizes. As a rule, joints which must be immobilized should be kept in a functional position. If, because of the nature of the fracture, the adjacent joint must be immobilized in an awkward position, it should be brought out of this position at the earliest possible moment. Prolonged casting with a foot needlessly in equinus may cause a permanent deformity. If ankylosis is to occur in a joint, it is far better that it take place in a position favorable for function of the extremity. Thus if, following an olecranon fracture, an elbow should become stiff in full extension, the patient would be far worse off than if ankylosis had taken place with the joint in a position of about 90 degrees of flexion.

As soon as adequate fracture healing has taken place and the cast has been removed, an active and intensive program of restoring function should begin. Unfortunately, it is too easy for both the patient and the doctor, pleased with excellent fracture healing and the end of a long period of immobilization, to consider the battle won. The third principle of fracture treatment, restoration of function, is as important as the first two. Its application varies widely. The child, on the one hand, usually carries out his own program of exercises; once out of a cast, it is impossible to keep him from exercising the extremity and restoring its function. At the other extreme is the older fracture patient suffering from chronic arthritis, who, after removal of the cast, has discomfort with every movement and will do little on his own to restore lost mobility. He must be instructed, begged, and coerced to carry out the exercise program.

Although many forms of physical treatments and devices have been promoted to help the patient regain the use of his injured extremity, by far the most important factor in the restoration of function is active exercise of the patient's own muscles. The extremity may be massaged and passively exercised, but unless the patient works actively at using his atrophic, contracted, and scarred muscles, little will be accomplished. Thus it is essential that the patient receive careful and detailed instruction in a series of graduated active exercises for the muscles that control motion in the stiffened joint. Early, the preliminary use of heat and gentle massage may facilitate the exercises. At first the exercises may be done most comfortably under warm water. The water supports the painful extremity, and the heat promotes a certain amount of relaxation. Hydrotherapy can be carried out in a therapeutic pool, Hubbard tank, whirlpool bath, or ordinary bath tub. A stiffened joint which is slow in recovery may be helped along by gentle assistive passive exercise; this must be carried out with great care, for if too vigorous it may do more harm than good. In difficult cases, the active exercise induced by occupational therapy may be of great help. The patient is given interesting jobs to do, which are specifically designed to make him use the affected muscles and joints over and over again.

Other forms of physical therapy may supplement the active exercise program. Heat can be applied in a number of ways. Moist heat in the form of hot packs may give relaxation and comfort, enabling the patient to move a painful joint more effectively. Heating of deeper tissues may be accomplished by means of shortwave or microwave diathermy or by ultrasonic therapy. The effect of such deep heat may be beneficial in the last phase of fracture treatment. There is no clear evidence that any form of deep heat speeds fracture healing.

For the severely incapacitated patient, physical therapy must go much farther than simple exercise, heat, and massage. Instructions in ambulation with walker, crutches, or cane are often needed, and after these aids have been discarded, further gait training may be required. When multiple injuries have been sustained, instruction in the activities of daily living are important. Such patients may require special devices to help them carry out activities such as feeding and toilet care. Teaching the more seriously handicapped patients such common functions as getting in and out of a bed or a chair can tax the ingenuity of the physician and the therapist. With care and perseverance the solution to many such problems can be found and will provide the severely crippled individual with a wider range of activity and enhance his ultimate recovery.

Although, especially in children, normal function may be regained a few weeks after immobilization has been discontinued, a much longer period is commonly required. Most of the functional return takes place in the first three to four months. After this period improvement is slow, but it may continue for a year or more. During this entire time the patient has a disability which may be considered either partial or total but which is improving. After maximum functional recovery has been reached, the patient may be left with a residual permanent disability. If the fracture is ununited or malunited, improvement may in some instances be gained by reconstructive surgery; this has been discussed in Chapter 14.

Today, many injuries are financially compensable through liability insurance or workmen's compensation insurance. It is the duty of the patient's physician to evaluate the disability in order that the patient may be recompensed for his loss of function. Accordingly the physician who treats fractures must be familiar with methods of evaluating disability. Excellent reference books and tables on disability evaluation are available through libraries and medical societies; several are listed in the bibliography (p. 502).

Open (compound) fractures

Open fractures are especially serious injuries from two standpoints. First, they are contaminated. The degree of contamination varies from minimal in the case of a clean puncture wound to severe in a wound filled with dirt, grease, and other foreign material. Second, compound fractures are usually associated with more soft tissue damage than are closed fractures. Muscles may be crushed, skin coverage lost, and vessels and nerves torn or severed. Severely injured soft tissue presents a favorable environment for the development of infection and may interfere with the process of bone healing. Osteomyelitis and nonunion are frequent complications of open fractures.

The principles of treating open fractures require emphasis. First is an attempt to minimize infection by early, thorough cleansing of the wound and careful removal of all nonviable tissue and foreign material. This is termed *debridement*. Open fractures are acute emergencies. The longer definitive treatment is delayed, the greater the incidence of serious infection. Only acute respiratory embarrassment, hemorrhage, and shock take precedence over treatment of the fracture; as soon as these factors have been controlled, thorough debridement should be carried out under appropriate anesthesia in the operating room. If the wound is clean and only several hours have elapsed from the time of injury, the wound may be closed primarily. Most contaminated wounds are best left open and then closed secondarily five or six days later, because, if infection develops, an open wound allows ready escape of pus which otherwise might dissect along the tissue planes of the limb. Prophylactic antibiotic therapy is generally recommended in the case of compound fractures. Tetanus antitoxin or toxoid is usually indicated. After the soft tissue wound has been cared for, treatment of the fracture follows the general principles outlined previously. The immediate use of internal fixation devices in open fractures, however, is generally contraindicated. After the soft tissues have healed and all signs of infection are absent, open reduction and internal fixation may be carried out if indicated.

Fractures in children

Fractures in children differ in several ways from their counterparts in adults. The most striking difference is their tendency to heal rapidly and to undergo spontaneous correction of mild and even moderate degrees of angulation or overriding. With the exception of a very few fractures about the elbow or hip, almost all children's fractures should be treated by closed methods. Nonunion in childhood is quite rare unless the fracture has been exposed surgically or has become infected.

Certain types of fractures are found exclusively or almost exclusively in children. Since the epiphyseal line closes with maturity, *epiphyseal fractures,* or *epiphyseal separations,* fall into this category. Fractures involving the epiphyseal plate occasionally cause premature fusion of the epiphysis, which may result in a progressive angulation or shortening of the affected limb; the degree of deformity is determined by the location and extent of the injury and the age at which it occurs. The *greenstick fracture* is peculiar to children; it is an incomplete fracture in which the angulating force bends the cortex on the compression side and breaks it on the distraction side. In children the *torus fracture* is frequently seen in the distal third of the radius, where mild angulation causes a buckling or bulging of the cortex on the compression side.

The bones of children are covered with a thick, active periosteum that accelerates the healing process described in Chapter 14. During the period of active bone growth, constant remodeling and replacement of normal bone structure takes place in accordance with Wolff's law. Thus it is possible for a fracture in a young child which heals in a position of moderate deformity to be so completely remodeled during subsequent bone growth that the deformity becomes corrected. An interesting phenomenon of overgrowth is noted in complete fractures of the long bones of children. A displaced fracture of the femur of a young child, if reduced to anatomic position, will often result in a bone that is ½ to 1 inch longer than the corresponding bone of the uninjured extremity. Frequently, therefore, it is advisable to allow femoral shaft fractures in young children to heal with slight overriding.

Bibliography

The following texts contain excellent reference material:

Adams, J. C.:	Outline of orthopedics, 4th edition	Baltimore, Williams & Wilkins Co., 1961.
Aegerter, E., and Kirkpatrick, J. A., Jr.:	Orthopedic diseases: physiology, pathology, radiology, 2nd edition	Philadelphia, W. B. Saunders Co., 1963.
American Academy of Orthopaedic Surgeons:	Instructional course lectures, vols. 1-15	Ann Arbor, J. W. Edwards, 1943-1958.
	Instructional course lectures, vols. 16-18	St. Louis, The C. V. Mosby Co., 1959-1961.
	Selective bibliography of orthopaedic surgery, including a cumulative index of instructional course lectures	St. Louis, The C. V. Mosby Co., 1962.
Angevine, D. M., and Ash, J. E.:	Atlas of orthopedic pathology	Washington, D. C., Army Medical Museum, 1943.
Bancroft, F. W., and Marble, H. C., editors:	Surgical treatment of the motor-skeletal system, 2nd edition	Philadelphia, J. B. Lippincott Co., 1951.
Banks, S. W., and Laufman, H.:	An atlas of surgical exposures of the extremities	Philadelphia, W. B. Saunders Co., 1953.
Bechtol, C. O., Ferguson, A. B., Jr., and Laing, P. G.:	Metals and engineering in bone and joint surgery	Baltimore, Williams & Wilkins Co., 1959.
Bierman, W., and Licht, S.:	Physical medicine in general practice, 3rd edition	New York, Paul B. Hoeber, Inc., 1952.
Bleck, E. E., Duckworth, N., and Hunter, N.:	Atlas of plaster cast techniques	Chicago, Year Book Publishers, Inc., 1956.
Brailsford, J. F.:	The radiology of bones and joints, 5th edition	London, J. & A. Churchill, Ltd., 1953.
Brown, J. B., and McDowell, F.:	Skin grafting, 3rd edition	Philadelphia, J. B. Lippincott Co., 1958.
Burrows, H. J., and Coltart, W. D.:	Treatment by manipulation	London, Eyre & Spottiswoode, Ltd., 1951.
Caffey, J.:	Pediatric x-ray diagnosis, 4th edition	Chicago, Year Book Medical Publishers, Inc., 1961.
Casagrande, P. A., and Frost, H. M., Jr.:	Fundamentals of clinical orthopedics	New York, Grune & Stratton, Inc., 1953.

Bibliography

Coleman, C. R., editor:	Basic science conference for orthopedic surgery	Columbus, Ohio State University, 1960.
Collins, D. H.:	The pathology of articular and spinal diseases	Baltimore, Williams & Wilkins Co., 1950.
Colonna, P. C.:	Principles of orthopaedic surgery	Boston, Little, Brown & Co., 1960.
DeLorimier, A. A., Moehring, H. G., and Hannan, J. R.:	Clinical roentgenology. Vol. I. Developmental and systemic conditions and local lesions in the extremities	Springfield, Ill., Charles C Thomas, Publisher, 1954.
Dunton, W. R., Jr., and Licht, S.:	Occupational therapy: principles and practice, 2nd edition	Springfield, Ill., Charles C Thomas, Publisher, 1957.
English, M.:	Plaster of paris technique	Edinburgh, E. & S. Livingstone, Ltd., 1957.
Fairbank, Sir H. A. T.:	An atlas of general affections of the skeleton	Baltimore, Williams & Wilkins Co., 1952.
Ferguson, A. B., Jr.:	Orthopedic surgery in infancy and childhood	Baltimore, Williams & Wilkins Co., 1957.
Geckeler, E. O.:	Plaster of paris technic, 2nd edition	Baltimore, Williams & Wilkins Co., 1948.
Gilfillan, C. W.:	Notes in orthopedic pathology	Los Angeles, College of Medical Evangelists, 1949.
Gilmer, W. S., Jr., Higley, G. B., Jr., and Kilgore, W. E.:	Atlas of bone tumors; including tumorlike lesions	St. Louis, The C. V. Mosby Co., 1963.
Greulich, W. W., and Pyle, S. I.:	Radiographic atlas of skeletal development of the hand and wrist, 2nd edition	Stanford, Calif., Stanford University Press, 1959.
Henry, A. K.:	Extensile exposure, 2nd edition	Baltimore, Williams & Wilkins Co., 1957.
Howorth, M. B.:	A textbook of orthopaedics	Philadelphia, W. B. Saunders Co., 1952.
Jones, R., and Lovett, R. W.:	Orthopedic surgery, 2nd edition	New York, William Wood & Co., 1929.
Köhler, A. (revised by E. A. Zimmer and translated by J. T. Case):	Borderlands of the normal and early pathologic in skeletal roentgenology, 10th edition	New York, Grune & Stratton, Inc., 1956.
Luck, J. V.:	Bone and joint diseases: pathology correlated with roentgenological and clinical features	Springfield, Ill., Charles C Thomas, Publisher, 1950.
McBride, E. D.:	Disability evaluation: principles of treatment of compensable injuries, 5th edition (revised)	Philadelphia, J. B. Lippincott Co., 1953.
McKusick, V. A.:	Hereditable disorders of connective tissue	St. Louis, The C. V. Mosby Co., 1956.
McMurray, T. P.:	A practice of orthopaedic surgery, 3rd edition	Baltimore, Williams & Wilkins Co., 1949.
Mercer, Sir W.:	Orthopaedic surgery, 5th edition	Baltimore, Williams & Wilkins Co., 1959.
Moore, F. D.:	Metabolic care of the surgical patient	Philadelphia, W. B. Saunders Co., 1959.
Moseley, H. F.:	An atlas of musculoskeletal exposures	Philadelphia, J. B. Lippincott Co., 1955.
Nicola, T.:	Atlas of surgical approaches to bones and joints	New York, The Macmillan Co., 1945.

O'Donoghue, D. H.:	Treatment of injuries to athletes	Philadelphia, W. B. Saunders Co., 1962.
Platt, Sir H., editor:	Modern trends in orthopaedics, 1st & 2nd editions	New York, Paul B. Hoeber, Inc., 1950 and 1956.
Raney, R. B.:	The prevention of deformity in childhood	Elyria, Ohio, National Society for Crippled Children, 1941.
Schmeisser, G., Jr.:	A clinical manual of orthopedic traction techniques	Philadelphia, W. B. Saunders Co., 1963.
Scuderi, C.:	Atlas of orthopedic traction procedures	St. Louis, The C. V. Mosby Co., 1954.
Shafer, S. J., and Compere, E. L.:	Basic sciences for orthopedics (Veterans Administration)	Washington, D. C., U. S. Government Printing Office, 1949.
Smith, W. C.:	Principles of disability evaluation	Philadelphia, J. B. Lippincott Co., 1959.
Speed, J. S., and Knight, R. A.:	Campbell's operative orthopaedics, 3rd edition	St. Louis, The C. V. Mosby Co., 1956.
Stein, I., Stein, R. O., and Beller, M. L.:	Living bone in health and disease	Philadelphia, J. B. Lippincott Co., 1955.
Steindler, A.:	Orthopedic operations: indications, technique, and end results	Springfield, Ill., Charles C Thomas, Publisher, 1947.
	Post-graduate lectures on orthopedic diagnosis and indications, vols. I-IV	Springfield, Ill., Charles C Thomas, Publisher, 1950.
	Kinesiology of the human body	Springfield, Ill., Charles C Thomas, Publisher, 1955.
Tracy, J. E.:	The doctor as a witness	Philadelphia, W. B. Saunders Co., 1957.
Turek, S. L.:	Orthopaedics: principles and their application	Philadelphia, J. B. Lippincott Co., 1959.
Wiles, P.:	Essentials of orthopaedics, 3rd edition	Boston, Little, Brown & Co., 1959.
Willard, H. S., and Spackman, C.:	Principles of occupational therapy, 2nd edition	Philadelphia, J. B. Lippincott Co., 1954.
Young, H. H., editor:	Year book of orthopedics and traumatic surgery	Chicago, Year Book Medical Publishers, Inc., 1960.

Chapter 1

Introduction

American Academy of Orthopaedic Surgeons:	Measuring and recording of joint motion	Chicago, American Academy of Orthopaedic Surgeons, 1961.
Anderson, C. E.:	The structure and function of cartilage	American Academy of Orthopaedic Surgeons Instructional Courses: J. Bone & Joint Surg. 44-A:777-786, 1962.
Andry, N.:	Orthopaedia: or the art of correcting and preventing deformities in children	Paris, 1741; London, 1743; Philadelphia, reproduced by J. B. Lippincott Co., 1961.
Barnett, C. H., Davies, D. V., and MacConaill, M. A.:	Synovial joints: their structure and mechanics	Springfield, Ill., Charles C Thomas, Publisher, 1961.
Bassett, C. A. L.:	Current concepts of bone formation	American Academy of Orthopaedic Surgeons Instructional Courses: J. Bone & Joint Surg. 44-A:1217-1244, 1962.

Bick, E. M.:	Source book of orthopaedics, 2nd edition	Baltimore, Williams & Wilkins Co., 1948.
	Surgical pathology of synovial tissue	J. Bone & Joint Surg. **12**:33-44, 1930.
Bourne, G. H.:	The biochemistry and physiology of bone	New York, Academic Press, Inc., 1956.
Cave, E. F., and Roberts, S. M.:	A method for measuring and recording joint function	J. Bone & Joint Surg. **18**:455-465, 1936.
Cohen, J., and Harris, W. H.:	The three-dimensional anatomy of haversian systems	J. Bone & Joint Surg. **40-A**:419-434, 1958.
Daniels, L., Williams, M., and Worthingham, C.:	Muscle testing: techniques of manual examination	Philadelphia, W. B. Saunders Co., 1956.
Davies, D. V.:	Synovial membrane and synovial fluid of joints	Lancet **2**:815-819, 1946.
Ferguson, A. B.:	Roentgen diagnosis of the extremities and spine, 2nd edition (enlarged)	New York, Paul B. Hoeber, Inc., 1949.
Fox, T. A., editor:	Manual of orthopaedic surgery, 4th edition	Chicago, American Orthopaedic Association and American Academy of Orthopaedic Surgeons, 1962.
Furey, J. G., Clark, W. S., and Brine, K. L.:	The practical importance of synovial-fluid analysis	J. Bone & Joint Surg. **41-A**:167-174, 1959.
Gardner, E.:	The development and growth of bones and joints	American Academy of Orthopaedic Surgeons Instructional Course Lectures, vol. XIII, Ann Arbor, J. W. Edwards, 1956, pp. 235-246.
Ghormley, R. K.:	Specialization in medicine; what is orthopaedic surgery?	J. Bone & Joint Surg. **31-A**:459-463, 1949.
Howorth, B.:	Examination and diagnosis of the spine and extremities	Springfield, Ill., Charles C Thomas, Publisher, 1962.
Jones, A. R.:	A review of orthopaedic surgery in Britain	J. Bone & Joint Surg. **38-B**:27-45, 1956.
Keith, A.:	Menders of the maimed	London, Oxford University Press, 1919, and Philadelphia, J. B. Lippincott Co., 1951.
Kendall, H. O., and Kendall, F. P.:	Muscles: testing and function	Baltimore, Williams & Wilkins Co., 1949.
Kessler, H. H.:	Rehabilitation of the physically handicapped	New York, Columbia University Press, 1953.
Little, E. M.:	Orthopaedics before Stromeyer (The Robert Jones Birthday Volume)	New York, Oxford University Press, 1928.
MacConaill, M. A.:	The movements of bones and joints: 1. Fundamental principles with particular reference to rotation movement	J. Bone & Joint Surg. **30-B**:322-326, 1948.
	The movements of bones and joints: 2. Function of the musculature	J. Bone & Joint Surg. **31-B**:100-104, 1949.
	The movements of bones and joints: 3. The synovial fluid and its assistants	J. Bone & Joint Surg. **32-B**:244-252, 1950.

Bibliography

McLean, F. C.:	The ultrastructure and function of bone	Science **127**:451-456, 1958.
McLean, F. C., and Urist, M. R.:	Bone: an introduction to the physiology of skeletal tissue, 2nd edition	Chicago, University of Chicago Press, 1961.
Meschan, I.:	Synopsis of roentgen signs	Philadelphia, W. B. Saunders Co., 1962.
Osgood, R. B.:	The evolution of orthopaedic surgery	St. Louis, The C. V. Mosby Co., 1925.
Pugh, D. G.:	The roentgenologic diagnosis of diseases of bones	Baltimore, Williams & Wilkins Co., 1954.
Raney, R. B.:	Andry and the orthopaedia	J. Bone & Joint Surg. **31-A**:675-682, 1949.
Robinson, R. A., and Cameron, D. A.:	The organic matrix of bone and epiphyseal cartilage	In De Palma, A. F., editor: Clinical orthopaedics, vol. 9, Philadelphia, J. B. Lippincott Co., 1957, pp. 16-29.
Rusk, H. A.:	Rehabilitation medicine	St. Louis, The C. V. Mosby Co., 1958.
Weinmann, J. P., and Sicher, H.:	Bone and bones: fundamentals of bone biology, 2nd edition	St. Louis, The C. V. Mosby Co., 1955.

Chapter 2

Congenital deformities

Congenital clubfoot

Bell, J. F., and Grice, D. S.:	Treatment of congenital talipes equinovarus with the modified Denis Browne splint	J. Bone & Joint Surg. **26**:799-811, 1944.
Browne, D.:	Talipes equino-varus	Lancet **2**:969-974, 1934.
Garceau, G. J.:	Congenital talipes equinovarus	American Academy of Orthopaedic Surgeons Instructional Course Lectures, vol. XVIII, St. Louis, The C. V. Mosby Co., 1961, pp. 178-183.
Garceau, G. J., and Manning, K. R.:	Transposition of the anterior tibial tendon in the treatment of recurrent congenital clubfoot	J. Bone & Joint Surg. **29**:1044-1048, 1947.
Irani, R. N., and Sherman, M. S.:	The pathological anatomy of club foot	J. Bone & Joint Surg. **45-A**:45-52, 1963.
Kite, J. H.:	Non-operative treatment of congenital clubfeet	South. M. J. **23**:337-345, 1930.
	Principles involved in the treatment of congenital club-foot	J. Bone & Joint Surg. **21**:595-606, 1939.
	The operative treatment of congenital clubfeet	American Academy of Orthopaedic Surgeons Instructional Course Lectures, vol. XII, Ann Arbor, J. W. Edwards, 1955, pp. 100-105.
Kuhlmann, R. F., and Bell, J. F.:	A clinical evaluation of operative procedures for congenital talipes equinovarus	J. Bone & Joint Surg. **39-A**:265-283, 1957.
MacEwen, G. D., Scott, D. J., Jr., and Shands, A. R., Jr.:	Follow-up survey of clubfoot	J.A.M.A. **175**:427-430, 1961.

McCauley, J. D., Jr.:	Treatment of clubfoot	American Academy of Orthopaedic Surgeons Instructional Course Lectures, vol. XVI, St. Louis, The C. V. Mosby Co., 1959, pp. 93-99.
Ponseti, I. V., and Smoley, E. N.:	Congenital club foot, the results of treatment	J. Bone & Joint Surg. **45-A**:261-275, 1963.
Stewart, S. F.:	Club-foot: its incidence, cause, and treatment	J. Bone & Joint Surg. **33-A**:577-590, 1951.

Other congenital deformities

Angle, C. R.:	Congenital bowing and angulation of long bones	Pediatrics **13**:257-268, 1954.
Arnold, W. D.:	Congenital absence of the fibula	In De Palma, A. F., editor: Clinical Orthopaedics, vol. 14, Philadelphia, J. B. Lippincott Co., 1959, pp. 20-29.
Badgley, C. E., O'Connor, S. J., and Kudner, D. F.:	Congenital kyphoscoliotic tibia	J. Bone & Joint Surg. **34-A**:349-371, 1952.
Barenberg, L. H., and Greenberg, B.:	Intrauterine amputations and constriction bands	Am. J. Dis. Child. **64**:87-92, 1942.
Barsky, A. J.:	Congenital anomalies of the hand	J. Bone & Joint Surg. **33-A**:35-64, 1951.
Blackfield, H. M., and Hause, D. P.:	Syndactylism	Plast. and Reconstruct. Surg. **16**:37-46, 1955.
Bonola, A.:	Surgical treatment of the Klippel-Feil syndrome	J. Bone & Joint Surg. **38-B**:440-449, 1956.
Böök, J. A., and Hesselvik, L.:	Acrocephalosyndactyly (Apert's syndrome)	Acta paediat. **42**:359-364, 1953.
Browne, D.:	Congenital deformities of mechanical origin	Arch. Dis. Childhood **30**:37-41, 1955.
Bryan, R. S., Lipscomb, P. R., and Chatterton, C. C.:	Orthopedic aspects of congenital hypertrophy	Am. J. Surg. **96**:654-659, 1958.
Coventry, M. B.:	Some skeletal changes in the Ehlers-Danlos syndrome	J. Bone & Joint Surg. **43-A**:855-860, 1961.
Coventry, M. B., and Johnson, E. W., Jr.:	Congenital absence of the fibula	J. Bone & Joint Surg. **34-A**:941-956, 1952.
Duraiswami, P. K.:	Experimental causation of congenital skeletal defects and its significance in orthopaedic surgery	J. Bone & Joint Surg. **34-B**:646-698, 1952.
Fahlstrom, S.:	Radio-ulnar synostosis	J. Bone & Joint Surg. **14**:395-403, 1932.
Farmer, A. W., and Laurin, C. A.:	Congenital absence of the fibula	J. Bone & Joint Surg. **42-A**:1-12, 1960.
Ferguson, A. D., and Scott, R. B.:	Congenital absence of the tibia, report of a case in a Negro infant	Am. J. Dis. Child. **84**:84-89, 1952.
Fishbein, M., editor:	First International Conference on Congenital Malformations	Philadelphia, J. B. Lippincott Co., 1961.
Frantz, C. H., and O'Rahilly, R.:	Congenital skeletal limb deficiencies	J. Bone & Joint Surg. **43-A**:1202-1224, 1961.
Fraser, F. C.:	Causes of congenital malformations in human beings	J. Chron. Dis. **10**:97-110, 1959.

Freund, E.:	Congenital defects of femur, fibula and tibia	Arch. Surg. 33:349-391, 1936.
Gordon, G. C.:	Congenital deformities	Baltimore, Williams & Wilkins Co., 1961.
Harris, L. E., and Steinberg, A. G.:	Abnormalities observed during the first six days of life in 8,716 live-born infants	Pediatrics 14:314-326, 1954.
Heyman, C. H.:	The diagnosis and treatment of congenital convex pes valgus or vertical talus	American Academy of Orthopaedic Surgeons Instructional Course Lectures, vol. XVI, St. Louis, The C. V. Mosby Co., 1959, pp. 117-126.
Heyman, C. H., Herndon, C. H., and Heiple, K. G.:	Congenital posterior angulation of the tibia with talipes calcaneus	J. Bone & Joint Surg. 41-A:476-488, 1959.
Jeannopoulos, C. L.:	Congenital elevation of the scapula	J. Bone & Joint Surg. 34-A:883-892, 1952.
Kahn, A. J., Jr., and Fulmer, J.:	Acrocephalosyndactylism (Apert's syndrome)	New England J. Med. 252:379-382, 1955.
Kelikian, H., and Doumanian, A.:	Congenital anomalies of the hand. Parts I and II	J. Bone & Joint Surg. 39-A:1002-1019, 1249-1266, 1957.
Kiskadden, W. S., Schechtman, A. M., and Brock, C.:	Theories of the etiology of congenital deformities	Internat. Abstr. Surg. 88:1-14, 1949.
Kite, J. H.:	Arthrogryposis multiplex congenita	South. M. J. 48:1141-1146, 1955.
	Congenital metatarsus varus; report of 300 cases	J. Bone & Joint Surg. 32-A:500-506, 1950.
	Torsion of the lower extremities in small children	J. Bone & Joint Surg. 36-A:511-520, 1954.
Lloyd-Roberts, G. C., and Spence, A. J.:	Congenital vertical talus	J. Bone & Joint Surg. 40-B:33-41, 1958.
Lyons, C. G., and Sawyer, J. G.:	Cleidocranial dysostosis	Am. J. Roentgenol. 51:215-219, 1944.
MacCollum, D. W.:	Webbed fingers	Surg., Gynec. and Obst. 71:782-789, 1940.
Madsen, E. T.:	Congenital angulations and fractures of the extremities	Acta orthop. scandinav. 25:242-280, 1956.
McCormick, D. W., and Blount, W. P.:	Metatarsus adductovarus, "skewfoot"	J.A.M.A. 141:449-453, 1949.
McIntosh, R., Merritt, K. K., Richards, M. R., Samuels, M. H., and Bellows, M. T.:	The incidence of congenital malformations: a study of 5,964 pregnancies	Pediatrics 14:505-522, 1954.
Mead, N. G., Lithgow, W. C., and Sweeney, H. J.:	Arthrogryposis multiplex congenita	J. Bone & Joint Surg. 40-A:1285-1309, 1958.
Miles, P. W.:	Cleidocranial dysostosis: a survey of six new cases and 126 from the literature	J. Kansas M. Soc. 41:462-468, 1940.
Murphy, D. P.:	Congenital malformations, 2nd edition	Philadelphia, J. B. Lippincott Co., 1947.
Peabody, C. W.:	Hemihypertrophy and hemiatrophy; congenital total unilateral somatic asymmetry	J. Bone & Joint Surg. 18:466-474, 1936.
Pygott, F.:	Arachnodactyly (Marfan's syndrome) with a report of two cases	Brit. J. Radiol. 28:26-29, 1955.

Rechtman, A. M., and Horwitz, M. T.:	Congenital synostosis of the cervicothoracic vertebrae (the Klippel-Feil syndrome)	Am. J. Roentgenol. **43**:66-73, 1940.
Ring, P. A.:	Congenital short femur	J. Bone & Joint Surg. **41-B**:73-79, 1959.
Riordan, D. C.:	Congenital absence of the radius	J. Bone & Joint Surg. **37-A**:1129-1140, 1955.
Ross, L. J.:	Arachnodactyly	Am. J. Dis. Child. **78**:417-436, 1949.
Russell, L. B., and Russell, W. L.:	Radiation hazards to the embryo and fetus	Radiology **58**:369-377, 1952.
Schrock, R. D.:	Congenital elevation of the scapula	J. Bone & Joint Surg. **8**:207-215, 1926.
	Congenital abnormalities at the cervicothoracic level	American Academy of Orthopaedic Surgeons Instructional Course Lectures, vol. VI, Ann Arbor, J. W. Edwards, 1949, pp. 229-236.
Shoul, M. I., and Ritvo, M.:	Clinical and roentgenological manifestations of the Klippel-Feil syndrome	Am. J. Roentgenol. **68**:369-385, 1952.
Soule, A. B., Jr.:	Mutational dysostosis (cleidocranial dysostosis)	J. Bone & Joint Surg. **28**:81-102, 1946.
Starr, D. E.:	Congenital absence of the radius; a method of surgical correction	J. Bone & Joint Surg. **27**:572-577, 1945.
Stevenson, S. S., Worcester, J., and Rice, R. G.:	677 congenitally malformed infants and associated gestational characteristics	Pediatrics **6**:37 - 50, 208 - 222, 1950.
Summer, G. K.:	The Ehlers-Danlos syndrome	Am. J. Dis. Child. **91**:419-428, 1956.
Thompson, T. C., Straub, L. R., and Arnold, W. D.:	Congenital absence of the fibula	J. Bone & Joint Surg. **39-A**:1229-1237, 1957.
Vinke, T. H.:	Re-evaluation of etiologic factors in congenital anomalies of the skeleton	In De Palma, A. F., editor, Clinical orthopaedics, vol. 8, Philadelphia, J. B. Lippincott Co., 1956, pp. 7-12.
Wallace, H. M., Baumgartner, L., and Rich, H.:	Congenital malformations and birth injuries in New York City	Pediatrics **12**:525-535, 1953.
Warkany, J.:	Production of congenital malformations by dietary measures	J.A.M.A. **168**:2020-2023, 1958.
Yamazaki, J. N., Wright, S. W., and Wright, P. M.:	Outcome of pregnancy in women exposed to the atomic bomb in Nagasaki	Am. J. Dis. Child. **87**:448-463, 1954.

Chapter 3

Congenital deformities—cont'd

Congenital dislocation of the hip

Anderson, M. E., and Bickel, W. H.:	Shelf operation for congenital subluxation and dislocation of the hip	J. Bone & Joint Surg. **33-A**:87-102, 1951.
Badgley, C. E.:	Etiology of congenital dislocation of the hip	J. Bone & Joint Surg. **31-A**:341-356, 1949.

Bost, F. C., Hagey, H., Schottstaedt, E. R., and Larsen, L. J.:	The results of treatment of congenital dislocation of the hip in infancy	J. Bone & Joint Surg. **30-A**:454-468, 1948.
Bosworth, D. M., Fielding, J. W., Ishizuka, T., and Ege, R.:	Hip-shelf operation in adults	J. Bone & Joint Surg. **43-A**:93-106, 1961.
Caffey, J., Ames, R., Silverman, W. A., Ryder, C. T., and Hough, G.:	Contradiction of the congenital dysplasia—predislocation hypothesis of congenital dislocation of the hip	Pediatrics **17**:632-641, 1956.
Chuinard, E. G.:	Early weight-bearing and the correction of anteversion in the treatment of congenital dislocation of the hip	J. Bone & Joint Surg. **37-A**:229-245, 1955.
Coleman, S. S.:	Diagnosis of congenital dysplasia of the hip in the newborn infant	J.A.M.A. **162**:548-554, 1956.
Colonna, P. C.:	Capsular arthroplasty for congenital dislocation of the hip	J. Bone & Joint Surg. **35-A**:179-197, 1953.
	Care of the infant with congenital subluxation of the hip	J.A.M.A. **166**:715-720, 1958.
	Congenital dislocation of the hip in children and adults	American Academy of Orthopaedic Surgeons Instructional Course Lectures, vol. VIII, Ann Arbor, J. W. Edwards, 1951, pp. 169-180.
Crego, C. H., Jr., and Schwartzmann, J. R.:	Follow-up study of the early treatment of congenital dislocation of the hip	J. Bone & Joint Surg. **30-A**:428-442, 1948.
Dunlap, K., Shands, A. R., Jr., Hollister, L. C., Jr., Gaul, J. S., Jr., and Streit, H. A.:	A new method for determination of torsion of the femur	J. Bone & Joint Surg. **35-A**:289-311, 1953.
Fairbank, Sir H. A. T.:	Congenital dislocation of the hip: with special reference to the anatomy	Brit. J. Surg. **17**:380-416, 1930.
Gill, A. B.:	Operation for old or irreducible congenital dislocation of the hip	J. Bone & Joint Surg. **10**:696-711, 1928.
	The end results of early treatment of congenital dislocation of the hip	J. Bone & Joint Surg. **30-A**:442-453, 1948.
Hart, V. L.:	Congenital dislocation of the hip in the newborn and in early postnatal life	J.A.M.A. **143**:1299-1303, 1950.
	Congenital dysplasia of the hip joint and sequelae	Springfield, Ill., Charles C Thomas, Publisher, 1952.
Hass, J.:	Congenital dislocation of the hip	Springfield, Ill., Charles C Thomas, Publisher, 1951.
Heubelin, G. W., Greene, G. S., and Conforti, V. P.:	Hip joint arthrography	Am. J. Roentgenol. **68**:736-748, 1952.
Hindenach, J. C. R.:	Early clinical diagnosis of congenital dislocation of hip	Lancet **1**:15-16, 1955.
Jakobsson, A.:	The shelf operation, an evaluation of results in congenital dysplasia, subluxation and dislocation of the hip joint	Acta orthop. scandinav. **23** (supp. 15):5-120, 1954.

Larson, R. L., Neumann, R. F., and Meredith, D. C.:	Congenital subluxation and dislocation of the hip	J.A.M.A. **178**:14-18, 1961.
MacKenzie, I. G., Seddon, H. J., and Trevor, D.:	Congenital dislocation of the hip	J. Bone & Joint Surg. **42-B**:689-705, 1960.
Massie, W. K.:	Vascular epiphyseal changes in congenital dislocation of the hip	J. Bone & Joint Surg. **33-A**:284-306, 1951.
Massie, W. K., and Howorth, M. B.:	Congenital dislocation of the hip, results of open reduction as seen in early adult period	J. Bone & Joint Surg. **33-A**:171-198, 1951.
McCarroll, H. R.:	Congenital dislocation of the hip after the age of infancy	American Academy of Orthopaedic Surgeons Instructional Course Lectures, vol. XII, Ann Arbor, J. W. Edwards, 1955, pp. 69-89.
	Congenital dysplasia and congenital dislocation of the hip in early infancy	American Academy of Orthopaedic Surgeons Instructional Course Lectures, vol. XIV, Ann Arbor, J. W. Edwards, 1957, pp. 183-195.
	Primary anterior congenital dislocation of the hip	J. Bone & Joint Surg. **30-A**:416-421, 1948.
McFarland, B.:	Some observations on congenital dislocation of the hip	J. Bone & Joint Surg. **38-B**:54-69, 1956.
Muller, G. M., and Seddon, H. J.:	Late results of treatment of congenital dislocation of the hip	J. Bone & Joint Surg. **35-B**:342-362, 1953.
Palm´n, K.:	Preluxation of the hip joint	Acta paediat. **50** (supp. 129): 1-71, 1961.
Platou, E.:	Luxatio coxae congenita, a follow-up study of 406 cases of closed reduction	J. Bone & Joint Surg. **35-A**:843-866, 1953.
Platt, Sir H.:	Congenital dislocation of the hip, its early recognition and treatment	Brit. J. Surg. **45**:438-442, 1958.
Plummer, G. W.:	Congenital dislocation of the hip, diagnosis and natural course	Pediatrics **11**:28-36, 1953.
Ponseti, I. V., and Frigerio, E. R.:	Results of treatment of congenital dislocation of the hip	J. Bone & Joint Surg. **41-A**:823-846, 1959.
Putti, V.:	Early treatment of congenital dislocation of the hip	J. Bone & Joint Surg. **15**:16-21, 1933.
Ring, P. A.:	The treatment of unreduced congenital dislocation of the hip in adults	J. Bone & Joint Surg. **41-B**:299-313, 1959.
Severin, E.:	Contribution to the knowledge of congenital dislocation of the hip joint	Acta chir. scandinav. **84** (supp. 63):1-142, 1941.
	Congenital dislocation of the hip, development of the joint after closed reduction	J. Bone & Joint Surg. **32-A**:507-518, 1950.
Shands, A. R., Jr., and Steele, M. K.:	Torsion of the femur	J. Bone & Joint Surg. **40-A**:803-816, 1958.
Somerville, E. W.:	Development of congenital dislocation of the hip	J. Bone & Joint Surg. **35-B**:568-577, 1953.
Somerville, E. W., and Scott, J. C.:	The direct approach to congenital dislocation of the hip	J. Bone & Joint Surg. **39-B**:623-640, 1957.

Wiberg, G.:	Shelf operation in congenital dysplasia of the acetabulum and in subluxation and dislocation of the hip	J. Bone & Joint Surg. **35-A**:65-80, 1953.

Congenital dislocation of other joints

Caravias, D. E.:	Some observations on congenital dislocation of the head of the radius	J. Bone & Joint Surg. **39-B**:86-90, 1957.
Cozen, L.:	Congenital dislocation of the shoulder and other anomalies	Arch. Surg. **35**:956-966, 1937.
McFarland, B. L.:	Congenital dislocation of the knee	J. Bone & Joint Surg. **11**:281-285, 1929.
Niebauer, J. J., and King, D. E.:	Congenital dislocation of the knee	J. Bone & Joint Surg. **42-A**:207-225, 1960.

Chapter 4
General affections of the skeleton

Albright, F., Burnett, C. H., Parson, W., Reifenstein, E. C., Jr., and Roos, A.:	Osteomalacia and late rickets	Medicine **25**:399-479, 1946.
Arkin, A. M., and Schein, A. J.:	Aseptic necrosis in Gaucher's disease	J. Bone & Joint Surg. **30-A**:631-641, 1948.
Avery, M. E., McAfee, J. G., and Guild, H. G.:	The course and prognosis of reticuloendotheliosis (eosinophilic granuloma, Schüller-Christian disease and Letterer-Siwe disease)	Am. J. Med. **22**:636-652, 1957.
Banks, S. W.:	Bone changes in acute and chronic scurvy	J. Bone & Joint Surg. **25**:553-565, 1943.
Blount, W. P.:	Tibia vara, osteochondrosis deformans tibiae	J. Bone & Joint Surg. **19**:1-29, 1937.
Bromer, R. S.	The roentgen-ray diagnosis of infantile scurvy	Am. J. Roentgenol. **19**:112-125, 1928.
Chaplin, H., Jr., Clark, L. D., and Ropes, M. W.:	Vitamin D intoxication	Am. J. M. Sc. **221**:369-378, 1951.
Crocker, A. C., and Farber, S.:	Niemann-Pick disease: a review of eighteen patients	Medicine **37**:1-95, 1958.
Danis, P. G., and Rossen, J. A.:	Renal rickets	J. Pediat. **18**:103-116, 1941.
Dent, C. E.:	Rickets and osteomalacia from renal tubule defects	J. Bone & Joint Surg. **34-B**:266-274, 1952.
Dent, C. E., and Harris, H.:	Hereditary forms of rickets and osteomalacia	J. Bone & Joint Surg. **38-B**:204-226, 1956.
Dickson, W., and Horrocks, R. H.:	Hypophosphatasia	J. Bone & Joint Surg. **40-B**:64-74, 1958.
Fisher, R. H.:	Multiple lesions of bone in Letterer-Siwe disease	J. Bone & Joint Surg. **35-A**:445-464, 1953.
Fourman, P.:	Calcium metabolism and the bone	Oxford, Blackwell Scientific Publications, 1960.
Geppert, T. V.:	Physiological knock-knee	Am. J. Dis. Child. **83**:154-155, 1952.
Green, W. T., and Farber, S.:	"Eosinophilic or solitary granuloma" of bone	J. Bone & Joint Surg. **24**:469-526, 1942.
Harrison, H. E.:	The Fanconi syndrome	J. Chron. Dis. **7**:346-355, 1958.

Holt, J. F., Latourette, H. B., and Watson, E. H.:	Physiological bowing of the legs in young children	J.A.M.A. **154**:390-394, 1954.
Hsia, D. Y. Y.:	Inborn errors in metabolism	Chicago, Year Book Publishers, Inc., 1959.
Hunter, T.:	Solitary eosinophilic granuloma of bone	J. Bone & Joint Surg. **38-B**:545-557, 1956.
Key, J. A., Elzinga, E., and Fischer, F.:	Local atrophy of bone, effect of immobilization and of operative procedures	Arch. Surg. **28**:936-942, 1934.
McGavran, M. H., and Spady, H. A.:	Eosinophilic granuloma of bone	J. Bone & Joint Surg. **42-A**:979-992, 1960.
Moe, P. J., and Hansen, A. E.:	Reticuloendothelial granuloma	Am. J. Dis. Child. **99**:175-184, 1960.
Morley, A. J. M.:	Knock-knee in children	Brit. M. J. **2**:976-979, 1957.
Nicholas, J. A., Saville, P. D., and Bronner, F.:	Osteoporosis, osteomalacia, and the skeletal system	American Academy of Orthopaedic Surgeons Instructional Course Lectures, J. Bone & Joint Surg. **45-A**:391-405, 1963.
Nordin, B. E. C.:	Osteomalacia, osteoporosis and calcium deficiency	In De Palma, A. F., editor: Clinical orthopaedics, vol. 17, Philadelphia, J. B. Lippincott Co., 1960, pp. 235-257.
Oliver, T. K., Jr.:	Chronic vitamin A intoxication	Am. J. Dis. Child. **95**:57-68, 1958.
Pease, C. N.:	Focal retardation and arrestment of growth of bones due to vitamin A intoxication	J.A.M.A. **182**:980-985, 1962.
Pedersen, H. E., and McCarroll, H. R.:	Vitamin-resistant rickets	J. Bone & Joint Surg. **33-A**:203-220, 1951.
Ponseti, I.:	Bone lesions in eosinophilic granuloma, Hand-Schüller-Christian disease, and Letterer-Siwe disease	J. Bone & Joint Surg. **30-A**:811-833, 1948.
Sherman, M. S.	Osteomalacia	J. Bone & Joint Surg. **32-A**:193-206, 1950.
	Physiologic bowing of the legs	South. M. J. **53**:830-836, 1960.
Shiers, J. A., Neuhauser, E. B. D., and Bowman, J. R.:	Idiopathic hypercalcemia	Am. J. Roentgenol. **78**:19-29, 1957.
Shorbe, H. B.:	Infantile scurvy	In De Palma, A. F., editor: Clinical orthopaedics, vol. 1, Philadelphia, J. B. Lippincott Co., 1953, pp. 49-55.
Silverman, F. N.:	The roentgen manifestations of unrecognized skeletal trauma in infants	Am. J. Roentgenol. **69**:413-427, 1953.
Thannhauser, S. J.:	Lipidoses, diseases of the intracellular lipid metabolism, 3rd edition	New York, Grune & Stratton, Inc., 1958.
Todd, R. M., and Keidan, S. E.:	Changes in the head of the femur in children suffering from Gaucher's disease	J. Bone & Joint Surg. **34-B**:447-453, 1952.
Winters, R. W., Graham, J. B., Williams, T. F., McFalls, V. W., and Burnett, C. H.:	A genetic study of familial hypophosphatemia and vitamin D resistant rickets with a review of the literature	Medicine **37**:97-142, 1958.

Wolbach, S. B.:	Vitamin-A deficiency and excess in relation to skeletal growth	J. Bone & Joint Surg. **29**:171-192, 1947.

Chapter 5

General affections of the skeleton—cont'd

Albright, F.:	Osteoporosis	Ann. Int. Med. **27**:861-882, 1947.
Albright, F., and Reifenstein, E. C., Jr.:	The parathyroid glands and metabolic bone disease	Baltimore, Williams & Wilkins Co., 1948.
Albright, F., Butler, A. M., Hampton, A. O., and Smith, P.:	Syndrome characterized by osteitis fibrosa disseminata, areas of pigmentation and endocrine dysfunction, with precocious puberty in females	New England J. Med. **216**:727-746, 1937.
Baker, L. D., and Jones, H. A.:	Osteopathia condensans disseminata, osteopoikilosis (spotted bones): report of a case	J. Bone & Joint Surg. **23**:164-169, 1941.
Bartter, F. C.:	Osteoporosis	Am. J. Med. **22**:797-806, 1957.
Bickel, W. H., Ghormley, R. K., and Camp, J. D.:	Osteogenesis imperfecta	Radiology **40**:145-154, 1943.
Brailsford, J. F.:	Chondro-osteo-dystrophy	J. Bone & Joint Surg. **34-B**:53-63, 1952.
Brooksaler, F., and Miller, J. E.:	Infantile cortical hyperostosis	J. Pediat. **48**:739-753, 1956.
Caffey, J.:	Gargoylism (Hunter-Hurler disease, dysostosis multiplex, lipochondrodystrophy)	Am. J. Roentgenol. **67**:715-731, 1952.
Caffey, J., and Silverman, W. A.:	Infantile cortical hyperostoses	Am. J. Roentgenol. **54**:1-16, 1945.
Campbell, C. S.:	Melorheostosis of the upper limb	J. Bone & Joint Surg. **37-B**:471-473, 1955.
Christensen, W. R., Lin, R. K., and Berghout, J.:	Dysplasia epiphysialis multiplex	Am. J. Roentgenol. **74**:1059-1067, 1955.
Cohen, J.:	Osteopetrosis	J. Bone & Joint Surg. **33-A**:923-938, 1951.
Daves, M. L., and Yardley, J. H.:	Fibrous dysplasia of bone	Am. J. M. Sc. **234**:590-606, 1957.
Dixon, T. F., Mulligan, L., Nassim, R., and Stevenson, F. H.:	Myositis ossificans progressiva	J. Bone & Joint Surg. **36-B**:445-449, 1954.
Drucker, W. R., Hubay, C. A., Holden, W. D., and Bukovnic, J. A.:	Pathogenesis of post-traumatic sympathetic dystrophy	Am. J. Surg. **97**:454-465, 1959.
Evans, J. A.:	Reflex sympathetic dystrophy; report on 57 cases	Ann. Int. Med. **26**:417-426, 1947.
Fairbank, T. J.:	Dysplasia epiphysialis hemimelica (tarso-epiphysial aclasis)	J. Bone & Joint Surg. **38-B**:237-257, 1956.
Gilbert, E. F., and Guin, G. H.:	Gargoylism	Am. J. Dis. Child. **95**:69-80, 1958.
Goldenberg, R. R.:	The skull in Paget's disease	J. Bone & Joint Surg. **33-A**:911-922, 1951.
Griffiths, D. Ll.:	Engelmann's disease	J. Bone & Joint Surg. **38-B**:313-326, 1956.
Hammarsten, J. F., and O'Leary, J.:	The features and significance of hypertrophic osteoarthropathy	Arch. Int. Med. **99**:431-441, 1957.

Harris, W. H., Dudley, H. R., Jr., and Barry, R. J.:	The natural history of fibrous dysplasia	J. Bone & Joint Surg. **44-A**:207-233, 1962.
Hasenhuttl, K.:	Osteopetrosis	J. Bone & Joint Surg. **44-A**:359-370, 1962.
Hess, W. E., and Street, D. M.:	Melorheostosis	J. Bone & Joint Surg. **32-A**:422-427, 1950.
Hinkel, C. L.:	Developmental affections of the skeleton characterized by osteosclerosis	In De Palma, A. F., editor: Clinical orthopaedics, vol. 9, Philadelphia, J. B. Lippincott Co., 1957, pp. 85-106.
Holling, H. E., and Brodey, R. S.:	Pulmonary hypertrophic osteoarthropathy	J.A.M.A. **178**:977-982, 1961.
Howat, T. W., and Ashurst, G. M.:	Pseudohypoparathyroidism	J. Bone & Joint Surg. **39-B**:39-44, 1957.
Hume, J. B.:	The causation of multiple exostoses	Brit. J. Surg. **17**:236-241, 1929.
Jackson, W. P. U., Albright, F., Drewry, G., Hanelin, J., and Rubin, M. I.:	Metaphyseal dysplasia, epiphyseal dysplasia, diaphyseal dysplasia, and related conditions (disorders of "bone remodeling")	Arch. Int. Med. **94**:871-910, 1954.
Jaffe, H. L.:	Primary and secondary (renal) hyperparathyroidism	S. Clin. North America **22**:621-639, 1942.
Karlen, A. G., and Cameron, J. A. P.:	Dysplasia epiphysialis punctata	J. Bone & Joint Surg. **39-B**:293-301, 1957.
Key, J. A.:	Brittle bones and blue sclera	Arch. Surg. **13**:523-567, 1926.
Lake, M.:	Studies of Paget's disease (osteitis deformans)	J. Bone & Joint Surg. **33-B**:323-335, 1951.
Lennon, E. A., Schechter, M. M., and Hornabrook, R. W.:	Engelmann's disease	J. Bone & Joint Surg. **43-B**:273-284, 1961.
Lichtenstein, L.:	Polyostotic fibrous dysplasia	Arch. Surg. **36**:874-898, 1938.
Lipschutz, A.:	Morquio's disease	J. Pediat. **46**:403-414, 1955.
McKusick, V. A.:	Hereditary disorders of connective tissue	Bull. New York Acad. Med. **35**:143-156, 1959.
McLean, F. C.:	The parathyroid hormone and bone	In De Palma, A. F., editor: Clinical orthopaedics, vol. 9, Philadelphia, J. B. Lippincott Co., 1957, pp. 46-57.
Mahorner, H. R.:	Dyschondroplasia	J. Pediat. **10**:1-26, 1937.
Mercer, W., and Duthie, R. B.:	Some observations on osteitis deformans of Paget	J. Roy. Coll. Surgeons, Edinburgh **1**:58-74, 1955.
Nicholas, J. A., and Wilson, P. D.:	Diagnosis and treatment of osteoporosis	J.A.M.A. **171**:2279-2284, 1959.
O'Connor, S. J., and Ivanoff, J. C.:	Infantile cortical hyperostosis	Ann. Surg. **145**:573-579, 1957.
Plewes, L. W.:	Sudeck's atrophy in the hand	J. Bone & Joint Surg. **38-B**:195-203, 1956.
Porretta, C. A., Dahlin, D. C., and Janes, J. M.:	Sarcoma in Paget's disease of bone	J. Bone & Joint Surg. **39-A**:1314-1329, 1957.
Reed, R. J.:	Fibrous dysplasia of bone, a review of 25 cases	Arch. Path. **75**:480-495, 1963.
Reifenstein, E. C., Jr., and Albright, F.:	Paget's disease: its pathologic physiology and the importance of this in the complications arising from fracture and immobilization	New England J. Med. **231**:343-355, 1944.

Riley, H. D., Jr., and Christie, A.:	Myositis ossificans progressiva	Pediatrics **8**:753-767, 1951.
Rosenkrantz, J. A., Wolf, J., and Kaicher, J. J.:	Paget's disease (osteitis deformans), review of 111 cases	Arch. Int. Med. **90**:610-633, 1952.
Simpson, S. L.:	Endocrinology and orthopaedics in fifty years	J. Bone & Joint Surg. **32-B**:730-740, 1950.
Singleton, E. B., Thomas, J. R., Worthington, W. W., and Hild, J. R.:	Progressive diaphyseal dysplasia (Engelmann's disease)	Radiology **67**:233-241, 1956.
Smith, E. B., Hempelmann, T. C., Moore, S., and Barr, D. P.:	Gargoylism (dysostosis multiplex): two adult cases with one autopsy	Ann. Int. Med. **36**:652-667, 1952.
Steindler, A.:	Osteoporosis	American Academy of Orthopaedic Surgeons Instructional Course Lectures, vol. XIII, Ann Arbor, J. W. Edwards, 1956, pp. 167-176.
Stewart, M. J., Gilmer, W. S., Jr., and Edmonson, A. S.:	Fibrous dysplasia of bone	J. Bone & Joint Surg. **44-B**:302-318, 1962.
Tampas, J. P., Van Buskirk, F. W., Peterson, O. S., Jr., and Soule, A. B.:	Infantile cortical hyperostosis	J.A.M.A. **175**:491-493, 1961.
Toumey, J. W.:	Reflex sympathetic dystrophy in orthopaedic surgery	American Academy of Orthopaedic Surgeons Instructional Course Lectures, vol. VII, Ann Arbor, J. W. Edwards, 1950, pp. 181-186.
Urist, M. R.:	The problem of osteoporosis	Clin. Res. **6**:377-385, 1958.
Vanzant, B. T., and Vanzant, F. R.:	Hereditary deforming chondrodysplasia	J.A.M.A. **119**:786-790, 1942.
Wakeley, C. P. G., and Atkinson, F. R. B.:	Acromegaly, a detailed report on two cases	Surgery **3**:8-20, 1938.
Warrick, C. K.:	Polyostotic fibrous dysplasia—Albright's syndrome	J. Bone & Joint Surg. **31-B**:175-183, 1949.
Wyatt, G. M., and Randall, W. S.:	Monostotic fibrous dysplasia	Am. J. Roentgenol. **61**:354-365, 1949.
Zellweger, H., Giaccai, L., and Firzli, S.:	Gargoylism and Morquio's disease	Am. J. Dis. Child. **84**:421-435, 1952.

Chapter 6

Infections of bones and joints (exclusive of tuberculosis)

Pyogenic infections of bones and joints

Altemeier, W. A., and Largen, T.:	Antibiotic and chemotherapeutic agents in infections of the skeletal system	J.A.M.A. **150**:1462-1468, 1952.
Blanche, D. W.:	Osteomyelitis in infants	J. Bone & Joint Surg. **34-A**:71-85, 1952.
Boger, W. P.:	Pneumococcic arthritis	J.A.M.A. **126**:1062-1065, 1944.
Brailsford, J. F.:	Brodie's abscess and its differential diagnosis	Brit. M. J. **2**:119-123, 1938.
Buchman, J.:	Osteomyelitis	American Academy of Orthopaedic Surgeons Instructional Course Lectures, vol. XVI, St. Louis, The C. V. Mosby Co., 1959, pp. 232-245.

Caldwell, G. A.:	Repair of bony defects associated with osteomyelitis	Ann. Surg. **123**:698-704, 1946.
Capener, N., and Pierce, K. C.:	Pathological fractures in osteomyelitis	J. Bone & Joint Surg. **14**:501-510, 1932.
Chartier, Y., Martin, W. J., and Kelly, P. J.:	Bacterial arthritis: experiences in the treatment of 77 patients	Ann. Int. Med. **50**:1462-1474, 1959.
Coventry, M. B., and Mitchell, W. C.:	Osteitis pubis, observations based on a study of 45 patients	J.A.M.A. **178**:898-905, 1961.
David, J. R., and Black, R. L.:	Salmonella arthritis	Medicine **39**:385-403, 1960.
Dennison, W. M.:	Unilateral limb lengthening associated with haematogenous osteitis in childhood	Arch. Dis. Child. **27**:54-59, 1952.
	Haematogenous osteitis in the newborn	Lancet **2**:474-476, 1955.
Downey, J. W., and Simon, H. E.:	Brodie's abscess, two case reports	Am. J. Surg. **70**:86-94, 1945.
Dunlop, D. M., and Murdoch, J. McC.:	The dangers of antibiotic treatment	Brit. M. Bull. **16**:67-72, 1960.
Eyre-Brook, A. L.:	Septic arthritis of the hip and osteomyelitis of the upper end of the femur in infants	J. Bone & Joint Surg. **42-B**:11-20, 1960.
Fett, H. C., O'Connor, J. J., and Johnson, J. A.:	Experiences in treatment of traumatic cavitation in the upper tibia	Am. J. Surg. **73**:11-21, 1947.
Fox, M. J., and Gilbert, J.:	Meningococcus infections with articular complications	Am. J. M. Sc. **208**:63-69, 1944.
Garcia, A., Jr., and Grantham, S. A.:	Hematogenous pyogenic vertebral osteomyelitis	J. Bone & Joint Surg. **42-A**:429-436, 1960.
Garrod, L. P., and Scowen, E. F.:	The principles of therapeutic use of antibiotics	Brit. M. Bull. **16**:23-28, 1960.
Gilmour, W. N.:	Acute haematogenous osteomyelitis	J. Bone & Joint Surg. **44-B**:841-853, 1962.
Green, M., Nyhan, W. L., Jr., and Fousek, M. D.:	Acute hematogenous osteomyelitis	Pediatrics **17**:368-382, 1956.
Hagemann, P. O., Hendin, A., Lurie, H. H., and Stein, M.:	Therapy of gonococcal arthritis	Ann. Int. Med. **36**:77-89, 1952.
Hampton, O. P., Jr.:	The management of penetrating wounds and suppurative arthritis of the knee joint in the Mediterranean Theater of Operations	J. Bone & Joint Surg. **28**:659-680, 1946.
Henson, S. W., and Coventry, M. B.:	Osteomyelitis of the vertebrae as the result of infection of the urinary tract	Surg., Gynec. & Obst. **102**:207-214, 1956.
Hook, E. W., Campbell, C. G., Weens, H. S., and Cooper, G. R.:	Salmonella osteomyelitis in patients with sickle-cell anemia	New England J. Med. **257**:403-407, 1957.
Horwitz, T., and Lambert, R. G.:	Chronic osteomyelitis complicating war compound fractures	Surg., Gynec. & Obst. **82**:573-578, 1946.
Howard, L. G., Anderson, D. G., Christophe, K., Potter, T. A., and Moore, R. L.:	Treatment of chronic osteomyelitis with penicillin and primary closure of operative wounds	Arch. Surg. **60**:112-124, 1950.
James, T.:	Acute osteomyelitis in infancy and early childhood	Brit. J. Surg. **41**:87-91, 1953.
Kelly, P. J., Martin, W. J., Schirger, A., and Weed, L. A.:	Brucellosis of the bones and joints	J.A.M.A. **174**:347-353, 1960.

Kernwein, G. A., and Capps, R. B.:	Typhoid osteomyelitis, case report	Am. J. Surg. 60:433-437, 1943.
Kitlowski, E. A.:	The treatment of chronic osteomyelitis with flaps	Am. J. Surg. 87:351-356, 1954.
Knight, M. P., and Wood, G. O.:	Surgical obliteration of bone cavities following traumatic osteomyelitis	J. Bone & Joint Surg. 27:547-556, 1945.
Kulowski, J.:	Management of hematogenous pyogenic osteomyelitis	Surgery 40:1094-1104, 1956.
Lame, E. L., and Chang, H. C.:	Pubic and ischial necrosis following cystostomy and prostatectomy (osteitis pubis)	Am. J. Roentgenol. 71:193-212, 1954.
Lovell, W. W., King, R. E., and Alldredge, R.:	Carcinoma in skin, sinuses and bone following chronic osteomyelitis	South. M. J. 50:266-271, 1957.
Mantle, J. A.:	Brucellar spondylitis	J. Bone & Joint Surg. 37-B:456-461, 1955.
Meyerding, H. W.:	Chronic sclerosing osteitis (Sclerosing non-suppurative osteomyelitis of Garré)	S. Clin. North America 24:762-779, 1944.
Moe, J. H.:	Prevention and treatment of infections in bone	Journal-Lancet 79:2-7, 1959.
Obletz, B. E.:	Acute suppurative arthritis of the hip in the neonatal period	J. Bone & Joint Surg. 42-A:23-30, 1960.
Orr, H. W.:	Osteomyelitis and compound fractures and other infected wounds	St. Louis, The C. V. Mosby Co., 1929.
Ortiz, A. C., and Miller, W. E.:	Treatment of a septic joint	South. M. J. 54:594-599, 1961.
Potter, C. M. C.:	Osteomyelitis in the new-born	J. Bone & Joint Surg. 36-B:578-583, 1954.
Reynolds, F. C., and Zaepfel, F.:	Management of chronic osteomyelitis secondary to compound fractures	J. Bone & Joint Surg. 30-A:331-338, 1948.
Ross, D. W.:	Acute suppurative arthritis of the hip in premature infants	J.A.M.A. 156:303-307, 1954.
Rowling, D. E.:	The positive approach to chronic osteomyelitis	J. Bone & Joint Surg. 41-B:681-688, 1959.
Silver, H. K., Simon, J. L., and Clement, D. H.:	Salmonella osteomyelitis and abnormal hemoglobin disease	Pediatrics 20:439-447, 1957.
Spitzer, N., and Steinbrocker, O.:	The treatment of gonorrheal arthritis with penicillin	Am. J. M. Sc. 218:138-144, 1949.
Trueta, J.:	The three types of acute haematogenous osteomyelitis	J. Bone & Joint Surg. 41-B:671-680, 1959.
Trueta, J., and Morgan, J. D.:	Late results in the treatment of 100 cases of acute haematogenous osteomyelitis	Brit. J. Surg. 41:449-457, 1954.
Watkins, M. B., Samilson, R. L., and Winters, D. M.:	Acute suppurative arthritis	J. Bone & Joint Surg. 38-A:1313-1320, 1956.
White, M., and Dennison, W. M.:	Acute haematogenous osteitis in childhood	J. Bone & Joint Surg. 34-B:608-623, 1952.
Wiltse, L. L., and Frantz, C. H.:	Non-suppurative osteitis pubis in the female	J. Bone & Joint Surg. 38-A:500-516, 1956.
Winters, J. L., and Cahen, I.:	Acute hematogenous osteomyelitis	J. Bone & Joint Surg. 42-A:691-704, 1960.
Zammit, F.:	Undulant fever spondylitis	Brit. J. Radiol. 31:683-690, 1958.

Fungous, parasitic, and syphilitic infections of bones and joints

Alfred, K. S., and Harbin, M.:	Blastomycosis of bone, report of a case	J. Bone & Joint Surg. **32-A**:887-892, 1950.
Allen, J. H., Jr.:	Bone involvement with disseminated histoplasmosis	Am. J. Roentgenol. **82**:250-254, 1959.
Borella, L., Goobar, J. E., and Clark, G. M.:	Synovitis of the knee joints in late congenital syphilis, Clutton's joints	J.A.M.A. **180**:190-192, 1962.
Carnesale, P. L., and Stegman, K. F.:	Blastomycosis of bone, report of 4 cases	Ann. Surg. **144**:252-257, 1956.
Colonna, P. C., and Gucker, T., III:	Blastomycosis of the skeletal system	J. Bone & Joint Surg. **26**:322-328, 1944.
Conaty, J. P., Biddle, M., and McKeever, F. M.:	Osseous coccidioidal granuloma	J. Bone & Joint Surg. **41-A**:1109-1122, 1959.
Cope, V. Z.:	Actinomycosis of bone with special reference to infection of the vertebral column	J. Bone & Joint Surg. **33-B**:205-214, 1951.
Cullen, C. H., and Sharp, M. E.:	Infection of wounds with actinomyces	J. Bone & Joint Surg. **33-B**:221-227, 1951.
Duran, R. J., Coventry, M. B., Weed, L. A., and Kierland, R. R.:	Sporotrichosis	J. Bone & Joint Surg. **39-A**:1330-1342, 1957.
Dykes, J., Segesman, J. K., and Birsner, J. W.:	Coccidioidomycosis of bone in children	Am. J. Dis. Child. **85**:34-42, 1953.
Ehrenpreis, B.:	Syphilis of bone in the adult	New York J. Med. **57**:3486-3488, 1957.
Faget, G. H., and Mayoral, A.:	Bone changes in leprosy: a clinical and roentgenologic study of 505 cases	Radiology **42**:1-13, 1944.
Helfet, A. J.:	Acute manifestations of yaws of bone and joint	J. Bone & Joint Surg. **26**:672-681, 1944.
Howorth, M. B.:	Echinococcosis of bone	J. Bone & Joint Surg. **27**:401-411, 1945.
Hutchison, W. F., Thompson, W. B., and Derian, P. S.:	Osseous hydatid (echinococcus) disease	J.A.M.A. **182**:81-83, 1962.
Kellsey, D. C., and Sproat, H. F.:	Echinococcus disease of bone	J. Bone & Joint Surg. **36-A**:1241-1248, 1954.
McMaster, P. E., and Gilfillan, C.:	Coccidioidal osteomyelitis	J.A.M.A. **112**:1233-1237, 1939.
Morton, J. J.:	Syphilis of bone	Urol. & Cutan. Rev. **43**:72-78, 1939.
Murray, R. O., and Haddad, F.:	Hydatid disease of the spine	J. Bone & Joint Surg. **41-B**:499-506, 1959.
Oyston, J. K.:	Madura foot	J. Bone & Joint Surg. **43-B**:259-267, 1961.
Reeves, R. J., and Pedersen, R.:	Fungous infection of bone	Radiology **62**:55-60, 1954.
Sotelo-Ortiz, F.:	Chronic coccidioidal synovitis of the knee joint	J. Bone & Joint Surg. **37-A**:49-56, 1955.
Thomason, H. A., and Mayoral, A.:	Syphilitic osteomyelitis	J. Bone & Joint Surg. **22**:203-206, 1940.
Thompson, W. F.:	Blastomycosis of bone, report of a case	J. Bone & Joint Surg. **35-A**:777-781, 1953.
Toone, E. C., Jr., and Kelly, J.:	Joint and bone disease due to mycotic infection	Am. J. M. Sc. **231**:263-273, 1956.

520 Bibliography

Webster, F. S., and Willander, D.:	Chronic sporotrichal synovitis of the knee	J. Bone & Joint Surg. **39-A**:207-215, 1957.
Wolfe, J. N., and Jacobson, G.:	Roentgen manifestations of torulosis (cryptococcosis)	Am. J. Roentgenol. **79**:216-227, 1958.

Chapter 7
Tuberculosis of bones and joints
General considerations

Allen, A. R., and Stevenson, A. W.:	The results of combined drug therapy and early fusion in bone tuberculosis	J. Bone & Joint Surg. **39-A**:32-42, 1957.
Allred, S. W., and Minear, W. L.:	Statistical study of tuberculosis of the bones and joints in children	Am. Surgeon **18**:58-65, 1952.
Bosworth, D. M.:	Treatment of bone and joint tuberculosis in children	J. Bone & Joint Surg. **41-A**:1255-1266, 1959.
	Treatment of tuberculosis of bone and joint	Bull. New York Acad. Med. **35**:167-177, 1959.
Bosworth, D. M., Wright, H. A., and Fielding, J. W.:	The treatment of bone and joint tuberculosis	J. Bone & Joint Surg. **34-A**:761-771, 1952.
Carrell, W. B., and Childress, H. M.:	Tuberculosis of the large long bones of the extremities	J. Bone & Joint Surg. **22**:569-588, 1940.
Crofton, J.:	The chemotherapy of tuberculosis	Brit. M. Bull. **16**:55-60, 1960.
Evans, D.:	The diagnosis and treatment of skeletal tuberculosis	Brit. J. Clin. Pract. **12**:811-820, 1958.
Girdlestone, G. R., and Somerville, E. W.:	Tuberculosis of bone and joint	New York, Oxford University Press, 1952.
Hartung, E. F.:	Tuberculous arthritis	J.A.M.A. **158**:818-821, 1955.
Hsieh, C. K., Miltner, L. J., and Chang, C. P.:	Tuberculosis of the shaft of the large long bones of the extremities	J. Bone & Joint Surg. **16**:545-563, 1934.
Katayama, R., Itami, Y., and Marumo, E.:	Treatment of hip and knee-joint tuberculosis, an attempt to retain motion	J. Bone & Joint Surg. **44-A**:897-917, 1962.
Kessler, A. D., Scott, R. B., Kelley, C. H., and Steinman, R.	Cystic tuberculosis of the bones in children, report of two cases	Am. J. Dis. Child. **88**:201-209, 1954.
Lipscomb, P. R., and McCaslin, F. E., Jr.:	Arthrodesis of the hip	J. Bone & Joint Surg. **43-A**:923-938, 1961.
Phemister, D. B.:	Changes in the articular surfaces in tuberculous arthritis	J. Bone & Joint Surg. **7**:835-848, 1925.
Pimm, L. H., and Waugh, W.:	Tuberculous tenosynovitis	J. Bone & Joint Surg. **39-B**:91-101, 1957.
Pomeranz, M. M.:	Roentgen diagnosis of bone and joint tuberculosis	Am. J. Roentgenol. **29**:753-762, 1933.
Poppel, M. H., Lawrence, L. R., Jacobson, H. G., and Stein, J.:	Skeletal tuberculosis, a roentgenographic survey with reconsideration of diagnostic criteria	Am. J. Roentgenol. **70**:936-963, 1953.
Stevenson, F. H.:	Chemotherapy and tuberculosis of bone and joint	Tubercle **38**:355-364, 1957.
Wilkinson, M. C.:	Synovectomy and curettage in the treatment of tuberculosis of joints	J. Bone & Joint Surg. **35-B**:209-223, 1953.
	Chemotherapy of tuberculosis of bones and joints	J. Bone & Joint Surg. **36-B**:23-35, 1954.
	Partial synovectomy in the treatment of tuberculosis of the knee	J. Bone & Joint Surg. **44-B**:34-41, 1962.

Tuberculosis of individual joints

Ahern, R. T.:	Tuberculosis of the femoral neck and greater trochanter	J. Bone & Joint Surg. **40-B**:406-419, 1958.
Albee, F. H.:	The bone-graft operation for tuberculosis of the spine: twenty years' experience	J.A.M.A. **94**:1467-1471, 1930.
Auerbach, O., and Stemmerman, M. G.:	The roentgen interpretation of the pathology in Pott's disease	Am. J. Roentgenol. **52**:57-63, 1944.
Bosworth, D. M.:	Femoro-ischial transplantation	J. Bone & Joint Surg. **24**:38-46, 1942.
Butler, R. W.:	Paraplegia in Pott's disease, with special reference to the pathology and etiology	Brit. J. Surg. **22**:738-768, 1935.
Charnley, J., and Baker, S. L.:	Compression arthrodesis of the knee	J. Bone & Joint Surg. **34-B**:187-199, 1952.
Cleveland, M., and Bosworth, D. M.:	The pathology of tuberculosis of the spine	J. Bone & Joint Surg. **24**:527-546, 1942.
Cleveland, M., Bosworth, D. M., Fielding, J. W., and Smyrnis, P.:	Fusion of the spine for tuberculosis in children	J. Bone & Joint Surg. **40-A**:91-106, 1958.
Cleveland, M., Bosworth, D. M., and Thompson, F. R.:	Pseudarthrosis in the lumbosacral spine	J. Bone & Joint Surg. **30-A**:302-312, 1948.
Ghormley, R. K.:	Use of the anterior superior spine and crest of ilium in surgery of the hip joint	J. Bone & Joint Surg. **13**:784-798, 1931.
Ghormley, R. K., and Brav, E. A.:	Resected knee joints	Arch. Surg. **26**:465-484, 1933.
Hatcher, C. H., and Phemister, D. B.:	The primary point of infection in tuberculosis of the hip joint	Surg., Gynec. & Obst. **65**:721-740, 1937.
Hibbs, R. A., and Risser, J. C.:	Treatment of vertebral tuberculosis by the spine fusion operation, a report of 286 cases	J. Bone & Joint Surg. **10**:805-815, 1928.
Hodgson, A. R., and Stock, F. E.:	Anterior spine fusion for the treatment of tuberculosis of the spine	J. Bone & Joint Surg. **42-A**:295-310, 1960.
Johnson, R. W., Jr., Hillman, J. W., and Southwick, W. O.:	The importance of direct surgical attack upon lesions of the vertebral bodies, particularly in Pott's disease	J. Bone & Joint Surg. **35-A**:17-25, 1953.
Karlén, A.:	Early drainage of paraspinal tuberculous abscesses in children	J. Bone & Joint Surg. **41-B**:491-498, 1959.
Mercer, W.:	The management of the tuberculous hip joint	J. Bone & Joint Surg. **36-A**:1123-1128, 1954.
Seddon, H. J.:	Pott's paraplegia	In Platt H., editor: Modern trends in orthopedics (second series), New York, Paul B. Hoeber, Inc., 1956, pp. 220-245.
Soholt, S. T.:	Tuberculosis of the sacro-iliac joint	J. Bone & Joint Surg. **33-A**:119-130, 1951.
Stevenson, F. H., Cholmeley, J. A., and Jory, H. I.:	Tuberculosis of the hip in children, seven years use of chemotherapy	Tubercle **38**:164-174, 1957.
	Tuberculosis of the knee: results with chemotherapy between 1948 and 1956	Tubercle **39**:1-6, 1958.

Weinberg, J. A.:	The surgical excision of psoas abscesses resulting from spinal tuberculosis	J. Bone & Joint Surg. **39-A**:17-27, 1957.
Wilkinson, M. C.:	Partial synovectomy and curettage in the treatment of tuberculosis of the hip	J. Bone & Joint Surg. **39-B**:66-79, 1957.
	Treatment of tuberculosis of the spine	Brit. M. J. **2**:280-282, 1959.
Wilson, J. N.:	Tuberculosis of the elbow	J. Bone & Joint Surg. **35-B**:551-560, 1953.

Chapter 8
Chronic arthritis

Adams, C. H., and Cecil, R. L.:	Gold therapy in early rheumatoid arthritis	Ann. Int. Med. **33**:163-173, 1950.
American Rheumatism Association Committee:	Primer on the rheumatic diseases	J.A.M.A. **171**:1205-1220, 1345-1356, 1680-1691, 1959.
	Diagnostic criteria for rheumatoid arthritis, 1958 revision	Ann. Rheumat. Dis. **18**:49-53, 1959.
Badgley, C. E.:	The orthopedic treatment of arthritis	American Academy of Orthopaedic Surgeons Instructional Course Lectures, vol. V, Ann Arbor, J. W. Edwards, 1948, pp. 314-322.
Bauer, W., and Bennett, G. A.:	Experimental and pathological studies in the degenerative type of arthritis	J. Bone & Joint Surg. **18**:1-18, 1936.
Copeman, W. S. C., editor:	Textbook of the rheumatic diseases, 2nd edition	Edinburgh, E. & S. Livingstone, Ltd., 1955.
Crain, D. C.:	The hands in arthritis	J.A.M.A. **170**:795-798, 1959.
Duthie, J. J. R., Brown, P. E., Knox, J. D. E. and Thompson, M.:	Course and prognosis in rheumatoid arthritis	Ann. Rheumat. Dis. **16**:411-424, 1957.
Empire Rheumatism Council:	Gold therapy in rheumatoid arthritis	Ann. Rheumat. Dis. **19**:95-119, 1960.
Forkner, C. E., Shands, A. R., and Poston, M. A.:	Synovial fluid in chronic arthritis	Arch. Int. Med. **42**:675-702, 1928.
Hart, F. D.:	Corticosteroids in treatment of rheumatic disorders	Brit. M. J. **1**:493-496, 1960.
Hench, P. S., and Rosenberg, E. F.:	Palindromic rheumatism	Arch. Int. Med. **73**:293-321, 1944.
Hollander, J. L.:	Intra-articular hydrocortisone in arthritis and allied conditions	J. Bone & Joint Surg. **35-A**:983-990, 1953.
Hollander, J. L., editor:	Arthritis and allied conditions, 6th edition	Philadelphia, Lea & Febiger, 1960.
Holman, H. R.:	The L. E. cell phenomenon	Ann. Rev. Med. **11**:231-242, 1960.
Johnson, L. C.:	Kinetics of osteoarthritis	Lab. Invest. **8**:1223-1241, 1959.
Johnson, N. J., and Dodd, K.:	Juvenile rheumatoid arthritis	M. Clin. North America **39**:459-487, 1955.
Kuhns, J. G.:	Management of osteoarthritis in the aged	J.A.M.A. **151**:98-102, 1953.
	Surgery in chronic arthritis	New England J. Med. **240**:605-610, 1949.

Bibliography

Laine, V. A. I., Sairanen, E., and Vainio, K.:	Finger deformities caused by rheumatoid arthritis	J. Bone & Joint Surg. **39-A**:527-533, 1957.
Larmon, W. A., and Kurtz, J. F.:	The surgical management of chronic tophaceous gout	J. Bone & Joint Surg. **40-A**:743-772, 1958.
Law, W. A.:	Surgical treatment of the rheumatic diseases	J. Bone & Joint Surg. **34-B**:215-225, 1952.
Lawrence, J. S.:	Prevalence of rheumatoid arthritis	Ann. Rheumat. Dis. **20**:11-17, 1961.
Lockie, L. M.:	Steroid therapy in rheumatoid diseases	J.A.M.A. **170**:1063-1066, 1959.
Lowman, E. W., Lee, P. R., and Rusk, H. A.:	Total rehabilitation of the rheumatoid arthritic cripple	J.A.M.A. **158**:1335-1344, 1955.
McEwen, C., Ziff, M., Carmel, P., DiTata, D, and Tanner, M.:	The relationship to rheumatoid arthritis of its so-called variants	Arthritis & Rheumatism **1**:481-496, 1958.
McKusick, V. A.:	Genetic factors in diseases of connective tissue	Am. J. Med. **26**:283-302, 1959.
Mellors, R. C., Nowoslawski, A., Korngold, L., and Sengson, B. L.:	Rheumatoid factor and the pathogenesis of rheumatoid arthritis	J. Exper. Med. **113**:475-484, 1961.
Montgomery, M. M., Pilz, C. G., and Aronson, A. R.:	Early diagnosis of arthritis and allied disorders	M. Clin. North America **44**:29-48, 1960.
Neustadt, D. H.:	Corticosteroid therapy in rheumatoid arthritis	J.A.M.A. **170**:1253-1260, 1959.
Polley, H. F., and Mason, H. L.:	Rheumatoid arthritis	J.A.M.A. **143**:1474-1481, 1950.
Portis, R. B.:	Pathology of chronic arthritis of children (Still's disease)	Am. J. Dis. Child. **55**:1000-1017, 1938.
Ragan, C. A., Jr.:	Steroid therapy in arthritis	American Academy of Orthopaedic Surgeons Instructional Course Lectures, vol. XV, Ann Arbor, J. W. Edwards, 1958, pp. 245-253.
Rhinelander, F. W.:	The effectiveness of splinting and bracing on rheumatoid arthritis	Arthritis & Rheumatism **2**:270-277, 1959.
Ropes, M. W., and Bauer, W.:	Synovial fluid changes in joint disease	Cambridge, Mass., Harvard University Press, 1953.
Sherman, M. S.:	Psoriatic arthritis	J. Bone & Joint Surg. **34-A**:831-852, 1955.
Short, C. L., Bauer, W., and Reynolds, W. E.:	Rheumatoid arthritis	Cambridge, Mass., Harvard University Press, 1957.
Small, J. C.:	The mechanics of deformities of the hands in atrophic arthritis, and a discussion of their prevention and correction	Ann. Int. Med. **32**:1087-1094, 1950.
Smyth, C. J.:	Rheumatism and arthritis: review of American and English literature of recent years (fourteenth rheumatism review)	Ann. Int. Med. **56**(supp. 1):1-152, 1962.
Smyth, C. J., Huffman, E. R., and Wilson, G. M.:	Treatment of gout	Arch. Int. Med. **97**:783-792, 1956.
Swaim, L. T., and Kuhns, J. G.:	The prevention of deformities in chronic arthritis	
	(1) The upper extremity	J.A.M.A. **93**:1853-1856, 1929.
	(2) The spine and the head	J.A.M.A. **94**:1123-1125, 1930.
	(3) The lower extremity	J.A.M.A. **94**:1743-1745, 1930.

Talbott, J. H.:	Gout	New York, Grune & Stratton, Inc., 1957.
Traut, E. F.:	Degenerative arthritis: its causes, recognition and management	M. Clin. North America **40**:63-78, 1956.
Vaughan, J. H., and Butler, V. P., Jr.:	Current status of the rheumatoid factor	Ann. Int. Med. **56**:1-11, 1962.
Weiss, T. E., and Segaloff, A.:	Gouty arthritis and gout	Springfield, Ill., Charles C Thomas, Publisher, 1959.

Chapter 9
Chronic arthritis of individual joints—ankylosis and arthroplasty

Chronic arthritis of individual joints

Bennett, G. A., Waine, H., and Bauer, W.:	Changes in the knee joint at various ages, with particular reference to the nature and development of degenerative joint disease	New York, The Commonwealth Fund, 1942.
Bick, E. M.:	Vertebral osteophytosis, pathologic basis of its roentgenology	Am. J. Roentgenol. **73**:979-983, 1955.
Blumberg, B., and Ragan, C.:	The natural history of rheumatoid spondylitis	Medicine **35**:1-31, 1956.
Boland, E. W., and Shebesta, E. M.:	Rheumatoid spondylitis: correlation of clinical and roentgenographic features	Radiology **47**:551-561, 1946.
Clayton, M. L.:	Surgery of the thumb in rheumatoid arthritis	J. Bone & Joint Surg. **44-A**:1376-1386, 1962.
Forestier, J., Jacqueline, F., and Rotes-Querol, J.:	Ankylosing spondylitis (translated from the French by A. U. Desjardins)	Springfield, Ill., Charles C Thomas, Publisher, 1956.
Geckeler, E. O., and Quaranta, A. V.:	Patellectomy for degenerative arthritis of the knee, late results	J. Bone & Joint Surg. **44-A**:1109-1114, 1962.
Golding, F. C.:	Spondylitis ankylopoietica	Brit. J. Surg. **23**:484-500, 1936.
Harrison, M. H. M., Schajowicz, F., and Trueta, J.:	Osteoarthritis of the hip: a study of the nature and evolution of the disease	J. Bone & Joint Surg. **35·B**:598-626, 1953.
Henderson, E. D., and Lipscomb, P. R.:	Surgical treatment of rheumatoid hand	J.A.M.A. **175**:431-436, 1961.
Howard, F. M.:	Surgical aid for arthritis of the hand and elbow	J. Internat. Coll. Surgeons **33**:336-341, 1960.
Kuhns, J. G.:	Orthopaedic treatment of hypertrophic arthritis of the hip	J. Bone & Joint Surg. **24**:547-554, 1942.
	Treatment of arthritic contractures of the knee	New England J. Med. **227**:975-980, 1942.
Law, W. A.:	Late results in vitallium-mold arthroplasty of the hip	J. Bone & Joint Surg. **44-A**:1497-1517, 1962.
Lloyd-Roberts, G. C.:	Osteoarthritis of the hip, a study of the clinical pathology	J. Bone & Joint Surg. **37-B**:8-47, 1955.
McMurray, T. P.:	Osteo-arthritis of the hip joint	J. Bone & Joint Surg. **21**:1-11, 1939.
Mulder, J. D.:	Denervation of the hip joint in osteoarthritis	J. Bone & Joint Surg. **30-B**:446-448, 1948.
Nicoll, E. A., and Holden, N. T.:	Displacement osteotomy in the treatment of osteoarthritis of the hip	J. Bone & Joint Surg. **43-B**:50-60, 1961.
Polley, H. F., and Slocumb, C. H.:	Rheumatoid spondylitis: a study of 1,035 cases	Ann. Int. Med. **26**:240-249, 1947.

Rhaney, K., and Lamb, D. W.:	The cysts of osteoarthritis of the hip	J. Bone & Joint Surg. **37-B**:663-675, 1955.
Rose, G. K.:	The surgical management of ankylosing spondylitis	Rheumatism **17**:63-69, 1961.
Shands, A. R., Jr., and Muehe, C. C.:	Rheumatoid arthritis in childhood, involvement of the hip	Delaware M. J. **32**:1-12, 1960.
Smith, C. F., Pugh, D. G., and Polley, H. F.:	Physiologic vertebral ligamentous calcification: an aging process	Am. J. Roentgenol. **74**:1049-1058, 1955.
Straub, L. R.:	The rheumatoid hand	In De Palma, A. F., editor: Clinical orthopaedics, vol. 15, Philadelphia, J. B. Lippincott, 1959, pp. 127-139.
Watson-Jones, R., and Robinson, W. C.:	Arthrodesis of the osteoarthritic hip joint	J. Bone & Joint Surg. **38-B**:353-377, 1956.
Wilkinson, M., and Bywaters, E. G. L.:	Clinical features and course of ankylosing spondylitis	Ann. Rheumat. Dis. **17**:209-228, 1958.

Ankylosis and arthroplasty

Aufranc, O. E.:	Constructive hip surgery with the Bitallium mold	J. Bone & Joint Surg. **39-A**:237-248, 1957.
	Constructive surgery of the hip	St. Louis, The C. V. Mosby Co., 1962.
Barr, J. S., Compere, E. L., Ghormley, R. K., Jergesen, F. H., Preston, R. L., and Thomson, J. E. M.:	A symposium on hip joint prostheses	American Academy of Orthopaedic Surgeons Instructional Course Lectures, vol. XV, Ann Arbor, J. W. Edwards, 1958, pp. 1-48.
Bennett, G. E.:	Lengthening of the quadriceps tendon	J. Bone & Joint Surg. **4**:279-316, 1922.
Campbell, W. C.:	The physiology of arthroplasty	J. Bone & Joint Surg. **13**:223-245, 1931.
Hammond, G., Crawford, H. R., and Haggart, G. E.:	Vitallium mold arthroplasty of hip, end result study	J.A.M.A. **158**:161-165, 1955.
Kelikian, H.:	A method of mobilizing the temporomandibular joint	J. Bone & Joint Surg. **32-A**:113-131, 1950.
Knight, R. A.:	Arthroplasty	In Carter, B. N., editor: Monographs on surgery, 1950-1952, Baltimore, Williams & Wilkins Co., 1952, pp. 253-309.
Knight, R. A., and Van Zandt, I. L.:	Arthroplasty of the elbow, an end-result study	J. Bone & Joint Surg. **34-A**:610-618, 1952.
Lambert, C. N., Straub, L. R., and King, D. E.:	Symposium on femoral-head replacement prostheses	J. Bone & Joint Surg. **38-A**:407-420, 1956.
Moore, A. T.:	The self-locking metal hip prosthesis	J. Bone & Joint Surg. **39-A**:811-827, 1957.
Schrock, R. D.:	Fixation position for optimum joint function	Nebraska M. J. **19**:211-214, 1934.
Smith-Petersen, M. N.:	Arthroplasty of the hip, a new method	J. Bone & Joint Surg. **21**:269-288, 1939.
	Evolution of mould arthroplasty of the hip joint	J. Bone & Joint Surg. **30-B**:59-75, 1948.
Speed, J. S., and Trout, P. C.:	Arthroplasty of the knee, a follow-up study	J. Bone & Joint Surg. **31-B**:53-60, 1949.

Stinchfield, F. E., and Carroll, R. E.:	Vitallium-cup arthroplasty of the hip joint	J. Bone & Joint Surg. **31-A**:628-638, 1949.
Thompson, T. C.:	Quadricepsplasty	Ann. Surg. **121**:751-755, 1945.

Chapter 10

Neuromuscular disabilities—poliomyelitis

American Orthopaedic Association, Research Committee:	A survey of end results on stabilization of the paralytic shoulder	J. Bone & Joint Surg. **24**:699-707, 1942.
Baker, A. B., and Cornwell, S.:	Poliomyelitis; the spinal cord	Arch. Path. **61**:185-206, 1956.
Blount, W. P.:	Unequal leg length	American Academy of Orthopaedic Surgeons Instructional Course Lectures, vol. XVII, St. Louis, The C. V. Mosby Co., 1960, pp. 218-245.
Campbell, W. C.:	Bone-block operation for dropfoot; analysis of end results	J. Bone & Joint Surg. **12**:317-324, 1930.
Clippinger, F. W., Jr., and Irwin, C. E.:	The opponens transfer, analysis of end results	South. M. J. **55**:33-36, 1962.
Colonna, P. C., and vom Saal, F.:	A study of paralytic scoliosis based on five hundred cases of poliomyelitis	J. Bone & Joint Surg. **23**:335-353, 1941.
Crego, C. H., Jr., and McCarroll, H. R.:	Recurrent deformities in stabilized paralytic feet	J. Bone & Joint Surg. **20**:609-620, 1938.
Davis, G. G.:	The treatment of hollow foot (pes cavus)	Am. J. Orthop. Surg. **11**:231-242, 1913.
Dickson, F. D.:	An operation for stabilizing paralytic hips	J. Bone & Joint Surg. **9**:1-7, 1927.
Drew, A. J.:	The late results of arthrodesis of the foot	J. Bone & Joint Surg. **33-B**:496-502, 1951.
Dunn, N.:	Stabilizing operations in the treatment of paralytic deformities of the foot	Proc. Roy. Soc. Med. (Sect. Orthop.) **15**:15-22, 1922.
Fitzgerald, F. P., and Seddon, H. J.:	Lambrinudi's operation for dropfoot	Brit. J. Surg. **25**:283-292, 1937.
Gill, A. B.:	Operation for correction of paralytic genu recurvatum	J. Bone & Joint Surg. **13**:49-53, 1931.
	A new operation for arthrodesis of the shoulder	J. Bone & Joint Surg. **13**:287-295, 1931.
	An operation to make a posterior bone block at the ankle to limit foot-drop	J. Bone & Joint Surg. **15**:166-170, 1933.
Green, W. T., and Anderson, M.:	Epiphyseal arrest for the correction of discrepancies in length of the lower extremities	J. Bone & Joint Surg. **39-A**:853-872, 1957.
	Experiences with epiphyseal arrest in correcting discrepancies in length of the lower extremities in infantile paralysis, a method of predicting the effect	J. Bone & Joint Surg. **29**:659-675, 1947.
Green, W. T., and Grice, D. S.:	The management of calcaneus deformity	American Academy of Orthopaedic Surgeons Instructional Course Lectures, vol. XIII, Ann Arbor, J. W. Edwards, 1956, pp. 135-149.

Grice, D. S.:	An extra-articular arthrodesis of the subastragalar joint for correction of paralytic flat feet in children	J. Bone & Joint Surg. **34-A**:927-940, 1952.
	Further experience with extra-articular arthrodesis of the subtalar joint	J. Bone & Joint Surg. **37-A**:246-259, 1955.
Grulee, C. G., Jr.:	Differential diagnosis of poliomyelitis	J.A.M.A. **152**:1587-1590, 1953.
Herndon, C. H.:	Tendon transplantation at the knee and foot	American Academy of Orthopaedic Surgeons Instructional Course Lectures, vol. XVIII, St. Louis, The C. V. Mosby Co., 1961, pp. 145-168.
Herndon, C. H., Strong, J. M., and Heyman, C. H.:	Transposition of the tibialis anterior in the treatment of paralytic talipes calcaneus	J. Bone & Joint Surg. **38-A**:751-760, 1956.
Hoke, M.:	An operation for stabilizing paralytic feet	J. Orthop. Surg. **3**:494-507, 1921.
Ingram, A. J., and Hundley, J. M.:	Posterior bone block of the ankle for paralytic equinus, an end-result study	J. Bone & Joint Surg. **33-A**:679-691, 1951.
Irwin, C. E.:	Transplants to the thumb to restore function of opposition: end results	South. M. J. **35**:257-262, 1942.
	Genu recurvatum following poliomyelitis, a controlled method of operative correction	J.A.M.A. **120**:277-280, 1942.
	Iliotibial band, its role in producing deformity in poliomyelitis	J. Bone & Joint Surg. **31-A**:141-146, 1949.
	The calcaneus foot	South. M. J. **44**:191-197, 1951.
Irwin, C. E., and Eyler, D. L.:	Surgical rehabilitation of the hand and forearm disabled by poliomyelitis	J. Bone & Joint Surg. **33-A**:825-835, 1951.
Kendall, H. O., and Kendall, F. P.:	Care during the recovery period in paralytic poliomyelitis	Public Health Bulletin No. 242, Public Health Service, Washington, D. C., United States Government Printing Office, revised 1939.
	Muscles, testing and function	Baltimore, Williams & Wilkins Co., 1949.
Kettelkamp, D. B., and Larson, C. B.:	Evaluation of the Steindler flexorplasty	J. Bone & Joint Surg. **45-A**:513-518, 1963.
Koprowski, H.:	Live poliomyelitis virus vaccines	J.A.M.A. **178**:1151-1155, 1961.
Kuhlmann, R. F., and Bell, J. F.:	A clinical evaluation of tendon transplantations for poliomyelitis affecting the lower extremities	J. Bone & Joint Surg. **34-A**:915-926, 1952.
Legg, A. T.:	Tensor fascia femoris transplantation in cases of weakened gluteus medius	New England J. Med. **209**:61-62, 1933.
Lenhard, R. E.:	Prognosis in poliomyelitis	J. Bone & Joint Surg. **32-A**:71-79, 1950.

Lowman, C. L.:	Fascial transplants in paralysis of abdominal and shoulder girdle muscles	American Academy of Orthopaedic Surgeons Instructional Course Lectures, vol. XIV, Ann Arbor, J. W. Edwards, 1957, pp. 300-304.
	The relation of the abdominal muscles to paralytic scoliosis	J. Bone & Joint Surg. 14:763-772, 1932.
Marchand, J. F.:	Care of respiratory paralysis from poliomyelitis	J.A.M.A. 155:1297-1302, 1954.
Mayer, L.:	The physiological method of tendon transplants reviewed after forty years	American Academy of Orthopaedic Surgeons Instructional Course Lectures, vol. XIII, Ann Arbor, J. W. Edwards, 1956, pp. 116-120.
	Further studies of fixed paralytic pelvic obliquity	J. Bone & Joint Surg. 18:87-100, 1936.
	Operative reconstruction of the paralyzed upper extremity	J. Bone & Joint Surg. 21:377-383, 1939
Mayer, L., and Green, W.:	Experiences with the Steindler flexorplasty at the elbow	J. Bone & Joint Surg. 36-A:775-789, 1954.
Mortens, J., and Pilcher, M. F.:	Tendon transplantation in the prevention of foot deformities after poliomyelitis in children	J. Bone & Joint Surg. 38-B:633-639, 1956.
Mustard, W. T.:	A follow-up study of iliopsoas transfer for hip instability	J. Bone & Joint Surg. 41-B:289-298, 1959.
Ober, F. R.:	An operation for the relief of paralysis of the gluteus maximus muscle	J.A.M.A. 88:1063-1064, 1927.
Patterson, R. L., Jr., Parrish, F. F., and Hathaway, E. N.:	Stabilizing operations on the foot, a study of the indications, techniques used, and end results	J. Bone & Joint Surg. 32-A:1-26, 1950.
Phemister, D. B.:	Operative arrestment of longitudinal growth of bones in the treatment of deformities	J. Bone & Joint Surg. 15:1-15, 1933.
Piszczek, E. A.:	Epidemiological aspects of poliomyelitis	American Academy of Orthopaedic Surgeons Instructional Course Lectures, vol. VIII, Ann Arbor, J. W. Edwards, 1951, pp. 255-261.
Reidy, J. A., Broderick, T. F., Jr., and Barr, J. S.:	Tendon transplantations in lower extremity: a review of end results in poliomyelitis; I. Tendon transplantations about the foot and ankle. II. Tendon transplantations at the knee	J. Bone & Joint Surg. 34-A:900-914, 1952.
Sabin, A. B., Michaels, R. H., Spigland, I., Pelon, W., Rhim, J. S., and Wehr, R. E.:	Community-wide use of oral poliovirus vaccine	Am. J. Dis. Child. 101:546-567, 1961.
Salk, J. E.:	Studies in human subjects on active immunization against poliomyelitis	J.A.M.A. 151:1081-1098, 1953.
Schottstaedt, E. R., Larsen, L. J., and Bost, F. C.:	The surgical reconstruction of the upper extremity paralyzed by poliomyelitis	J. Bone & Joint Surg. 40-A:633-643, 1958.

Schwartzmann, J. R., and Crego, C. H., Jr.:	Hamstring-tendon transplantation for the relief of quadriceps femoris paralysis in residual poliomyelitis, a follow-up study of 134 cases	J. Bone & Joint Surg. **30-A**:541-549, 1948.
Segal, A., Seddon, H. J., and Brooks, D. M.:	Treatment of paralysis of the flexors of the elbow	J. Bone & Joint Surg. **41-B**:44-50, 1959.
Sharrard, W. J. W.:	Muscle recovery in poliomyelitis	J. Bone & Joint Surg. **37-B**:63-79, 1955.
Sofield, H. A., Blair, S. J., and Millar, E. A.:	Leg-lengthening	J. Bone & Joint Surg. **40-A**:311-322, 1958.
Steindler, A.:	The pathomechanics of the paralytic gait	American Academy of Orthopaedic Surgeons Instructional Course Lectures, vol. XII, Ann Arbor, J. W. Edwards, 1955, pp. 189-200.
	Tendon transplantation in the upper extremity	Am. J. Surg. **44**:260-271, 1939.
Stinchfield, A. J., Reidy, J. A., and Barr, J. S.:	Prediction of unequal growth of lower extremities in anterior poliomyelitis	J. Bone & Joint Surg. **31-A**:478-486, 1949.
Straub, L. R., Harvey, J. P., Jr., and Fuerst, C. E.:	A clinical evaluation of tendon transplantation in the paralytic foot	J. Bone & Joint Surg. **39-A**:1-16, 1957.
Straub, L. R., Thompson, T. C., and Wilson, P. D.:	Results of epiphyseodesis and femoral shortening in relation to equalization of limb length	J. Bone & Joint Surg. **27**:254-266, 1945.
Thompson, C. F.:	Fusion of the metacarpals of the thumb and index finger to maintain functional position of the thumb	J. Bone & Joint Surg. **24**:907-911, 1942.
Thompson, T. C.:	Astragalectomy and the treatment of calcaneovalgus	J. Bone & Joint Surg. **21**:627-647, 1939.
	A modified operation for opponens paralysis	J. Bone & Joint Surg. **24**:632-640, 1942.
Thompson, T. C., Straub, L. R., and Campbell, R. D.:	An evaluation of femoral shortening with intramedullary nailing	J. Bone & Joint Surg. **36-A**:43-56, 1954.
Watkins, M. B., Jones, J. B., Ryder, C. T., Jr., and Brown, T. H., Jr.:	Transplantation of the posterior tibial tendon	J. Bone & Joint Surg. **36-A**:1181-1189, 1954.
Westin, G. W., and Hall, C. B.:	Subtalar extra-articular arthrodesis	J. Bone & Joint Surg. **39-A**:501-512, 1957.
White, J. W.:	Femoral shortening for equalization of leg length	J. Bone & Joint Surg. **17**:597-604, 1935.
Yount, C. C.:	The role of the tensor fasciae femoris in certain deformities of the lower extremities	J. Bone & Joint Surg. **8**:171-193, 1926.

Chapter 11
Neuromuscular disabilities (exclusive of poliomyelitis)—involvement of the brain and spinal cord

Cerebral palsy

Anderson, G. W., Hicks, S. P., Palmer, M. F., Hughes, J. G., Arey, J. B., Yakovlev, P. I., Unna, K. R., and Byers, R. K.:	Symposium on cerebral palsy	J. Pediat. **40**:340-375, 489-524, 606-633, 1952.

Bibliography

Baker, L. D.:	A rational approach to the surgical needs of the cerebral palsy patient	J. Bone & Joint Surg. 38-A:313-323, 1956.
Baker, L. D., and Dodelin, R. A.:	Extra-articular arthrodesis of the subtalar joint (Grice procedure), results in seventeen patients with cerebral palsy	J.A.M.A. 168:1005-1008, 1958.
Banks, H. H., and Green, W. T.:	Adductor myotomy and obturator neurectomy for the correction of adduction contracture of the hip in cerebral palsy	J. Bone & Joint Surg. 42-A:111-126, 1960.
	The correction of equinus deformity in cerebral palsy	J. Bone & Joint Surg. 40-A:1359-1379, 1958.
Barnett, H. E.:	Orthopedic surgery in cerebral palsy	J.A.M.A. 150:1396-1398, 1952.
Benda, C. E.:	Developmental disorders of mentation and cerebral palsies	New York, Grune & Stratton, Inc., 1952.
Chandler, F. A.:	Surgical procedures commonly used in correcting the deformities of spastic paralysis	Clinics 2:992-1001, 1943.
Cooper, W.:	The diagnosis and treatment of cerebral palsy	American Academy of Orthopaedic Surgeons Instructional Course Lectures, vol. XIV, Ann Arbor, J. W. Edwards, 1957, pp. 293-299.
Crothers, B., and Paine, R. S.:	The natural history of cerebral palsy	Cambridge, Mass., Harvard University Press, 1959.
Deaver, G. G.:	Cerebral palsy: methods of treating the neuromuscular disabilities	Arch. Phys. Med. & Rehab. 37:363-367, 1956.
Denhoff, E., Holden, R. H., and Silver, M. L.:	Prognostic studies in children with cerebral palsy	J.A.M.A. 161:781-784, 1956.
Eggers, G. W. N.:	Selective surgery for the cerebral palsy patient	American Academy of Orthopaedic Surgeons Instructional Course Lectures, vol. XII, Ann Arbor, J. W. Edwards, 1955, pp. 221-231.
	Transplantation of hamstring tendons to femoral condyles in order to improve hip extension and to decrease knee flexion in cerebral spastic paralysis	J. Bone & Joint Surg. 34-A:827-830, 1952.
Goldner, J. L.:	Reconstructive surgery of the hand in cerebral palsy and spastic paralysis resulting from injury to the spinal cord	J. Bone & Joint Surg. 37-A:1141-1154, 1955.
Green, W. T., and Banks, H. H.:	Flexor carpi ulnaris transplant and its use in cerebral palsy	J. Bone & Joint Surg. 44-A:1343-1352, 1962.
Green, W. T., and McDermott, L. J.:	Operative treatment of cerebral palsy of spastic type	J.A.M.A. 118:434-440, 1942.
Heyman, C. H.:	The surgical treatment of spastic paralysis	Surg., Gynec. & Obst. 68:792-800, 1939.
Hohman, L. B.:	Intelligence levels in cerebral palsied children	Am. J. Phys. Med. 32:282-290, 1953.

Irish, C. W.:	Cerebral vascular lesions in newborn infants and young children	J. Pediat. 15:64-74, 1939.
Keats, S.:	Surgery of the extremities in treatment of cerebral palsy	J.A.M.A. 174:1266-1268, 1960.
Kirman, B. H.:	Epilepsy and cerebral palsy	Arch. Dis. Child. 31:1-7, 1956.
Koven, L. J., and Lamm, S. S.:	The athetoid syndrome in cerebral palsy, clinical aspects	Pediatrics 14:181-192, 1954.
Levitt, S., and Perlstein, M. A.:	Physiotherapy in cerebral palsy	Springfield, Ill., Charles C Thomas, Publisher, 1962.
Miller, E., and Rosenfeld, G. B.:	The psychologic evaluation of children with cerebral palsy and its implications in treatment	J. Pediat. 41:613-621, 1952.
Minear, W. L.:	A classification of cerebral palsy	Pediatrics 18:841-852, 1956.
Penfield, W.:	Ablation of abnormal cortex in cerebral palsy	J. Neurol., Neurosurg. & Psychiat. 15:73-78, 1952.
Perlstein, M. A., and Hood, P. N.:	Infantile spastic hemiplegia I. Incidence II. Laterality of involvement III. Intelligence IV. Birth weights V. Oral language and motor development	Pediatrics 14:436-441, 1954; Am. J. Phys. Med. 34:457-466, 1955; Pediatrics 15:676-682, 1955; Pediatrics 16:470-477, 1955; Pediatrics 17:58-62, 1956.
Phelps, W. M.:	Classification of athetosis with special reference to the motor classification	Am. J. Phys. Med. 35:24-31, 1956.
	Description and differentiation of types of cerebral palsy	Nerv. Child 8:107-127, 1949.
	Long-term results of orthopaedic surgery in cerebral palsy	J. Bone & Joint Surg. 39-A:53-59, 1957.
Pohl, J. F.:	Cerebral palsy	St. Paul, Bruce Publishing Co., 1950.
Pollock, G. A.:	Surgical treatment of cerebral palsy	J. Bone & Joint Surg. 44-B:68-81, 1962.
Putnam, T. J.:	Results of treatment of athetosis by section of extrapyramidal tracts in the spinal cord	Arch. Neurol. & Psychiat. 39:258-275, 1938.
Roberts, W. M., and Adams, J. P.:	The patellar-advancement operation in cerebral palsy	J. Bone & Joint Surg. 35-A:958-966, 1953.
Saturen, P., and Tobis, J. S.:	Evaluation and management of motor disturbance in brain-damaged children	J.A.M.A. 175:588-591, 1961.
Schwartz, P.:	Birth injuries of the newborn: morphology, pathogenesis, clinical pathology and prevention	New York, Hafner Publishing Co., Inc., 1961.
Silver, C. M., and Simon, S. D.:	Gastrocnemius-muscle recession (Silfverskiold operation) for spastic equinus deformity in cerebral palsy	J. Bone & Joint Surg. 41-A:1021-1028, 1959.
Stamp, W. G.:	Bracing in cerebral palsy	American Academy of Orthopaedic Surgeons Instructional Courses: J. Bone & Joint Surg. 44-A:1457-1476, 1962.
Strayer, L. M., Jr.:	Gastrocnemius recession	J. Bone & Joint Surg. 40-A:1019-1030, 1958.

Bibliography

Author	Title	Source
Towbin, A.:	The pathology of cerebral palsy	Springfield, Ill., Charles C Thomas, Publisher, 1961.

Other neuromuscular disabilities (exclusive of poliomyelitis) from involvement of the brain or spinal cord

Author	Title	Source
Aring, C. D., and Cobb, S.:	The muscular atrophies and allied disorders	Medicine **14**:77-118, 1935.
Bluestone, S. S., and Deaver, G. G.:	Habilitation of the child with spina bifida and myelomeningocele	J.A.M.A. **161**:1248-1251, 1956.
Burdick, W. F., Whipple, D. V., and Freeman, W.:	Amyotonia congenita (Oppenheim), report of 5 cases with necropsy	Am. J. Dis. Child. **69**:295-307, 1945.
Cameron, A. H.:	The spinal cord lesion in spina bifida cystica	Lancet **2**:171-174, 1956.
Covalt, D. A., Cooper, I. S., Hoen, T. I., and Rusk, H. A.:	Early management of patients with spinal cord injury	J.A.M.A. **151**:89-94, 1953.
Delano, P. J.:	The pathogenesis of Charcot's joint	Am. J. Roentgenol. **56**:189-200, 1946.
Ford, F. R.:	Diseases of the nervous system in infancy, childhood and adolescence, 3rd edition	Springfield, Ill., Charles C Thomas, Publisher, 1952.
Jaeger, R.:	Congenital spinal meningocele	J.A.M.A. **153**:792-795, 1953.
Kessler, H.:	Traumatic paraplegia—rationale of therapy	Ann. Int. Med. **40**:905-923, 1954.
Lamm, S. S.:	Pediatric neurology	New York, Landsberger Medical Books, Inc., 1959.
Lawyer, T., Jr., and Netsky, M. G.:	Amyotrophic lateral sclerosis, a clinicoanatomic study of fifty-three cases	Arch. Neurol. & Psychiat. **69**:171-192, 1953.
Luck, J. V.:	Psychosomatic problems in military orthopaedic surgery	J. Bone & Joint Surg. **28**:213-228, 1946.
Makin, M.:	The surgical management of Friedreich's ataxia	Ann. Roy. Coll. Surgeons England **22**:1-10, 1958.
Myerson, A.:	Hysterical paralysis and its treatment	J.A.M.A. **105**:1565-1567, 1935.
Perret, G.:	Diagnosis and treatment of diastematomyelia	Surg., Gynec. & Obst. **105**:69-83, 1957.
Pomeranz, M. M., and Rothberg, A. S.:	A review of 58 cases of tabetic arthropathy	Am. J. Syph., Gonor. & Ven. Dis. **25**:103-119, 1941.
Samilson, R. L., Sankaran, B., Bersani, F. A., and Smith, A. D.:	Orthopedic management of neuropathic joints	Arch. Surg. **78**:115-121, 1959.
Schwidde, J. T.:	Spina bifida, survey of 225 encephaloceles, meningoceles, and myelomeningoceles	Am. J. Dis. Child. **84**:35-51, 1952.
Shands, A. R., Jr.:	Neuropathies of the bones and joints, report of a case of an arthropathy of the ankle due to a peripheral nerve lesion	Arch. Surg. **20**:614-636, 1930.
Smith, R. S.:	Orthopedic considerations in the treatment of spina bifida	Surg., Gynec. & Obst. **62**:218-227, 1936.
Soto-Hall, R., and Haldeman, K. O.:	The diagnosis of neuropathic joint disease (Charcot joint), an analysis of forty cases	J.A.M.A. **114**:2076-2078, 1940.

Taylor, R. G., and Gleave, J. R. W.:	Incomplete spinal cord injuries, with Brown-Séquard phenomena	J. Bone & Joint Surg. **39-B**:438-450, 1957.
Walton, J. N.:	Amyotonia congenita, a follow-up study	Lancet **1**:1023-1027, 1956.

Chapter 12

Neuromuscular disabilities (exclusive of poliomyelitis)—involvement of peripheral nerves and of muscles

Peripheral nerve injuries

Barnes, R.:	Traction injuries of the brachial plexus in adults	J. Bone & Joint Surg. **31-B**:10-16, 1949.
	Peripheral nerve injuries	In Platt, Sir H., editor: Modern trends in orthopaedics, second series, New York, Paul B. Hoeber, Inc., 1956, Chap. 2, pp. 36-64.
Bateman, J. E.:	Peripheral nerve injuries	American Academy of Orthopaedic Surgeons Instructional Course Lectures, vol. XIII, Ann Arbor, J. W. Edwards, 1956, pp. 85-100.
	Trauma to nerves in limbs	Philadelphia, W. B. Saunders Co., 1962.
Bonney, G.:	Prognosis in traction lesions of the brachial plexus	J. Bone & Joint Surg. **41-B**:4-35, 1959.
Childress, H. M.:	Recurrent ulnar-nerve dislocation at the elbow	J. Bone & Joint Surg. **38-A**:978-984, 1956.
Clawson, D. K., and Seddon, H. J.:	The results of repair of the sciatic nerve	J. Bone & Joint Surg. **42-B**:205-212, 1960.
Combes, M. A., Clark, W. K., Gregory, C. F., and James, J. A.:	Sciatic nerve injury in infants, recognition and prevention of impairment resulting from intragluteal injections	J.A.M.A. **173**:1336-1339, 1960.
Cullen, C. H.:	Causalgia, diagnosis and treatment	J. Bone & Joint Surg. **30-B**:467-477, 1948.
Gay, J. R., and Love, J. G.:	Diagnosis and treatment of tardy paralysis of the ulnar nerve	J. Bone & Joint Surg. **29**:1087-1097, 1947.
Goldner, J. L., and Kelley, J. M.:	Radial nerve injuries	South. M. J. **51**:873-883, 1958.
Haymaker, W.:	The pathology of peripheral nerve injuries	Mil. Surgeon **102**:448-459, 1948.
Haymaker, W., and Woodhall, B.:	Peripheral nerve injuries, principles of diagnosis, 2nd edition	Philadelphia, W. B. Saunders Co., 1953.
Hendry, A. M.:	The treatment of residual paralysis after brachial plexus injuries	J. Bone & Joint Surg. **31-B**:42-49, 1949.
Howard, F. M.:	Ulnar-nerve palsy in wrist fractures	J. Bone & Joint Surg. **43-A**:1197-1201, 1961.
Johnson, J. T. H., and Kendall, H. O.:	Isolated paralysis of the serratus anterior muscle	J. Bone & Joint Surg. **37-A**:567-574, 1955.
King, T., and Morgan, F. P.:	Late results of removing the medial humeral epicondyle for traumatic ulnar neuritis	J. Bone & Joint Surg. **41-B**:51-55, 1959.
Larsen, R. D., and Posch, J. L.:	Nerve injuries in the upper extremity	Arch. Surg. **77**:469-482, 1958.

Littler, J. W.:	Tendon transfers and arthrodeses in combined median and ulnar nerve paralysis	J. Bone & Joint Surg. **31-A**:225-234, 1949.
Lyons, W. R., and Woodhall, B.:	Atlas of peripheral nerve injuries	Philadelphia, W. B. Saunders Co., 1949.
McGowan, A. J.:	The results of transposition of the ulnar nerve for traumatic ulnar neuritis	J. Bone & Joint Surg. **32-B**:293-301, 1950.
Overpeck, D. O., and Ghormley, R. K.:	Paralysis of serratus magnus muscle, caused by lesions of long thoracic nerve	J.A.M.A. **114**:1994-1996, 1940.
Parry, C. B. W.:	Electrodiagnosis	J. Bone & Joint Surg. **43-B**:222-236, 1961.
Phalen, G. S.:	The carpal tunnel syndrome	American Academy of Orthopaedic Surgeons Instructional Course Lectures, vol. XIV, Ann Arbor, J. W. Edwards, 1957, pp. 142-148.
Riordan, D. C.:	Surgery of the paralytic hand	American Academy of Orthopaedic Surgeons Instructional Course Lectures, vol. XVI, St. Louis, The C. V. Mosby Co., 1959, pp. 79-90.
Rosenthal, A. M.:	Electrodiagnostic testing in neuromuscular disease	J.A.M.A. **177**:829-833, 1961.
Sakellarides, H.:	A follow-up study of 172 peripheral nerve injuries in the upper extremity in civilians	J. Bone & Joint Surg. **44-A**:140-148, 1962.
Scuderi, C.:	Tendon transplants for irreparable radial nerve paralysis	Surg., Gynec. & Obst. **88**:643-651, 1949.
Shumacker, H. B., Jr., Speigel, I. J., and Upjohn, R. H.:	Causalgia, I. The rôle of sympathetic interruption in treatment	Surg., Gynec. & Obst. **86**:76-86, 1948.
	Causalgia, II. The signs and symptoms, with particular reference to vasomotor disturbances	Surg., Gynec. & Obst. **86**:452-460, 1948.
Stern, W. E.:	Recognition and treatment of peripheral nerve injuries in civilian practice	J.A.M.A. **178**:462-467, 1961.
Stookey, B.:	Meralgia paraesthetica, etiology and surgical treatment	J.A.M.A. **90**:1705-1707, 1928.
Sunderland, S.:	Course and rate of regeneration of motor fibers following lesions of the radial nerve	Arch. Neurol. & Psychiat. **56**:133-157, 1946.
Tanzer, R. C.:	The carpal-tunnel syndrome, a clinical and anatomical study	J. Bone & Joint Surg. **41-A**:626-634, 1959.
Tracy, J. F., and Brannon, E. W.:	Management of brachial-plexus injuries (traction type)	J. Bone & Joint Surg. **40-A**:1031-1042, 1958.
Versaci, A. D.:	Tendon transfers in ulnar-nerve injuries	New England J. Med. **262**:801-804, 1960.
Woodhall, B.:	Common injuries of peripheral nerves	American Academy of Orthopaedic Surgeons Instructional Course Lectures, vol. XI, Ann Arbor, J. W. Edwards, 1954, pp. 269-273.

Yeoman, P. M., and Seddon, H. J.:	Brachial plexus injuries: treatment of the flail arm	J. Bone & Joint Surg. **43-B**:493-500, 1961.

Obstetric paralysis

Kleinberg, S.:	Reattachment of the capsule and external rotators of shoulder for obstetric paralysis	J.A.M.A. **98**:294-298, 1932.
L'Episcopo, J. B.:	Tendon transplantation in obstetrical paralysis	Am. J. Surg. **25**:122-125, 1934.
Sever, J. W.:	Obstetrical paralysis	Surg., Gynec. & Obst. **44**:547-549, 1927.
Wickstrom, J., Haslam, E. T., and Hutchinson, R. H.:	The surgical management of residual deformities of the shoulder following birth injuries of the brachial plexus	J. Bone & Joint Surg. **37-A**:27-36, 1955.

Neuritis

Bardenwerper, H. W.:	Serum neuritis from tetanus antitoxin	J.A.M.A. **179**:763-766, 1962.
Haymaker, W., and Kernohan, J. W.:	The Landry-Guillain-Barré syndrome, a clinicopathologic report of 50 fatal cases and a critique of the literature	Medicine **28**:59-141, 1949.
Magee, K. R., and DeJong, R. N.:	Paralytic brachial neuritis, discussion of clinical features with review of 23 cases	J.A.M.A. **174**:1258-1262, 1960.
Peterman, A. F., Daly, D. D., Dion, F. R., and Keith, H. M.:	Infectious neuronitis (Guillain-Barré syndrome) in children	Neurology **9**:533-539, 1959.
Von Hagen, K. O., and Baker, R. N.:	Infectious neuronitis, present concepts of etiology and treatment	J.A.M.A. **151**:1465-1472, 1953.
Young, F.:	Peripheral nerve paralyses following the use of various serums, report of a case and review of the literature	J.A.M.A. **98**:1139-1143, 1932.

Involvement of muscles

Adams, R. D., Denny-Brown, D., and Pearson, C. M.:	Diseases of muscle, 2nd edition	New York, Paul B. Hoeber, Inc., 1962.
Geschickter, C. F., and Maseritz, I. H.:	Affections of muscles	J. Bone & Joint Surg. **21**:576-594, 1939.
Jacobs, J. E., and Carr, C. R.:	Progressive muscular atrophy of the peroneal type (Charcot-Marie-Tooth disease), orthopaedic management and end-result study	J. Bone & Joint Surg. **32-A**:27-38, 1950.
Ramsey, R. H., and McCarroll, H. R.:	Problem of muscular dystrophies	J.A.M.A. **150**:659-662, 1952.
Ross, A. T.:	The myopathies and the atrophies	American Academy of Orthopaedic Surgeons Instructional Course Lectures, vol. XIII, Ann Arbor, J. W. Edwards, 1956, pp. 71-78.
Vignos, P. J., Jr., Spencer, G. E., Jr., and Archibald, K. C.:	Management of progressive muscular dystrophy of childhood	J.A.M.A. **184**:89-96, 1963.

Bibliography

Voshell, A. F.: Progressive pseudohypertrophic muscular dystrophy — South. M. J. **26**:156-166, 1933.

Chapter 13

Tumors

Tumors and tumorlike affections of bone

Ackerman, L. V., and Spjut, H. J.:	Tumors of bone and cartilage	Washington, D. C., Armed Forces Institute of Pathology, 1962.
Alldredge, R. H.:	Localized fibrocystic disease of bone, results of treatment in one hundred and fifty-two cases	J. Bone & Joint Surg. **24**:795-804, 1942.
Baker, P. L., Dockerty, M. B., and Coventry, M. B.:	Adamantinoma (so-called) of the long bones, review of the literature and a report of three new cases	J. Bone & Joint Surg. **36-A**:704-720, 1954.
Bremner, R. A., and Jelliffe, A. M.:	The management of pathological fracture of the major long bones from metastatic cancer	J. Bone & Joint Surg. **40-B**:652-659, 1958.
Campbell, C. J., and Harkess, J.:	Fibrous metaphyseal defect of bone	Surg., Gynec. & Obst. **104**:329-336, 1957.
Chandler, F. A., and Kaell, H. I.:	Osteoid-osteoma	Arch. Surg. **60**:294-304, 1950.
Changus, G. W., Speed, J. S., and Stewart, F. W.:	Malignant angioblastoma of bone, a reappraisal of adamantinoma of long bone	Cancer **10**:540-559, 1957.
Coley, B. L.:	Neoplasms of bone and related conditions, 2nd edition	New York, Paul B. Hoeber, Inc., 1960.
Coley, B. L., and Higinbotham, N. L.:	Conservative surgery in tumors of bone with special reference to segmental resection	Ann. Surg. **127**:231-242, 1948.
Compere, C. L., and Coleman, S. S.:	Nonosteogenic fibroma of bone	Surg., Gynec. & Obst. **105**:588-598, 1957.
Copeland, M. M.:	Benign tumors of bone	Surg., Gynec. & Obst. **90**:697-712, 1950.
Copeland, M. M., and Geschickter, C. F.:	The treatment of parosteal osteoma of bone	Surg., Gynec. & Obst. **108**:537-548, 1959.
Coventry, M. B., and Dahlin, D. C.:	Osteogenic sarcoma	J. Bone & Joint Surg. **39-A**:741-758, 1957.
Cunningham, J. B., and Ackerman, L. V.:	Metaphyseal fibrous defects	J. Bone & Joint Surg. **38-A**:797-808, 1956.
Dahlin, D. C.:	Bone tumors	Springfield, Ill., Charles C Thomas, Publisher, 1957.
	Chondromyxoid fibroma of bone, with emphasis on its morphological relationship to benign chondroblastoma	Cancer **9**:195-203, 1956.
Dahlin, D. C., and Henderson, E. D.:	Chondrosarcoma, a surgical and pathological problem	J. Bone & Joint Surg. **38-A**:1025-1038, 1956.
Dahlin, D. C., Coventry, M. B., and Scanlon, P. W.:	Ewing's sarcoma	J. Bone & Joint Surg. **43-A**:185-192, 1961.
Dahlin, D. C., Besse, B. E., Jr., Pugh, D. G., and Ghormley, R. K.:	Aneurysmal bone cysts	Radiology **64**:56-65, 1955.

Donaldson, W. F., Jr.:	Aneurysmal bone cyst	J. Bone & Joint Surg. **44-A**:25-40, 1962.
Dwinnell, L. A., Dahlin, D. C., and Ghormley, R. K.:	Parosteal (juxtacortical) osteogenic sarcoma	J. Bone & Joint Surg. **36-A**:732-744, 1954.
Francis, K. C.:	Prophylactic internal fixation of metastatic osseous lesions	Cancer **13**:75-76, 1960.
Freiberger, R. H., Loitman, B. S., Helpern, M., and Thompson, T. C.:	Osteoid osteoma, a report on 80 cases	Am. J. Roentgenol. **82**:194-205, 1959.
Garceau, G. J., and Gregory, C. F.:	Solitary unicameral bone cyst	J. Bone & Joint Surg. **36-A**:267-280, 1954.
Geschickter, C. F., and Copeland, M. M.:	Tumors of bone, 3rd edition	Philadelphia, J. B. Lippincott Co., 1949.
Geschickter, C. F., and Maseritz, I. H.:	Skeletal metastasis in cancer	J. Bone & Joint Surg. **21**:314-322, 1939.
Ghormley, R. K., and Adson, A. W.:	Hemangioma of vertebrae	J. Bone & Joint Surg. **23**:887-895, 1941.
Gilmer, W. S., Jr., Higley, G. B., and Kilgore, W. E.:	Atlas of bone tumors; including tumorlike lesions	St. Louis, The C. V. Mosby Co., 1963.
Golding, J. S. R.:	The natural history of osteoid osteoma	J. Bone & Joint Surg. **36-B**:218-229, 1954.
Greenwald, C. M., Meaney, T. F., and Hughes, C. R.:	Chordoma—uncommon destructive lesion of cerebrospinal axis	J.A.M.A. **163**:1240-1244, 1957.
Haggart, G. E., Johnston, D. O., and Creeden, F.:	Supervoltage radiation for sarcomata of the pelvis and lower extremities	J. Bone & Joint Surg. **40-A**:870-876, 1958.
Hayles, A. B., Dahlin, D. C., and Coventry, M. B.:	Osteogenic sarcoma in children	J.A.M.A. **174**:1174-1177, 1960.
Jaffe, H. L.:	Osteogenic sarcoma of bone	In De Palma, A. F., editor: Clinical orthopaedics, vol. 7, Philadelphia, J. B. Lippincott Co., 1956, pp. 27-40.
	Tumors and tumorous conditions of the bones and joints	Philadelphia, Lea & Febiger, 1958.
Jaffe, H. L., and Lichtenstein, L.:	Osteoid-osteoma	J. Bone & Joint Surg. **22**:645-682, 1940.
	Solitary benign enchondroma of bone	Arch. Surg. **46**:480-493, 1943.
	Solitary unicameral bone cyst, with emphasis on the roentgen picture, the pathologic appearance and the pathogenesis	Arch. Surg. **44**:1004-1025, 1942.
Johnson, E. W., Jr.:	Intramedullary fixation of pathological fractures	J.A.M.A. **163**:417-419, 1957.
Johnson, E. W., Jr., and Dahlin, D. C.:	Treatment of giant-cell tumor of bone	J. Bone & Joint Surg. **41-A**:895-904, 1959.
Kenny, J. J., and Moloney, W. C.:	Multiple myeloma: diagnosis and management in a series of 57 cases	Ann. Int. Med. **46**:1079-1091, 1957.
Kunkel, M. G., Dahlin, D. C., and Young, H. H.:	Benign chondroblastoma	J. Bone & Joint Surg. **38-A**:817-826, 1956.
Lichtenstein, L.:	Aneurysmal bone cyst	J. Bone & Joint Surg. **39-A**:873-882, 1957.
	Bone tumors, 2nd edition	St. Louis, The C. V. Mosby Co., 1959.

Bibliography

Lichtenstein, L., and Jaffe, H. L.:	Chondrosarcoma of bone	Am. J. Path. **19**:553-574, 1943.
	Ewing's sarcoma of bone	Am. J. Path. **23**:43-78, 1947.
Lumb, G., and Mackenzie, D. H.:	Round-cell tumours of bone	Brit. J. Surg. **43**:380-389, 1956.
Lumb, G., and Prossor, T. M.:	Plasma cell tumours	J. Bone & Joint Surg. **30-B**:124-152, 1948.
Marbrey, R. E.:	Chordoma: a study of 150 cases	Am. J. Cancer **25**:501-517, 1935.
McCarroll, H. R.:	Practical considerations in the management of malignant bone tumors	J.A.M.A. **152**:297-300, 1953.
Magnus, H. A., and Wood, H. L.-C.:	Primary reticulo-sarcoma of bone	J. Bone & Joint Surg. **38-B**:258-278, 1956.
Morton, J. J., and Mider, G. B.:	Chondrosarcoma	Ann. Surg. **126**:895-931, 1947.
Phalen, G. S.:	Hodgkin's disease of bone	In De Palma, A. F., editor: Clinical orthopaedics, vol. 13, Philadelphia, J. B. Lippincott Co., 1959, pp. 234-244.
Ralph, L. L.:	Chondromyxoid fibroma of bone	J. Bone & Joint Surg. **44-**□:7-24, 1962.
Scaglietti, O., and Calandriello, B.:	Ossifying parosteal sarcoma	J. Bone & Joint Surg. **44-A**:635-647, 1962.
Schajowicz, F.:	Giant-cell tumors of bone (osteoclastoma)	J. Bone & Joint Surg. **43-A**:1-29, 1961.
Selby, S.:	Metaphyseal cortical defects in the tubular bones of growing children	J. Bone & Joint Surg. **43-A**:395-400, 1961.
Sherman, M. S.:	Osteoid osteoma, review of the literature and report of thirty cases	J. Bone & Joint Surg. **29**:918-930, 1947.
Sherman, R. S., and Soong, K. Y.:	Ewing's sarcoma: its roentgen classification and diagnosis	Radiology **66**:529-539, 1956.
Staley, C. J.:	Skeletal metastases in cancer of the breast	Surg., Gynec. & Obst. **102**:683-688, 1956.
Thomas, G. L.:	Metastasis to bone in gastrointestinal malignancy	S. Clin. North America **26**:692-694, 1946.
Thomson, A. D., and Turner-Warwick, R. T.:	Skeletal sarcomata and giant-cell tumour	J. Bone & Joint Surg. **37-B**:266-303, 1955.
Troup, J. B., and Bickel, W. H.:	Malignant disease of the extremities treated by exarticulation, analysis of 264 consecutive cases with survival rates	J. ̄one & Joint Surg. **42-A**:1041-1050, 1960.
Tudway, R. C.:	The place of external irradiation in the treatment of osteogenic sarcoma	J. Bone & Joint Surg. **35-B**:9-21, 1953.
Turner, J. W., and Jaffe, H. L.:	Metastatic neoplasms, a clinical and roentgenological study of involvement of skeleton and lungs	Am. J. Roentgenol. **43**:479-492, 1940.
Weinfeld, M. S., and Dudley, H. R., Jr.:	Osteogenic sarcoma	J. Bone & Joint Surg. **44-A**:269-276, 1962.
Windeyer, B. W.:	Chordoma	Proc. Roy. Soc. Med. **52**:1088-1100, 1959.

Tumors of soft tissues

Bennett, G. A.:	Malignant neoplasms originating in synovial tissues (synoviomata)	J. Bone & Joint Surg. 29:259-291, 1947.
Berger, L.:	Synovial sarcomas in serous bursae and tendon sheaths	Am. J. Cancer 34:501-539, 1938.
Cobey, M. C.:	Hemangioma of joints	Arch. Surg. 46:465-468, 1943.
De Santo, D. A., and Wilson, P. D.:	Xanthomatous tumors of joints	J. Bone & Joint Surg. 21:531-558, 1939.
Dockerty, M. B.:	Synovial sarcomas	American Academy of Orthopaedic Surgeons Instructional Course Lectures, vol. XI, Ann Arbor, J. W. Edwards, 1954, pp. 45-49.
Galloway, J. D. B., Broders, A. C., and Ghormley, R. K.:	Xanthoma of tendon sheaths and synovial membranes, a clinical and pathologic study	Arch. Surg. 40:485-538, 1940.
Geschickter, C. F., and Lewis, D.:	Tumors of tendon sheaths, joints, and bursae	Am. J. Cancer 22:96-126, 1934.
Ghormley, R. K.:	Soft-tissue tumors of the extremities exclusive of skin and lymphatics	Arch. Surg. 72:817-823, 1956.
Haagensen, C. D., and Stout, A. P.:	Synovial sarcoma	Ann. Surg. 120:826-842, 1944.
Hunt, J. C., and Pugh, D. G.:	Skeletal lesions in neurofibromatosis	Radiology 76:1-20, 1961.
Ivins, J. C.:	Fibrosarcoma of the soft tissues of the extremities	American Academy of Orthopaedic Surgeons Instructional Course Lectures, vol. XI, Ann Arbor, J. W. Edwards, 1954, pp. 18-22.
Jenkins, S. A.:	Solitary tumours of peripheral nerve trunks	J. Bone & Joint Surg. 34-B:401-411, 1952.
Johnson, E. W., Jr., Ghormley, R. K., and Dockerty, M. B.:	Hemangiomas of the extremities	Surg., Gynec. & Obst. 102:531-538, 1956.
King, E. S. J.:	Concerning the pathology of tumours of tendon-sheaths	Brit. J. Surg. 18:594-617, 1931.
Lawrence, E. A., Dickey, J. W., and Vellios, F.:	Malignant tumors of the soft tissues of the extremities	Arch. Surg. 67:392-401, 1953.
Lichtenstein, L.:	Tumors of synovial joints, bursae and tendon sheaths	Cancer 8:816-830, 1955.
Mason, M. L., and Woolston, W. H.:	Isolated giant cell xanthomatic tumors of the fingers and hand	Arch. Surg. 15:499-529, 1927.
McCarroll, H. R.:	Soft-tissue neoplasms associated with congenital neurofibromatosis	J. Bone & Joint Surg. 38-A:717-731, 1956.
Pack, G. T.:	End results in the treatment of sarcomata of the soft somatic tissues	J. Bone & Joint Surg. 36-A:241-263, 1954.
Pinkel, D., and Pickren, J.:	Rhabdomyosarcoma in children	J.A.M.A. 175:293-298, 1961.
Shallow, T. A., Eger, S. A., and Wagner, F. B., Jr.:	Primary hemangiomatous tumors of skeletal muscle	Ann. Surg. 119:700-740, 1944.
Sharpe, J. C., and Young, R. H.:	Recklinghausen's neurofibromatosis, clinical manifestations in 31 cases	Arch. Int. Med. 59:299-328, 1937.

Soule, E. H.:	Lipomatous tumors: classification, pathology, and diagnosis	American Academy of Orthopaedic Surgeons Instructional Course Lectures, vol. XIV, Ann Arbor, J. W. Edwards, 1957, pp. 311-320.
	Myomatous tumors of the extremities: classification and pathology	American Academy of Orthopaedic Surgeons Instructional Course Lectures, vol. XIV, Ann Arbor, J. W. Edwards, 1957, pp. 321-328.
Stout, A. P.:	Tumors of the peripheral nervous system	Washington, D. C., Armed Forces Institute of Pathology, 1949.
	Tumors of the soft tissues	Washington, D. C., Armed Forces Institute of Pathology, 1953.
Sullivan, C. R., Dahlin, D. C., and Bryan, R. S.:	Lipoma of the tendon sheath	J. Bone & Joint Surg. **38-A**:1275-1280, 1956.
Tillotson, J. F., McDonald, J. R., and Janes, J. M.:	Synovial sarcomata	J. Bone & Joint Surg. **33-A**:459-473, 1951.

Chapter 14

Fracture deformities

General problems of bone formation and repair

Bassett, C. A. L.:	Current concepts of bone formation	American Academy of Orthopaedic Surgeons Instructional Courses; J. Bone & Joint Surg. **44-A**:1217-1244, 1962.
Bourne, G. H.:	The biochemistry and physiology of bone	New York, Academic Press, Inc., 1956.
Eggers, G. W. N., Shindler, T. O., and Pomerat, C. M.:	Influence of contact-compression factor on osteogenesis in surgical fractures	J. Bone & Joint Surg. **31-A**:693-716, 1949.
Haldeman, K. O.:	Factors determining the deposition and demineralization of bone	J. Bone & Joint Surg. **32-A**:596-600, 1950.
Ham, A. W.:	Some histophysiological problems peculiar to calcified tissues	J. Bone & Joint Surg. **34-A**:701-728, 1952.
Howard, J. E.:	Some current concepts on the mechanism of calcification	J. Bone & Joint Surg. **33-A**:801-806, 1951.
Johnson, R. W., Jr.:	A physiological study of the blood supply of the diaphysis	J. Bone & Joint Surg. **9**:153-184, 1927.
Leriche, R., and Policard, A.:	The normal and pathological physiology of bone	St. Louis, The C. V. Mosby Co., 1928.
Lorch, I. J.:	Alkaline phosphatase and the mechanism of ossification	J. Bone & Joint Surg. **31-B**:94-99, 1949.
Martland, M., and Robison, R.:	The possible significance of hexose-phosphoric esters in ossification, the bone phosphatase	Biochem. J. **21**:665-674, 1927.
McLean, F. C., and Budy, A. M.:	Radioisotopes in the study of bone	In De Palma, A. F., editor: Clinical orthopaedics, vol. 24, Philadelphia, J. B. Lippincott Co., 1962, pp. 178-197.

Phemister, D. B.:	Repair of bone in the presence of aseptic necrosis resulting from fractures, transplantations, and vascular obstruction	J. Bone & Joint Surg. **12**:769-787, 1930.
Robinson, R. A.:	An electron-microscopic study of the crystalline inorganic component of bone and its relationship to the organic matrix	J. Bone & Joint Surg. **34-A**:389-435, 1952.

Delayed union, malunion, and nonunion

Abbott, L. C., Schottstaedt, E. R., Saunders, J. B. De C. M., and Bost, F. C.:	The evaluation of cortical and cancellous bone as grafting material	J. Bone & Joint Surg. **29**:-381 414, 1947.
Barr, J. S., et al.:	Fracture of the carpal navicular (scaphoid) bone, an end-result study in military personnel	J. Bone & Joint Surg. **35-A**:609-625, 1953.
Bickel, W. H.:	Bone repair, delayed union, nonunion, and malunion	In Cyclopedia of medicine, surgery, specialties, vol. 5, Philadelphia, F. A. Davis Co., 1951, pp. 843-888.
Blount, W. P.:	Proximal osteotomies of the femur	American Academy of Orthopaedic Surgeons Instructional Course Lectures, vol. IX, Ann Arbor, J. W. Edwards, 1952, pp. 1-29.
Bonfiglio, M., and Bardenstein, M. B.:	Treatment by bone-grafting of aseptic necrosis of the femoral head and non-union of the femoral neck (Phemister technique)	J. Bone & Joint Surg. **40-A**:1329-1346, 1958.
Boyd, H. B.:	Avascular necrosis of the head of the femur	American Academy of Orthopaedic Surgeons Instructional Course Lectures, vol. XIV, Ann Arbor, J. W. Edwards, 1957, pp. 196-204.
Boyd, H. B., and Brindley, H. H.:	Nonunion of the neck of the femur, study of 347 cases	Arch. Surg. **65**:169-180, 1952.
Boyd, H. B., and Lipinski, S. W.:	Causes and treatment of nonunion of the shafts of the long bones	American Academy of Orthopaedic Surgeons Instructional Course Lectures, vol. XVII, St. Louis, The C. V. Mosby Co., 1960, pp. 165-183.
Boyd, H. B., and Sage, F. P.:	Congenital pseudarthrosis of the tibia	J. Bone & Joint Surg. **40-A**:1245-1270, 1958.
Boyd, H. B., Lipinski, S. W., and Wiley, J. H.:	Observations on non-union of the shafts of the long bones, with a statistical analysis of 842 patients	J. Bone & Joint Surg. **43-A**:159-168, 1961.
Brav, E. A., and Blair, J. D.:	Reconstruction procedures for forearm bone defects	Am. J. Surg. **86**:139-144, 1953.
Campbell, W. C.:	Malunited fractures and unreduced dislocations about the elbow	J.A.M.A. **92**:122-128, 1929.
	Malunited Colles' fractures	J.A.M.A. **109**:1105-1108, 1937.
	Onlay bone graft for ununited fractures	Arch. Surg. **38**:313-327, 1939.

Capener, N.:	Reconstructive surgery of the hip joint	In Platt, Sir H., editor: Modern trends in orthopaedics, second series, New York, Paul B. Hoeber, Inc., 1956, Chap. 1, pp. 1-35.
Carr, C. R., and Hyatt, G. W.:	Clinical evaluation of freeze-dried bone grafts	J. Bone & Joint Surg. 37-A:549-566, 1955.
Cave, E. F.:	The healing of fractures and non-union of bone	S. Clin. North America 43:337-349, 1963.
Charnley, J.:	Congenital pseudarthrosis of the tibia treated by the intramedullary nail	J. Bone & Joint Surg. 38-A:283-290, 1956.
Cleveland, M., and Fielding, J. W.:	A continuing end-result study of intracapsular fracture of the neck of the femur	J. Bone & Joint Surg. 36-A:1020-1030, 1954.
Cleveland, M., and Winant, E. M.:	Treatment of non-union in compound fractures with infection	J. Bone & Joint Surg. 34-A:554-563, 1952.
Colonna, P. C.:	The trochanteric reconstruction operation for ununited fractures of the upper end of the femur	J. Bone & Joint Surg. 42-B:5-10, 1960.
Connelly, J. R.:	Plastic surgery in bone problems	Plast. & Reconstruct. Surg. 17:129-167, 1956.
Cooper, W.:	Aseptic (avascular) necrosis of the femoral head in adults	In Carter, B. N., editor: Monographs on surgery for 1952, Baltimore, Williams & Wilkins Co., 1952, pp. 214-252.
Coventry, M. B.:	The Phemister bone graft in ununited fractures of the long bones	In De Palma, A. F., editor: Clinical orthopaedics, vol. 2, Philadelphia, J. B. Lippincott Co., 1953, pp. 194-202.
Dickson, J. A.:	The high geometric osteotomy, with rotation and bone graft, for ununited fractures of the neck of the femur	J. Bone & Joint Surg. 29:1005-1018, 1947.
	The "unsolved" fracture	J. Bone & Joint Surg. 35-A:805-822, 1953.
Dineen, J. R., and Gresham, R. B.:	Rib osteoperiosteal grafts	J. Bone & Joint Surg. 44-A:1653-1658, 1962.
Durman, D. C.:	An operation for correction of deformities of the wrist following fracture	J. Bone & Joint Surg. 17:1014-1016, 1935.
Flanagan, J. J., and Burem, H. S.:	Reconstruction of defects of the tibia and femur with apposing massive grafts from the affected bone	J. Bone & Joint Surg. 29:587-597, 1947.
Garber, C. Z., and Bush, L. F.:	The bone bank and the use of homogenous bone	In Carter, B. N., editor: Monographs on surgery for 1950, New York, Thos. Nelson & Sons, 1950, pp. 383-407.
Gibson, A., and Loadman, B.:	The bridging of bone defects	J. Bone & Joint Surg. 30-A:381-396, 1948.
Green, W. T., and Rudo, N.:	Pseudarthrosis and neurofibromatosis	Arch. Surg. 46:639-651, 1943.
Hallock, H.:	Arthrodesis of the ankle joint for old painful fractures	J. Bone & Joint Sugr. 27:49-58, 1945.

Bibliography

Herndon, C. H.:	Principles of bone graft surgery—different methods of operative procedure and indications for each	American Academy of Orthopaedic Surgeons Instructional Course Lectures, vol. XVII, St. Louis, The C. V. Mosby Co., 1960, pp. 149-164.
Higgs, S. L.:	The use of cancellous chips in bone-grafting	J. Bone & Joint Surg. 28:15-18, 1946.
Horwitz, T., and Lambert, R. G.:	Massive iliac bone grafts in the treatment of ununited fractures and large defects of long bones; the combined bone graft-metallic plate technique	Surg., Gynec. & Obst. 84:435-450, 1947.
Jackson, R. W., and Macnab, I.:	Fractures of the shaft of the tibia, a clinical and experimental study	Am. J. Surg. 97:543-557, 1959.
King, D., and Secor, C.:	Bow elbow (cubitus varus)	J. Bone & Joint Surg. 33-A:572-576, 1951.
Leadbetter, G. W.:	A treatment for fracture of the neck of the femur	J. Bone & Joint Surg. 15:931-940, 1933.
MacAusland, W. R.:	Total patellectomy	Am. J. Surg. 87:221-226, 1954.
Mazet, R., Jr., and Hohl, M.:	Fractures of the carpal navicular	J. Bone & Joint Surg. 45-A:82-112, 1963.
McCarroll, H. R.:	The surgical management of ununited fractures of the tibia	J.A.M.A. 175:578-583, 1961.
McFarland, B.:	Pseudarthrosis of the tibia in childhood	J. Bone & Joint Surg. 33-B:36-46, 1951.
McKeever, F. M.:	Fractures of tarsal and metatarsal bones	Surg., Gynec. & Obst. 90:735-745, 1950.
Milch, H.:	Fractures of the external humeral condyle	J.A.M.A. 160:641-646, 1956.
Moore, J. R.:	Cartilaginous-cup arthroplasty in ununited fractures of the neck of the femur	J. Bone & Joint Surg. 30-A:313-330, 1948.
	Congenital pseudarthrosis of the tibia	American Academy of Orthopaedic Surgeons Instructional Course Lectures, vol. XIV, Ann Arbor, J. W. Edwards, 1957, pp. 222-237.
Phemister, D. B.:	Treatment of ununited fractures by onlay bone grafts without screw or tie fixation and without breaking down of the fibrous union	J. Bone & Joint Surg. 29:946-960, 1947.
Reich, R. S.:	Treatment of ununited fractures of the neck of the femur	American Academy of Orthopaedic Surgeons Instructional Course Lectures, vol. XVII, St. Louis, The C. V. Mosby Co., 1960, pp. 68-77.
Reynolds, F. C., and Oliver, D. R.:	Experimental evaluation of homogenous bone grafts	J. Bone & Joint Surg. 32-A:283-297, 1950.
Salner, N. P., and Pendergrass, E. P.:	Roentgenologic considerations in fractures of the neck of the femur, a review of pertinent aspects of diagnosis and treatment	Am. J. Roentgenol. 67:732-756, 1952.

Schumm, H. C.:	The Schanz osteotomy for fractures of the neck of the femur	J. Bone & Joint Surg. **19**:955-963, 1937.
Shands, A. R., Jr.:	Malunited fractures of lower end of humerus	Am. J. Surg. **36**:679-693, 1937.
Sherman, M. S., and Phemister, D. B.:	The pathology of ununited fractures of the neck of the femur	J. Bone & Joint Surg. **29**:19-40, 1947.
Smith-Petersen, M. N.:	Treatment of fractures of the neck of the femur by internal fixation	Surg., Gynec. & Obst. **64**:287-295, 1937.
Speed, J. S., and Knight, R. A.:	The treatment of malunited Colles' fractures	J. Bone & Joint Surg. **27**:361-367, 1945.
Speed, J. S., and Smith, H.:	Trochanteric osteotomy for ununited fractures of the neck of the femur	South. M. J. **34**:798-806, 1941.
Stewart, M. J.:	Fractures of the carpal navicular (scaphoid), a report of 436 cases	J. Bone & Joint Surg. **36-A**:998-1006, 1954.
Stewart, M. J., and Wells, R. E.:	Osteotomy and osteotomy combined with bone-grafting for non-union following fracture of the femoral neck	J. Bone & Joint Surg. **38-A**:33-49, 1956.
Taylor, L. W.:	Principles of treatment of fractures and non-union of the shaft of the femur	American Academy of Orthopaedic Surgeons Instructional Courses; J. Bone & Joiut Surg. **45-A**:191-198, 1963.
Urist, M. R.:	Bone: transplants, implants, derivatives, and substitutes—a survey of research of the past decade	American Academy of Orthopaedic Surgeons Instructional Course Lectures, vol. XVII, St. Louis, The C. V. Mosby Co., 1960, pp. 184-195.
Urist, M. R., Mazet, R., Jr., and McLean, F. C.:	The pathogenesis and treatment of delayed union and non-union, a survey of 85 ununited fractures of the shaft of the tibia and 100 control cases with similar injuries	J. Bone & Joint Surg. **36-A**:931-968, 1954.
Watson-Jones, R., and Coltart, W. D.:	Slow union of fractures, with a study of 804 fractures of the shafts of the tibia and femur	Brit. J. Surg. **30**:260-276, 1943.
Wilson, P. D.:	Fracture of the lateral condyle of the humerus in childhood	J. Bone & Joint Surg. **18**:301-318, 1936.
	Experience with the use of refrigerated homogenous bone	J. Bone & Joint Surg. **33-B**:301-315, 1951.

Chapter 15

Amputations, prostheses, and braces

Amputations

Aitken, G. T., and Frantz, C. H.:	Management of the child amputee	American Academy of Orthopaedic Surgeons Instructional Course Lectures, vol. XVII, St. Louis, The C. V. Mosby Co., 1960, pp. 246-295.
	The juvenile amputee	J. Bone & Joint Surg. **35-A**:659-664, 1953.

Bibliography

Alldredge, R. H.:	Amputations and artificial limbs	In Christopher, F., editor: textbook of surgery, ed. 6, Philadelphia, W. B. Saunders Co., 1956, pp. 1240-1256.
	Major amputations	Surg., Gynec. & Obst. 84:759-764, 1947.
Bailey, R. W., and Stevens, D. B.:	Radical exarticulation of the extremities for the curative and palliative treatment of malignant neoplasms	J. Bone & Joint Surg. 43-A:845-854, 1961.
Boyd, H. B.:	Amputation of the foot, with calcaneotibial arthrodesis	J. Bone & Joint Surg. 21:997-1000, 1939.
Brav, E. A., et al.:	Cineplasty	J. Bone & Joint Surg. 39-A:59-76, 1957.
Compere, C. L., and Thompson, R. G.:	Amputations and modern prosthetics	S. Clin. North America 37:103-118, 1957.
Dale, R. H.:	Electrical accidents, a discussion with illustrative cases	Brit. J. Plast. Surg. 7:44-66, 1954.
Falconer, M. A.:	Surgical treatment of intractable phantom-limb pain	Brit. M. J. 1:299-304, 1953.
Gillis, L.:	Amputations	London, William Heinemann, Ltd., 1954.
Hall, C. B., Brooks, M. B., and Dennis, J. F.:	Congenital skeletal deficiencies of the extremities, classification and fundamentals of treatment	J.A.M.A. 181:590-599, 1962.
Harris, R. I.:	Syme's amputation	J. Bone & Joint Surg. 38-B:614-632, 1956.
Kelly, P. J., and Janes, J. M.:	Criteria for determining the proper level of amputation in occlusive vascular disease	J. Bone & Joint Surg. 39-A:883-891, 1957.
Lambert, C. N., and Novotny, A. J.:	Amputations and amputees—adult and juvenile	S. Clin. North America 37:119-134, 1957.
Mazet, R., Jr.:	Cineplasty	J. Bone & Joint Surg. 40-A:1389-1400, 1958.
Mazet, R., Jr., Taylor, C. L., and Bechtol, C. O.:	Upper-extremity amputation surgery and prosthetic prescription	J. Bone & Joint Surg. 38-A:1185-1198, 1956.
Mercer, W.:	Syme's amputation	Artificial Limbs 6:1-3, 1961.
Morris, H. D.:	Amputations for congenital anomalies of the lower extremities	American Academy of Orthopaedic Surgeons Instructional Course Lectures, vol. XV, Ann Arbor, J. W. Edwards, 1958, pp. 255-261.
Moseley, H. F.:	The forequarter amputation	Philadelphia, J. B. Lippincott Co., 1957.
Pack, G. T.:	Major exarticulations for malignant neoplasms of the extremities	J. Bone & Joint Surg. 38-A:249-262, 1956.
Pedersen, H. E.:	Lower extremity amputations for gangrene	American Academy of Orthopaedic Surgeons Instructional Course Lectures, vol. XV, Ann Arbor, J. W. Edwards, 1958, pp. 262-281.
Russell, W. R., and Spalding, J. M. K.:	Treatment of painful amputation stumps	Brit. M. J. 2:68-73, 1950.

Slocum, D. B.:	Amputations of the fingers and the hand	In DePalma, A. F., editor: Clinical orthopaedics, vol. 15, Philadelphia, J. B. Lippincott Co., 1959, pp. 35-59.
	An atlas of amputations	St. Louis, The C. V. Mosby Co., 1949.
Smith, B. C.:	A twenty-year follow-up in fifty below knee amputations for gangrene in diabetics	Surg., Gynec. & Obst. **103**:625-630, 1956.
Zanoli, R.:	Krukenberg - Putti amputation - plasty	J. Bone & Joint Surg. **39-B**:230-232, 1957.

Prostheses

American Academy of Orthopaedic Surgeons, Office of the Surgeon General of the U. S. Army, and the Veterans Administration:	Orthopaedic appliances atlas, vol. 2: Artificial limbs	Ann Arbor, J. W. Edwards, 1960.
Anderson, M. H., Bechtol, C. O., and Sollars, R. E.:	Clinical prosthetics for physicians and therapists	Springfield, Ill., Charles C Thomas, Publisher, 1959.
Bechtol, C. O., and Compere, C. L.:	The above-knee suction-socket artificial leg	American Academy of Orthopaedic Surgeons Instructional Course Lectures, vol. IX, Ann Arbor, J. W. Edwards, 1952, pp. 247-249.
Bunnell, S.:	The management of the nonfunctional hand—reconstruction vs. prosthesis	Artificial Limbs **4**:76-102, 1957.
Klopsteg, P. E., and Wilson, P. D.:	Human limbs and their substitutes	New York, McGraw-Hill Book Co., Inc., 1954.
Lambert, C. N.:	Upper-extremity prostheses in juvenile amputees	J. Bone & Joint Surg. **38-A**:421-426, 1956.
McKenzie, D. S.:	The prosthetic management of congenital deformities of the extremities	J. Bone & Joint Surg. **39-B**:233-247, 1957.
Murphy, E. F., and Wilson, A. B.:	Anatomical and physiological considerations in below-knee prosthetics	Artificial Limbs **6**:4-15, 1962.
Thorndike, A., and Eberhart, H. D.:	Suction socket prosthesis for above-knee amputations	Am. J. Surg. **80**:727-731, 1950.
Tosberg, W. A.:	Upper and lower extremity prostheses	Springfield, Ill., Charles C Thomas, Publisher, 1962.

Braces

Alldredge, R. H., and Snow, B. M.:	Principles of ambulatory bracing of the lower extremity	American Academy of Orthopaedic Surgeons Instructional Course Lectures, vol. X, Ann Arbor, J. W. Edwards, 1953, pp. 293-298.
American Academy of Orthopaedic Surgeons, Office of the Surgeon General of the U. S. Army, and the Veterans Administration:	Orthopaedic appliances atlas, Vol. 1: Braces, splints, shoe alterations	Ann Arbor, J. W. Edwards, 1952.

Anderson, M. H.:	Functional bracing of the upper extremities	Springfield, Ill., Charles C Thomas, Publisher, 1958.
Bunnell, S.:	Splinting the hand	American Academy of Orthopaedic Surgeons Instructional Course Lectures, vol. IX, Ann Arbor, J. W. Edwards, 1952, pp. 233-243.
Deaver, G. G., and Brittis, A. L.:	Braces, crutches, wheelchairs	New York, Institute of Physical Medicine and Rehabilitation, 1953.
Schottstaedt, E. R., and Robinson, G. B.:	Functional bracing of the arm	J. Bone & Joint Surg. **38-A**:477-499, 841-856, 1956.
Street, D. M.:	Paraplegic bracing	American Academy of Orthopaedic Surgeons Instructional Course Lectures, vol. XIV, Ann Arbor, J. W. Edwards, 1957, pp. 336-341.
Thomas, A.:	Braces for the spine and trunk	American Academy of Orthopaedic Surgeons Instructional Course Lectures, vol. X, Ann Arbor, J. W. Edwards, 1953, pp. 298-302.

Chapter 16

Affections of the spine and thorax

Affections of the spine

American Orthopaedic Association, Research Committee:	End-result study of the treatment of idiopathic scoliosis	J. Bone & Joint Surg. **23**:963-977, 1941.
Bingold, A. C.:	Congenital kyphosis	J. Bone & Joint Surg. **35-B**:579-583, 1953.
Blount, W. P., Schmidt, A. C., Keever, E. D., and Leonard, E. T.:	The Milwaukee brace in the operative treatment of scoliosis	J. Bone & Joint Surg. **40-A**:511-525, 1958.
Cobb, J. R.:	Technique, after-treatment, and results of spine fusion for scoliosis	American Academy of Orthopaedic Surgeons Instructional Course Lectures, vol. IX, Ann Arbor, J. W. Edwards, 1952, pp. 65-70.
Compere, E. L., Johnson, W. E., and Coventry, M. B.:	Vertebra plana (Calvé's disease) due to eosinophilic granuloma	J. Bone & Joint Surg. **36-A**:969-980, 1954.
Edelstein, J. M.:	Adolescent kyphosis	Brit. J. Surg. **22**:119-133, 1934.
Epstein, B. S.:	The spine, a radiological text and atlas, 2nd edition	Philadelphia, Lea & Febiger, 1962.
Goldthwait, J. E., Brown, L. T., Swaim, L. T., and Kuhns, J. G.:	Essentials of body mechanics in health and disease, 4th edition	Philadelphia, J. B. Lippincott Co., 1945.
Harrington, P. R.:	Treatment of scoliosis, correction and internal fixation by spine instrumentation	J. Bone & Joint Surg. **44-A**:591-610, 1962.
Hellebrandt, F. A., and Franseen, E. B.:	Physiological study of the vertical stance of man	Physiol. Rev. **23**:220-255, 1943.
Hibbs, R. A., Risser, J. C., and Ferguson, A. B.:	Scoliosis treated by the fusion operation, an end-result study of 360 cases	J. Bone & Joint Surg. **13**:91-104, 1931.

Hodgen, J. T., and Frantz, C. H.:	Juvenile kyphosis	Surg., Gynec. & Obst. 72:798-806, 1941.
Howorth, B.:	Dynamic posture	J.A.M.A. 131:1398-1404, 1946.
James, J. I. P.:	Idiopathic scoliosis, the prognosis, diagnosis, and operative indications related to curve patterns and the age at onset	J. Bone & Joint Surg. 36-B:36-49, 1954.
	Paralytic scoliosis	J. Bone & Joint Surg. 38-B:660-685, 1956.
James, J. I. P., Lloyd-Roberts, G. C., and Pilcher, M. F.:	Infantile structural scoliosis	J. Bone & Joint Surg. 41-B:719-735, 1959.
Keegan, J. J.:	Alterations of the lumbar curve related to posture and seating	J. Bone & Joint Surg. 35-A:589-603, 1953.
Keith, A.:	Man's posture: its evolution and disorders	Brit. M. J. 1:451-454, 1923.
Kuhns, J. G., and Hormell, R. S.:	Management of congenital scoliosis, review of 170 cases	Arch. Surg. 65:250-263, 1952.
Lowman, C. L., and Young, C. H.:	Postural fitness: significance and variances	Philadelphia, Lea & Febiger, 1960.
MacGowan, T. J. B. A.:	Adolescent kyphosis	Lancet 1:211-214, 1944.
McKenzie, K. G., and Dewar, F. P.:	Scoliosis with paraplegia	J. Bone & Joint Surg. 31-B:162-174, 1949.
Moe, J. H.:	A critical analysis of methods of fusion for scoliosis	J. Bone & Joint Surg. 40-A:529-554, 1958.
	The management of paralytic scoliosis	South. M. J. 50:67-81, 1957.
Morgan, T. H., and Scott, J. C.:	Treatment of infantile idiopathic scoliosis	J. Bone & Joint Surg. 38-B:450-457, 1956.
Nassim, R., and Burrows, H. J., editors:	Modern trends in diseases of the vertebral column	New York, Paul B. Hoeber, Inc., 1959.
Nathan, L., and Kuhns, J. G.:	Epiphysitis of the spine	J. Bone & Joint Surg. 22:55-62, 1940.
Osgood, R. B.:	Body mechanics and posture	J.A.M.A. 96:2032-2035, 1931.
Outland, T., and Snedden, H. E.:	Juvenile dorsal kyphosis	In De Palma, A. F., editor: Clinical orthopaedics, vol. 5, Philadelphia, J. B. Lippincott Co., 1955, pp. 155-163.
Phelps, W. M., Kiphuth, R. J. H., and Goff, C. W.:	The diagnosis and treatment of postural defects, 2nd edition	Springfield, Ill., Charles C Thomas, Publisher, 1956.
Ponseti, I. V., and Friedman, B.:	Prognosis in idiopathic scoliosis	J. Bone & Joint Surg. 32-A:381-395, 1950.
	Changes in the scoliotic spine after fusion	J. Bone & Joint Surg. 32-A:751-766, 1950.
Risser, J. C.:	Scoliosis	American Academy of Orthopaedic Surgeons Instructional Course Lectures, vol. XIV, Ann Arbor, J. W. Edwards, 1957, pp. 91-105.
	The iliac apophysis: an invaluable sign in the management of scoliosis	In DePalma, A. F., editor: Clinical orthopaedics, vol. 11, Philadelphia, J. B. Lippincott Co., 1958, pp. 111-119.
Risser, J. C., and Norquist, D. M.:	A follow-up study of the treatment of scoliosis	J. Bone & Joint Surg. 40-A:555-569, 1958.
Roaf R.:	Paralytic scoliosis	J. Bone & Joint Surg. 38-B:640-659, 1956.

Saunders, J. B. de C. M., Inman, V. T., and Eberhart, H. D.:	The major determinants in normal and pathological gait	J. Bone & Joint Surg. **35-A**:543-558, 1953.
Schmorl, G., and Junghanns, H.:	The human spine in health and disease	New York, Grune & Stratton, Inc., 1959.
Schwartz, R. P., and Heath, A. L.:	The definition of human locomotion on the basis of measurement	J. Bone & Joint Surg. **29**:203-214, 1947.
Shands, A. R., Jr., and Eisberg, H. B.:	The incidence of scoliosis in the state of Delaware, a study of 50,000 minifilms of the chest made during a survey for tuberculosis	J. Bone & Joint Surg. **37-A**:1243-1249, 1955.
Smith, A. DeF., Butte, F. L., and Ferguson, A. B.:	Treatment of scoliosis by the wedging jacket and spine fusion	J. Bone & Joint Surg. **20**:825-838, 1938.
Steindler, A.:	On biomechanics (presidential address)	J. Bone & Joint Surg. **15**:567-573, 1933.
	Diseases and deformities of the spine and thorax	St. Louis, The C. V. Mosby Co., 1929.
	Mechanics of normal and pathological locomotion in man	Springfield, Ill., Charles C Thomas, Publisher, 1935.
Weston, W. J., and Goodson, G. M.:	Vertebra plana (Calvé)	J. Bone & Joint Surg. **41-B**:477-485, 1959.
Willis, T. A.:	Structure and development of the spine	J.A.M.A. **125**:407-412, 1944.

Deformities of the thorax

Chin, E. F.:	Surgery of funnel chest and congenital sternal prominence	Brit. J. Surg. **44**:360-376, 1957.
King, F. G.:	Surgical correction of funnel chest	Ann. Surg. **136**:798-810, 1952.
Lester, C. W.:	Pigeon breast, funnel chest, and other congenital deformities of the chest	J.A.M.A. **156**:1063-1067, 1954.
Sutherland, I. D.:	Funnel chest	J. Bone & Joint Surg. **40-B**:244-251, 1958.

Chapter 17

Affections of the low back

Abbott, K. H., and Retter, R. H.:	Protrusions of thoracic intervertebral disks	Neurology **6**:1-10, 1956.
Adkins, E. W. O.:	Spondylolisthesis	J. Bone & Joint Surg. **37-B**:48-62, 1955.
Aitken, A. P.:	Rupture of the intervertebral disc in industry, further observations on the end results	Am. J. Surg. **84**:261-267, 1952.
Andrew, J.:	Sacralization: an aetiological factor in lumbar intervertebral disk lesions, and a cause of misleading focal signs	Brit. J. Surg. **42**:304-311, 1954.
Armstrong, J. R.:	Lumbar disc lesions: pathogenesis and treatment of low back pain and sciatica, 2nd edition	Baltimore, Williams & Wilkins Co., 1958.
Barr, J. S.:	Low-back and sciatic pain, results of treatment	J. Bone & Joint Surg. **33-A**:633-649, 1951.

Bibliography

Barr, J. S., Hampton, A. O., and Mixter, W. J.:	Pain low in the back and "sciatica," due to lesions of the intervertebral disks	J.A.M.A. 109:1265-1270, 1937.
Bosworth, D. M.:	Surgery of the spine	American Academy of Orthopaedic Surgeons Instructional Course Lectures, vol. XIV, Ann Arbor, J. W. Edwards, 1957, pp. 39-55.
Bosworth, D. M., Fielding, J. W., Demarest, L., and Bonaquist, M.:	Spondylolisthesis, a critical review of a consecutive series of cases treated by arthrodesis	J. Bone & Joint Surg. 37-A:767-786, 1955.
Brav, E. A.:	An analysis of orthopedic causes of low back and sciatic pain	Am. J. Surg. 87:235-240, 1954.
Bucy, P. C.:	Neuroanatomical and neurosurgical aspects of herniated intervertebral discs	American Academy of Orthopaedic Surgeons Instructional Course Lectures, vol. XVIII, St. Louis, The C. V. Mosby Co., 1961, pp. 21-34.
Cain, J. P., Jr.:	Low-back pain, evaluation of disability	Arch. Industr. Health 19:593-595, 1959.
Camp, J. D.:	Contrast myelography past and present	Radiology 54:477-506, 1950.
Chandler, F. A.:	Lesions of the "isthmus" (pars interarticularis) of the laminae of the lower lumbar vertebrae and their relation to spondylolisthesis	Surg., Gynec. & Obst. 53:273-306, 1931.
Cloward, R. B.:	Vertebral body fusion for ruptured lumbar discs, a roentgenographic study	Am. J. Surg. 90:969-976, 1955.
Colonna, P. C.:	Spondylolisthesis, analysis of 201 cases	J.A.M.A 154:398-402, 1954.
Colonna, P. C., and Friedenberg, Z. B.:	Disc syndrome, results of conservative care of patients with positive myelograms	J. Bone & Joint Surg. 31-A:614-618, 1949.
Compere, E. L.:	Origin, anatomy, physiology, and pathology of the intervertebral disc	American Academy of Orthopaedic Surgeons Instructional Course Lectures, vol. XVIII, St. Louis, The C. V. Mosby Co., 1961, pp. 15-20.
Coventry, M. B., Ghormley, R. K., and Kernohan, J. W.:	The intervertebral disc, its microscopic anatomy and pathology	J. Bone & Joint Surg. 27:105-112, 233-247, 460-474, 1945.
Craig, W. M., Svien, H. J., Dodge, H. W., Jr., and Camp, J. D.:	Intraspinal lesions masquerading as protruded lumbar intervertebral disks	J.A.M.A. 149:250-253, 1952.
Danforth, M. S., and Wilson, P. D.:	The anatomy of the lumbo-sacral region in relation to sciatic pain	J. Bone & Joint Surg. 7:109-160, 1925.
Davis, L., Martin, J., and Goldstein, S. L.:	Sensory changes with herniated nucleus pulposus	J. Neurosurg. 9:133-138, 1952.
Deyerle, W. M., and May, V. R., Jr.:	Sciatic tension test	South. M. J. 49:999-1005, 1956.
Duncan, W. S.:	The relation of the prostate gland to orthopaedic problems	J. Bone & Joint Surg. 18:101-104, 1936.
Feffer, H. L., and Adams, J. P.:	Sacro-iliac changes associated with dysfunction of the spine	South. M. J. 51:986-993, 1958.

Ferguson, A. B.:	The clinical and roentgenographic interpretation of lumbosacral anomalies	Radiology 22:548-558, 1934.
Filtzer, D. L., and Bahnson, H. T.:	Low back pain due to arterial obstruction	J. Bone & Joint Surg. 41-B:244-247, 1959.
Ford, L. T., and Key, J. A.:	An evaluation of myelography in the diagnosis of intervertebral-disc lesions in the low back	J. Bone & Joint Surg. 32-A:257-266, 1950.
Friberg, S.:	Studies on spondylolisthesis	Acta chir. scandinav., supp. 55, 1939.
Friedman, J., and Goldner, M. Z.:	Discography in evaluation of lumbar disk lesions	Radiology 65:653-662, 1955.
Ghormley, R. K.:	The problem of multiple operations on the back	American Academy of Orthopaedic Surgeons Instructional Course Lectures, vol. XIV, Ann Arbor, J. W. Edwards, 1957, pp. 56-63.
Greenwood, J., Jr., McGuire, T. H., and Kimbell, F.:	A study of the causes of failure in the herniated intervertebral disc operation, an analysis of 67 reoperated cases	J. Neurosurg. 9:15-20, 1952.
Haggart, G. E., and Grannis, W. R.:	Pantopaque myelography in low back and sciatic pain	S. Clin. North America 32:695-703, 1952.
Harris, R. I., and Macnab, I.:	Structural changes in the lumbar intervertebral discs, their relationship to low back pain and sciatica	J. Bone & Joint Surg. 36-B:304-322, 1954.
Hibbs, R. A., and Swift, W. E.:	Developmental abnormalities at the lumbosacral juncture causing pain and disability	Surg., Gynec. & Obst. 48:604-612, 1929.
Hitchcock, H. H.:	Spondylolisthesis, observations on its development, progression, and genesis	J. Bone & Joint Surg. 22:1-16, 1940.
Howorth, B.:	The painful coccyx	In DePalma, A. F., editor: Clinical orthopaedics, vol. 14, Philadelphia, J. B. Lippincott Co., 1959, pp. 145-161.
Isley, J. K., Jr., and Baylin, G. J.:	Prognosis in osteitis condensans ilii	Radiology 72:234-237, 1959.
Jostes, F. A.:	Place of manipulative procedures in the over-all treatment rationale for painful back conditions	Arch. Phys. Therapy 25:716-720, 1944.
Key, J. A.:	Operative treatment of coccygodynia	J. Bone & Joint Surg. 19:759-764, 1937.
Krusen, E. M., and Ford, D. E.:	Compensation factor in low back injuries	J.A.M.A. 166:1128-1133, 1958.
Lansche, W. E., and Ford, L. T.:	Correlation of the myelogram with clinical and operative findings in lumbar disc lesions	J. Bone & Joint Surg. 42-A:193-206, 1960.
Laurent, L. E.:	Spondylolisthesis, a study of 53 cases treated by spine fusion and 32 cases treated by laminectomy	Acta orthop. scandinav., supp. 35, 1958.

Bibliography

Love, J. G., and Rivers, M. H.:	Spinal cord tumors simulating protruded intervertebral disks	J.A.M.A. **179**:878-881, 1962.
McBride, E. D.:	The conservative treatment of backache	Am. Surgeon **18**:504-512, 1952.
McConville, B. E.:	Conservative management of low back pain	Am. J. Surg. **85**:335-338, 1953.
McCracken, W. J.:	Low back disability	Canad. M. A. J. **80**:331-336, 1959.
Mensor, M. C.:	Non-operative treatment, including manipulation, for lumbar intervertebral disc syndrome	J. Bone & Joint Surg. **37-A**:925-936, 1955.
Meyerding, H. W.:	Spondylolisthesis: surgical treatment and results	J. Bone & Joint Surg. **25**:65-77, 1943.
Millikan, C. H.:	The problem of evaluating treatment of protruded lumbar intervertebral disk, observations of results of conservative and surgical treatment in 429 cases	J.A.M.A. **155**:1141-1143, 1954.
Morgan, F. P., and King, T.:	Primary instability of lumbar vertebrae as a common cause of low back pain	J. Bone & Joint Surg. **39-B**:6-22, 1957.
Morris, J. M., Lucas, D. B., and Bresler, B.:	Role of the trunk in stability of the spine	J. Bone & Joint Surg. **43-A**:327-351, 1961.
Mutch, J., and Walmsley, R.:	The aetiology of cleft vertebral arch in spondylolisthesis	Lancet **1**:74-77, 1956.
Newman, P. H.:	Sprung back	J. Bone & Joint Surg. **34-B**:30-37, 1952.
Newman, P. H., and Stone, K. H.:	The etiology of spondylolisthesis	J. Bone & Joint Surg. **45-B**:39-59, 1963.
O'Connell, J. E. A.:	Involvement of the spinal cord by intervertebral disk protrusions	Brit. J. Surg. **43**:225-247, 1955.
Pietra, A. D.:	Stabilizing spinal fusion following herniated disk removal without fusion	J.A.M.A. **157**:701-702, 1955.
Pyper, J. B.:	Excision of the coccyx for coccydynia	J. Bone & Joint Surg. **39-B**:733-737, 1957.
Raney, R. B.:	Isthmus defects of the fifth lumbar vertebra	South. M. J. **38**:166-176, 1945.
Research Committee of the American Orthopaedic Association (I. W. Nachlas, chairman):	End-result study of the treatment of herniated nucleus pulposus by excision with fusion and without fusion	J. Bone & Joint Surg. **34-A**:981-988, 1952.
Reynolds, F. C., McGinnis, A. E., and Morgan, H. C.:	Surgery in the treatment of low-back pain and sciatica	J. Bone & Joint Surg. **41-A**:223-235, 1959.
Rhodes, M. P., and Colangelo, C.:	Spondylolysis and its relation to spondylolisthesis	Am. J. Surg. **72**:20-25, 1946.
Rojkó, A., and Farkas, K.:	Osteitis condensans ossis ilii	Acta orthop. scandinav. **29**:108-120, 1959.
Rose, G. K.:	Backache and the disc	Lancet **1**:1143-1149, 1954.
Runge, C. F.:	Roentgenographic examination of the lumbosacral spine in routine pre-employment examinations	J. Bone & Joint Surg. **36-A**:75-84, 1954.

Schneider, C. C.:	Diagnosis, treatment, and rehabilitation of the industrial low back cripple	American Academy of Orthopaedic Surgeons Instructional Course Lectures, vol. XVI, St. Louis, The C. V. Mosby Co., 1959, pp. 173-183.
	Trends in disability evaluation, with particular reference to the low back	American Academy of Orthopaedic Surgeons Instructional Course Lectures, vol. XIII, Ann Arbor, J. W. Edwards, 1956, pp. 293-298.
Sell, L. S.:	Misdiagnosis and mismanagement of early intervertebral disk lesions	J.A.M.A. **150**:987-990, 1952.
Shaw, E. G., and Taylor, J. G.:	The results of lumbo-sacral fusion for low back pain	J. Bone & Joint Surg. **38-B**:485-497, 1956.
Shutkin, N. M.:	Syndrome of the degenerated intervertebral disc	Am. J. Surg. **84**:162-171, 1952.
Splithoff, C. A.:	Lumbosacral junction, roentgenographic comparison of patients with and without backaches	J.A.M.A. **152**:1610-1613, 1953.
Stinchfield, F. E., and Sinton, W. A.:	Criteria for spine fusion with use of "H" bone graft following disc removal, results in 100 cases	Arch. Surg. **65**:542-550, 1952.
Sullivan, C. R., Bickel, W. H., and Svien, H. J.:	Infections of vertebral interspaces after operations on intervertebral disks	J.A.M.A. **166**:1973-1977, 1958.
Sullivan, J. E.:	Backache due to visceral lesions of the chest and the abdomen	In DePalma, A. F., editor: Clinical orthopaedics, vol. 26, Philadelphia, J. B. Lippincott Co., 1963, pp. 67-73.
Thiele, G. H.:	Coccygodynia, the mechanism of its production and its relationship to anorectal disease	Am. J. Surg. **79**:110-116, 1950.
Toumey, J. W., Poppen, J. L., and Hurley, M. T.:	Cauda equina tumors as a cause of the low-back syndrome	J. Bone & Joint Surg. **32-A**:249-256, 1950.
Von Werssowetz, O. F.:	Back braces and supports	In DePalma, A. F., editor: Clinical orthopaedics, vol. 5, Philadelphia, J. B. Lippincott Co., 1955, pp. 169-183.
Williams, P. C.:	Lesions of the lumbosacral spine. Part I: Acute traumatic destruction of the lumbosacral intervertebral disc; Part II: Chronic traumatic (postural) destruction of the lumbosacral intervertebral disc	J. Bone & Joint Surg. **19**:343-363, 690-703, 1937.
	The conservative management of lesions of the lumbosacral spine	American Academy of Orthopaedic Surgeons Instructional Course Lectures, vol. X, Ann Arbor, J. W. Edwards, 1953, pp. 90-121.
Willis, T. A.:	Man's back	Springfield, Ill., Charles C Thomas, Publisher, 1953.
Wiltse, L. L.:	The etiology of spondylolisthesis	J. Bone & Joint Surg. **44-A**:539-560, 1962.

Young, H. H.:	Non-neurological lesions simulating protruded intervertebral disk	J.A.M.A. **148**:1101-1105, 1952.
Young, H. H., and Love, J. G.:	End results of removal of protruded lumbar intervertebral discs with and without fusion	American Academy of Orthopaedic Surgeons Instructional Course Lectures, vol. XVI, St. Louis, The C. V. Mosby Co., 1959, pp. 213-216

Chapter 18
Affections of the hip
Arterial supply of the femoral head

Howe, W. W., Jr., Lacey, T., II, and Schwartz, R. P.:	A study of the gross anatomy of the arteries supplying the proximal portion of the femur and the acetabulum	J. Bone & Joint Surg. **32-A**:856-866, 1950.
Trueta, J.:	The normal vascular anatomy of the human femoral head during growth	J. Bone & Joint Surg. **39-B**:358-394, 1957.
Trueta, J., and Harrison, M. H. M.:	The normal vascular anatomy of the femoral head in adult man	J. Bone & Joint Surg. **35-B**:442-461, 1953.
Tucker, F. R.:	Arterial supply to the femoral head and its clinical importance	J. Bone & Joint Surg. **31-B**:82-93, 1949.

Coxa plana

Carpenter, E. B., and Powell, D. O.:	Osteochondrosis of capital epiphysis of femur (Legg-Calvé-Perthes disease)	J.A.M.A. **172**:525-527, 1960.
Evans, D. L.:	Legg-Calvé-Perthes' disease, a study of late results	J. Bone & Joint Surg. **40-B**:168-181, 1958.
Evans, D. L., and Lloyd-Roberts, G. C.:	Treatment in Legg-Calvé-Perthes' disease	J. Bone & Joint Surg. **40-B**:182-189, 1958.
Ferguson, A. B., and Howorth, M. B.:	Coxa plana and related conditions at the hip	J. Bone & Joint Surg. **16**:781-803, 1934.
Gill, A. B.:	Legg-Perthes disease of the hip: its early roentgenographic manifestations and its cyclical course	J. Bone & Joint Surg. **22**:1013-1047, 1940.
Goff, C. W.:	Legg-Calvé-Perthes syndrome and related osteochondroses of youth	Springfield, Ill., Charles C Thomas, Publisher, 1954.
Hauge, M. F.:	The treatment of coxa plana	Acta orthop. scandinav. **26**:53-65, 1956.
Herndon, C. H., and Heyman, C. H.:	Legg-Perthes disease, an evaluation of treatment by traction and ischial weight-bearing brace	J. Bone & Joint Surg. **34-A**:25-46, 1952.
Katz, J. F.:	Legg-Calvé-Perthes disease—results of treatment	In DePalma, A. F., editor: Clinical orthopaedics, vol. 10, Philadelphia, J. B. Lippincott Co., 1957, pp. 61-78.
Kreuz, F. P., and Shands, A. R., Jr.:	Some congenital and developmental problems of the hip joint in infancy and childhood	In Carter, B. N., editor: Monographs on surgery, 1951, New York, Thos. Nelson & Sons, 1950, pp. 327-392.

Legg, A. T.:	An obscure affection of the hip-joint	Boston M. & S. J. **162**:202-204, 1910.
Maudsley, R. H.:	Dysplasia epiphysialis multiplex	J. Bone & Joint Surg. **37-B**:228-240, 1955.
Mindell, E. R., and Sherman, M. S.:	Late results in Legg-Perthes disease	J. Bone & Joint Surg. **33-A**:1-23, 1951.
O'Garra, J. A.:	The radiographic changes in Perthes' disease	J. Bone & Joint Surg. **41-B**:465-476, 1959.
Pedersen, H. E., and McCarroll, H. R.:	Treatment in Legg-Perthes disease	J. Bone & Joint Surg. **33-A**:591-600, 1951.
Ponseti, I. V.:	Legg-Perthes disease, observations on pathological changes in two cases	J. Bone & Joint Surg. **38-A**:739-750, 1956.
Ralston, E. L.:	Legg-Calvé-Perthes disease—factors in healing	J. Bone & Joint Surg. **43-A**:249-260, 1961.
Ratliff, A. H. C.:	Pseudocoxalgia, a study of late results in the adult	J. Bone & Joint Surg. **38-B**:498-512, 1956.
Shephard, E.:	Multiple epiphysial dysplasia	J. Bone & Joint Surg. **38-B**:458-467, 1956.
Stamp, W. G., Canales, G., and Odell, R. T.:	Late results in osteochondrosis of capital epiphysis of femur (Legg-Calvé-Perthes disease)	J.A.M.A. **169**:1443-1446, 1959.
Wansbrough, R. M., Carrie, A. W., Walker, N. F., and Ruckerbauer, G.:	Coxa plana, its genetic aspects and results of treatment with the long Taylor walking caliper	J. Bone & Joint Surg. **41-A**:135-146, 1959.

Congenital coxa vara

Amstutz, H. C., and Wilson, P. D., Jr.:	Dysgenesis of the proximal femur (coxa vara) and its surgical management	J. Bone & Joint Surg. **44-A**:1-24, 1962.
Babb, F. S., Ghormley, R. K., and Chatterton, C. C.:	Congenital coxa vara	J. Bone & Joint Surg. **31-A**:115-131, 1949.
Duncan, G. A.:	Congenital and developmental coxa vara	Surgery **3**:741-765, 1937.
Finby, N., Jacobson, H. G., and Poppel, M. H.:	Idiopathic coxa vara in childhood	Radiology **67**:10-16, 1956.
Le Mesurier, A. B.:	Developmental coxa vara	J. Bone & Joint Surg. **30-B**:595-605, 1948.
Zadek, I.:	Congenital coxa vara	Arch. Surg. **30**:62-102, 1935.

Slipping of the capital femoral epiphysis

Badgley, C. E., Isaacson, A. S., Wolgamot, J. C., and Miller, J. W.:	Operative therapy for slipped upper femoral epiphysis, an end-result study	J. Bone & Joint Surg. **30-A**:19-30, 1948.
Billing, L., and Severin, E.:	Slipping epiphysis of the hip	Acta radiol., supp. 174, 1959.
Cleveland, M., Bosworth, D. M., Daly, J. N., and Hess, W. E.:	Study of displaced capital femoral epiphyses	J. Bone & Joint Surg. **33-A**:955-967, 1951.
Compere, C. L.:	Correction of deformity and prevention of aseptic necrosis in late cases of slipped femoral epiphysis	J. Bone & Joint Surg. **32-A**:351-362, 1950.
Durbin, F. C.:	Treatment of slipped upper femoral epiphysis	J. Bone & Joint Surg. **42-B**:289-302, 1960.

Heyman, C. H.:	The treatment of slipping of the upper femoral epiphysis	American Academy of Orthopaedic Surgeons Instructional Course Lectures, vol. XIII, Ann Arbor, J. W. Edwards, 1956, pp. 45-60.
Heyman, C. H., Herndon, C. H., and Strong, J. M.:	Slipped femoral epiphysis with severe displacement	J. Bone & Joint Surg. 39-A:293-303, 1957.
Klein, A., Joplin, R. J., and Reidy, J. A.:	Treatment of slipped capital femoral epiphysis	J.A.M.A. 136:445-451, 1948.
Klein, A., Joplin, R. J., Reidy, J. A., and Hanelin, J.:	Roentgenographic changes in nailed slipped capital femoral epiphysis	J. Bone & Joint Surg. 31-A:1-22, 1949.
Lacroix, P., and Verbrugge, J.:	Slipping of the upper femoral epiphysis, a pathological study	J. Bone & Joint Surg. 33-A:371-381, 1951.
Meyer, L. C., Stelling, F. H., and Wiese, F.:	Slipped capital femoral epiphysis	South. M. J. 50:453-459, 1957.
Ponseti, I. V., and McClintock, R.:	The pathology of slipping of the upper femoral epiphysis	J. Bone & Joint Surg. 38-A:71-83, 1956.
Tachdjian, M. O., and Minear, W. L.:	Hip dislocation in cerebral palsy	J. Bone & Joint Surg. 38-A:1358-1364, 1956.
Wilson, P. D.:	The treatment of slipping of the upper femoral epiphysis with minimal displacement	J. Bone & Joint Surg. 20:379-399, 1938.

Other affections of the hip

Adams, J. P.:	Coxa magna	South. M. J. 49:604-607, 1956.
Bryson, A. F.:	Treatment of pathological dislocation of the hip joint after suppurative arthritis in infants	J. Bone & Joint Surg. 30-B:449-453, 1948.
Dickinson, A. M.:	Bilateral snapping hip	Am. J. Surg. 6:97-101, 1929.
Ferguson, A. B., and Howorth, M. B.:	Coxa magna, a condition of the hip related to coxa plana	J.A.M.A. 104:808-812, 1935.
Finder, J. G.:	Iliopectineal bursitis	Arch. Surg. 36:519-538, 1938.
Gellman, M.:	Arthrokatadysis of the hip joint	South. M. J. 27:215-219, 1934.
Gilmour, J.:	Adolescent deformities of the acetabulum, an investigation into the nature of protrusio acetabuli	Brit. J. Surg. 26:670-699, 1939.
Golding, F. C.:	Protrusio acetabuli (central luxation)	Brit. J. Surg. 22:56-62, 1934.
Gordon, E. J.:	Trochanteric bursitis and tendinitis	In DePalma, A. F., editor: Clinical orthopaedics, vol. 20, Philadelphia, J. B. Lippincott Co., 1961, pp. 193-202.
Jones, G. B.:	Paralytic dislocation of the hip	J. Bone & Joint Surg. 44-B:573-587, 1962.
Simril, W. A.:	Roentgen manifestations of hip disease in children	American Academy of Orthopaedic Surgeons Instructional Course Lectures, vol. XVIII, St. Louis, The C. V. Mosby Co., 1961, pp. 187-206.
Smith-Petersen, M. N.:	A new supra-articular subperiosteal approach to the hip joint	Am. J. Orthop. Surg. 15:592-595, 1917.
Spear, I. M., and Lipscomb, P. R.:	Noninfectious trochanteric bursitis and peritendinitis	S. Clin. North America 32:1217-1224, 1952.

White, H.:	Hip diseases in children, the roentgenographic findings	American Academy of Orthopaedic Surgeons Instructional Course Lectures, vol. XV, Ann Arbor, J. W. Edwards, 1958, pp. 283-294.

Chapter 19

Affections of the knee

Internal derangements

Abbott, L. C., Saunders, J. B. DeC. M., Bost, F. C., and Anderson, C. E.:	Injuries to the ligaments of the knee joint	J. Bone & Joint Surg. 26:503-521, 1944.
Bennett, G. E.:	Internal derangement of the knee joint	Am. J. Surg. 42:670-678, 1938.
Bonnin, J. G.:	Cysts of the semilunar cartilages of the knee-joint	Brit. J. Surg. 40:558-565, 1953.
Brantigan, O. C., and Voshell, A. F.:	The mechanics of the ligaments and menisci of the knee joint	J. Bone & Joint Surg. 23:44-66, 1941.
Brewer, B. J.:	Injuries to the knee	American Academy of Orthopaedic Surgeons Instructional Course Lectures, vol. XVI, St. Louis, The C. V. Mosby Co., 1959, pp. 29-34.
Cave, E. F.:	Internal derangements of the knee	In Carter, B. N., editor: Monographs on surgery, 1951, New York, Thos. Nelson & Sons, 1950, pp. 443-470.
DeLorme, T. L.:	Restoration of muscle power by heavy-resistance exercises	J. Bone & Joint Surg. 27:645-667, 1945.
DePalma, A. F.:	Diseases of the knee: management in medicine and surgery	Philadelphia, J. B. Lippincott Co., 1954.
du Toit, G. T.:	Internal derangement of the knee	American Academy of Orthopaedic Surgeons Instructional Course Lectures, vol. XII, Ann Arbor, J. W. Edwards, 1955, pp. 9-34.
Fairbank, H. A. T.:	Osteo-chondritis dissecans	Brit. J. Surg. 21:67-82, 1933.
Green, W. T., and Banks, H. H.:	Osteochondritis dissecans in children	J. Bone & Joint Surg. 35-A:26-47, 1953.
Haldeman, K. O.:	Internal derangements of the knee	American Academy of Orthopaedic Surgeons Instructional Course Lectures, vol. XVI, St. Louis, The C. V. Mosby Co., 1959, pp. 161-169.
Helfet, A. J.:	Mechanism of derangements of the medial semilunar cartilage and their management	J. Bone & Joint Surg. 41-B:319-336, 1959.
Hughston, J. C.:	Acute knee injuries in athletes	In DePalma, A. F., editor: Clinical orthopaedics, vol. 23, Philadelphia, J. B. Lippincott Co., 1962, pp. 114-133.
Jaffe, H. L., Lichtenstein, L., and Sutro, C. J.:	Pigmented villonodular synovitis, bursitis and tenosynovitis	Arch. Path. 31:731-765, 1941.

Kaplan, E. B.:	Discoid lateral meniscus of the knee joint	J. Bone & Joint Surg. **39-A**:77-87, 1957.
	Injuries and afflictions of the menisci of the knee	American Academy of Orthopaedic Surgeons Instructional Course Lectures, vol. XVI, St. Louis, The C. V. Mosby Co., 1959, pp. 153-160.
King, D.:	The healing of semilunar cartilages	J. Bone & Joint Surg. **18**:333-342, 1936.
	The function of semilunar cartilages	J. Bone & Joint Surg. **18**:1069-1076, 1936.
Lannin, D. R.:	Rehabilitation of knee meniscus injury with associated malacia of the patella	J.A.M.A. **171**:1662-1664, 1959.
Lewin, P.:	The knee and related structures: injuries, deformities, diseases, disabilities	Philadelphia, Lea & Febiger, 1952.
Lipscomb, P. R., and Henderson, M. S.:	Internal derangements of the knee	J.A.M.A. **135**:827-831, 1947.
MacAusland, W. R.:	A study of derangement of semilunar cartilages based on 850 cases	Surg., Gynec. & Obst. **77**:141-152, 1943.
Mauck, H. P.:	A new operative procedure for instability of the knee	J. Bone & Joint Surg. **18**:984-990, 1936.
McMaster, P. E.:	Pigmented villonodular synovitis with invasion of bone, report of six cases	J. Bone & Joint Surg. **42-A**:1170-1183, 1960.
Meyers, M. H., and McKeever, F. M.:	Fracture of the intercondylar eminence of the tibia	J. Bone & Joint Surg. **41-A**:209-222, 1959.
Murdoch, G.:	Errors of diagnosis revealed at meniscectomy	J. Bone & Joint Surg. **39-B**:502-507, 1957.
Murphy, F. P., Dahlin, D. C., and Sullivan, C. R.:	Articular synovial chondromatosis	J. Bone & Joint Surg. **44-A**:77-86, 1962.
Mussey, R. D., Jr., and Henderson, M. S.:	Osteochondromatosis	J. Bone & Joint Surg. **31-A**:619-627, 1949.
O'Donoghue, D. H.:	Surgical repair of knee ligament injuries	American Academy of Orthopaedic Surgeons Instructional Course Lectures, vol. XV, Ann Arbor, J. W. Edwards, 1958, pp. 105-115.
	Surgical treatment of fresh injuries to the major ligaments of the knee	J. Bone & Joint Surg. **32-A**:721-738, 1950.
	An analysis of end results of surgical treatment of major injuries to the ligaments of the knee	J. Bone & Joint Surg. **37-A**:1-13, 1955.
Peabody, C. W., and Walsh, F. P.:	Lesions of patellar cartilage as a cause of internal derangements of the knee	Arch. Surg. **57**:589-598, 1948.
Phemister, D. B.:	The causes of and changes in loose bodies arising from the articular surface of the joint	J. Bone & Joint Surg. **6**:278-315, 1924.
Shafer, S. J., and Larmon, W. A.:	Pigmented villonodular synovitis, a report of seven cases	Surg., Gynec. & Obst. **92**:574-580, 1951.

Shands, A. R., Jr., Hutchison, J. L., and Ziv, L.:	Derangements of the semilunar cartilages of the knee, a clinical and experimental study	South. M. J. **29**:1045-1050, 1936.
Smillie, I. S.:	Observations on the regeneration of the semilunar cartilages in man	Brit. J. Surg. **31**:398-401, 1944.
	The congenital discoid meniscus	J. Bone & Joint Surg. **30-B**:671-682, 1948.
	Osteochondritis dissecans	Baltimore, Williams & Wilkins Co., 1960.
	Injuries of the knee joint, 3rd edition	Edinburgh, E. & S. Livingstone, Ltd., 1962.
Steindler, A.:	Synovectomy and fat pad removal in the knee	J.A.M.A. **84**:16-20, 1925.

Other affections of the knee

Bronitsky, J.:	Chondromalacia patellae	J. Bone & Joint Surg. **29**:931-945, 1947.
Burleson, R. J., Bickel, W. H., and Dahlin, D. C.:	Popliteal cyst, a clinicopathological survey	J. Bone & Joint Surg. **38-A**:1265-1274, 1956.
Cave, E. F., and Rowe, C. R.:	The patella, its importance in derangement of the knee	J. Bone & Joint Surg. **32-A**:542-553, 1950.
Cohen, B., and Wilkinson, R. W.:	The Osgood-Schlatter lesion	Am. J. Surg. **95**:731-742, 1958.
DePalma, A. F., and Cotler, J.:	Hemophilic arthropathy	In DePalma, A. F., editor: Clinical orthopaedics, vol. 8, Philadelphia, J. B. Lippincott Co., 1956, pp. 163-190.
Ehrenborg, G.:	The Osgood-Schlatter lesion	Acta chir. scandinav., supp. 288, 1962.
Ghormley, R. K., and Clegg, R. S.:	Bone and joint changes in hemophilia, with report of cases of so-called hemophilic pseudotumor	J. Bone & Joint Surg. **30-A**:589-600, 1948.
Haggart, G. E.:	Synovial cysts of the popliteal space; clinical significance and treatment	Ann. Surg. **118**:438-444, 1943.
Heywood, A. W. B.:	Recurrent dislocation of the patella	J. Bone & Joint Surg. **43-B**:508-517, 1961.
Hughes, E. S. R.:	Osgood-Schlatter's disease	Surg., Gynec. & Obst. **86**:323-328, 1948.
Johnson, J. B., Davis, T. W., and Bullock, W. H.:	Bone and joint changes in hemophilia, a long-term study in 12 Negro subjects	Radiology **63**:64-71, 1954.
Key, J. A.:	Hemophilic arthritis (bleeder's joints)	Ann. Surg. **95**:198-225, 1932.
Kulowski, J.:	Post-traumatic para-articular ossification of the knee joint (Pellegrini-Stieda's disease)	Am. J. Roentgenol. **47**:392-404, 1942.
Macnab, I.:	Recurrent dislocation of the patella	J. Bone & Joint Surg. **34-A**:957-967, 1952.
McCarroll, H. R., and Schwartzmann, J. R.:	Lateral dislocation of the patella, correction by simultaneous transplantation of the tibial tubercle and semitendinosus tendon	J. Bone & Joint Surg. **27**:446-452, 1945.

Nachlas, I. W.:	The Pellegrini-Stieda para-articular calcification	In DePalma, A. F., editor: Clinical orthopaedics, vol. 3, Philadelphia, J. B. Lippincott Co., 1954, pp. 121-127.
Osgood, R. B.:	Lesions of the tibial tubercle occurring during adolescence	Boston M. & S. J. **148**:114-117, 1903.
Rapp, I. H., and Lazerte, G.:	Clinical pathological correlation in Osgood-Schlatter's disease	South. M. J. **51**:909-912, 1958.
Scuderi, C.:	Ruptures of the quadriceps tendon, study of twenty tendon ruptures	Am. J. Surg. **95**:626-635, 1958.
Voshell, A. F., and Brantigan, O. C.:	Bursitis in the region of the tibial collateral ligament	J. Bone & Joint Surg. **26**:793-798, 1944.
Weiner, A. D., and Ghormley, R. K.:	Periodic benign synovitis, idiopathic intermittent hydrarthrosis	J. Bone & Joint Surg. **38-A**:1039-1055, 1956.
West, F. E., and Soto-Hall, R.:	Recurrent dislocation of the patella in the adult	J. Bone & Joint Surg. **40-A**:386-394, 1958.
Wiles, P., Andrews, P. S., and Devas, M. B.:	Chondromalacia of the patella	J. Bone & Joint Surg. **38-B**:95-113, 1956.
Wilson, P. D.:	Posterior capsuloplasty in certain flexion contractures of the knee	J. Bone & Joint Surg. **11**:40-58, 1929.
Wilson, P. D., Eyre-Brook, A. L., and Francis, J. D.:	A clinical and anatomical study of the semimembranosus bursa in relation to popliteal cyst	J. Bone & Joint Surg. **20**:963-984, 1938.

Chapter 20

Affections of the ankle and foot

Arner, O., and Lindholm, A.:	Subcutaneous rupture of the achilles tendon, a study of 92 cases	Acta chir. scandinav., supp. 239, 1959.
Bernstein, A., and Stone, J. R.:	March fracture	J. Bone & Joint Surg. **26**:743-750, 1944.
Bingold, A. C., and Collins, D. H.:	Hallux rigidus	J. Bone & Joint Surg. **32-B**:214-222, 1950.
Blockey, N. J.:	Peroneal spastic flat foot	J. Bone & Joint Surg. **37-B**:191-202, 1955.
Bonney, G., and Macnab, I.:	Hallux valgus and hallux rigidus, a critical survey of operative results	J. Bone & Joint Surg. **34-B**:366-385, 1952.
Burman, M.:	Stenosing tendovaginitis of the foot and ankle	Arch. Surg. **67**:686-698, 1953.
Chandler, F. A.:	Children's feet, normal and presenting common abnormalities	Am. J. Dis. Child. **63**:1136-1146, 1942.
Cleveland, M., and Winant, E. M.:	An end-result study of the Keller operation	J. Bone & Joint Surg. **32-A**:163-175, 1950.
Cole, W. H.:	The treatment of claw-foot	J. Bone & Joint Surg. **22**:895-908, 1940.
Crego, C. H., Jr., and Ford, L. T.:	An end-result study of various operative procedures for correcting flat feet in children	J. Bone & Joint Surg. **34-A**:183-195, 1952.
Dickson, F. D., and Diveley, R. L.:	Functional disorders of the foot: their diagnosis and treatment, 2nd edition	Philadelphia, J. B. Lippincott Co., 1944.

Dwight, T.:	A clinical atlas, variations of the bones of the hands and feet	Philadelphia, J. B. Lippincott Co., 1907.
Freiberg, A. H.:	The so-called infractions of the second metatarsal bone	J. Bone & Joint Surg. 8:257-261, 1926.
Freiberg, J. A.:	The diagnosis and treatment of common painful conditions of the foot	American Academy of Orthopaedic Surgeons Instructional Course Lectures, vol. XIV, Ann Arbor, J. W. Edwards, 1957, pp. 238-247.
Friedman, B., and Smith, E. E.:	Foot problems in infants and children, rotational deviations of lower extremities	J. Pediat. 46:573-580, 1955.
Garceau, G. J., and Brahms, M. A.:	A preliminary study of selective plantar-muscle denervation for pes cavus	J. Bone & Joint Surg. 38-A:553-562, 1956.
Graham, J.:	Weak foot: pathogenesis and treatment	Am. J. Surg. 35:486-508, 1937.
Haines, R. W., and McDougall, A.:	The anatomy of hallux valgus	J. Bone & Joint Surg. 36-B:272-293, 1954.
Hammond, G.:	The operative treatment of hallux valgus and metatarsus primus varus	S. Clin. North America 32:733-745, 1952.
Harris, R. I.:	Peroneal spastic flatfoot	American Academy of Orthopaedic Surgeons Instructional Course Lectures, vol. XV, Ann Arbor, J. W. Edwards, 1958, pp. 116-134.
	Rigid valgus foot due to talocalcaneal bridge	J. Bone & Joint Surg. 37-A:169-183, 1955.
Harris, R. I., and Beath, T.:	Army foot survey	Ottawa, Canada National Research Council, 1947.
	Hypermobile flat-foot with short tendo achillis	J. Bone & Joint Surg. 30-A:116-140, 1948.
	The short first metatarsal, its incidence and clinical significance	J. Bone & Joint Surg. 31-A:553-565, 1949.
Hartley, J. B.:	"Stress" or "fatigue" fractures of bone	Brit. J. Radiol. 16:225-262, 1943.
Hauser, E. D. W.:	Diseases of the foot, 2nd edition	Philadelphia, W. B. Saunders Co., 1950.
Hughes, E. S. R.:	Painful heels in children	Surg., Gynec. & Obst. 86:64-68, 1948.
Hutter, C. G., Jr., and Scott, W.:	Tibial torsion	J. Bone & Joint Surg. 31-A:511-518, 1949.
Jack, E. A.:	Bone anomalies of the tarsus in relation to "peroneal spastic flat foot"	J. Bone & Joint Surg. 36-B:530-542, 1954.
Jones, E.:	Operative treatment of chronic dislocation of the peroneal tendons	J. Bone & Joint Surg. 14:574-576, 1932.
Joplin, R. J.:	Some common foot disorders amenable to surgery	American Academy of Orthopaedic Surgeons Instructional Course Lectures, vol. XV, Ann Arbor, J. W. Edwards, 1958, pp. 144-158.

Karp, M. G.:	Köhler's disease of the tarsal scaphoid, an end-result study	J. Bone & Joint Surg. **19**:84-96, 1937.
Keith, A.:	The history of the human foot and its bearing on orthopaedic practice	J. Bone & Joint Surg. **11**:10-32, 1929.
Keller, W. L.:	Further observations on the surgical treatment of hallux valgus and bunions	New York M. J. **95**:696-698, 1912.
Kendrick, J. I.:	Treatment of calcaneonavicular bar	J.A.M.A. **172**:1242-1244, 1960.
Kidner, F. C.:	The prehallux (accessory scaphoid) in its relation to flat-foot	J. Bone & Joint Surg. **11**:831-837, 1929.
Kite, J. H.:	Torsion of the lower extremities in small children	J. Bone & Joint Surg. **36-A**:511-520, 1954.
Kohler, A.:	Typical disease of the second metatarsophalangeal joint	Am. J. Roentgenol. **10**:705-710, 1923.
Lake, N. C.:	The foot, 4th edition	Baltimore, Williams & Wilkins Co., 1952.
Lapidus, P. W.:	Spastic flat-foot	J. Bone & Joint Surg. **28**:126-136, 1946.
Lawrence, G. H., Cave, E. F., and O'Connor, H.:	Injury to the Achilles tendon, experience at the Massachusetts General Hospital, 1900-1954	Am. J. Surg. **89**:795-802, 1955.
Lewin, P.:	The foot and ankle; their injuries, diseases, deformities and disabilities, 4th edition	Philadelphia, Lea & Febiger, 1959.
McBride, E. D.:	Hallux valgus bunion deformity	American Academy of Orthopaedic Surgeons Instructional Course Lectures, vol. IX, Ann Arbor, J. W. Edwards, 1952, pp. 334-346.
McDougall, A.:	The os trigonum	J. Bone & Joint Surg. **37-B**:257-265, 1955.
McElvenny, R. T.:	The etiology and surgical treatment of intractable pain about the fourth metatarsophalangeal joint (Morton's toe)	J. Bone & Joint Surg. **25**:675-679, 1943.
Meyerding, H. W., and Stuck, W. G.:	Painful heels among children (apophysitis)	J.A.M.A. **102**:1658-1660, 1934.
Miller, O. L.:	A plastic flat foot operation	Lectures on peace and war orthopedic surgery, American Academy of Orthopaedic Surgeons Instructional Course Lectures, vol. I, Ann Arbor, J. W. Edwards, 1943, pp. 224-225.
Mitchell, C. L., Fleming, J. L., Allen, R., Glenney, C., and Sanford, G. A.:	Osteotomy-bunionectomy for hallux valgus	J. Bone & Joint Surg. **40-A**:41-60, 1958.
Morton, D. J.:	The human foot; its evolution, physiology and functional disorders	New York, Columbia University Press, 1935.
Nissen, K. I.:	Plantar digital neuritis, Morton's metatarsalgia	J. Bone & Joint Surg. **30-B**:84-94, 1948.

O'Donoghue, D. H.:	Impingement exostoses of the talus and tibia	J. Bone & Joint Surg. **39-A**:835-852, 1957.
O'Rahilly, R.:	A survey of carpal and tarsal anomalies	J. Bone & Joint Surg. **35-A**:626-642, 1953.
Saunders, J. T.:	Etiology and treatment of clawfoot	Arch. Surg. **30**:179-198, 1935.
Schwartz, R. P., and Heath, A. L.:	Conservative treatment of functional disorders of the feet in the adolescent and adult	J. Bone & Joint Surg. **31-A**:501-510, 1949.
Shands, A. R., Jr.:	The accessory bones of the foot	South. Med. & Surg. **93**:326-334, 1931.
Shands, A. R., Jr., and Wentz, I. J.:	Congenital anomalies, accessory bones, and osteochondritis in the feet of 850 children	S. Clin. North America **33**:1643-1666, 1953.
Silver, D.:	The operative treatment of hallux valgus	J. Bone & Joint Surg. **5**:225-232, 1923.
Steindler, A.:	Stripping of the os calcis	J. Orthop. Surg. **2**:8-12, 1920.
	The pathomechanics of the static disabilities of foot and ankle	American Academy of Orthopaedic Surgeons Instructional Course Lectures, vol. IX, Ann Arbor, J. W. Edwards, 1952, pp. 327-334.
Wang, C. C., Lowrey, C. W., and Severance, R. L.:	Fatigue fracture of the pelvis and the lower extremity	New England J. Med. **260**:958-962, 1959.
Waugh, W.:	The ossification and vascularisation of the tarsal navicular and their relation to Köhler's disease	J. Bone & Joint Surg. **40-B**:765-777, 1958.
Webster, F. S., and Roberts, W. M.:	Tarsal anomalies and peroneal spastic flatfoot	J.A.M.A. **146**:1099-1104, 1951.
Wells, P. O.:	March fracture of the tibia	Radiology **58**:714-719, 1952.
Williams, A. A.:	Tenosynovitis of the tendo achillis	Brit. M. J. **2**:377-378, 1941.
Zadek, I., and Gold, A. M.:	The accessory tarsal scaphoid	J. Bone & Joint Surg. **30-A**:957-968, 1948.

Chapter 21

Affections of the neck, shoulder, and jaw

Torticollis

Adson, A. W., Young, H. H., and Ghormley, R. K.:	Spasmodic torticollis	J. Bone & Joint Surg. **28**:299-308, 1946.
Chandler, F. A.:	Congenital muscular torticollis	American Academy of Orthopaedic Surgeons Instructional Course Lectures, vol. VI, Ann Arbor, J. W. Edwards, 1949, pp. 236-242.
Coventry, M. B., and Harris, L. E.:	Congenital muscular torticollis in infancy	J. Bone & Joint Surg. **41-A**:815-822, 1959.
Hulbert, K. F.:	Congenital torticollis	J. Bone & Joint Surg. **32-B**:50-59, 1950.
Kiesewetter, W. B., Nelson, P. K., Palladino, V. S., and Koop, C. E.:	Neonatal torticollis	J.A.M.A. **157**:1281-1285, 1955.

Middleton, D. S.:	The pathology of congenital torticollis	Brit. J. Surg. **18**:188-204, 1930.
Rugh, J. T.:	Spasmodic torticollis: its cause and treatment	Am. J. Surg. **49**:490-495, 1940.

Cervical root syndrome, cervical rib, and scalenus syndrome

Adson, A. W.:	Surgical treatment for symptoms produced by cervical ribs and the scalenus anticus muscle	Surg., Gynec. & Obst. **85**:687-700, 1947.
Adson, A. W., and Coffey, J. R.:	Cervical rib	Ann. Surg. **85**:839-857, 1927.
Clarke, E.:	Cervical myelopathy, a common neurological disorder	Lancet **1**:171-176, 1955.
Friedenberg, Z. B., Broder, H. A., Edeiken, J. E., and Spencer, H. N.:	Degenerative disk disease of cervical spine, clinical and roentgenographic study	J.A.M.A. **174**:375-380, 1960.
Gage, M., and Parnell, H.:	Scalenus anticus syndrome	Am. J. Surg. **73**:252-268, 1947.
Hadley, L. A.:	The covertebral articulations and cervical foramen encroachment	J. Bone & Joint Surg. **39-A**:910-920, 1957.
Jackson, R.:	The cervical syndrome	American Academy of Orthopaedic Surgeons Instructional Course Lectures, vol. X, Ann Arbor, J. W. Edwards, 1953 pp. 65-90.
McGowan, J. M.:	Cervical rib: the rôle of the clavicle in occlusion of the subclavian artery	Ann. Surg. **124**:71-89, 1946.
Michelsen, J. J., and Mixter, W. J.:	Pain and disability of shoulder and arm due to herniation of the nucleus pulposus of cervical intervertebral disks	New England J. Med. **231**:279-287, 1944.
Odom, G. L., Finney, W., and Woodhall, B.:	Cervical disk lesions	J.A.M.A. **166**:23-28, 1958.
Raaf, J.:	Surgery for cervical rib and scalenus anticus syndrome	J.A.M.A. **157**:219-223, 1955.
Rosati, L. M., and Lord, J. W.:	Neurovascular compression syndromes of the shoulder girdle	New York, Grune & Stratton, Inc., 1961.
Smith, G. W., and Robinson, R. A.:	The treatment of certain cervical-spine disorders by anterior removal of the intervertebral disc and interbody fusion	J. Bone & Joint Surg. **40-A**:607-624, 1958.
Steindler, A.:	The cervical pain syndrome	American Academy of Orthopaedic Surgeons Instructional Course Lectures, vol. XIV, Ann Arbor, J. W. Edwards, 1957, pp. 1-10.
Telford, E. D., and Mottershead, S.:	Pressure at the cervico-brachial junction, an operative and anatomical study	J. Bone & Joint Surg. **30-B**:249-265, 1948.

The shoulder

Adams, J. C.:	Recurrent dislocation of the shoulder	J. Bone & Joint Surg. **30-B**:26-38, 1948.
Badgley, C. E.:	Sports injuries of the shoulder girdle	J.A.M.A. **172**:444-448, 1960.

Bibliography

Bankart, A. S. B.:	An operation for recurrent dislocation (subluxation) of the sternoclavicular joint	Brit. J. Surg. **26**:320-323, 1938.
	The pathology and treatment of recurrent dislocation of the shoulder joint	Brit. J. Surg. **26**:23-29, 1938.
Bateman, J. E.:	The shoulder and environs	St. Louis, The C. V. Mosby Co., 1955.
Bost, F. C., and Inman, V. T.:	The pathological changes in recurrent dislocation of the shoulder, a report of Bankart's operative procedure	J. Bone & Joint Surg. **24**:595-613, 1942.
Bosworth, B. M.:	Calcium deposits in the shoulder and subacromial bursitis, a survey of 12,122 shoulders	J.A.M.A. **116**:2477-2482, 1941.
Bosworth, D. M.:	The supraspinatus syndrome, symptomatology, pathology and repair	J.A.M.A. **117**:422-428, 1941.
Brav, E. A.:	Recurrent dislocation of the shoulder, ten years' experience with the Putti-Platt reconstruction procedure	Am. J. Surg. **100**:423-430, 1960.
Caldwell, G. A., and Unkauf, B. M.:	Results of treatment of subacromial bursitis in 340 cases	Ann. Surg. **132**:432-442, 1950.
Codman, E. A.:	The shoulder; rupture of the supraspinatus tendon and other lesions in or about the subacromial bursa	Boston, Thomas Todd Co., 1934.
Conwell, H. E.:	Subcutaneous rupture of the biceps flexor cubiti	J. Bone & Joint Surg. **10**:788-790, 1928.
Cubbins, W. R., Callahan, J. J., and Scuderi, C. S.:	The reduction of old or irreducible dislocations of the shoulder joint	Surg., Gynec. & Obst. **58**:129-135, 1934.
DePalma, A. F.:	Bicipital tenosynovitis	S. Clin. North America **33**:1693-1702, 1953.
	Frozen shoulder	American Academy of Orthopaedic Surgeons Instructional Course Lectures, vol. IX, Ann Arbor, J. W. Edwards, 1952, pp. 313-325.
	Surgery of the shoulder	Philadelphia, J. B. Lippincott Co., 1950.
Dickson, J. A., Humphries, A. W., and O'Dell, H. W.:	Recurrent dislocation of the shoulder	Baltimore, Williams & Wilkins Co., 1953.
Gilcreest, E. L.:	The common syndrome of rupture, dislocation and elongation of the long head of the biceps brachii, an analysis of 100 cases	Surg., Gynec. & Obst. **58**:322-340, 1934.
Haggart, G. E., Dignam, R. J., and Sullivan, T. S.:	Management of the "frozen" shoulder	J.A.M.A. **161**:1219-1222, 1956.
Henry, M. O.:	Acromio-clavicular dislocations	Minnesota Med. **12**:431-433, 1929.
Hitchcock, H. H., and Bechtol, C. O.:	Painful shoulder, observations on role of the tendon of the long head of the biceps brachii in its causation	J. Bone & Joint Surg. **30-A**:263-273, 1948.

Howorth, M. B.:	Calcification of the tendon cuff of the shoulder	Surg., Gynec. & Obst. **80**:337-345, 1945.
Inman, V. T., Saunders, J. B. deC. M., and Abbott, L. C.:	Observations on the function of the shoulder joint	J. Bone & Joint Surg. **26**:1-30, 1944.
Keyes, E. L.:	Observations on rupture of the supraspinatus tendon, based upon the study of 73 cadavers	Ann. Surg. **97**:849-856, 1933.
Lazcano, M., Anzel, S. H., and Kelly, P. J.:	Complete dislocation and subluxation of the acromioclavicular joint, end result in seventy-three cases	J. Bone & Joint Surg. **43-A**:379-391, 1961.
Lloyd-Roberts, G. C., and French, P. R.:	Periarthritis of the shoulder, a study of the disease and its treatment	Brit. M. J. **1**:1569-1571, 1959.
MacAusland, W. R.:	Recurrent anterior dislocation of the shoulder	Am. J. Surg. **91**:323-331, 1956.
McLaughlin, H. L.:	Lesions of the musculotendinous cuff of the shoulder: I. the exposure and treatment of tears with retraction	J. Bone & Joint Surg. **26**:31-51, 1944.
	II. Differential diagnosis of rupture	J.A.M.A. **128**:563-568, 1945.
	III. Observations on the pathology, course and treatment of calcific deposits	Ann. Surg. **124**:354-362, 1946.
McLaughlin, H. L., and Asherman, E. G.:	Lesions of the musculotendinous cuff of the shoulder: IV. Some observations based upon the results of surgical repair	J. Bone & Joint Surg. **33-A**:76-86, 1951.
McMaster, P. E.:	Tendon and muscle ruptures, clinical and experimental studies on the causes and location of subcutaneous ruptures	J. Bone & Joint Surg. **15**:705-722, 1933.
Moseley, H. F.:	Recurrent dislocation of the shoulder	Edinburgh, E. & S. Livingstone, Ltd., 1961.
	Ruptures of the rotator cuff	Springfield, Ill., Charles C Thomas, Publisher, 1952.
	Shoulder lesions, 2nd edition	New York, Paul B. Hoeber, Inc., 1953.
Neviaser, J. S.:	Arthrography of the shoulder joint, study of the findings in adhesive capsulitis of the shoulder	J. Bone & Joint Surg. **44-A**:1321-1330, 1962.
Nicola, T.:	Recurrent anterior dislocation of the shoulder, a new operation	J. Bone & Joint Surg. **11**:128-132, 1929.
	Recurrent dislocation of the shoulder	Am. J. Surg. **86**:85-91, 1953.
Norwich, I.:	Calcification of the supraspinatus tendon: infiltration therapy with local anesthesia and multiple needling	Surg., Gynec. & Obst. **86**:183-191, 1948.
O'Donoghue, D. H.:	Injuries to the shoulder girdle	American Academy of Orthopaedic Surgeons Instructional Course Lectures, vol. XVII, St. Louis, The C. V. Mosby Co., 1960, pp. 392-405.

Osmond-Clarke, H.:	Habitual dislocation of the shoulder, the Putti-Platt operation	J. Bone & Joint Surg. **30-B**:19-25, 1948.
Rowe, C. R.:	Prognosis in dislocations of the shoulder	J. Bone & Joint Surg. **38-A**:957-977, 1956.
Samilson, R. L., et al.:	Shoulder arthrography	J.A.M.A. **175**:773-778, 1961.
Steinbrocker, O., Spitzer, N., and Friedman, H. H.:	The shoulder-hand syndrome in reflex dystrophy of the upper extremity	Ann. Int. Med. **29**:22-52, 1948.
Steindler, A.:	Interpretation of pain in the shoulder	American Academy of Orthopaedic Surgeons Instructional Course Lectures, vol. XV, Ann Arbor, J. W. Edwards, 1958, pp. 159-171.
	The traumatic deformities and disabilities of the upper extremity	Springfield, Ill., Charles C Thomas, Publisher, 1946.
Young, B. R.:	The roentgen treatment of bursitis of the shoulder	Am. J. Roentgenol. **56**:626-630 1946.

The jaw

Burman, M., and Sinberg, S. E.:	Condylar movement in the study of internal derangement of the temporomandibular joint	J. Bone & Joint Surg. **28**:351-373, 1946.
Gerry, R. G., and Rowan, R. L.:	Temporomandibular joint disease, abnormal mandibular function as basis	Arch. Surg. **69**:635-645, 1954.
Kazanjian, V. H.:	Ankylosis of the temporomandibular joint	Surg., Gynec. & Obst. **67**:333-348, 1938.
Sarnat, B. G., and Laskin, D. M.:	Diagnosis and surgical management of diseases of the temporomandibular joint	Springfield, Ill., Charles C Thomas, Publisher, 1962.
Schwartz, L.:	Disorders of the temporomandibular joint	Philadelphia, W. B. Saunders Co., 1959.
Silver, C. M., and Simon, S. D.:	Meniscus injuries of the temporomandibular joint	J. Bone & Joint Surg. **45-A**:113-124, 1963.
	Operative treatment for recurrent dislocation of the temporomandibular joint	J. Bone & Joint Surg. **43-A**:211-218, 1961.

Chapter 22
Affections of the elbow, wrist, and hand

The elbow

Ackerman, L. V.:	Extra-osseous localized non-neoplastic bone and cartilage formation (so-called myositis ossificans)	J. Bone & Joint Surg. **40-A**:279-298, 1958.
Campbell, W. C.:	Malunited fractures and unreduced dislocations about the elbow	J.A.M.A. **92**:122-128, 1929.
Conacher, C.:	Volkmann's ischaemic contracture of the forearm	M. J. Australia **2**:383-386, 1954.
Dobbie, R. P.:	Avulsion of the lower biceps brachii tendon, analysis of fifty-one previously unreported cases	Am. J. Surg. **51**:662-683, 1941.

Foisie, P. S.:	Volkmann's ischaemic contracture, an analysis of its proximate mechanism	New England J. Med. **226**:671-679, 1942.
Garden, R. S.:	Tennis elbow	J. Bone & Joint Surg. **43-B**:100-106, 1961.
Geschickter, C. F., and Maseritz, I. H.:	Myositis ossificans	J. Bone & Joint Surg. **20**:661-674, 1938.
Griffin, M. E.:	Subluxation of the head of the radius in young children	Pediatrics **15**:103-106, 1955.
Griffiths, D. Ll.:	Volkmann's ischaemic contracture	Brit. J. Surg. **28**:239-260, 1940.
Hart, G. M.:	Subluxation of the head of the radius in young children	J.A.M.A. **169**:1734-1736, 1959.
Laurent, L. E., and Lindström, B. L.:	Osteochondrosis of the capitulum humeri (Panner's disease)	Acta orthop. scandinav. **26**:111-119, 1956.
Lipscomb, P. R.:	The etiology and prevention of Volkmann's ischaemic contracture	Surg., Gynec. & Obst. **103**:353-361, 1956.
March, H. C.:	Osteochondritis of the capitellum (Panner's disease)	Am. J. Roentgenol. **51**:682-684, 1944.
Osgood, R. B.:	Radiohumeral bursitis, epicondylitis, epicondylalgia (Tennis elbow)	Arch. Surg. **4**:420-433, 1922.
Seddon, H. J.:	Volkmann's contracture: treatment by excision of the infarct	J. Bone & Joint Surg. **38-B**:152-174, 1956.
Smith, F. M.:	Surgery of the elbow	Springfield, Ill., Charles C Thomas, Publisher, 1954.
Speed, J. S.:	An operation for unreduced posterior dislocation of the elbow	South. M. J. **18**:193-198, 1925.
Spencer, G. E., Jr., and Herndon, C. H.:	Surgical treatment of epicondylitis	J. Bone & Joint Surg. **35-A**:421-424, 1953.

The wrist and hand

Anton, J. I., Reitz, G. B., and Spiegel, M. B.:	Madelung's deformity	Ann. Surg. **108**:411-439, 1938.
Bickel, W. H., Kimbrough, R. F., and Dahlin, D. C.:	Tuberculous tenosynovitis	J.A.M.A. **151**:31-35, 1953.
Boyes, J. H.:	Dupuytren's contracture, notes on the age at onset and the relationship to handedness	Am. J. Surg. **88**:147-154, 1954.
Boyes, J. H., Wilson, J. N., and Smith, J. W.:	Flexor-tendon ruptures in the forearm and hand	J. Bone & Joint Surg. **42-A**:637-646, 1960.
Britt, L. P.:	Principles of hand rehabilitation	South. M. J. **47**:205-209, 1954.
Buchman, J.:	Traumatic osteoporosis of the carpal bones	Ann. Surg. **87**:892-910, 1928.
Bunnell, S.:	Surgery of the hand, 3rd edition	Philadelphia, J. B. Lippincott Co., 1956.
Butler, E. D., Hamill, J. P., Seipel, R. S., and de Lorimier, A. A.:	Tumors of the hand, a 10-year survey and report of 437 cases	Am. J. Surg. **100**:293-302, 1960.
Carroll, R. E., Sinton, W., and Garcia, A.:	Acute calcium deposits in the hand	J.A.M.A. **157**:422-426, 1955.
Conway, H.:	Dupuytren's contracture	Am. J. Surg. **87**:101-119, 1954.
Dwight, T.:	A clinical atlas: variations of the bones of the hands and feet	Philadelphia, J. B. Lippincott Co., 1907.

Bibliography

Fahey, J. J., and Bollinger, J. A.:	Trigger-finger in adults and children	J. Bone & Joint Surg. **36-A**:1200-1218, 1954.
Gillespie, H. S.:	Excision of the lunate bone in Kienbock's disease	J. Bone & Joint Surg. **43-B**:245-249, 1961.
Goldner, J. L.:	Deformities of the hand incidental to pathological changes of the extensor and intrinsic muscle mechanisms	J. Bone & Joint Surg. **35-A**:115-131, 1953.
Goldsmith, R.:	Kienböch's disease of the semilunar bone	Ann. Surg. **81**:857-862, 1925.
Harris, C., Jr., and Riordan, D. C.:	Intrinsic contracture in the hand and its surgical treatment	J. Bone & Joint Surg. **36-A**:10-20, 1954.
Holm, C. L., and Embick, R. P.:	Anatomical considerations in the primary treatment of tendon injuries of the hand	J. Bone & Joint Surg. **41-A**:599-608, 1959.
Howard, L. D., Jr.:	Contracture of the thumb web	J. Bone & Joint Surg. **32-A**:267-273, 1950.
Kanavel, A. B.:	Infections of the hand, 7th edition	Philadelphia, Lea & Febiger, 1939.
Kaplan, E. B.:	Anatomy, injuries and treatment of the extensor apparatus of the hand and the digits	In DePalma, A. F., editor: Clinical orthopaedics, vol. 13, Philadelphia, J. B. Lippincott Co., 1959, pp. 24-41.
	Functional and surgical anatomy of the hand	Philadelphia, J. B. Lippincott Co., 1953.
Kelly, A. P., Jr.:	Primary tendon repairs, a study of 789 consecutive tendon severances	J. Bone & Joint Surg. **41-A**:581-598, 1959.
Koch, S. L.:	Acquired contractures of the hand	Am. J. Surg. **9**:413-423, 1930.
Lamphier, T. A., Long, N. G., and Dennehy, T.:	DeQuervain's disease, an analysis of 52 cases	Ann. Surg. **138**:832-841, 1953.
Lapidus, P. W., and Fenton, R.:	Stenosing tenovaginitis at the wrist and fingers, report of 423 cases in 369 patients with 354 operations	Arch. Surg. **64**:475-487, 1952.
Larsen, R. D., and Posch, J. L.:	Dupuytren's contracture	J. Bone & Joint Surg. **40-A**:773-792, 1958.
Littler, J. W.:	The severed flexor tendon	S. Clin. North America **39**:435-447, 1959.
Loomis, L. K.:	Variations of stenosing tenosynovitis at the radial styloid process	J. Bone & Joint Surg. **33-A**:340-346, 1951.
Luck, J. V.:	Dupuytren's contracture	J. Bone & Joint Surg. **41-A**:635-664, 1959.
Moorhead, J. J.:	Trauma and Dupuytren's contracture	Am. J. Surg. **85**:352-358, 1953.
Nichols, H. M.:	Manual of hand injuries, 2nd edition	Chicago, Year Book Publishers, Inc., 1955.
O'Rahilly, R.:	A survey of carpal and tarsal anomalies	J. Bone & Joint Surg. **35-A**:626-642, 1953.
Patterson, D. C., and Jones, E. K.:	DeQuervain's disease, stenosing tendovaginitis at the radial styloid	Am. J. Surg. **67**:296-301, 1945.

Peacock, E. E., Jr., and Hartrampf, C. R.:	The repair of flexor tendons in the hand	Internat. Absts. Surg. **113**:411-432, 1961.
Pedersen, H. E., and Day, A. J.:	Dupuytren's disease of the foot	J.A.M.A. **154**:33-35, 1954.
Piver, J. D., and Raney, R. B.:	De Quervain's tendovaginitis	Am. J. Surg. **83**:691-694, 1952.
Posch, J. L.:	Tumors of the hand	J. Bone & Joint Surg. **38-A**:517-540, 1956.
Pulvertaft, R. G.:	Tendon grafts for flexor tendon injuries in the fingers and thumb	J. Bone & Joint Surg. **38-B**:175-194, 1956.
Rhode, C. M.:	Treatment of hand infections	Am. Surgeon **27**:85-115, 1961.
Rhodes, R. L.:	Tenosynovitis of the forearm	Am. J. Surg. **73**:248-251, 1947.
Riordan, D. C.:	Dupuytren's contracture	South. M. J. **54**:1391-1394, 1961.
Smith, F. M.:	Late rupture of extensor pollicis longus tendon following Colles' fracture	J. Bone & Joint Surg. **28**:49-59, 1946.
Stark, H. H., Boyes, J. H., and Wilson, J. N.:	Mallet finger	J. Bone & Joint Surg. **44-A**:1061-1068, 1962.
Straub, L. R., and Wilson, E. H., Jr.:	Spontaneous rupture of extensor tendons in the hand associated with rheumatoid arthritis	J. Bone & Joint Surg. **38-A**:1208-1217, 1956.

Appendix

Fracture principles

Adams, J. C.:	Outline of fractures, including joint injuries, 3rd edition	Baltimore, Williams & Wilkins Co., 1960.
Altemeier, W. A., Culbertson, W. R., Vetto, M., and Cole, W.:	Problems in the diagnosis and treatment of gas gangrene	Arch. Surg. **74**:839-845, 1957.
Aufranc, O. E.:	Care of the patient with multiple injuries	J.A.M.A. **168**:2091-2094, 1958.
Barker, W. F.:	Treatment of shock: practical aspects	American Academy of Orthopaedic Surgeons Instructional Courses; J. Bone & Joint Surg. **44 - A** : 767 - 776, 1962.
Bechtol, C. O., Ferguson, A. B., Jr., and Laing, P. G.:	Metals and engineering in bone and joint surgery	Baltimore, Williams & Wilkins Co., 1959.
Blount, W. P.:	Fractures in children	Baltimore, Williams & Wilkins Co., 1954.
Böhler, L.:	The treatment of fractures, 5th edition, vols. 1-3	New York, Grune & Stratton, Inc., 1956.
Bowers, W. F.:	Surgery of trauma	Philadelphia, J. B. Lippincott Co., 1953.
Brav, E. A.:	The management of open fractures of the extremities	American Academy of Orthopaedic Surgeons Instructional Course Lectures, vol. XIII, Ann Arbor, J. W. Edwards, 1956, pp. 227-233.
Cave, E. F., editor:	Fractures and other injuries	Chicago, Year Book Publishers, Inc., 1958.
Charnley, J.:	The closed treatment of common fractures, 3rd edition	Baltimore, Williams & Wilkins Co., 1958.
Clowes, G. H. A., Jr.:	Metabolic responses to injury	J. Trauma **3**:149-175, 1963.

Bibliography

Cobb, C. A., Jr., and Hillman, J. W.:	Fat embolism	American Academy of Orthopaedic Surgeons Instructional Course Lectures, vol. XVIII, St. Louis, The C. V. Mosby Co., 1961, pp. 122-129.
Collins, D. H.:	Structural changes around nails and screws in human bones	J. Path. & Bact. **65:**109-121, 1953.
Committee on Trauma, American College of Surgeons:	The management of fractures and soft tissue injuries	Philadelphia, W. B. Saunders Co., 1960.
Compere, E. L., Banks, S. W., and Compere, C. L.:	Pictorial handbook of fracture treatment, 5th edition	Chicago, Year Book Medical Publishers, Inc., 1963.
Conwell, H. E., and Reynolds, F. C.:	Key and Conwell's management of fractures, dislocations and sprains, 7th edition	St. Louis, The C. V. Mosby Co., 1961.
Eggers, G. W. N.:	Internal contact splint	J. Bone & Joint Surg. **30-A:**40-52, 1948.
	The internal fixation of fractures of the shafts of long bones	In Carter, B. N., et al., editors: Monographs on surgery, 1952, Baltimore, Williams & Wilkins Co., 1952, pp. 130-178.
Estes, W. L., Jr.:	The surgeon's responsibility in rehabilitation of the injured	Surg., Gynec. & Obst. **100:**619-621, 1955.
Filler, R. M., and Ellerbeck, W.:	Tetanus prophylaxis	J.A.M.A. **174:**1-4, 1960.
Frankel, C. J., Bateman, J. E., Eaton, G. O., Kessler, H. H., and McBride, E. D.:	Symposium on disability evaluation	American Academy of Orthopaedic Surgeons Instructional Course Lectures, vol. XVII, St. Louis, The C. V. Mosby Co., 1960, pp. 331-350.
Godfrey, J. D.:	Major and extensive soft-tissue injuries complicating skeletal fractures	American Academy of Orthopaedic Surgeons Instructional Courses; J. Bone & Joint Surg. **44-A:**753-766, 1962.
Gurd, F. N., et al.:	A symposium on shock	J. Trauma **2:**355-423, 1962.
Harris, W. R.:	Epiphyseal injuries	American Academy of Orthopaedic Surgeons Instructional Course Lectures, vol. XV, Ann Arbor, J. W. Edwards, 1958, pp. 206-214.
Hoover, N. W., and Ivins, J. C.:	Wound debridement	Arch. Surg. **79:**701-710, 1959.
Howard, J. M.:	Fluid replacement in shock and hemorrhage	J.A.M.A. **173:**516-518, 1960.
Hughes, C. W., and Bowers, W. F.:	Traumatic lesions of peripheral vessels	Springfield, Ill., Charles C Thomas, Publisher, 1961.
Liebenson, H. A.:	The doctor in personal injury cases	Chicago, Year Book Publishers, Inc., 1956.
McCarroll, H. R.:	Orthopedic management of the severely injured patient	J.A.M.A. **165:**1913-1916, 1957.
McLaughlin, H. L.:	Internal fixation of fractures	Surgery **39:**892-899, 1956.
	Trauma	Philadelphia, W. B. Saunders Co., 1959.
Moore, J. R.:	The closed fracture of the long bones	J. Bone & Joint Surg. **42-A:**869-874, 1960.
Moyer, C. A.:	Fluid balance and trauma	American Academy of Orthopaedic Surgeons Instructional Course Lectures, vol. XI, Ann Arbor, J. W. Edwards, 1954, pp. 275-278.

Owens, J. C.:	The management of arterial trauma	S. Clin. North America **43**:371-385, 1963.
Peterson, L. T.:	Principles of internal fixation with plates and screws	Arch. Surg. **64**:345-354, 1952.
Rifkind, D.:	The diagnosis and treatment of gas gangrene	S. Clin. North America **43**:511-517, 1963.
Schmeisser, G., Jr.:	A clinical manual of orthopedic traction techniques	Philadelphia, W. B. Saunders Co., 1963.
Scuderi, C.:	Atlas of orthopedic traction procedures	St. Louis, The C. V. Mosby Co., 1954.
Seeley, S. F.:	Emergency care of wounds	J.A.M.A. **173**:518-521, 1960.
Steel, H. H.:	Surgical infections—orthopaedic considerations	American Academy of Orthopaedic Surgeons Instructional Course Lectures, vol. XVIII, St. Louis, The C. V. Mosby Co., 1961, pp. 288-293.
Stein, A. H., Jr.:	Diagnosis of arterial injury in the extremities	American Academy of Orthopaedic Surgeons Instructional Course Lectures, vol. XVII, St. Louis, The C. V. Mosby Co., 1960, pp. 47-60.
Stetler, C. J., and Moritz, A. R.:	Doctor and patient and the law, 4th edition	St. Louis, The C. V. Mosby Co., 1962.
Stokes, J. M.:	Surgical management of vascular injuries associated with long bone fracture	American Academy of Orthopaedic Surgeons Instructional Course Lectures, vol. XVII, St. Louis, The C. V. Mosby Co., 1960, pp. 61-67.
Street, D. M.:	Medullary nailing of the femur, comparative study of skeletal traction, dual plating and medullary nailing	J.A.M.A. **143**:709-714, 1950.
Strode, J. E.:	Postoperative wound infections	Arch. Surg. **79**:141-143, 1959.
Teschan, P. E.:	Management of patients with posttraumatic renal insufficiency	J. Trauma **3**:181-188, 1963.
Venable, C. S., and Stuck, W. G.:	Electrolysis controlling factor in the use of metals in treating fractures	J.A.M.A. **111**:1349-1352, 1938.
	The internal fixation of fractures	Springfield, Ill., Charles C Thomas, Publisher, 1947.
Watson-Jones, Sir R.:	Fractures and joint injuries, 4th edition	Baltimore, Williams & Wilkins Co., 1952-55.
Wiles, P.:	Fractures, dislocations and sprains	Boston, Little, Brown & Co., 1960.

Index

A

Abnormalities of fingers and toes, congenital, 53
Abscess, Brodie's, 140
 cold, 150
 psoas, 156
 tuberculous, 150, 155
Absence, congenital, of individual bones, 49
Accessory bones of foot, 436
 navicular, 436
 of hand and wrist, 483
 nerve, injury of, 246
Achilles bursa, posterior, 433
 tendon, lengthening of, in poliomyelitis, 215
 rupture of, 434
 shortening of, 421
 tenosynovitis of, 433
Achondroplasia, 104
Aclasis, diaphyseal or metaphyseal, 104
Acrocephaly-syndactyly, 53
Acromegaly, 121
Acromioclavicular dislocation, old, 459
Actinomycosis, 146
Acute suppurative tenosynovitis, 475
Adamantinoma, 264
Adductor tenotomy in cerebral palsy, 231
Adhesive capsulitis of shoulder, 452
Adolescent coxa vara, 381
 kyphosis, 338
 rickets, 95
Adult rickets, 98
 round back, 341
Affections of skeleton, 81-132
Albee bone peg operation, 299
 inlay bone graft, 295
 technic of spinal fusion, 158
Albers-Schönberg disease, 116
Albright's syndrome, 113
Albuminuria, Bence Jones, in multiple myeloma, 278
Allis' sign, 67
Amputation, 314-323
 Boyd, 319
 Callander, 321
 Chopart, 319
 cineplastic, 317
 congenital, 56, 316, 321
 Gritti-Stokes, 321
 in children, 321
 indications for, 314
 Kirk, 321

Amputation—cont'd
 Krukenberg, 318
 Lisfranc, 319
 neuroma, 323
 of lower extremity, 318
 of upper extremity, 316
 Pirogoff, 319
 Slocum, 321
 stump disabilities, 322
 Syme, 319
Amyoplasia congenita, 57
Amyotonia congenita, 233
Amyotrophic lateral sclerosis, 233
Anatomy of bones and joints, 22-26
 of wrist and hand, 471
Andry's L'Orthopédie, 21
Aneurysmal bone cyst, 264
Angioma of muscle or fascia, 283
Angle, lumbosacral, 357
Ankle, ankylosis of, optimum position for, 200
 arthrodesis of, after old injury, 306
 in poliomyelitis, 218
 malunion of fracture in region of, 305
 reconstruction of, after old injury, 306
Ankylosing arthritis, 183
Ankylosis, 194-200
 in pyogenic arthritis, 142
 in rheumatoid arthritis, 167
 of jaw, 461
 optimum positions for, 197
Annulus fibrosus, 362
Anomaly, congenital (*see* Deformity, congenital)
Anserina bursa, 412
Anterior bowleg, 89
 heel, Cook, 426
 metatarsalgia, 425
 poliomyelitis, 203
 spina bifida, 238
Anteversion of femur, 66, 75
Apert's syndrome, 53
Apophysitis of calcaneus, 433
 of tibial tuberosity, 405
Arachnodactyly, 56
Aran-Duchenne type of paralysis, 233
Arch supports, 418, 426
Arches of foot, 415
Arnold-Chiari malformation, 238
Arrest of epiphyseal growth, 223
Arthritis, atrophic, 167
 Brucella, 145

573

574   Index

Arthritis—cont'd
   chronic, 166-181
   climacteric, 176
   degenerative (see Osteoarthritis), 175-179
   gonococcal, 144
   gummatous, 148
   incidence, 166
   menopausal, 176
   osteoarthritis, 175-179
      of hip, 189
      of knee, 192
      of spine, 186
      treatment, 178
   pneumococcal, 144
   proliferative, 167
   psoriatic, 170
   pyogenic, 142-144
      of hip in infants, 144
   rheumatoid, 167-175
      juvenile, 170
      of knee, 192
      of spine, 182
      rheumatoid factor in, 171
      treatment, 172
      variants of, 169
   Salmonella, 145
   Strümpell-Marie type of, 183
      treatment, 188
   suppurative, 142-144
   syphilitic, 146
   tuberculous, 149-165
      of hip, 161-164
      of sacroiliac joint, 160
      of spine, 154-160
Arthrodesis after poliomyelitis, 218
   in cerebral palsy, 232
   in treatment of tuberculosis, 153
   ischiofemoral, 164
   of ankle, after old injury, 306
      in poliomyelitis, 218
   of foot, in cerebral palsy, 232
      in clawfoot, 424
      in hereditary muscular atrophy, 260
      in poliomyelitis, 218
      in rigid flatfoot, 421
   of hip, in malum coxae senilis, 192
      in pathologic dislocation, 388
      in poliomyelitis, 218
      in tuberculosis, 162
   of knee, in poliomyelitis, 218
   of lumbosacral joint, for low back pain, 354
   of sacroiliac joint, in tuberculosis, 161
   of shoulder, in poliomyelitis, 220
   of spine, after old injury, 316
      Albee method, 158
      for low back pain, 354
      Hibbs method, 157
      in scoliosis, 335
      in spondylolisthesis, 360
      in tuberculosis, 157
   of wrist, in cerebral palsy, 232
      in poliomyelitis, 222
   optimum positions for, 197
   subtalar, 218
   triple, 219
Arthrogryposis multiplex congenita, 57
Arthrokatadysis, 388
Arthropathy, neuropathic, 235

Arthroplasty, 200-202
   of elbow, after old injury, 309
   of hip, after old injury, 305
      Colonna, for congenital dislocation, 76
      in chronic arthritis, 192
      in malum coxae senilis, 192
      replacement, 202
      Smith-Petersen cup, 201
   of knee, in chronic arthritis, 194
Ascorbic acid and bone changes, 84
Aseptic necrosis, 27
   of capital femoral epiphysis, 374
   of carpal bones, 481
   of metatarsal head, 428
   of tarsal navicular, 424
Astragalectomy, for calcaneal foot, 220
Asymmetrical development of body, 56
Ataxia, Friedreich's, 234
   in cerebral palsy, 228
Athetosis, in cerebral palsy, 228
Atrophic arthritis, 167
Atrophy, bone, 81
   hereditary muscular, of peroneal type, 260
   infantile spinal muscular, 233
   progressive muscular, 233
      of Aran-Duchenne type, 233
      of Charcot-Marie-Tooth type, 260
   Sudeck's, 132
Avascular necrosis of capital femoral epiphysis, 374
   of carpal bones, 481
   of metatarsal head, 428
   of tarsal navicular, 424
Axillary nerve, injuries of, 251
Axonotmesis, 243

B

Back, adult round, 341
   hollow, 343
   knee (see Genu recurvatum)
   pain (see Low back pain)
   round, 338
   strain of (see Low back, affections of)
Backache (see Low back pain)
Baker's cyst, 412
Bamberger-Marie disease, 129
Bankart operation for recurrent shoulder dislocation, 457
Barton tongs, 494
Baseball finger, 473
Belt, lumbosacral, 353
Bence Jones albuminuria, 278
Benign chondroblastoma, 264
   congenital hypotonia, 233
Bennett fracture, malunited, 311
   operation for lengthening quadriceps tendon, 197
Biceps brachii, rupture of, 455
Bicipital tenosynovitis, 451
Bicipitoradial bursitis, 465
Bifurcation operation in congenital dislocation of hip, 78
Biophysics of locomotor system, 345
Bipartite patella, 52
Birth palsy, 247
Blastomycosis, 146
Blount brace for scoliosis, 335
   epiphyseal stapling, 223

Blount—cont'd
  hip osteotomy, 300
Blount's disease, 89
Blue sclerae in osteogenesis imperfecta, 111
Bodies, loose, 401
Body, asymmetrical development of, 56
Bone abscess, Brodie's, 140
  actinomycosis of, 146
  atrophy of, 81
  bank, 293
  block operations in paralytic talipes, 222
    in recurrent dislocation of jaw, 461
  brittle, 111
  cyst, 356
    aneurysmal, 264
    in echinococcus infection, 146
    in hyperparathyroidism, 123
  felon, 476
  functional adaptations of, 81
  fungus infection of, 146
  grafts of, 293-295
  healing of, 286
  hypertrophy of, 81
  lengthening operations upon, 222
  neuropathic disease of, 235
  omovertebral, 60
  plate, 495
  pyogenic infection of (see Osteomyelitis)
  regeneration of, after fracture, 286
  rider's, 468
  Salmonella infection of, 145
  shortening operations upon, 223
  spotted, 117
  syphilis of, 146
  tuberculosis of (see Tuberculosis of bones and joints)
  tumors of (see Tumors of bone)
  typhoid infection of, 145
  von Recklinghausen's disease of (see Hyperparathyroidism)
Bones, accessory, of foot, 436
  of hand, 483
  brittle (see Osteogenesis imperfecta)
  marble, 116
  sesamoid, of foot, 436
  spotted, 117
Bosworth femoro-ischial transplantation, 164
Bowleg, 89
  anterior, 89
Boyd amputation, 319
  dual graft, 295
Brace, ankle, 326
  foot drop, 245, 326
  functional, 326
  in cerebral palsy, 229
  in clubfoot, 42
  in genu valgum, 93
  in genu varum, 92
  in low back affections, 323
  in peripheral nerve injury, 245
  in poliomyelitis, 211, 215
  in scoliosis, Blount or Milwaukee, 335
  in tuberculosis of spine, 158
  ischial weight-bearing, 323
  knee, after internal derangement, 397
  neck, 326
  prescription of, 326
  principles of, 323
  shoulder, 215, 323

Brachial plexus, injury of, 247
  by birth trauma (see Paralysis, obstetric)
  by cervical rib (see Rib, cervical)
  in dislocation of shoulder, 247
Breast, pigeon, 346
Brittain, hip fusion, 164
Brittle bones (see Osteogenesis imperfecta)
Brodie's abscess, 140
Brucella arthritis and osteomyelitis, 145
Bryant's line, 32
  traction, 492
Buck's extension, 492
  traction, 492
Bumper fractures and genu valgum, 93
Bunion, 428
Bunionette, 435
Bunnell dynamic splints, 326
  operation for opponens pollicis paralysis, 217
Bursa, 26
  adventitious, in clubfoot, 40
    in hallux valgus, 430
  anserina, 412
  beneath tibial collateral ligament, 412
  of elbow, 463
  of heel, 433
  of hip, 389
  of knee, 411
  of shoulder, 448
  tumors of, 282
Bursitis, Achilles, posterior, 433
  bicipitoradial, 465
  calcaneal, superficial, 433
  gastrocnemio-semimembranosus, 412
  iliopectineal, 389
  iliopsoas, 389
  infrapatellar, deep, 411
  ischiogluteal, 391
  olecranon, 463
  popliteal, 412
  prepatellar, 411
  pretibial, superficial, 412
  radiohumeral, 464
  retrocalcaneal, 433
  subacromial, 448
  subcoracoid, 451
  subdeltoid, 448
  trochanteric, deep, 390
    superficial, 391

C

C, vitamin, in scurvy, 84, 94
Caffey's disease, 130
Calcaneal bursa, superficial, 433
  epiphysitis, 433
Calcaneonavicular bar, 421
Calcaneus, apophysitis of, 433
  deformity, 39, 45
  epiphysitis of, 433
  inflammation or injury under, 434
  malunited fracture of, 307
  periostitis of, 433
  spurs of, 434
Calcific tendinitis, 476
Calcification in fracture healing, 289
Callander amputation, 321
Callus, exuberant, 468
  formation of, 287
  in fracture healing, 288
Calot jacket in tuberculosis of spine, 159

Calvé, disease of spine, 341
  on avascular necrosis of upper femoral epiphysis, 374
Campbell operation, for drop foot, 222
  for genu recurvatum, 214
  for hip flexion contracture, 214
Cancellous graft, 295
Capsulitis, adhesive, of shoulder, 452
Capsuloplasty, in contracture of knee, 175
Carcinoma, metastatic, of bone, 279
Carpal bones, avascular necrosis of, 481
  ununited fracture of, 302
  tunnel syndrome, 250
Cartilage, discoid type, 398
  semilunar, of knee, cysts of, 398
    injury of, 393
      treatment of, 396
Casts, plaster, 490
Cauda equina, injury of, 255
  syndrome, 255
Causalgia, 244
Cavus deformity in clawfoot, 422
Cells, Gaucher, 102
Central extensor slip, rupture of, 473
Cerebral palsy, 224-240
Cervical coxa vara, 380
  rib, 444
  root syndrome, 441
  spine, synostosis of, 61
Chandler operation for knee flexion, 231
Charcot-Marie-Tooth type of progressive muscular atrophy, 260
Charcot's joints, 235
Check operations in paralytic talipes, 222
Chest, deformity of, in rickets, 86
  in scoliosis, 331
  flat, 345
  funnel, 346
Chondroblastoma, benign, 264
Chondrodystrophia foetalis, 104
Chondroma, 265
Chondromalacia of patella, 408
Chondromas, synovial, 404
Chondromyxoid fibroma, 264
Chondro-osteodystrophy, 109
Chondrosarcoma, 275
Chopart amputation, 319
Chordoma, 264
Christian's syndrome, 101
Chronic sclerosing osteitis, 141
Cineplastic amputations, 317
Circulation in bone, 25
  of femoral head, 372
Clavicle, congenital deficiency of, in cleidocranial dysostosis, 58
  malunited fracture of, 307
  ununited fracture of, 301
Clawfoot, 421
  in hereditary muscular atrophy, 260
  in spina bifida, 240
Clawhand, in cervical rib, 445
  in hereditary muscular atrophy, 260
  in progressive muscular atrophy, 233
  in ulnar nerve injury, 253
Cleft foot, 55
  hand, 55
Cleidocranial dysostosis, 58

Climacteric arthritis, 176
Clubbed fingers, 129
Clubfoot, congenital, 39-46
  in spina bifida, 240
Clubhand, 47
Clutton's joints, 147
Coccidioidomycosis, 146
Coccygodynia, 369
Coccyx, excision of, 370
Cock-up splint in radial nerve injury, 252
Codman's tumor, 264
Cold abscess, 150
  treatment of, 154
Collar, Thomas, 336, 443
Collateral ligaments of knee, ossification of, 409
  rupture of, 399
Colles' fracture, malunited, 310
Colonna, hip arthroplastic operation, 76
Comminuted fracture, 485
Common peroneal nerve, injuries of, 256
Compound fractures, 500
Congenital amyotonia, 233
  deformity (see Deformity, congenital)
  fractures, 296
  hypotonia, benign, 233
Constriction, congenital, 56
Contact-compression in fracture healing, 495
Contracted foot (see Clawfoot)
Contracture, congenital, 53
  Dupuytren's, 479
  hip flexion, examination for, 32
    in poliomyelitis, 213
  of fingers, 478
  of hand, 478
  of palmar fascia (see Dupuytren's contracture)
  of skin, 478
  Volkmann's ischemic, 466
Conus medullaris, injury of, 255
  syndrome, 256
Cook anterior heel, 426
Cord involvement, in poliomyelitis, 204
  in spastic paralysis, 227
  in spina bifida, 338
  in tuberculosis of spine, 156
Cortisone in treatment of rheumatoid arthritis, 173
Coxa plana, 374
  valga, 387
  vara, 378
    adolescent, 381
    cervical, 380
    congenital, 380
    epiphyseal, 381
Craniotabes in rickets, 87
Cretinism, 122
Chronic arthritis, 166-181
Cross-legged progression in spastic paralysis, 227
Cruciate ligaments, rupture of, 400
Crutch palsy, 251, 258
Crutchfield tongs, 494
Cubitus valgus and varus after fracture of humeral condyles, 308
Curvature of spine, anteroposterior, 338-346
  lateral (see Scoliosis)
Cyst, Baker's 412
  bone, 271
    aneurysmal, 264

Cyst—cont'd
  echinococcus, of bone, 146
  of bone in hyperparathyroidism, 123
  of semilunar cartilages of knee, 398

D

D, vitamin, in rickets, 85
Dactylitis, tuberculous, 165
Debridement in open fractures, 500
Deep trochanteric bursitis, 390
Defects, congenital, of individual bones, 49
  massive, of long bones, 297
Deformity, congenital, 37-62
  abnormalities of fingers and toes, 53-56
  absence of individual bones, 49-52
  amputation, 56, 316, 321
  asymmetrical development of body, 56
  cervical rib, 444
  cleft foot, 55
    hand, 55
  clubfoot, 41
  clubhand, 47
  constriction, 56
  contracture, 52
  coxa valga, 387
    vara, 380
  defects of individual bones, 49-52
  dislocation, of elbow, 80
    of hip, 63-79
    of knee, 79
    of patella, 80
    of shoulder, 80
    of wrist, 80
  elevation of scapula, 59
  etiology of, 37
  fracture, 296
  hemihypertrophy, 56
  high scapula, 59
  in arthrogryposis multiplex congenita, 57
  in cleidocranial dysostosis, 58
  in Klippel-Feil syndrome, 61
  "lobster claw" hand and foot deformity, 55
  macrodactyly, 54
  Madelung's, 483
  metatarsus varus, 46
  of low back, 354
  of thorax, 346
  of vertebrae, 354
    scoliosis from, 328
  phocomelia, 50
  polydactyly, 54
  radioulnar synostosis, 52
  spina bifida, 237
  Sprengel's, 59
  syndactyly, 53
  synostosis of cervical spine, 61
  talipes, equinovarus, 38-46 (see also Clubfoot, congenital)
    of other types, 38, 45
    vertical talus, 47
  in fractures, 488
Degeneration of nerve after injury, 243
Degenerative arthritis, 175-179
  disk disease, 363
  joint disease, 175-179
Delayed traumatic ulnar neuritis, 253
  union of fractures, 289

Deltoid paralysis in axillary nerve injury, 251
  in poliomyelitis, 217
    Mayer operation in, 217
    Ober operation in, 217
Denis Browne splint, for clubfoot, 42
  for talipes calcaneovalgus, 45
De Quervain's tenosynovitis, 475
Derangement, internal, of knee, 393
Diagnosis of orthopaedic patient, 27-34
Diaphyseal aclasis, 105
  dysplasia, progressive, 117
Diastematomyelia, 238
Dickson operation for paralysis of gluteus maximus, 216
  for ununited hip fracture, 299
Disability evaluation after fractures, 499
Disarticulation, 316
Discography, 463
Discoid semilunar cartilage, 398
Disease, Albers-Schönberg, 116
  Albright's, 113
  Bamberger-Marie, 129
  Blount's 89
  Caffey's, 130
  Calvé's, 341
  Charcot-Marie-Tooth, 260
  degenerative, of disks, 363
    of joints, 175
  Engelmann's, 117
  Freiberg's, 428
  Gaucher's, 102
  Haglund's, 433
  Hand-Schüller-Christian, 101
  Hurler's, 110
  Kienböck's, 481
  Köhler's, 424
  Legg-Calvé-Perthes, 374
  Letterer-Siwe, 102
  Little's, 228
  Morquio's, 109
  neuropathic, of bones and joints, 235
  Niemann-Pick, 102
  Ollier's, 107
  Oppenheim's, 233
  Osgood-Schlatter, 405
  Paget's, 124
  Pellegrini-Stieda, 409
  Perthes', 374
  Pott's, 155 (see also Tuberculosis of spine)
  Preiser's, 481
  Scheuermann's, 338
  Schüller-Christian, 101
  Still's, 170
  von Recklinghausen's, of bones, 123
    of nerves, 285
  Werdnig-Hoffmann, 233
Disk, intervertebral, anatomy and pathology of, 360
  degenerative disease of, 363
  lesions of, in adult round back, 342
  lumbar, lesions of, 360
  protrusion of, causing sciatic pain, 360
  rupture of, 363
Dislocation, acromioclavicular, old, 459
  of elbow, congenital, 80
    old traumatic, 465
  of hip, congenital, 63-79
    in poliomyelitis, 213

Dislocation of hip—cont'd
  pathologic, 387
 of jaw, recurrent, 460
 of knee, congenital, 79
 of lunate bone, old, 482
 of patella, congenital, 80
 of peroneal tendons, 436
 of shoulder, congenital, 80
  old traumatic, 458
  paralysis following, 250
  recurrent, 457
 of temporomandibular joint, recurrent, 460
 of ulnar nerve, recurrent, 253
 of wrist, congenital, 80
 pathologic, of hip, 387
 sternoclavicular, old, 459
Displacement of peroneal tendons, 436
 of semilunar cartilage, 393
 of toes, 432
Disuse atrophy, 81
Divided scaphoid bone, 483
Dropped finger, 473
 foot, 256 (see also Foot drop)
 wrist, 252 (see also Wrist drop)
Dunn's tarsal arthrodesis, 219
Dupuytren's contracture, 479
Dwarfism, hypopituitary, 120
 in achondroplasia, 104
 in cretinism, 122
 renal, 97
Dyschondroplasia, 105
Dysostosis, cleidocranial, 58
Dysplasia, acetabular, 64
 diaphyseal, progressive, 117
 epiphyseal, multiple, 375
 fibrous, 113
  monostotic, 115
  of hip, 63
  polyostotic, 113
Dystrophy, facioscapulohumeral, paralysis in, 261
 Landouzy-Déjerine type of, 261
 posttraumatic, sympathetic, 132
 progressive muscular, 260
 pseudohypertrophic muscular, 260
 reflex sympathetic, 132

E

Echinococcus cyst of bone, 146
Eggers operation for knee flexion, 231
 slotted plates, 495
Ehlers-Danlos syndrome, 56
Elbow, affections of, 462-470
 ankylosis of, optimum position for, 198
 arthroplasty of, after old injury, 309
 bursae in region of, 463
 bursitis, bicipitoradial, 465
  olecranon, 463
  radiohumeral, 464
 congenital dislocation of, 80
 deformity of, after fracture of humerus, 307
 malunion of fracture in region of, 308
 miner's, 464
 nursemaid's, 465
 old dislocation of, 465
 sprain of, 463
 strain in region of, 462
 tendon transplantation in region of, 217

Elbow—cont'd
 tennis, 464
Elevation of scapula, congenital, 59
Embryology, 22
Enchondroma, 265
 multiple, 265
Engelmann's disease, 117
Eosinophilic granuloma, 100
Epicondylitis, 464
Epiphyseal arrest, 223
 coxa vara, 381
 dysplasia, multiple, 375
 fractures, 500
 stapling, 223
Epiphyseodesis, 223
Epiphysis, capital femoral, avascular necrosis of, 374
 slipping of, 381
 operative fusion of, 223
 ossification of, 24
 separation of, traumatic, 501
Epiphysitis, calcaneal, 433
 vertebral, 338
Equalization of length of legs, 222
Equinus, definition of, 39
Erb-Duchenne type of obstetric paralysis, 247
Etiology of orthopaedic affections, 26
Ewing's sarcoma, 276
 tumor, 276
Examination of orthopaedic patient, 29
Exostoses, hereditary multiple cartilaginous, 107
 osteocartilaginous, 266
Exostosis, about knee joint, symptoms from, 405
 definition of, 265
 of bones of foot, 435
 subungual, 435
Extensor pollicis longus tendon, rupture of, 472
Exuberant callus, 468

F

Facets, lumbosacral, variations of, 357
Facioscapulohumeral paralysis, 261
Fanconi's syndrome, 97
Fascia lata, in arthroplasty, 201
 in reconstruction of ligaments, 401
Fasciotomy, for flexion contracture of hip, 214
Fat, herniation in low back, 367
 pad, infrapatellar, hypertrophy of, 404
Fatigue fracture, 428
Faulty posture, 343
 treatment, 345
Felon, bone, 476
Felty's syndrome, 170
Femoral nerve, injuries of, 257
Femur, congenital defects of, 51
 head of, blood supply to, 372
 malunited fracture of, 303
 ununited fracture of neck of, 298
 of shaft of, 300
Fibroma, chondromyxoid, 264
 nonossifying or nonosteogenic, 268
 of joints and tendon sheaths, 282
 of muscles and fasciae, 283
Fibrosarcoma, of fascia, 283
Fibrous dysplasia, monostotic, 113, 115
 polyostotic, 113
Fibula, congenital defects of, 51
 malunited fracture of, 305

Fibula—cont'd
  ununited fracture of, 300
Finger, baseball or mallet, 473
  clubbed, 129
  congenital anomalies of, 53-55
  contracture of, 478
  dropped, 473
  snapping or trigger, 475
  spider, 56
  webbed, 53
Finkelstein test, 475
Fixation, internal, 495
  intramedullary, 495
  of joints, optimum position for, 197
Flail joint, arthrodesis of, 218
Flat chest, 345
  foot, flexible, 418
    spastic, 419
Foot, accessory bones of, 435
  affections of, 415-436
  arches of, 415
  arthrodesis of, in cerebral palsy, 232
    in clawfoot, 424
    in hereditary muscular atrophy, 260
    in poliomyelitis, 218
    in spastic flatfoot, 421
  claw, 421
    in hereditary muscular atrophy, 424
    in spina bifida, 240
  cleft, 55
  club, congenital, 38-47
  contracted, 421 (see also Clawfoot)
  drop, in peripheral nerve injury, 256
    in poliomyelitis, 206
    steppage gait in, 256
    treatment of, 215
      Campbell operation in, 222
      Gill operation in, 222
  exostoses of bones of, 435
  flat, flexible, 418
    spastic, 419
  function of, 415
  "lobster claw," 55
  strain, 417
  supernumerary bones of, 436
  tendon transplantation in region of, 216
  terminology of motion of, 415
Forearm, bones of, congenital synostosis of, 52
  malunited fracture of, 309
  ununited fracture of, 302
Fracture, acute hemorrhage in, 486
  bumper, and genu valgum, 93
  Colles', malunion of, 310
  comminuted, 485
  compound, 500
  congenital, nonunion of, 296
  definitions of, 485
  deformities, 286-313
  deformity in, 488
  delayed union of, 289-291
  disability evaluation after, 499
  epiphyseal, 500
  greenstick, 501
  in children, 500
  malunion of, 303-312
  manipulation for, 489
  march, 428
  Monteggia, malunion of, 309

Fracture—cont'd
  nonunion of, 291-303
  of tibial spine, 401
  open, 500
    reduction of, 490
  overgrowth after, 501
  pathologic, in bone cyst, 271
    in hyperparathyroidism, 123
    in metastatic tumor of bone, 280
    in multiple myeloma, 278
    in neuropathic osteopathy, 235
    in osteitis deformans, 127
    in osteogenesis imperfecta, 111
    in osteomalacia, 99
    in osteomyelitis, 136
  physical therapy for, 498, 499
  reduction of, 489
  repair of, 286
  respiratory difficulty in, 486
  shock in, 486
  stiffness after, 497
  torus, 501
  traction for, 491
  types of, 485
  ununited, 291-303
Fragilitas ossium, 111
Freiberg's disease of metatarsal head, 428
Frejka abduction pillow splint, 72
Friedreich's ataxia, 234
Frozen shoulder, 452
Functional adaptations of bone, 81
  bracing, 326
  paralysis, 232
Fungus infections of bone, 146
Funnell chest, 346
Fusion, lumbosacral, 354
  in spondylolisthesis, 360
  of epiphysis, surgical, 223
  spinal, Albee's method in, 158
    Hibbs' method in, 157
    in scoliosis, 335
    in tuberculosis, 157

G

Gait, in bilateral coxa vara, 380
  in cerebral palsy, 227
  in congenital clubfoot, 40
  in dislocation of hip, 67
  in Friedreich's ataxia, 234
  in genu valgum, 93
    varum, 92
  in hereditary muscular atrophy, 260
  in paralysis of dorsiflexors of ankle, 206, 256
    of gluteus maximus, 206
    of gluteus medius, 206
    of quadriceps, 206
  scissors, in spastic paraplegia, 227
  steppage, in foot drop, 206, 256
Ganglion of tendon sheath, 477
Gargoylism, 110
Garré's osteitis, 141
Gas gangrene, amputation in, 315
Gastrocnemio-semimembranosus bursa, affections of, 412
Gaucher's cells, 102
  disease, 102
Generalized osteitis fibrosa cystica, 123

Genu recurvatum, congenital, 80
    in poliomyelitis, 214
        Campbell operation for, 214
        Gill operation for, 214
    valgum, 92
    varum, 89
Giant cell tumor of bone, 270
    of tendon sheath, 282
Gigantism, 121
Gill operation for arthrodesis of shoulder, 221
    for calcaneus foot, 222
    for foot drop, 222
    for genu recurvatum, 214
Gluteus maximus, paralysis of, in poliomyelitis, 216
    medius, paralysis of, in poliomyelitis, 216
Goniometer, use of, 30
Gonococcal arthritis, 144
Gout, 179-181
Gowers' sign, 261
Grafts, bone, 293-295
Granuloma, eosinophilic, 100
Greenstick fracture, 501
Grice operation for arthodesis of foot, 220
Gritti-Stokes amputation, 321
Groove, Harrison's, 86
Growth, asymmetrical, 56
    operation for arresting, 223
Guillain-Barré syndrome, 259
Gummatous arthritis, 148

H

Haglund's disease, 433
Hallux rigidus, 431
    valgus, 428
    varus, 431
Hammer toe, 431
Hamstring muscles, transplantation of, in poliomyelitis, 216
Hand, accessory bones of, 483
    affections of, 470-484
    anatomy of, 471
    claw, in cervical rib, 445
        in progressive muscular atrophy, 233
        in ulnar nerve injury, 253
    cleft, 55
    club, 47
    contracture of, 478
        intrinsic, 479
            plus or minus, 479
    infections of, 475
    "lobster claw," 55
    malunited fractures in region of, 311
    supernumerary bones of, 483
    tendon transplantation in region of, 217
    tenosynovitis in region of, 474
    trident, in achondroplasia, 104
Hand-Schüller-Christian disease, 101
Harrison's groove, in rickets, 86
Haversian system, 24
Heart-shaped pelvis, in osteomalacia, 98
Heberden's nodes, 176
Heel, affections of, 433
    bursitis in region of, 433
    Cook anterior, 426
    inflammation or injury under, 434
    orthopaedic, 418
    spurs of, 434

Heel—cont'd
    Thomas, 418
Hemangioma of bone, 264
    of joint, 282
Hematoma of sternocleidomastoid muscle, 437
    ossifying, 468
Hemihypertrophy, congenital, 56
Hemimacrosomia, 56
Hemiplegia in cerebral palsy, 224
    gait in, 227
Hemophilia, joint involvement in, 412
Hereditary multiple cartilaginous exostoses, 107
    muscular atrophy of peroneal type, 260
Herniation of fascial fat, 367
    of nucleus pulposus, 363
Hibbs' method of spinal fusion, 157
High scapula, congenital, 60
Hip, affections of, 372-391
    ankylosis of, optimum position for, 198
    arthrodesis of, in malum coxae senilis, 192
        in poliomyelitis, 218
        in tuberculosis, 163
        Smith-Petersen cup, 201
    arthrokatadysis of, 388
    arthroplasty of, after old injury, 303
        in malum coxae senilis, 192
        replacement, 202
    bursitis in region of, 389
    chronic arthritis of, 189-192
    congenital dislocation of, 65-79
        dysplasia of, 63
        subluxation of, 64
    deformities of, in poliomyelitis, 213
    dislocation of, congenital, 65-79
        in poliomyelitis, 213
        pathologic, 387
    dysplasia of, congenital, 63
    flexion contracture of, Campbell operation for, 214
        examination for, 32
        in poliomyelitis, 213
        Soutter fasciotomy for, 214
        Yount operation for, 214
    malunited fracture of, 303
    osteoarthritis of, 189
    pathologic dislocation of, 387
    prosthesis, 202
    pyogenic arthritis of, in infants, 144
    rheumatoid arthritis of, 189
    snapping, 391
    subluxation of, congenital, 64
    transient synovitis of, 389
    tuberculosis of, 161-164
    ununited fracture of, 298
Histiocytosis, 100
History of orthopaedics, 21
History taking, 27, 486
Hoke operation for stabilization of foot, 219
Hollow back, 343
Horizontal sacrum, 357
Horner's syndrome in obstetric paralysis, 248
Housemaid's knee, 411
Humerus, congenital defects of, 50
    malunited fracture of, 307
    ununited fracture of, 302
        step-cut operation in, 302
Hurler's syndrome, 110
Hydarthrosis, intermittent, 170, 410

Index 581

Hydatid cyst, 146
Hydrocephalus, 239
Hyperostosis, infantile cortical, 130
Hyperparathyroidism, 123
Hyperpituitarism, 121
Hypertrophic pulmonary osteoarthropathy, secondary, 129
Hypertrophy of bone, 81
  of infrapatellar fat pad, 404
  of synovial membrane, 405
Hypervitaminosis A, 84
  D, 85
Hypopituitary dwarfism, 120
Hypothyroidism, 122
Hypotonia, benign, congenital, 233
Hysterical paralysis, 232
  torticollis, 440

I

Idiopathic osteopsathyrosis, 111
  scoliosis, 328
Iliopectineal or iliopsoas bursitis, 389
Inequality of leg length, 222
Infantile cortical hyperostosis, 130
  paralysis, 203-223 (see also Poliomyelitis)
  rickets, 85
  spinal muscular atrophy, 233
Infections of hand, 475
Infraclavicular lesions of brachial plexus, 250
Infrapatellar bursitis, deep, 411
  fat pad, hypertrophy and pinching of, 404
Injury of peripheral nerves, 241
Inlay bone graft, 295
Intermittent hydrarthrosis or synovitis, 170, 410
Internal derangement of knee, 393
  fixation of fractures, 495
Intervertebral disk, anatomy and pathology, 360
  degenerative disease of, 363
  lumbar, lesions of, 360
  protrusion of, causing sciatic pain, 360
  rupture of, 363
Intramedullary fixation, 495
Intrapelvic protrusion of acetabulum, 388
Intrinsic contracture of hand, 479
  plus or minus hand, 479
Involucrum, in osteomyelitis, 135
Irwin osteotomy for genu recurvatum, 214
Ischemic contracture of Volkmann, 466
Ischiofemoral arthrodesis, 164
Ischiogluteal bursitis, 391
Isthmus defects, 358

J

Jacket, Calot, in tuberculosis of spine, 159
  Risser turnbuckle, in scoliosis, 335
Jaw, affections of, 460-461
  ankylosis of, 461
  recurrent dislocation of, 460
  snapping, 460
Joint, anatomy of, 26
  ankylosis of, 194-200
  Charcot's, 235
  Clutton's, 147
  etiology of disease of, 26
  examination of, 30
  fixation, optimum positions for, 197
  gonococcus infection of, 144
  hemophilic involvement of, 412

Joint—cont'd
  hysterical affections of, 232
  mice, 401
  motion, terminology of, 30
  neuropathic disease of, 235
  pneumococcus infection of, 144
  pyogenic infection of, 142
  septic (see Joint, pyogenic infection of)
  syphilis of, 146
  tuberculosis of (see Tuberculosis of bones and joints)
  tumors of, 282
Juvenile rheumatoid arthritis, 170

K

Kanavel on infections of hand, 470
Keller operation in hallux valgus, 430
Kernicterus in cerebral palsy, 226
Kernig's sign in poliomyelitis, 205
Kidner operation for long arch depression, 436
Kienböch's disease, 481
Kirk amputation, 321
Kirschner wire, 493
Klippel-Feil syndrome, 61
Klumpke type of obstetric paralysis, 248
Knee, affections of, 392-414
  ankylosis, optimum position for, 198
  arthritis of, 192
  arthrodesis of, in poliomyelitis, 218
  arthroplasty of, in chronic arthritis, 194
  brace, after internal derangement, 397
  bursitis in region of, 411
  cartilages of, discoid type, 398
    semilunar, 393
      cysts of, 398
      excision of, 397
      injury of, 393
        treatment of, 396
  collateral ligaments of, rupture of, 399
  congenital dislocation of, 79
  cruciate ligaments of, rupture of, 400
  cysts of semilunar cartilages of, 398
  deformities of, in poliomyelitis, 214
  exostoses in region of, 405
  flexion contracture of, in poliomyelitis, 214
  hemophilic involvement of, 412
  housemaid's, 411
  hypertrophy of infrapatellar fat pad of, 404
    of synovial villi of, 405
  intermittent hydrarthrosis of, 170, 410
  internal derangements of, 393
  lateral ligaments of, rupture of, 399
  loose bodies in, 401
  meniscus (see Knee, semilunar cartilage)
  Osgood-Schlatter disease of, 405
  ossification in tibial collateral ligament of, 409
  osteochondritis dissecans of, 402
  osteochondromatosis of, 404
  pigmented villonodular synovitis of, 405
  pinching of infrapatellar fat pad of, 404
  recurvatum of, congenital, 79
    in poliomyelitis, 214
  semilunar cartilages, cysts of, 398
    excision of, 397
    injuries of, 393
  snapping, 410
  synovial chondromatosis of, 404
  tendon transplantation in region of, 216

Index

Knee—cont'd
    tibial spine fracture in, 401
Knock-knee, 92
    in poliomyelitis, 214
Köhler's disease of tarsal navicular, 424
Krukenberg operation, 318
Küntscher rod, 495
Kyphosis, 338
    adolescent, 338
    in adult round back, 341
    in Morquio's disease, 110
    in osteochondritis, 341
    in tuberculosis of spine, 155
    in vertebral epiphysitis, 338
    senile, 341

L

Laboratory diagnosis, 34
Lambrinudi operation for arthrodesis of foot, 220
Laminectomy, in tuberculosis of spine, 158
Landouzy-Déjerine type of progressive muscular dystrophy, 261
Lane technic, 495
Lasègue's sign, 351
Late median nerve palsy, 255
    rickets, 95
    traumatic ulnar neuritis, 253
Lateral curvature of spine (see Scoliosis)
    ligaments of knee, rupture of, 399
    sclerosis, amyotrophic, 233
Law, Wolff's, 81
Leadbetter hip maneuver, 386
Leg length, equalization of, 222
    measurement of, 32
Legg operation for paralysis of gluteus medius, 216
Legg-Calvé-Perthes disease, 374
Lengthening of bones, 222
Letterer-Siwe disease, 102
Ligament, collateral, of knee, rupture of, 399
    cruciate, rupture of, 400
    patellar, rupture of, 409
    tibial collateral, ossification of, 409
Limb, phantom, 323
Limp (see Gait)
Line, Bryant's, 32
    Nélaton's, 32
    Shenton's, 68
    white, of scurvy, 94
Lipochondro-osteodystrophy, 110
Lipoma, of bone, 264
    of fascia, 283
    of joint, 282
    of muscle, 283
Lisfranc amputation, 319
Little's disease, 228
"Lobster claw" deformity of hand or foot, 55
Locking, in internal derangement of knee, 395
Locomotor system, biophysics of, 345
Long thoracic nerve, injuries of, 251
Longitudinal arch of foot, 415
Loose bodies in joints, 401
Looser's zones, 99
Lordosis, 343
Lorenz bifurcation operation, 78
    on treatment of congenital dislocation of hip, 65

Low back, acquired skeletal lesions of, 367
    affections of, 348-371
        classification, 348
        diagnosis, 352
        etiology, 348
        intervertebral disk rupture, 360
        myofascitis, 367
        osteoarticular lesions, 367
        pain in, 349
        posture in, 350
        roentgenograms in, 352
        tests of passive mobility in, 351
        treatment, 352
            conservative, 352
            manipulative, 366
            surgical, 354
    bony anomalies of, 354
    fascial fat herniations in, 367
    ligamentous injuries of, 349
    muscular injuries of, 349
    pain, classification of causes of, 349
Lowman operation for paralyzed abdominals, 215, 338
Lumbosacral angle, variations of, 357
    corset, 353
    facets, variations of, 357
    joint, affections of, 349 (see also Low back, affections of)
        anomalies of, 354
        arthrodesis of, for low back pain, 354
        in spondylolisthesis, 358
    plexus, injury of, 255
    sprain, 349
Lunate bone, old dislocation of, 482

M

Macrodactyly, 54
Madelung's deformity, 80
Main en trident in achondroplasia, 104
Malformation, congenital (see Deformity, congenital)
Malignant tumors of bone, 272-282
Mallet finger, 473
Malum coxae senilis, 189
Malunion of fractures, 303
Manipulation in ankylosis, 196
    in disk disorders, 366
    in malunited Colles' fracture, 311
        Pott's fracture, 306
    in semilunar cartilage injury, 396
    in talipes equinovarus, 41
    of fractures, 489
Marble bones, 116
March fracture, 428
Marfan's syndrome, 56
Marie's pulmonary osteoarthropathy, 129
Marie-Strümpell arthritis, 183
Maternal obstetric palsy, 255
Mauck's operation, 399
Mayer operation, for deltoid paralysis, 217
    for recurrent dislocation of jaw, 461
McMurray hip osteotomy, 192, 300
    sign, 395
Measurement of extremities, 32
    of range of joint motion, 30
Median nerve, injury of, 254
    late palsy of, 255
Melorheostosis, 117
Membrana reuniens in spina bifida, 239

Index 583

Membrane, synovial, 26
    hypertrophy of, 405
Meningocele, 239
Meniscus of knee (*see* Semilunar cartilages)
Menopausal arthritis, 176
Mental impairment in cerebral palsy, 228
    in cretinism, 122
Meralgia paraesthetica, 258
Metabolic disorders, 27
  simulating rickets, 95
Metacarpal bones, malunited fracture of, 311
  ununited fracture of, 303
Metaphyseal aclasis, 105
Metastatic tumors of bone, 279
Metatarsal arch of foot, 415
  bar, 426
  bone, Freiberg's disease of, 428
    malunited fracture of, 307
    march fracture of, 428
Metatarsalgia, anterior, 425
Metatarsus adductus, 46
  atavicus, 423
  varus, 46
Milwaukee brace for scoliosis, 335
Miner's elbow, 464
Monoplegia, in cerebral palsy, 224
Monostotic fibrous dysplasia, 115
Monteggia fracture, malunion of, 309
Morquio-Brailsford chondro-osteodystrophy, 109
Morquio's disease, 109
Morton's toe, 427
Motion in joint, measurement of, 30
  terminology of, 30
Motor education in cerebral palsy, 229
Multiple cartilaginous exostoses, 107
    enchondromas, 265
    epiphyseal dysplasia, 375
    myeloma, 277
    neuritis, 257
    neurofibroma, 285
Mumford operation for acromioclavicular dislocation, 307
Muscle, biceps brachii, rupture of, 455
  injuries causing low back pain, 349
  operations upon, in cerebral palsy, 231
    in poliomyelitis, 215
  testing, 34
  training, in cerebral palsy, 229
  transplantation, in poliomyelitis, 215
  tumors of, 283
Muscle-sliding operation of Page, 468
Muscular atrophy, infantile spinal, 233
    of Aran-Duchenne type, 233
    of Charcot-Marie-Tooth type, 260
    progressive, 233
  dystrophy, progressive, 260
    pseudohypertrophic, 260
Musculotendinous cuff, tears of, 453
Mycotic arthritis and osteomyelitis, 146
Myelocele, 239
Myelography, 366
Myeloma, multiple, 277
Myelomeningocele, 239
Myoblastoma, 283
Myofascitis, 367
Myopathy, primary, 260
Myositis ossificans, progressive, 119
    traumatic, 468

Myotomy in cerebral palsy, 231
  in congenital torticollis, 440

N

Navicular bone, accessory, 436
  Köhler's disease of, 424
Neck, affections of, 437-446
  web, 62
  wry, 437 (*see also* Torticollis)
Necrosis, avascular, 27
  of capital femoral epiphysis, 374 (*see also* Coxa plana)
  of carpal bones, 481
  of metatarsal head, 428
  of tarsal navicular, 424
Nélaton's line, 32
Neoplasms (*see* Tumor)
Nerve, anatomy of, 241
  degeneration after injury of, 243
  graft, 245
  injuries of, 241-257
    accessory, 246
    axillary, 251
    brachial plexus, 247
    cauda equina, 255
    cervical sympathetic, 442
    classification of, 243
    common peroneal, 256
    conus medullaris, 255
    degeneration in, 243
    femoral, 257
    following dislocation of shoulder, 250
    infraclavicular nerve trunks, 250
    lateral femoral cutaneous, 258
    long thoracic, 251
    lumbosacral plexus, 255
    mechanism of, 242
    median, 254
    obturator, 257
    pathology of, 242
    radial, 251
    reaction of degeneration in, 243
    regeneration after, 243
    root syndrome in, 441
    sciatic, 256
    supraclavicular, 250
    tibial, 257
    Tinel's sign in, 244
    treatment of, 244
    ulnar, 252
  neurolysis in constriction of, 246
  roots, of brachial plexus, syndrome after injury of, 247
  section of, in cerebral palsy, 230
  suture of, 245
  tumors of, 284
  von Recklinghausen's disease of, 373
Neuralgia, 259
Neurapraxia, 243
Neurectomy, in cerebral palsy, 230
  in malum coxae senilis, 191
  obturator, 231
  Stöffel, 230
Neuritis, 257
  multiple, 257
  serum, 258
  toxic, 258

Index

Neuritis—cont'd
  traumatic, 257
  late, of ulnar nerve, 253
Neurofibroma, 284
  after nerve injury, 242
Neurofibromatosis, 285
Neurofibrosarcoma, 284
Neurologic disorders, 203-262
Neurolysis, 246
Neuroma, 284
  after division of nerve, 242
  amputation, 323
  in continuity, 243
  plantar, 427
Neuropathic disease of bones and joints, 235
Neurosis, joint disabilities due to, 232
Neurotmesis, 244
Neutral zero joint position, 32
Nicola operation for recurrent dislocation of shoulder, 458
Niemann-Pick disease, 102
"No man's land" of tendon suture in palm, 471
Nodes, Heberden's, 176
  Schmorl's, 340, 342
Nonossifying fibroma, 268
Nonosteogenic fibroma, 268
Nonunion of fractures, 291
Nucleus pulposus, 361
  herniation of, 363
Nun's knee, 411
Nursemaid's elbow, 465

O

Ober's operation for paralysis of deltoid, 217
  for paralysis of gluteus maximus, 216
  sign for contracture of iliotibial band, 351
Obstetric paralysis, 247
  Erb-Duchenne type of, 247
  Klumpke type of, 248
  maternal, 255
Obturator nerve, injury of, 257
Occupational therapy, after amputation, 322
  after fracture, 499
  in cerebral palsy, 230
Ocular torticollis, 441
Olecranon bursitis, 463
Ollier's disease, 107
Omovertebral bone, 60
Onlay bone graft, 294
Open fractures, 500
  reduction of fractures, 490
Operation, Bankart, in recurrent dislocation of shoulder, 457
  Bennett, for quadriceps contracture, 197
  Bunnell, in paralysis of opponens pollicis, 217
  Campbell, for footdrop, 222
    for genu recurvatum, 214
    for hip flexion contracture, 214
  Colonna, for hip dislocation, 76
  Dickson, in gluteus maximus paralysis, 216
  Dunn, for stabilizing foot, 219
  Eggers, for knee flexion, 231
  Gill, for calcaneus foot, 222
    for footdrop, 222
    for genu recurvatum, 214
    shoulder arthrodesis, 221
  Grice, for arthrodesis of foot, 220
  Hoke, for stabilizing foot, 219
  Keller, in hallux valgus, 430

Operation—cont'd
  Lambrinudi, for arthrodesis of foot, 220
  Legg, in gluteus medius paralysis, 216
  Lorenz hip bifurcation, 78
  Lowman, in paralyzed abdominals, 215, 338
  Mayer, in deltoid paralysis, 217
    in recurrent dislocation of jaw, 461
  muscle-sliding, of Page, 468
  Nicola, in recurrent dislocation of shoulder, 458
  Ober, in deltoid paralysis, 217
    in gluteus maximus paralysis, 216
  Putti-Platt, in recurrent dislocation of shoulder, 458
  Schanz, in hallux valgus, 430
  Sever, in obstetric paralysis, 249
  shelf, 77
  Silver, in hallux valgus, 430
  Soutter, in hip flexion contracture, 214
  Steindler, in paralysis of elbow flexors, 217
  step-cut, 302
  Stöffel, in cerebral palsy, 230
  Thompson, for knee extension contracture, 197
  Yount, in hip flexion contracture, 214
Oppenheim's disease, 233
Orr method in treatment of osteomyelitis, 139
Orthopaedic heel, 418
  surgery, definition of, 22
    history of, 21
Ortolani's sign, 64
Os calcis (see Calcaneus)
  peroneale, 436
  tibiale, 436
  trigonum, 436
Osgood-Schlatter disease, 405
Ossification, of tibial collateral ligament, 409
  physiology of, in repair of fracture, 286
Ossifying hematoma, 468
Osteitis, chronic sclerosing, 141
  condensans ilii, 368
  deformans, 124
  fibrosa cystica, generalized, 123 (see also Hyperparathyroidism)
  of Garré, 141
  pubis, 141
  traumatic, of carpal bones, 481
Osteoarthritis, 175-179
  of hip, 189
  of knee, 192
  of spine, 186
Osteoarthropathy, neuropathic, 235
  secondary hypertrophic pulmonary, 129
Osteocartilaginous exostoses, 266
Osteochondritis dissecans, 402
  of metatarsal head, 428
  of navicular bone, 424
  syphilitic, 147
  vertebral, 341
Osteochondroma, 266
Osteochondromatosis, 282, 404
Osteoclasis, 88
Osteoclastoma, 270
Osteodystrophy, renal, 97
Osteogenesis imperfecta, 111
Osteogenic sarcoma, 272
Osteoid-osteoma, 267
Osteoma, 265
Osteomalacia, 98

Index 585

Osteomyelitis, 133-140
  Brodie's abscess in, 140
  chronic sclerosing, 139
  cloacae in, 135
  due to brucellosis, 145
  due to coccidioides infection, 146
  due to echinococcus infestation, 146
  due to fungus infection, 146
  involucrum in, 135
  of Garré, 141
  pathologic fracture in, 136
  pyogenic, 133-139
  Salmonella, 145
  sequestrum in, 135
  suppurative, 133-139
  syphilitic, 146
  typhoid, 145
Osteone, 24
Osteopathia striata, 116
Osteoperiosteal bone graft, 295
Osteoperiostitis, syphilitic, 147
Osteopetrosis, 116
Osteophytes in osteoarthritis, 176
Osteopoikilosis, 117
Osteoporosis, disuse, 81
  of carpal bones, traumatic, 481
  painful posttraumatic, 132
  senile, 127
Osteopsathyrosis, idiopathic, 111
Osteosarcoma, 272
Osteosclerosis, 116
Osteotomy, 89
  bifurcation, of Lorenz, 78
  in genu valgum, 94
    varum, 92
  in malum coxae senilis, 192
  Irwin, for genu recurvatum, 214
  subtrochanteric, of Schanz, 77
  wedge, in clubfoot, 44
Osteotomy-osteoclasis of Moore, 89
Otto pelvis, 388
Overflow, in spastic paralysis, 227
Overgrowth after fracture, 501
Overlapping of toes, 432

P

Pad, for longitudinal arch, 418
  for metatarsal arch, 426
Page muscle-sliding operation, 468
Paget's disease, 124
Pain, low back (see Low back pain)
Painful coccyx, 369
Palindromic rheumatism, 170
Palmar fascia, contracture of, 479
Palsy, birth, 247 (see also Obstetric paralysis)
  cerebral, 224-240
  crutch, 251, 258
  late median nerve, 255
    ulnar nerve, 253
  maternal obstetric, 255
Pannus, in rheumatoid arthritis, 167
Paralysis, Aran-Duchenne type of, 233
  cerebral spastic, 224-232
  Charcot-Marie-Tooth type of, 260
  facioscapulohumeral, 261
  following dislocation of shoulder, 250
    injection of serum, 258
  hysterical, 232
  in Friedreich's ataxia, 234

Paralysis—cont'd
  in spina bifida, 237
  in tuberculosis of spine, 156
  infantile, 203-223 (see also Poliomyelitis)
  ischemic, of Volkmann, 466
  Landouzy-Déjerine type of, 261
  obstetric, 247
  pseudohypertrophic muscular, 260
  spastic, 227
  Volkmann's ischemic, 466
Paralytic scoliosis, 328
Paraplegia, in cerebral palsy, 224
  in tuberculosis, 156
Parathyroid adenoma in hyperparathyroidism, 123
Patella, bipartite, 52
  chondromalacia of, 408
  congenital absence of, 52
    defects of, 52
  dislocation of, 80
  malunited fracture of, 303
  recurrent dislocation of, 407
  slipping, 407
  ununited fracture of, 300
Patellar ligament, rupture of, 409
Patellectomy in osteoarthritis of knee, 194
Pathologic dislocation of hip, 387
  fracture, in bone cyst, 271
  in hyperparathyroidism, 123
  in metastatic tumor of bone, 280
  in multiple myeloma, 278
  in neuropathic osteopathy, 235
  in osteitis deformans, 127
  in osteogenesis imperfecta, 111
  in osteomalacia, 99
  in osteomyelitis, 136
Pearson attachment, 493
Pectus carinatum, 346
  excavatum, 346
Pellegrini-Stieda disease, 409
Pelvis, heart-shaped, 98
  malunited fracture of, 212
  Otto, 488
Periarthritis of shoulder, 449, 452
Periostitis ossificans, 147
  syphilitic, 147
Peripheral nerve injuries, 241-257 (see also Nerve, injuries of)
Peroneal tendons, displacement of, 436
  type of hereditary muscular atrophy, 260
Perthes' disease, 374
Pes planus, 418
Phantom limb, 323
Phemister onlay graft, 295
Phocomelia, 50
Phosphatase in repair of fractures, 289
Physical diagnosis of fracture patient, 486
  of orthopaedic patient, 27-34
  therapy, in cerebral palsy, 229
    in faulty posture, 345
    in fibrous ankylosis, 195
    in osteoarthritis, 178
    in peripheral nerve injuries, 245
    in poliomyelitis, 210
    in psychosomatic syndromes, 232
    in rheumatoid arthritis, 173
    in scoliosis, exercises, 334
    in shoulder affections, 450, 453

Physical therapy—cont'd
    in treatment of fractures, 498, 499
Physiology of bones and joints, 22
Pigeon breast, 346
    toe, 432
Pigmented villonodular synovitis, 405
Pinching of infrapatellar fat pad, 404
    of synovial membrane, 404
Pirogoff amputation, 319
Plantar neuroma, 427
Plantaris tendon, rupture of, 434
Plaster jacket, in treatment of scoliosis, 335
    of tuberculosis of spine, 158
  of Paris, 490
  shell, in treatment of tuberculosis of spine, 157
Plexus, brachial, injury of, 247
    by dislocation of shoulder, 250
  lumbosacral, injury of, 255
Pneumococcal arthritis, 144
Poliomyelitis, acute stage of, 205
  anterior, 203
  cerebrospinal fluid in, 205
  clinical picture, 204
  convalescent stage, 206
  diagnosis, 206
  etiology, 203
  gait in, 206
  Kernig's sign in, 205
  nonparalytic, 206
  pathology, 204
  prognosis, 208
  scoliosis in, 215
  treatment, 209
    arthrodesis in, 218
    bone block operations in, 222
    of acute stage, 209
    of convalescent stage, 210
    of established deformities in, 213
    of residual stage, 212
    of respiratory paralysis, 210
    physical therapy in, 210
    prophylactic, 209
    surgical, 213
    tendon and muscle transplantation in, 215
  types of, 204
  vaccines for, 204
  viruses in, 203
Poliovirus, 203
Polydactyly, 54
Polyneuritis, 257
Polyostotic fibrous dysplasia, 113
Popliteal bursae, affections of, 412
Positions of joint fixation, optimum, 197
Posttraumatic painful osteoporosis, 132
  sympathetic dystrophy, 132
Posture, faulty, 343
  treatment of, 345
Pott's disease, 155 (see also Tuberculosis of spine)
  fracture, malunited, 305
Preiser's disease, 481
Prepatellar bursitis, 411
Prespondylolisthesis, 358
Pretibial bursitis, superficial, 412
Primary myopathy, 260
"Prize-fighter's knuckle," 312
Progressive diaphyseal dysplasia, 117

Progressive—cont'd
  muscular atrophy, 233
    of Aran-Duchenne type, 233
    of Charcot-Marie-Tooth type, 260
  dystrophy, 260
    facioscapulohumeral paralysis in, 261
    Landouzy-Déjerine type of, 261
  myositis ossificans, 119
Proliferative arthritis, 167
Pronator syndrome, 254
Prostheses, 323
  suction socket, 321
Protrusio acetabuli, 388
Protrusion of intervertebral disk, 360
Pseudarthrosis, after fracture, 291
  congenital, 296
Pseudofracture, in osteomalacia, 99
Pseudohypertrophic muscular dystrophy, 260
Pseudoneuroma after nerve injury, 243
Pseudoparalysis, syphilitic, 147
Pseudospondylolisthesis, 359
Psoas abscess, 156
Psoriatic arthritis, 170
Psychologic disorders, 27
Psychosomatic syndromes, 232
Pterygium colli, 62
Pull syndrome, 465
Pulmonary osteoarthropathy of Marie, 129
Putti abduction splint in congenital dislocation of hip, 72
Putti-Platt operation for recurrent dislocation of shoulder, 458
Pyogenic arthritis, 142-144
  of hip in infants, 144
    treatment of, 143
  osteomyelitis, 133-140
    clinical picture, 136
    cloacae in, 135
    diagnosis, 137
    etiology, 133
    involucrum in, 136
    pathologic fracture in, 136
    pathology of, 133
    prognosis in, 137
    roentgenograms in, 137
    sequestrum in, 136
    treatment of, 137
      closure of cavities in, 139
      Orr method, 139

Q

Quadriceps muscle, paralysis of, in poliomyelitis, 216
  in injury of femoral nerve, 257
  tendon, Bennett lengthening of, 197
    rupture of, 409
Quadriplegia, in cerebral palsy, 224

R

Rachischisis, 239
Rachitic craniotabes, 87
  genu valgum, 92
    varum, 89
  rosary, 86
  scoliosis, 87, 328
Radial head subluxation, 465
  nerve, injury of, 251

Radiohumeral bursitis, 464
Radioulnar synostosis, after fracture, 310
    congenital, 52
Radius, congenital defects of, 50
    malunited fracture of, 309
    ununited fracture of, 302
Recurrent dislocation of jaw, 460
    of patella, 407
    of peroneal tendons, 436
    of shoulder, 457
    of ulnar nerve, 253
Reduction of fractures, 489
    open, 490
Re-education of muscles in cerebral palsy, 229
Reflex sympathetic dystrophy, 132
Reflexes, in cerebral palsy, 227
    in poliomyelitis, 205
Regeneration of bone after fracture, 286
    of nerve after injury, 243
Rehabilitation, 36
Reiter's syndrome, 170
Renal dwarfism, 97
    lesions in hyperparathyroidism, 123
    osteodystrophy, 97
    rickets, 97
Repair of fractures, 286
Respirator in treatment of poliomyelitis, 210
Restoration of function after fracture, 497
Reticuloendotheliosis, 100
Retrocalcaneal bursitis, 433
Rhabdomyosarcoma, 283
Rheumatism, palindromic, 170
Rheumatoid arthritis, 167-175
    juvenile, 170
    of knee, 192
    of spine, 182
    treatment, 244
    variants of, 169
    factor, 171
Rib, cervical, 444
Rickets, 85-89
    adolescent or late, 95
    adult, 98
    infantile, 85-89
    renal, 97
    vitamin-resistant, 95
Rider's bone, 468
Rigid flatfoot, 419
Risser, localizer cast in scoliosis, 335
    on roentgenograms in scoliosis, 332
    turnbuckle jacket in scoliosis, 335
Robison on repair of fracture, 289
Rocker-bottom foot, 42
Roentgentherapy, in giant cell tumor, 271
    in Ewing's sarcoma, 277
    in metastatic tumors of bone, 281
    in multiple myeloma, 279
    in osteogenic sarcoma, 275
    in Strümpell-Marie arthritis, 188
Roentgenograms in diagnosis, 34
    in fracture diagnosis, 489
Root syndrome, cervical, 441
Rosary, rachitic, 86
Round back, 338
    adult, 341
    shoulders, 345
Rupture, of Achilles tendon, 434
    of biceps brachii, 455
    of central extensor slip, 473

Rupture—cont'd
    of collateral ligaments of knee, 399
    of cruciate ligaments of knee, 400
    of extensor pollicis longus, 472
    of intervertebral disk, 363
    of patellar ligament, 409
    of plantaris tendon, 434
    of quadriceps tendon, 409
    of supraspinatus tendon, 453
    of tendons, 472
Russell's traction, 492

S

Saber shin, 147
Sabin vaccine for poliomyelitis, 209
Sacralization of last lumbar vertebra, 355
Sacroiliac joint, sprain of, 349
    tuberculosis of, 160
Sacrum, horizontal, 357
Salk vaccine for poliomyelitis, 209
Salmonella arthritis and osteomyelitis, 145
Sarcoma, Ewing's, 276
    osteogenic, 272
    synovial, 282
Sartorius muscle transplantation in paralysis of quadriceps, 216
Saucerization, in osteomyelitis, 139
Scalenus anticus syndrome, 444
Scaphoid, divided, 483
    ununited fracture of, 302
    tarsal (see Navicular bone)
Scapula, congenital elevation of, 59
    malunited fracture of, 307
Schanz operation for hallux valgus, 430
    subtrochanteric osteotomy, 77
Scheuermann's disease, 338
Schmorl's nodes in adult round back, 342
    in vertebral epiphysitis, 340
Schrock on transplantation of scapula, 61
Schüller-Christian disease, 101
Sciatic nerve, injury of, 256
    scoliosis, 350, 365
Scissors gait, in spastic paralysis, 227
Sclerae, blue, in osteogenesis imperfecta, 111
Sclerosing osteitis, 141
Sclerosis, amyotrophic lateral, 233
    subacute combined, 234
Scoliosis, 327-338
    classification of, etiologic, 327
        regional, 329
    clinical picture, 331
    congenital, 328
        idiopathic, 328
    definition of, 327
    diagnosis, 332
    etiology, 327
    functional, 327
    idiopathic, 328
    in poliomyelitis, 215, 328
    incidence of, 327
    paralytic, 328
    pathology of, 329
    postural, 327
    prognosis of, 332
    rachitic, 328
    rotation of vertebrae in, 331
    sciatic, 350, 365
    structural, 327
    thoracic deformity in, 331

Scoliosis—cont'd
　treatment, 334
　　arthrodesis of spine, 335
　　Blount or Milwaukee brace, 335
　　corrective exercises, 334
　　prophylactic, 334
　　Risser localizer cast, 335
　　　turnbuckle jacket, 335
　　surgical, 335
　types of curvature in, 329
Scurvy, 94
Secondary hypertrophic pulmonary osteoarthropathy, 129
Semilunar bone (see Lunate bone)
　cartilages of knee, cysts of, 398
　　excision of, 397
　　injury of, 393
Senile kyphosis, 341
　osteoporosis, 127
Sequestra, in osteomyelitis, 135
Sequestrectomy, in osteomyelitis, 139
Serratus anterior muscle, paralysis of, 251
Serum neuritis, 258
Sesamoid bones of foot, 436
Sever's operation in obstetric paralysis, 249
Shaffer's nondeforming clubfoot, 422
Sharpey's fibers, 24
Shelf operation in congenital dislocation of hip, 77
　in pathologic dislocation of hip, 388
Shells, plaster, in treatment of tuberculosis of spine, 157
Shenton's line, 68
Shock, in fracture patient, 486
Shoe, clubfoot, 43
　in causation of foot disabilities, 417
　in treatment of foot disabilities, 418
Shortening, actual and apparent, 32
　of Achilles tendon, 421
　of leg, operative treatment of, 222
Shoulder, affections of, 446-460
　ankylosis of, optimum position for, 198
　arthrodesis of, in poliomyelitis, 220
　bursitis in region of, 448
　　subacromial, 448
　　subcoracoid, 451
　dislocation, congenital, 80
　　old, 458
　　paralysis following, 250
　　recurrent, 457
　frozen, 452
　musculotendinous cuff tear, 453
　periarthritis of, 452
　round, 345
　snapping, 456
　sprain of, 447
　Sprengel's deformity of, 59
　strain of, 447
　supraspinatus tendon, rupture of, 453
　synovitis of, 447
Shoulder-hand syndrome, 455
Sign, Allis', 67
　Gowers', in muscular dystrophy, 261
　Kernig's, in poliomyelitis, 205
　Lasègue's, 351
　McMurray's, in knee cartilage injury, 395
　Ober, 352
　Ortolani, 64
　Tinel's, in nerve regeneration, 244

Sign—cont'd
　Trendelenburg's, in congenital dislocation of hip, 68
Silver operation for hallux valgus, 430
Skeletal traction, 492
Skeleton, general affections of, 81-103
Skewfoot, 46
Skin contracture, 478
Slipping of capital femoral epiphysis, 381
　patella, 407
Slocum amputation, 321
Smith-Petersen nail for hip fracture, 486
Snapping finger, 475
　hip, 391
　jaw, 460
　knee, 410
　shoulder, 456
　thumb, 475
Solitary bone cyst, 271
　neurofibroma, 285
Soutter fasciotomy, 214
Spasmodic torticollis, 441
Spastic flatfoot, 419
　paralysis, 227
"Spider fingers and toes," 56
Spina bifida, 237
　anterior, 238
　deformities in, 240
　manifesta, 239
　occulta, 239, 356
Spinal cord, birth injury of, 227
　involvement in poliomyelitis, 204
　in spastic paralysis, 227
　in spina bifida, 238
　in tuberculosis of spine, 156
　fusion (see Spine, arthrodesis of)
Spine, affections of, 327-346
　Albee tibial graft of, 158
　ankylosis of, optimum position for, 197
　anteroposterior deformities of, 338-345
　arthritis of, 182-189
　　osteoarthritis, 186
　　rheumatoid, 182
　　Strümpell-Marie, 183
　　treatment of, 188
　arthrodesis of, 157
　　Albee's method in, 158
　　Hibbs' method in, 157
　　in scoliosis, 335
　　in tuberculosis, 157
　cervical, congenital synostosis of, 61
　deformities of, in poliomyelitis, 215
　fracture, malunited, of vertebra, 312
　Hibbs' arthrodesis of, 157
　intervertebral disks of, anatomy of, 361
　　lesions of, in adult round back, 342
　　rupture of, causing sciatic pain, 360
　lateral curvature of (see Scoliosis)
　malunited fracture of, 312
　osteoarthritis of, 186
　Pott's disease of (see Spine, tuberculosis of)
　rheumatoid arthritis of, 182
　spondylosis or spondylophytosis of, 186
　Strümpell-Marie arthritis of, 183
　　treatment, 188
　telescoped, in osteomalacia, 98
　tibial, fracture of, 401
　tuberculosis of, 154-160

Spine, tuberculosis of—cont'd
  Albee's arthrodesis in, 158
  Hibbs' arthrodesis in, 157
  neurologic involvement in, 156
    treatment, 158
  pathology, 155
Spinous processes, variations of, 356
Splint, abduction, in deltoid paralysis, 215
  cock-up, in wrist drop, 215
  Denis Browne, 42
  for fresh fractures, 488
  Frejka, 72
  Putti triangular, 72
  Thomas, 488
Spondylolisthesis, 358
  articular, 359
  pseudo, 359
  reverse, 359
Spondylolysis, 358
Spondylophytes, 186
Spondylophytosis, 363
Spondylosis, 186, 363
Spotted bones, 117
Sprain, lumbosacral, 349
  of elbow, 463
  of shoulder, 447
  sacroiliac, 349
Sprengel's deformity, 59
Spurs of calcaneus, 434
Stapling, epiphyseal, 223
Steindler's operation in paralysis of flexors of elbow, 217
Steppage gait, 206, 256
Sternoclavicular dislocation, old, 459
Still's disease, 170
Stöffel's operation in cerebral palsy, 230
Straight leg-raising test, 351, 365
Strain, muscular, lumbosacral, 349
  of elbow region, 462
  of foot, 417
  of shoulder region, 447
  sacroiliac, 349
Steinmann pin, 493
Stenosing tenosynovitis, 475
Stress fracture, 428
Stretch reflex, 227
Strümpell-Marie arthritis, 183
  treatment of, 188
Stump, amputation, disabilities of, 322
Subacromial bursitis, 448
Subacute combined sclerosis, 234
Subcoracoid bursitis, 451
Subdeltoid bursitis, 448
Subluxation of head of radius, 465
  of hip, congenital, 64
  of shoulder in poliomyelitis, 215
  of tibia in arthritis of knee, 192
  of wrist, congenital, 80
Subtalar arthrodesis, 218, 232
Subtrochanteric osteotomy of Schanz, 77
Subungual exostosis, 435
Suction socket prosthesis, 321
Sudeck's atrophy, 132
Sulfur granules in actinomycosis, 146
Superficial trochanteric bursa, 391
Supernumerary bones of foot, 436
Supports for arches of foot, 418, 426

Suppurative arthritis, 142-144
  tenosynovitis, 475
Supraclavicular nerve injuries, 250
Suprapatellar bursa, 392
Supraspinatus tendon, rupture of, 453
Syme amputation, 319
Symmetrical serous synovitis, 147
Sympathetic reflex dystrophy, 132
Syndactyly, 53
Syndrome, Apert, 53
  carpal tunnel, 254
  cauda equina, 255
  cervical root, 441
  Christian's, 101
  conus, 256
  Ehlers-Danlos, 56
  Fanconi's, 97
  Felty's, 170
  Guillain-Barré, 259
  Horner's, 248
  Hurler's, 110
  Klippel-Feil, 61
  Marfan's, 56
  pronator, 254
  pull, 465
  Reiter's, 170
  root, cervical, 441
  scalenus anticus, 444
  shoulder-hand, 455
Synostosis of cervical spine, congenital, 61
  radioulnar, after fracture, 310
    congenital, 52
Synovectomy in arthritis of knee, 193
  in rheumatoid arthritis, 175
  in synovial chondromatosis, 404
  in tumor of synovium, 282
Synovial chondromatosis, 404
  fluid, 26
  membrane, 26
    hypertrophy and pinching of, 405
  sarcoma, 282
Synovioma, 282
Synovitis, gummatous, 148
  intermittent, of knee, 170, 410
  of hip, transient, 389
  of shoulder, 447
  pigmented villonodular, 405
  symmetrical serous, 147
  syphilitic, 146
  tuberculous, 150
Syphilis of bones and joints, 146-148
Syringomyelia, neuropathic disease of bones and joints in, 235
Syringomyelocele, 239

T

Tabes dorsalis, neuropathic disease of bones and joints in, 235
Talipes, calcaneovalgus, congenital, 45
  calcaneus, congenital, 39-45
  cavus, 421 (see also Clawfoot)
  congenital, 38
  definition of, 38
  equinovarus, congenital, 39-45
  equinus, congenital, 45
  paralytic, in poliomyelitis, 215
    arthrodesis in, 218

Talipes, paralytic, in poliomyelitis—cont'd
    bone block operations in, 222
    transplantation of tendons in, 216
  spastic, in cerebral palsy, 228
  valgus, congenital, 45
  varus, congenital, 45
Talocalcaneal bridge, 421
Talus, excision of, 220
  malunited fracture of, 306
  vertical, congenital, 47
Tarsal bones, malunited fracture of, 306
Telescoped spine, in osteomalacia, 98
Temporomandibular joint, affections of, 460 (*see also* Jaw, affections of)
Tendinitis, acute calcific, 476
Tendon, Achilles, rupture of, 434
    shortening of, 421
    tenosynovitis of, 433
  biceps brachii, rupture of, 455
  extensor pollicis longus, rupture of, 472
  laceration of, 471
  lengthening, of quadriceps, 197
  peroneal, displacement of, 436
  plantaris, rupture of, 434
  quadriceps, Bennett lengthening of, 197
    rupture of, 409
  rupture of Achilles, 434
    of biceps brachii, 455
    of extensor pollicis longus, 472
    of plantaris, 434
    of quadriceps, 409
    of supraspinatus, 453
  sheath, affections of, 471
    ganglion of, 477
    inflammation of (*see* Tenosynovitis)
    tumors of, 282
  supraspinatus, rupture of, 453
  transplantation, in cerebral palsy, 231
    in clawfoot, 423
    in clubfoot, 45
    in poliomyelitis, 215
  tumors of, 282
Tennis elbow, 464
Tenosynovitis, acute, suppurative, 475
  bicipital, 451
  chronic stenosing, 475
  de Quervain type of, 475
  of Achilles tendon, 433
  of tendons of hand, 474
  stenosing, 475
  traumatic, 474
  tuberculous, 476
Tenotomy, in cerebral palsy, 231
  in congenital torticollis, 440
Tenovaginitis (*see* Tenosynovitis)
Tension, in cerebral palsy, 227
Tensor fasciae latae, transplantation of, 216
Terminology of joint motion, 30
Test, Trendelenburg, 68
  Finkelstein, 475
Therapy, occupational, after amputation, 322
  after fracture, 499
  physical (*see* Physical therapy)
Thomas collar, 336, 443
  heel, 418
  splint, 488
  wrench in malunited Pott's fracture, 306

Thompson operation for contracture of quadriceps tendon, 197
Thorax, deformities of, 346
  in rickets, 86
  in scoliosis, 331
Thumb, operations to restore opposition of, 217
  snapping, 475
Tibia, adamantinoma of, 264
  apophysitis of tuberosity of, 405
  congenital defects of, 51
  fracture of spine of, 401
  malunited fracture of, 304
  partial separation of tuberosity of, 405
  subluxation of, in arthritis of knee, 192
  ununited fracture of, 300
  vara, 89
Tibial collateral ligament, ossification of, 409
  nerve, injury of, 257
  spine, fracture of, 401
  torsion, 40
  tuberosity, apophysitis of, 405
    partial separation of, 405
Tinel's sign in regeneration of nerve, 244
Toe, congenital abnormalities of, 53
  displacement of, 432
  hammer, 431
  Morton's, 427
  overlapping of, 432
  pigeon, 432
  spider, 56
  webbed, 53
Tophi, in gout, 180
Torticollis, 437
  acquired, 440
    acute, 440
  congenital, 437
  spasmodic, 441
Torus fracture, 501
Toxic neuritis, 258
Traction, balanced, 494
  Bryant's, 492
  Buck's, 492
  in fracture treatment, 491
  Russell's, 492
  skeletal, 492
  skull, 494
Transfixation screw, 495
Transient synovitis of hip, 389
Transplantation of iliac crest, in contracture of hip, 214
  of muscle, in poliomyelitis, 215
  of nerve, in traumatic injury, 246
  of tendon, in cerebral palsy, 231
    in clawfoot, 423
    in clubfoot, 45
    in poliomyelitis, 215
Transposition of ulnar nerve, 254
Transverse vertebral processes, variations of, 355
Traumatic myositis ossificans, 309
  neuritis, 257
    of ulnar nerve, 253
  osteitis of carpal bones, 481
  osteoporosis of carpal bones, 481
  tenosynovitis, 474
Treatment of fresh fractures, 489
  orthopaedic, 35
Tremor in cerebral palsy, 227
Trendelenburg test in congenital dislocation of hip, 68

Trident hand in achondroplasia, 104
Trigger finger, 475
    knee, 396
Triple arthrodesis of tarsus, 219
Trochanteric bursitis, deep, 390
        superficial, 391
Trumble hip fusion, 164
Tuberculin test, 152
Tuberculosis of bones and joints, 149-165
        abscess in, 150
        clinical picture, 150
        dactylitis, 165
        diagnosis, 151
            tuberculin test in, 152
        drug therapy of, 153
        incidence, 149
        of hip, 161-164
            arthrodesis in, 163
        of sacroiliac joint, 160
        of spine, 154-160
            arthrodesis in, 157
        of synovial membrane, 150
        of tendon sheath, 476
        pathology, 149
        prognosis, 154
        roentgenograms in, 151
        treatment, 152
            of tuberculous abscess, 154
            surgical, 153
Tuberculous abscess, 150
    dactylitis, 165
    tenosynovitis, 476
Tuberosity of tibia, apophysitis of, 405
    Osgood-Schlatter disease of, 405
    partial separation of, 405
Tumor, Codman's, 264
    Ewing's, 276
    of bone, 263-282
        benign, 265
            giant cell, 270
        classification of, 263
        Ewing's, 276
        malignant, 272
        metastatic, 279
    of bursae, 282
    of fasciae, 283
    of joints, 282
    of muscles, 283
    of nerves, 284
    of tendon sheaths, 282
    of tendons, 282
Turnbuckle jacket, Risser's, in scoliosis, 335
Typhoid infections of bone, 145

U

Ulna, congenital defects of, 50
    malunited fracture of, 309
    ununited fracture of, 302
Ulnar nerve, injury of, 252
        clawhand deformity in, 253
        recurrent dislocation of, 253
        transposition of, 254
        traumatic neuritis of, late, 253
Unequal leg length, 222
Union of fracture, delayed, 289
Ununited fracture, 291 (*see also* Fracture, nonunion of)
    of femur, 300

Ununited fracture—cont'd
    of fibula, 300
    of hip, 298
    of humerus, 302
    of patella, 300
    of radius, 302
    of tibia, 300
    of ulna, 302
Upper femoral epiphysis, avascular necrosis of, 374
    slipping of, 381

V

Vaccines for poliomyelitis, 209
Varus, metatarsus, 46
Vertebra, epiphysitis of, 338
    malunited fracture of, 312
    osteochondritis of, 341
    plana, 341
    tuberculosis of (*see* Tuberculosis of spine)
Viruses in poliomyelitis, 203
Visceral lesions causing low back pain, 368
Vitallium cup, in hip arthroplasty, 201
Vitamin disturbances, skeletal changes in, 84
Vitamin-resistant rickets, 95
Volkmann's canals, 24
    ischemic contracture, 466
Von Recklinghausen's disease of bone, 123
    of nerves, 285

W

Wallerian degeneration, 243
Weaver's bottom, 391
Webbed fingers and toes, 53
    neck, 62
Wedging of casts, in clubfoot, 42
Werdnig-Hoffmann disease, 233
Whitman abduction treatment of fracture of neck of femur, 496
    astragalectomy, 220
Wiles on posture, 344
Wolff's law, 81
Wrist, accessory bones of, 483
    affections of, 470
    anatomy of, 471
    ankylosis of, optimum position for, 198
    arthrodesis of, in cerebral palsy, 232
        in poliomyelitis, 222
    congenital dislocation of, 80
    drop, in radial palsy, 252
    ganglion of, 477
    Madelung's deformity of, 483
    malunited fracture in region of, 310
    necrosis of carpal bones, 481
    tenosynovitis in region of, 474
Wry neck, 437 (*see also* Torticollis)

X

X-ray therapy (*see* Roentgentherapy)
X-rays in diagnosis, 34
    in fracture diagnosis, 489

Y

Yount operation for hip flexion contracture, 214

Z

Zone, Looser's, 99